Computed Tomography of the Cardiovascular System

Computed Tomography of the Cardiovascular System

Edited by

Thomas C Gerber MD
Mayo Clinic, Jacksonville, FL, USA

Birgit Kantor MD
Mayo Clinic, Rochester, MN, USA

Eric E Williamson MD
Mayo Clinic, Rochester, MN, USA

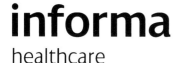

First published in the United Kingdom in 2007 by Informa Healthcare, Telephone House,
69-77 Paul Street, London EC2A 4LQ. Informa Healthcare is a trading division of Informa UK Ltd.
Registered Office: 37/41 Mortimer Street, London W1T 3JH. Registered in England and Wales
number 1072954.

Tel: +44 (0)20 7017 5000
Fax: +44 (0)20 7017 6699
Website: www.informahealthcare.com

A CIP record for this book is available from the British Library.
Library of Congress Cataloging-in-Publication Data

Data available on application

ISBN-10: 1 84184 625 2
ISBN-13: 978 1 84184 625 5

Composition by Cepha Imaging Private Ltd., Bangalore, India
Printed and bound in India by Replika Press Pvt. Ltd.

Contents

Contributors

Philip A Araoz MD
Mayo Clinic
Rochester, MN, USA

Soenke H Bartling MD
Molecular Imaging Junior Group
German Cancer Research Center
Heidelberg, Germany

Christoph Becker MD
University Hospital Grosshadern
Munich, Germany

Edwin JR van Beek MD
Carver College of Medicine
University of Iowa
Iowa City, IA, USA

Daniel S Berman MD
Cedars-Sinai Medical Center
Los Angeles, CA, USA

Lawrence Boxt MD
Manhasset, NY, USA

Peter A Brady MD
Mayo Clinic
Rochester, MN, USA

Thomas J Brady MD
Massachusetts General Hospital
Boston, MA, USA

Harald Brodoefel MD
Eberhard-Karls-University Tuebingen
Tuebingen, Germany

Arno Bücker MD
University Hospital
Hamburg, Germany

Matthew J Budoff MD
Harbor-UCLA Medical Center
Torrance, CA, USA

Christof Burgstahle MD
Eberhard-Karls-University Tuebingen
Tuebingen, Germany

Filippo Cademartiri MD PhD
Erasmus Medical Center
CA, Rotterdam, The Netherlands

Felix E Diehn MD
Mayo Clinic
Rochester, MN, USA

Yue Dong MD
Mayo Clinic
Rochester, MN, USA

Raimund Erbel MD
West German Heart Center Essen
University Essen-Duisburg
Essen, Germany

Pim J de Feyter MD PhD
Erasmus Medical Center
CA, Rotterdam, The Netherlands

Roman Fischbach MD
Department of Radiology
Neuroradiology and Nuclear Medicine
Asklepios Klinik Altona
Hamburg, Germany

Elliot K Fishman MD
Johns Hopkins Medical Institutions
Baltimore, MD, USA

Mario Garcia MD
Cleveland Clinic Foundation
Cleveland, OH, USA

Richard T George MD
Johns Hopkins Hospital
Jefferson, Baltimore, MD, USA

Thomas C Gerber MD
Mayo Clinic
Jacksonville, FL, USA

Robert C Gilkeson MD
University Hospitals of Cleveland
CWRU Medical School
Cleveland, OH, USA

James F Glocker MD
Mayo Clinic
Rochester, MN, USA

Rajiv Gupta PhD MD
Massachusetts General Hospital
Boston, MA, USA

Walter Heindel MD
University of Muenster
Muenster, Germany

Jeffrey C Hellinger MD
The Children's Hospital of Philadelphia
University of Philadelphia School of Medicine
Philadelphia, PA, USA

Martin Heuschmid MD
Eberhard-Karls-University Tuebingen
Tuebingen, Germany

Udo Hoffmann MD
Massachusetts General Hospital
Harvard Medical School
Boston, MA, USA

Karen M Horton MD
Johns Hopkins Medical Institutions
Baltimore, MD, USA

Kai Uwe Juergens MD
Institut fur Klinische Radiologie
Universitatsklinikum Munster
Munster, Germany

Marc Kachelrieß MD PhD
Institute of Medical Physics
Friedrich-Alexander-University of Erlangen-Nurnberg
Erlangen, Germany

Mannudeep K Kalra MD
Massachusetts General Hospital
Boston, MA, USA

Andreas Knez MD
Medical Hospital
Ludwig-Maximilians-University
München, Germany

Andreas F Kopp MD
Eberhard-Karls-University Tuebingen
Tuebingen, Germany

Gabriel P Krestin MD PhD
Erasmus Medical Center
CA Rotterdam, The Netherlands

Ronald S Kuzo MD
Mayo Clinic
Jacksonville, FL, USA

Alexander C Langheinrich MD
Justus-Liebig-University
Giessen, Germany

Albert C Lardo PhD
Johns Hopkins Hospital
Jefferson, Baltimore, MD, USA

Joao A C Lima MD
Johns Hopkins Hospital
Jefferson Baltimore, MD, USA

Paul Lindell MD
Mayo Clinic
Rochester, MN, USA

Andreas H Mahnken MD MBA
University Hospital
RWTH Aachen University
Aachen, Germany

Martin Lipton MD
Sausalito, CA, USA

David Maintz MD
University of Muenster
Munster, Germany

Amgad N Makaryus MD
Columbia University School of Medicine
New York, NY, USA

Cynthia McCollough MD
Mayo Clinic College of Medicine
Rochester, MN, USA

Michael McNitt-Gray MD
David Geffen School of Medicine, UCLA
Los Angeles, CA, USA

Willem B Meijboom MD
Erasmus Medical Center
CA Rotterdam, The Netherlands

Dylan V Miller MD
Mayo Clinic
Rochester, MN, USA

Nico R Mollet MD PhD
Erasmus Medical Center
CA Rotterdam, The Netherlands

Gareth Morgan-Hughes MD
Plymouth NHS Trust
Plymouth, United Kingdom

Fabian Bamberg MD
Massachusetts General Hospital
Harvard Medical School
Boston, MA, USA

Koen Nieman MD PhD
Erasmus Medical Center
CA Rotterdam, The Netherlands

Niels Van Pelt MD
Erasmus Medical Center
CA Rotterdam, The Netherlands

Paolo Raggi MD
Emory University School of Medicine
Atlanta, GA, USA

Anja Reimann MD
Eberhard-Karls-University Tuebingen
Tuebingen, Germany

Erik L Ritman MD
Mayo Clinic
Rochester, MN, USA

Alan Rozanski MD
St. Luke's Roosevelt Hospital Center
New York NY, USA

Klaus Schäfers MD
Institut fur Klinische Radiologie
Universitatsklinikum Munster
Munster, Germany

Axel Schmermund PhD
Cardioangiologisches Centrum Bethanien
Frankfurt, Germany

Bernhard Schmidt MD
Siemens Medical Solutions
Forchheim, Germany

Paul Schoenhagen MD FAHA
Cleveland Clinic Foundation
Cleveland, OH, USA

Stephen Schroeder MD
Eberhard-Karls-University Tuebingen
Tuebingen, Germany

Leslee J Shaw PhD
Emory University School of Medicine
Atlanta, GA, USA

Ernest S Siwik MD
University Hospitals of Cleveland
CWRU Medical School
Cleveland, OH, USA

Shawn DeWayne Teague MD
Indiana University Hospital
Indianapolis, IN, USA

Brad Thompson MD
Carver College of Medicine
University of Iowa, Iowa City, IA, USA

Kalpathi L Venkatachalam
Mayo Clinic
Rochester, MN, USA

Eric E Walser MD
Mayo Clinic
Jacksonville, FL, USA

Annick Weustink MD
Erasmus Medical Center
CA Rotterdam, The Netherlands

Erik E Williamson MD
Mayo Clinic
Rochester, MN, USA

Phillip Young MD
Mayo Clinic
Jacksonville, FL, USA

Kenneth G Zahka MD
University Hospitals of Cleveland
CWRU Medical School
Cleveland, OH, USA

Foreword

The use and acceptance of computed tomography (CT) in the clinical workup of patients with known or suspected cardiovascular disease is increasing rapidly. In particular, coronary CT angiography has become robust and accurate within the last few years. With CT technology evolving rapidly, coronary CT angiography has developed from the stage of "proof of principle" into a stable imaging modality that is clinically useful for many patients. All the same, uncertainties remain, and in order to use coronary CT angiography in the clinically most useful manner, detailed knowledge of its potential and limitations is required.

As more and more clinicians are considering the use of cardiovascular CT in their clinical practice, and as more and more researchers contribute to the evidence base for the use of this technology, students and users of cardiovascular CT must assimilate a large amount of information. Since the advantages and limitations of CT in clinical practice are closely related to how the images are generated, a solid understanding of the technical principles underlying cardiovascular CT is essential. Knowledge of cardiac anatomy needs be revisited from the perspective of cross-sectional and three-dimensional imaging. Practioners of cardiovascular CT must understand imaging protocols and algorithms in detail to be able to adapt them to individual clinical questions. The usefulness and accuracy of CT imaging for a wide range of diagnostic problems in cardiovascular disease needs to be understood and finally, with the field of cardiovascular CT moving forward rapidly, one should have an idea of what the near future holds in terms of technological developments and new clinical applications.

The magnificent book *Computed Tomography of the Cardiovascular System,* edited by Drs Gerber, Kantor and Williamson effortlessly covers this wide range of information and addresses all relevant areas with contributions from renowned experts in the field. This book is a rich source of information for both new and experienced users of cardiovascular CT and successfully puts current and future applications into technical and clinical context. The editors are to be commended for providing the medical community with such a complete but very readable account at a time when the need for reliable and concise yet thorough information is immense.

I congratulate Drs. Gerber, Kantor, and Williamson, along with their authors, for bringing this book to life. Without a doubt it will be a tremendously important resource to healthcare providers who order, perform or interpret cardiovascular CT studies and who must understand which patients and clinical scenarios benefit most from its use. As such, the book will be not only a wonderful and lasting reference but, because of its balanced approach to cardiovascular CT, will also make an important contribution to the rational growth of this field.

Stephan Achenbach MD
Professor of Medicine
University of Erlangen
Erlangen, Germany

Preface

This book is a labor of love by imaging enthusiasts from all over the world, meant for individuals interested in mastering cardiovascular computed tomography (CT). Two ideas have guided the development of its content: 1. both cardiologists and radiologists can become expert readers of cardiovascular CT studies and 2. the cardiovascular system is not separated at the aortic valve into two entirely disparate parts. To emphasize these points, we have invited cardiologists as well as radiologists as contributors, and have included a large section on vascular radiology which is missing from most current textbooks on cardiac CT.

Cardiovascular CT in its current, widely embraced form is a relatively young field. As a result, the evidence base for its use is still being developed, and there is controversy about the appropriateness of cardiovascular CT imaging in specific clinical situations. To address such concerns, we have included chapters on clinical context and on the relationship between CT and more established cardiovascular imaging techniques. Cardiovascular CT is evolving rapidly, and in order to avoid publishing material that is obsolete by the time it appears in print, we have placed great emphasis on discussing principles that are as much as possible independent of type and generation of CT scanners.

We have organized the book to progress from a discussion of basic concepts in cardiovascular CT, over descriptions of a wide array of clinical applications, to uses of CT that are currently considered investigational but are clearly on the horizon for the clinical realm and that contribute to the understanding of clinical problems in cardiology. Placing chapters on general issues next to chapters on specific aspects of cardiovascular CT has created minor overlaps that are intentional and that allow each chapter in the book to stand alone and be easily read and understood by itself.

We are very proud of, and grateful to, the many experts in CT from the U.S. and from abroad who have generously agreed to devote their time to contributing articles and who have made this book a unique and complete account of the current status of cardiac, vascular, and investigational applications of cardiovascular CT. We trust that readers will find it a valuable resource as they study the clinical use and the future potential of cardiovascular CT.

Thomas C Gerber
Birgit Kantor
Eric E Williamson

Acknowledgments

For Freya and Maximilian, who teach us as much about being good as we are teaching them.
B.K. and T.C.G.

To my parents, Eva and Hermann Gerber, in deep gratitude.
T.C.G.

To Geoff Rubin, Dominik Fleischmann and Jerry Breen who continue to teach me about cardiovascular CT. To Mary Jo who has supported me in every way possible, and to Alex and Katherine – the most fascinating people I know.
E.E.W

History of Cardiovascular Computed Tomography

Martin J. Lipton

1 INTRODUCTION

Historically, the diagnosis of heart disease has depended largely upon radiographic methods. This chapter describes the key requirements for imaging the heart using conventional X-ray methods and with Computed Tomography (CT) when it became available; it describes the feasibility and validation studies which formed the basis for modern clinical cardiac CT.

2 X-RAY IMAGING FROM 1895–1972 – PRE-CT ERA

The discovery of X-rays by W. Conrad Roentgen in 1895 had a dramatic and immediate impact in two fields. Not only did it create a new medical specialty called Roentgenology, named in honor of its founder, but also it profoundly changed the thinking of physicists of that time regarding the nature of atomic structure. Industry became heavily involved in the X-ray field from the beginning, because high vacuum tubes and more powerful generators were essential for the production of X-rays. Progressive improvements also occurred in all aspects of X-ray imaging, which became a big business driven by the diagnostic needs of physicians.[1]

Diseases of the heart and blood vessels represent one of the most challenging problems for advanced diagnostic imaging systems. The history of radiographic diagnosis over the decades following Roentgen's discovery explain to some extent the philosophic and practical differences between cardiology and radiology. Radiologists are traditionally trained to observe and recognize the broad range of normal anatomy and pathology. Since diagnostic imaging of most organs relies primarily on structural findings, industry responded by providing higher spatial and contrast resolution. Cardiologists, however, are primarily concerned with cardiac function, and use imaging methods routinely to quantitate cardiac indicees. This explains why dedicated and specialized equipment with high temporal resolution is necessary for every modality for cardiac imaging. Cardiac catheterization with haemodynamic recording and angiocardiography emerged as the most useful and reliable technique for evaluating patients prior to cardiac surgery. This generally has remained the practice despite remarkable advances in the established noninvasive fields of echocardiography and nuclear medicine. Cine-angiocardiography provides high temporal resolution in excess of 30 images per second without the need for ECG-gating. It does, however, require selective catheterization and contrast media injections. All conventional X-ray projection imaging methods suffer from the limitation of overlapping structures and, therefore, multiple angiographic projections are necessary, each of which requires an additional injection of contrast media. Nevertheless, invasive angiocardiography became established as the gold standard for identifying the site and severity of coronary artery disease, and for evaluating left ventricular function.

3 TOMOGRAPHIC IMAGING

It was to overcome the limitation of overlapping structures inherent in conventional X-ray projection imaging that linear and, later, almost as a precursor of CT, that rotational X-ray tomography was developed over 50 years ago by Takahashi.[2]

In this technique the X-ray tube and radiographic film was positioned, as shown in Figure 1.1, almost perpendicular and rotated around the patient. A single cross sectional slice was exposed at one level as shown in Figure 1.2. The X-ray projections for each angle were recorded on the radiographic film and summated. The resulting axial image is illustrated in Figure 1.3, and can be seen to be blurred. This is because simple back projection imaging of this type is only a first order solution. The complete solution requires two steps, the second of which had to wait until a computer was

incorporated into the X-ray system. Table 1.1 identifies the stages of development resulting in the first commercially available CT scanner in 1972, for which, like Roentgen, Godfrey Hounsfield and Alan Cormack were awarded the Nobel Prize for Physics in 1979. The appropriate convolution algorithms and filtering is described in Chapter 2.

4 THE CT ERA FROM 1972 ONWARDS

In Godfrey Hounsfield's Nobel acceptance speech in 1979, he said the following: 'Although it is barely 8 years since the first brain scanner was constructed computed tomography is now relatively widely used and been extensively demonstrated. At the present time the new system is operating in some 1,000 hospitals throughout the world. The technique has successfully overcome many of the limitations which are inherent in conventional X-ray technology.

When we consider the capabilities of conventional X-ray methods, three main limitations become obvious.

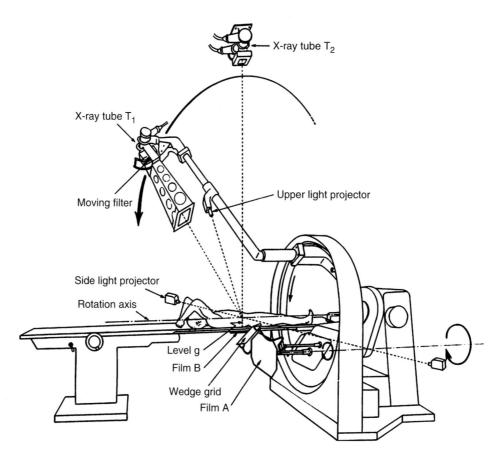

Figure 1.1   Diagram of an axial tomography machine designed for whole body scanning, which became commercially available and was designed by Takahasi. The X-ray tube was almost perpendicular to the X-ray film and rotated around the patient exposing a single cross sectional slice.

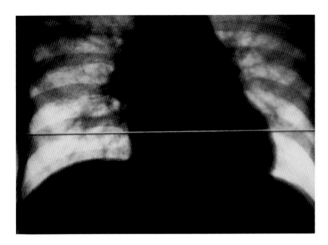

Figure 1.2 A localizing slice level though the heart in a patient.

Table 1.1	Development of computed tomography	
Year	Development	Inventor
1947	Axial tomography (AT)	Takahashi
1964 to 1966	Computed tomography	*Cormack /Kuhl
1972	First fan beam scanner	Boyd
1972	First commercial scanner	*Hounsfield
1973	5 minute CT scanner	
1976	20 second EMI scanner	
1977	5 second body scanner	
1978	Proposed cardiac scanners	
	**DSR	Ritman
	+CVCT	Boyd
	++EB CT	

*Nobel prize 1979.
**Dynamic Spatial Reconstructor (DSR)
+CVCT = cine computed tomographic C-100 scanner or
++Electron Beam (EB CT)

Firstly, it is impossible to display within the framework of a two-dimensional X-ray, a three-dimensional scene under view. Objects situated in depth, i.e. in the third dimension, superimpose, causing confusion to the viewer.

Secondly, conventional X-ray cannot distinguish between soft tissues. In general, a radiogram differentiates only between bone and air, as in the lungs. Variation in soft tissues such as the liver and pancreas are not discernible at all and certain other organs may be rendered visible only through the use of radio-opaque dyes.

Thirdly, when conventional X-ray methods are used, it is not possible to measure in a quantitative way the separate densities of the individual substances through which the X-ray has passed. The radiogram records the mean absorption by all the various tissues which the X-ray has penetrated. This is of little use for quantitative measurement.

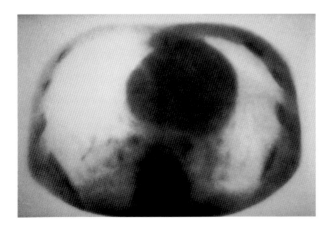

Figure 1.3 An example of the image obtained by axial tomography. Note that this blurring is due to simple back projection radiography and although quite useful has limitations.

Computed tomography, on the other hand, measures the attenuation of X-ray beams passing through sections of the body from hundreds of different angles, and then, from the evidence of these measurements, a computer is able to reconstruct pictures of the body's interior.

Pictures are based on the separate examination of a series of contiguous cross sections, as though we looked at the body separated into a series of thin 'slices.' By doing so, we virtually obtain total three-dimensional information about the body.'[3]

The era of digital imaging began with CT, and has since been applied to many other imaging modalities. CT has a density range of 2,000 shades of gray. The human eye can only recognize 11–21 approximately. Because the sensitivity of CT for density is over 1% and so much more sensitive than conventional X-ray film combinations, intravenous enhancement of the blood volume, combined with cross sectional imaging, provides sufficient contrast for angiography and avoids the need for arterial injections.

Early studies of CT for cardiovascular imaging explore the capability of CT to overcome the 3 major limitations of conventional X-ray. However, CT cannot yet match the resolution of conventional X-ray imaging, nor its exposure speed, or cost. However, as CT develops it will no doubt eventually replace almost all types of X-ray imaging.

The first CT scanners required 1–5 seconds to acquire a single slice. However, this was adequate for diagnozing most organ systems, because temporal resolution was not critical. These machines were designed initially for the head, and later for whole body. The impact of this new modality was dramatic, for example in neuroradiology the need for invasive angiography fell by almost 50%, and CT virtually replaced diagnostic nuclear scintigraphy in the brain. As Godfrey Housfield implied, within a few years CT dominated head imaging. Early CT studies of the heart however were confined to exploring morphology.[4–7]

5 CT ESTIMATES OF VENTRICULAR VOLUMES, WALL THICKNESS AND MASS

A critical measurement for evaluating cardiac function is left ventricular ejection fraction. Biplane angiography provided the most accurate and reproducible results.[8] One of the first cardiac quantitative studies explored the capability of CT for accurate volume measurements of postmortem silastic casts of the human left ventricle. The effect of cast shape and orientation on volume measurements was evaluated. Results were compared with those obtained by biplane radiography and by Archimedes principle.[9] Cast angulation was precisely measured for each technique, as illustrated in Figures 1.4 and 1.5. The true cast volume for validation was obtained for each cast using a Mettler balance to measure dry cast weight in air, and a torsion balance for each cast submerged in distilled water. Air trapped in the casts while submerged between trabecular and papillary muscles which can cause significant errors, was eliminated by degassing under water. The results are given in Figures 1.6 and 1.7 and were calculated by dividing the difference between the dry and submerged weight of each cast by the density of water at a recorded temperature. This study demonstrated

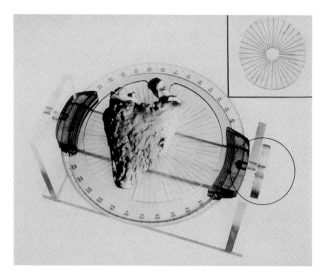

Figure 1.5   Casts were placed on a Plexiglas goniometer, which enables precise cast orientation in three planes insuring accurate positioning for computed tomographic volume measurements. Plexiglas does not interfere with computed tomographic reconstruction. (From ref. 10 with permission)

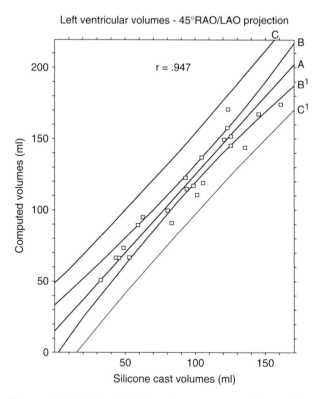

Left ventricular volumes - 45°RAO/LAO projection

r = .947

Computed volumes (ml)

Silicone cast volumes (ml)

Figure 1.6   Left ventricular volumes measured by radiography in the anteroposterior-lateral projections plotted against actual cast volumes. Ninety-five percent confidence limits for the regression lines are indicated by line BB[1], and 95% confidence limits for individual measurements are indicated by lines CC[1]. (From ref. 10 with permission)

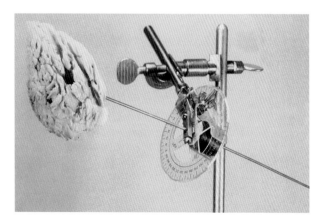

Figure 1.4   Ventricular cast in a stand which allows it to be positioned in any orientation for biplane volume measurement. (From ref. 10 with permission)

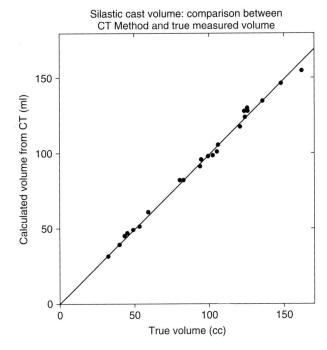

Figure 1.7 Calculated computed tomographic volumes plotted against true cast volumes. The regression line practically coincides with the line of identity. The correlation coefficient is 0.998. (From ref. 10 with permission)

the superiority of cross sectional 3-dimensional CT of the heart and raised several issued which are generic, including methods for edge detection, the influence on accuracy of CT windowing and level and the question of how many axial images and therefore slices are required to provide precise volume estimates for a given cardiac chamber. It also became apparent that, for each type of new scanner, such calibration issues would need to be addressed.[10,11]

6 MYOCARDIAL WALL DIMENSIONS AND MASS

The potential of CT for quantitative assessment of inter-ventricular septal wall thickness was evaluated in vivo in dogs. Fourteen pedigreed beagle puppies of both sexes comprised this study population. Seven underwent aortic banding at 6–8 weeks, so that the supravalve aortic circum-ference was reduced 25–40%. All the dogs were followed and scanned at 7–9 months. The study was performed using a General Electric CT/T 7800 Research Scanner (modified GE whole body scanner). This unit could per-form rapid sequential scanning, acquiring up to 12, 360° scans in 40 seconds; each having a 2.4 second exposure time.

This scanner was among the first to produce a projection 'scout view' or computed radiograph by pulsing the X-ray tube with the detector array in a stationary position, while the subject is moved through the X-ray field. The lateral scout view was used in this study to locate the cardiac apex, and all subsequent scans were indexed to this reference level, which was precisely identified under computer/oper-ator control. Until this view became available, surface land-marks had to be used and scanning levels could not be reliably reproduced. Today such localizing aids with lasers are taken for granted, and universally supplied with every CT scanner. Figure 1.8 illustrates one typical pair of CT scans from this study, and demonstrated the marked left ventricular hypertrophy compared with a litter matched control. A linear regression line for septal wall thickness was obtained by plotting the CT estimates derived from regions of interest (ROI), like the one seen in Figure 1.8, which includes both ventricles, against direct autopsy measurements, as shown in Figure 1.9. The corre-lation coefficient was 0.92 for the 14 experiments. Non-ECG-gated CT underestimated the autopsy values by 10–20%. However, this was a consistent underestimation. At that time, a paper pixel print out map had to be obtained of the ROI, as shown in Figure 1.10. Edge detection is critical for measurements. A boundary CT number was defined as the CT number halfway between the mean CT number of the ventricular cavities and the midpoint of the septal wall, from which the mean width is calculated.[12]

A study of left ventricular mass using 22 dogs and the same scanner was also performed. This research scanner was installed in UCSF in 1977 and was continuously modi-fied for cardiac applications. The gantry of this single slice machine, like all early CT scanners, had to be rotated in opposite directions between scan sequences, since the power cables would twist, limiting rotation and resulting in long interscan delay times. The CT data analysis involved two methods, a semi-automated computer technique and a manual tracing technique to define the myocardial boundary. Both methods showed similar results[13] (Figure 1.11). Such non ECG-gated CT feasibility studies are logical nec-essary steps in developing new clinical tools. However, extrapolating results to patients must be guarded. Nevertheless, this study showed that CT provides accurate dimensional measurements. Furthermore, in the presence of asymmetrical hypertrophy or abnormal chamber config-urations or both, CT, unlike echocardiography, should be superior, because no geometric assumptions are necessary later, Feiring measured LV mass by EBCT concerning its accuracy and precision.

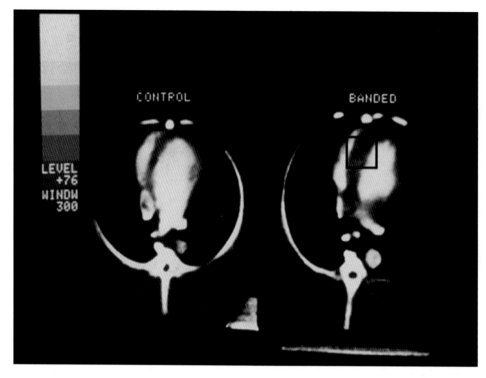

Figure 1.8 (a) Nongated, 1-cm thick computed transmission tomographic scan through the ventricular cavities of a non-banded control beagle after intravenous injection of contrast medium. (b) A similar scan at the same level is seen in a matched litter mate 7 months after banding. The myocardial wall is symmetrically hypertrophied and the relatively smaller contrast-enhanced left ventricular cavity is apparent. A region of interest has been selected to include a portion of both the right and left ventricular cavities.

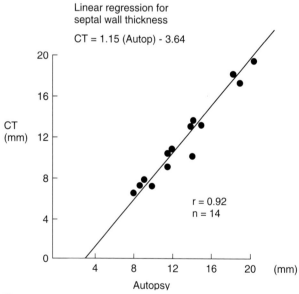

Figure 1.9 Linear regression for septal wall thickness; along the abscissa are measurements (mm) obtained at autopsy and corresponding computed transmission tomographic estimates lie on the ordinate. (From ref. 12 with permission)

7 ECG-GATED COMPUTED TOMOGRAPHIC

An exciting prospect for CT is quantitation of cardiac chamber and myocardial wall thickening dynamics for which ECG-gated CT was explored in a number of centers with single slice scanners in 1979 and 1980s.[14–18] This technique is one method of overcoming the problem of cardiac motion and is critical in obtaining quantitative dimensional data, ejection fractions and also for measuring the extent of wall thickening during the cardiac cycle.

Gated CT differs significantly from standard computed tomographic scanning. It was well realized 25 years ago that to obtain a reconstructed image of a stationary object by standard computed tomography, a full complement of angular X-ray data must be obtained over the full scanning circle from 0 to 360° without significant gaps in the angular data set, although some gating programs use only 180° plus the fan beam angle. However, no gaps are permitted in this data.

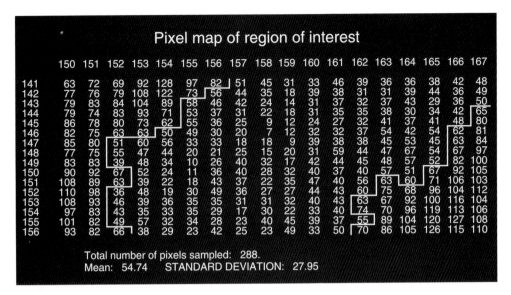

Figure 1.10 Computer printout of absolute computed transmission tomographic (CT) numbers present within the same region of interest as described in Figure 1.8. Each pixel is 1.3 × 1.3 mm. Lines demarcate all pixels with absolute CT numbers of 60 or less, thus defining the interventricular septum. This boundary CT number was defined as the CT number that was halfway between the mean CT number of the cavities and the mean CT number of the midportion of the septal wall. Scale drawing of the septum then defined the septal boundary within the region of interest, from which the mean width is calculated.

Therefore, multiple scans are required to obtain the necessary angular data to reconstruct a gated image of the heart.

8 RETROSPECTIVE VERSUS PROSPECTIVE GATING

Two gating techniques were utilized: retrospective[19] and prospective[18] gating. With retrospective gating, the computed tomographic scan data and the electrocardiogram are simultaneously recorded, and the CT data is binned to correspond with selected ECG windows. The prospective gating system allowed preselection of a fraction of the electrocardiographic RR interval width to be monitored.[18] The biologic window width sets the fraction of the cardiac cycle to be represented by each image. Prospective gating assures the even distribution of the R waves throughout the scanning circle in the minimal number of scans. This is accomplished by launching the X-ray tube at the appropriate time relative to the R wave on the electrocardiographic input, such that one of the following R waves falls in the largest gap in the already acquired angular X-ray data. In our studies, the width of the biologic window was set at 10% of the RR interval. Since the heart rate was maintained between 100 and 120 beats/min in dogs, each frame represents 0.05 to 0.06 second. With the biologic window set at 10% of the RR interval, approximately eight scans were

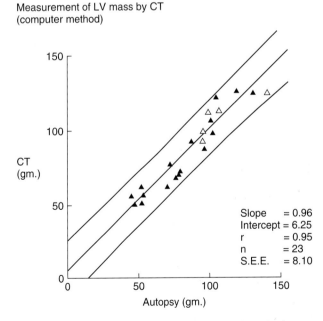

Figure 1.11 Relation between autopsy values and computed tomographic (CT) estimates of left ventricular (LV) mass. Results for the computer method. Filled triangles represent normotensive dogs; open triangles represent the beagles with left ventricular hypertrophy. The lines on either side of the regression line indicate the 95 percent confidence limits. (From ref. 13 with permission)

Table 1.2 Limitations of whole body scanners in 1980s

1) Exposure time is too long (1 to 5 seconds).
2) Repetition rate is too slow (0.5 to 2 second delay).
3) Single slice capability.
4) Heat load limitations of X-ray tube severely restricts the number of scans in dynamic sequence.
5) EKG gating is cumbersome.
6) Breath holding requirements are excessive for gating.
7) Requires relatively large volumes of contrast medium.
8) Quantitation of many functions is limited.

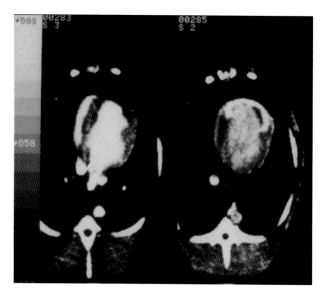

Figure 1.12 Two contrast enhanced CT scans acquired with a conventional whole body single slice scanner at the same level in a dog with an acute myocardial infarction in the antero-septal wall. The left image is during the first pass of an intravenous bolus of contrast agent. Note the myocardial enhancement void in the infarct area. The image on the right was obtained 10 minutes later after contrast washout has occurred. The infarct zone is seen as a bright, horseshoe area of delayed enhancement.

required to obtain a full complement of ECG-gated angular data, requiring approximately 45 seconds of breath-holding. The limitations of CT during this early period are summarized in Table 1.2.

9 CT EVALUATION OF MYOCARDIAL ISCHEMIA AND INFARCTION

Early CT studies of acute myocardial infarction (AMI) were performed in several centers on ex situ or arrested dog hearts.[4–7] The group at UCSF explored the detection and quantitation of myocardial injury in vivo using intracoronary and intravenous contrast media.[20–21] While the attenuation of infarcted myocardium was less than normal tissue and could be detected, it was much easier to identify with contrast enhancement.

10 CONTRAST ENHANCEMENT OF ACUTE MYOCARDIAL INFARCTION

Contrast material produces temporally distinct phases of enhancement of normal and ischemically damaged myocardium. During the perfusion phase, normal myocardium is maximally enhanced (maximum increase in X-ray attention value), whereas the area of damage is nonenchanced or minimally enhanced (Figure 1.12). Ten minutes after administration of the contrast material, enhancement of normal myocardium has declined and the damaged myocardium is nearly maximally enhanced. In the perfusion phase, the ischemically damaged area appears as a 'negative image' within the myocardium, whereas in the later phase, it appears as a 'positive image.' The early CT appearances reflect reduced tissue perfusion, while later, after more prolonged occlusion, it was thought to be related to necrosis and scar formation. Both iodinated contrast material and ^{99m}Tc-pyrophosphate were shown to be markers of myocardial necrosis. In some infarcts, both substances had a high concentration within the center, periphery, and margin of the infarct, whereas in others, the concentration of both substances was low in the center and high in the periphery and margin of the infarct. Measurement of regional myocardial blood flow with indium-111-labeled microspheres indicated that the accumulation of both contrast material and ^{99m}Tc-pyrophosphate in the center of the infarct occurred when residual blood flow was at least 3% of normal myocardial blood flow. Neither substance accumulates in the region of infarcted myocardium with a residual blood flow of less than 3% of normal. These studies inferred that contrast enhancement of ischemically damaged tissue is a marker of myocardial necrosis, but its occurrence is dependent upon the presence of a threshold level of residual myocardial perfusion.[22–24]

Doherty et al. performed an vivo AMI study with 28 dogs and showed that the distribution of contrast enhancement was not only similar to technetium-^{99m}

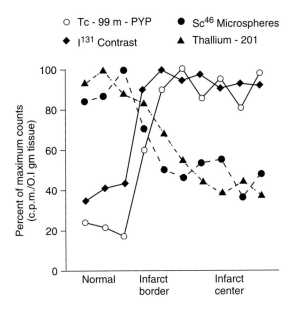

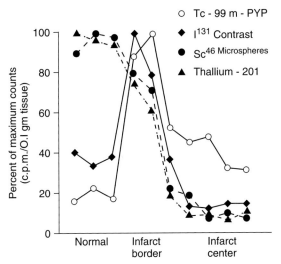

Figure 1.13 Distribution of pyrophosphate, thallium, microspheres and contrast material in (A) epicardial and (B) endocardial samples for a representative transmural anterior infarct. (A) The abscissa goes from normal tissue through an admixture of infarct foci in the normal tissue (labeled infarct border) and continues in the epicardial layer overlying the infarct center. (B) The progression is from normal tissue through the border zone into the homogenous necrotic core. (From ref. 21 with permission)

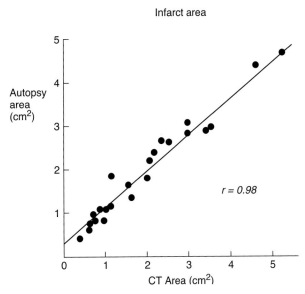

Figure 1.14 Comparison of computerized transmission tomography (CTT) and autopsy in the measurement of infarct area in individual tomographic slices from intact living dogs. The excellent correlation is attributable, in part, to the use of only transmural infarctions, which simplifies the task of boundary placement for area calculations by both CTT and autopsy. Infarct volume can be determined by summating the areas in contiguous 1-cm slices. (From ref. 21 with permission)

pyrophosphate in the border zone of the infarct in infusion studies, but also with bolus injections it behaves more like thallium–201 (Figure 1.13). Figure 1.14 shows a good correlation between CT and autopsy measures of infarct size.[21] However, delayed enhancement was only seen consistently 24 hours after coronary artery obstruction, and was not seen during transient occlusion for up to 10 minutes.[25]

Similar appearances occurred in patients with AMI, as seen in Figure 1.15, and in chronic infarction and remodeling (Figure 1.16). Their observations were confirmed in more recent studies with Multidetector CT (MDCT) scanners in animals and patients.[26–27] Kramer et al. used single slice nongated CT to study a series of 19 patients with CT elevation and myocardial infarction within 1 month of the event and confirmed these findings.[28] More recently Koyama, obtaining similar results with Multidetector CT, also reported similar findings in patients.[29]

II CT SCANNERS PROPOSED FOR IMAGING THE HEART

The requirements for imaging the heart with CT are listed in Table 1.3. Several methods were developed to overcome limited temporal resolution. Ritman and CT collaborators built a CT research machine using multiple X-ray tubes and image intensifiers for dynamic spatial reconstruction of the heart.[30–31] This pioneered many aspects of cardiac CT, but this scanner was never duplicated. A more practical

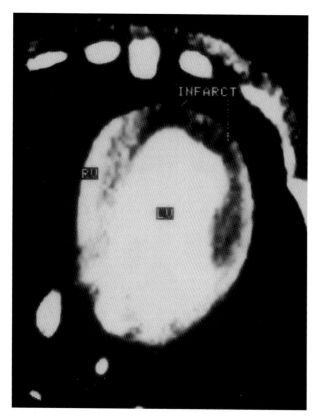

Figure 1.15 A 1 cm thick CT scan following a 20 ml bolus of intravenous contrast in a patient with a 36 hour antero septal myocardial infarct. Note the negative perfusion defect in the infarcted territory and normal enhanced myocardium elsewhere during the first passage of contrast. RV = right ventricle and LV = left ventricle.

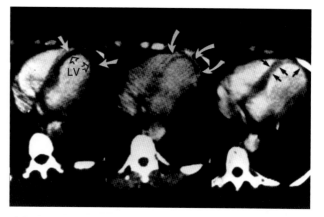

Figure 1.16 Contrast enhanced CT scan left panel in a patient 72 hours after acute myocardial infarction. The image on the left demonstrates hypoenhancement (straight white arrows) in the anteroseptal regions of ischemic injury after contrast infusion (white arrows). A second scan middle panel, at the same level, shows delayed enhancement of this zone at 10 mins. (curved arrows) after contrast has washed out of normal myocardium and the cardiac chambers. The right panel is the same patient 3 months later demonstrating left ventricular (LV) remodeling with thinning of the infarcted walls (black arrows). Left ventricular aneurysm formation and some compensatory hypertrophy of the free LV wall is present.

scanner was proposed by Douglas Boyd in 1978, employing a scanning electron beam.[32–33] This device is now very familiar and, known as EBCT, remains the only CT scanner designed specifically for millisecond cardiac CT scanning. The first machine was built and installed at UCSF. This scanner was introduced commercially in 1984. Since then new models appeared in 1988 and 2003 offering dual 1.5 mm slices and multilevel scanning at exposure speeds of 33 m sec. The capability of EBCT is summarized in Table 1.4. Approximately 300 EBCT scanners were installed world wide, representing only 1.5% of the entire CT market. ECG-gating was unnecessary with EBCT although CT acquisition could be triggered to the ECG.

The concept of improving mechanical scanners by ECG-gating methods found poor clinical utility with single slice machines. One solution for shortening exposure times and breath holding requirements was proposed by Redington.[34] This involved adding multiple X-ray tubes (3 or more) with opposed detectors arrays. This idea has also been introduced recently in dual source multidector CT (MDCT).

The concept of continuous spiral scanning began in the 1980s using slip-ring technology to transfer power continuously during rotation. With the advent of smaller, high frequency power units, this type of scanner became practical.[35] In 2000, Willi Kalendar, using a slip-ring scan, demonstrated the value of spiral CT.[36] Within a few years 8 then 16 and 64 slice MDCT machines became available, allowing

Table 1.3 Requirements for computed tomographic scanning of the heart

1) Rapid scan time, 33 to 100 ms or less with repeatability.
2) Multislice capability, eight or more simultaneously.
3) Repeat multislice study at 1 second during passage of contrast bolus.
4) Scan registration using computed radiography for slice localization.
5) Three-dimensional transformations into sagittal, coronal and oblique images.
6) Software for quantitative analysis.
7) Contrast medium enhancement (contrast medium with 40% iodine concentration)

Table 1.4 EBCT capability

1) Rapid scan time (50 ms).
2) Multislice capability (8 or more simultaneously).
3) Repeat multislice at 1 second (or faster) during passage of contrast bolus.
4) Three-dimensional transformation into sagittal, coronal, and oblique images.
5) Quantitative analysis software.
6) Subtraction.
7) Functional imaging analysis and display.

many benefits, including isotropic resolution, which is important for 3D image processing. It preserves image quality during multiplanar reconstruction from the original CT acquisition plane. The combination of 16 slice MDCT and ECG-gating methods made cardiac imaging feasible for the first time with mechanical CT scanners. It was now possible to acquire a volume of contiguous 0.5 mm thick slices in 10 seconds, with a significant reduction in contrast medium requirements as well as breath holdings time. The coronary arteries could be imaged even though scan speed remains at 300 m sec for a partial scan reconstruction; however with ECG-gating it was lowered by a factor of 2 to 150 m sec or 75 m sec by integrating CT data acquired during 2 or 4 consecutive heart beats.

EBCT enabled accurate quantitation of coronary calcification, and could display the coronary arteries with contrast enhancement as well as the pulmonary veins. An example is seen in Figure 1.17. This image was obtained in the early 1980s. EBCT demonstrated the value of post

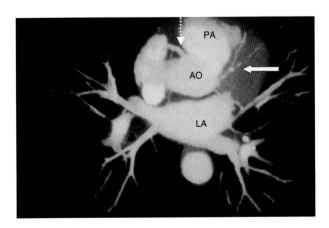

Figure 1.17 Post processed subtracted EBCT axial image demonstrating the right (dotted arrow) and left coronary arteries. There is calcification and beading of the left anterior descending artery (solid arrow). PA = pulmonary artery, AO – aorta, LA = Left atrium with 4 draining pulmonary veins.

processing techniques long before they became routine clinical tools and also the potential for CT angiography (CTA).[37–38] It seemed likely then, that once higher CT temporal resolution became widely available, measurements of all these structures and CTA would become routine in everyday clinical care. However, few were convinced at that time.

12 LEFT VENTRICULAR REMODELING

Myocardial infarction may result in compensatory hypertrophy, wall thinning and /or decreased myocardial thickening. This was well demonstrated by CT with conventional ECG-gating CT and with EBCT. Figure 1.18 illustrates a series of contrast-enhanced images during one cardiac cycle. The EBCT scanner table was designed to angulate and can therefore directly image the short axis plane without loss of CT image resolution in the acquired transaxial plane by 3D reconstruction. Endocardial and epicardial borders can be defined and segmented, hence ventricular indices could therefore be obtained at each scan level from the cardiac apex to base. The CT results compared favorably with established methods, as shown Figure 1.19. CT can therefore be used to evaluate patients in longitudinal studies. Reiter validated the accuracy of EBCT for left and right stroke volume measurements against implanted calibrated electrodes in dogs and also by thermodilution an excellent correlation was found, as seen in Figure 1.20. Simultaneous measures of right and left ventricular volumes were obtained from the same CT data acquisitions.[39] Caputo and Roig et al. in separate studies demonstrated the feasibility of performing exercise stress CT.[40–42] Lanzer et al.[43] demonstrated the feasibility of performing CT with pharmacological interventions.[44–45] The effect of pacing can also be assessed by CT, as shown in Figure 1.21. Further physiological animal studies were performed with EBCT to explore the pressure and volume effects of pericardial effusion on cardiac function involving LV failure.[44–45]

13 CT MEASUREMENT OF BLOOD FLOW

Single slice CT and later EBCT was also used to explore the potential of CT to measure blood flow in vessels, cardiac chambers and tissues. Jashke et al. used indicator dilation theory to study CT in a phantom.[46] Later blood flow was measured by CT in non-moving organs, notably the spleen,

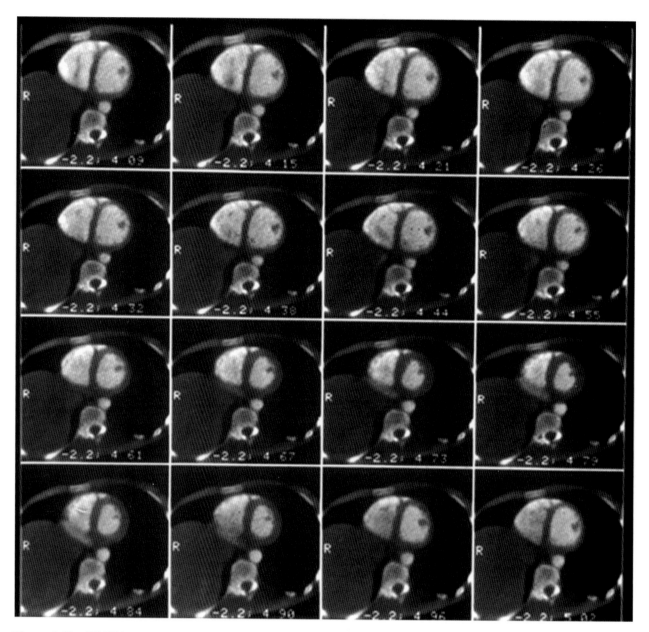

Figure 1.18 EBCT images acquired at 100 m sec interval in the short axis plane demonstrating the typical appearances of the right and left ventricular cavities through the cardiac cycle.

liver and kidney.[47] In the myocardium a gamma variant fit can be obtained from the first passage of a short intravenous contrast medium bolus, as shown in Figure 1.22. This was used by Gould et al. to study myocardial blood flow at rest and during maximum vasodilatation, and obtained a good correlation on a regional basis with microspheres, as can be seen for one dog in Figure 1.23, and for a series of 9 dogs in Figure 1.24. Other early feasibility studies showed similar results; more recently ECG-gated MDCT also appears to validate this earlier work with similar studies.[48–50]

 Ringertz showed reciprocal changes in blood flow in one carotid artery during contralateral occlusion and stenosis.[51]

The results were validated by electromagnetic flow probes on each carotid artery. One approach is illustrated in Figure 1.25 where the peak arrival time at multiple levels along the vessel can be measured by CT time-density curves and from this, the velocity is calculated. Measurements of the vessel area obtained from the axial CT images provide an area and velocity which is a useful measure of blood flow. The area under the time-density curve reflects cardiac output, and this too was validated against thermodilution, initially with a single slice scanner and later EBCT.[52–53] The linear regression line for CT density in Housfield numbers against iodine concentration is excellent over a wide range. Coronary artery by-pass

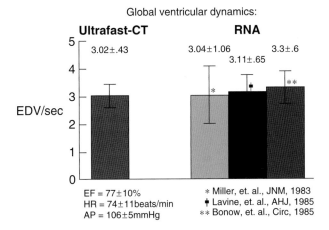

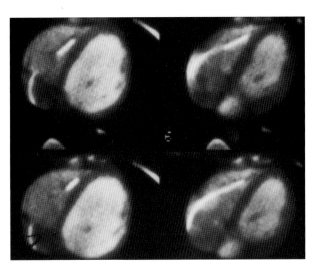

Figure 1.19 Global ventricular dynamics by EBCT in a patient series, compared with established values by radionuclide methods. A good correlation can be seen.

Figure 1.21 Contrast enhanced 8 mm thick EBCT scans at the same level during one cardiac cycle demonstrated the position of a pacing catheter in the right heart. Motion degradation due to pacemaker artifacts is not a significant problem.

graft patency with CT was first reported in a patient series by Brudage et al. and W. Stanford.[54–55] Measurements of graft flow were explored by Rumberger et al.[56–57]

14 CONGENITAL HEART DISEASE AND CT

The utility of CT for identifying intracardiac shunts was measured by Garrett et al. in a dog model, in which a variable shunt was created between the left atrium and pulmonary artery. CT measurements of shunt flow, using the recirculation time/density curves (similar to nuclear medicine studies) derived from an ROI over the atrium, showed excellent correlation with measurements of oxygen saturation curves.[58]

A large patient series with congenital heart has also been studied with EBCT by Eldrige et al.[59]

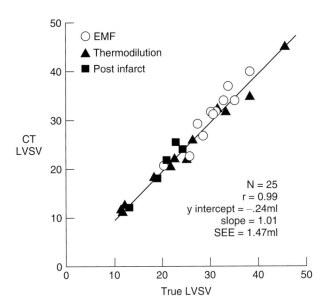

Figure 1.20 CT-derived left ventricular stoke volume (LVSV) compared with true LVSV determined by electromagnetic flow probe (EMF) or thermodilution cardiac output. Precision of measurements of right and left ventricular volume by cine computed tomography. (From ref. 39 with permission)

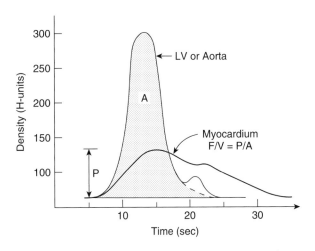

Figure 1.22 Myocardial perfusion curve generated over a myocardial region of interest. Curve analysis provides peak height. Blood flow (F/V) in any myocardial region can be calculated as the ratio of the peak of the time density curve in that area (P) to the area under the aorta or left ventricle time density curve (A), which is representative of cardiac output. HU = Hounsfield units.

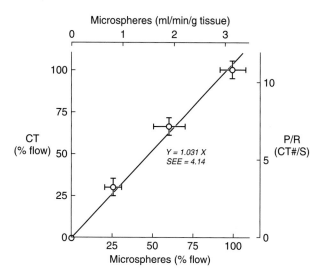

Figure 1.23 Comparison of EBCT and radiolabeled microsphere measurements of global myocardial flow in a mongrel dog. The dotted line is the line of unity.

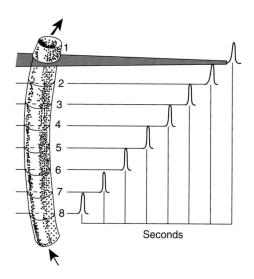

Figure 1.25 Illustration of the CT time density curves generated at eight contiguous levels from a multilevel EBCT flow sequence. The diagram represents a vessel-like carotid artery. The peak arrival time is given for each flow curve; hence, the velocity profile can be measured in cm per sec. Blood flow can be estimated from the velocity if the vessel area is known. This is readily calculated from the many cross-sectional CT images.

15 PULMONARY HYPERTENSION

Pulmonary embolism was also evaluated by CT in acute and chronic patients in the early part of the 1980s.[60–62]

16 SUMMARY

Many individuals have contributed to the development of CT for cardiac applications. The early studies described here suggest that CT still has a great deal to offer patients with heart disease. Feasibility studies are important, but now there is good evidence that MDCT, which is widely available, will have the critical mass of proponents to pursue it on a larger scale. Quantitation of cardiac function by CT can be considered in two major categories. The first is by motion versus time, in which endsystolic and diastolic images provide linear, area and /or volume measurements of arteries, cardiac chambers and myocardial walls over time intervals.

The second method is by obtaining CT images during a fixed phase of the cardiac cycle, usually diastole on every heart beat or every other, and measuring the flow of contrast (density) versus time, using indicator dilution principles.

CT has only been available for the past 30 years. Many factors are involved in determining which diagnostic study is preferred for a given patient with heart disease. These include proven efficacy, robustness, reliability and accuracy, additionally the comfort and confidence of the referring physician, as well as patients' is important. Availability and cost are also relevant issues, as well as competing studies, which are far more established and accepted than newer techniques.

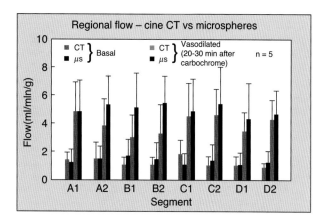

Figure 1.24 Comparison of EBCT measurements of regional myocardial perfusion with micropheres in a series of dogs. Four areas of interest were identified at two LV levels on CT images during sequential scans triggered at end diastole to minimize motion. Chromonar was administered to provide data for each 8 regions at rest and during maximal vasodilatation. The microspheres were injected simultaneously and the results graphed as illustrated in pairs for resting and stress states by region. The error bars illustrate the excellent correlation achieved. Measurement of regional myocardial blood flow in dogs by ultrafast CT. (From ref. 48 with permission).

This historical review of feasibility and validation studies should provide a broad base and encouragement for those more recently involved in cardiac CT. The early studies were designed to evaluate the potential of CT with the expectation that it would one day become the success for the heart that it has been for other organ systems. To this end the literature referenced can be considered in four main categories, ranging progressively from: (1) mathematical simulations, (2) Phantom experiments, (3) animal studies, and (4) patient pilot studies and clinical trials.

The chapters which follow expand greatly on the current and future clinical applications of CT for cardiovascular diagnosis.

REFERENCES

1. Rosenbusch G, Odkerk M, Amman E. Radiology in Medical Diagnostics – Evolution of X-ray application 1895–1995. Blackwell Science, Berlin, 1990.
2. Takashi S. Rotational Radiography. Society for the Promotion of Science, Tokyo, Japan, 1957.
3. Hounsfield GN, Computed Medical Imaging. Nobel lecture, December 8, 1979. Computed medical imaging. Med Phys. 1980; 7(4): 283–90.
4. Adams DF, Hessel SJ, Judy PF, et al. Computed Tomography of the Normal and Infarcted myocardium. Am J Roentgenol 1976; 126(4): 786–91.
5. Wittenberg J, Powell WJ, Jr., Dinsmore RF, et al. Computerized tomography of ischemic myocardium: Quantitation of extent and severity of edema in an in vitro canine model. Invest. Radiol. 1977; 12: 215–23.
6. Gray WR., Jr, Parkey RW, Buja IM., et al. Computed tomography: In vitro evaluation of myocardial infarction. Radiol. 1977; 122: 511–13.
7. Powell WJ, Jr., Wittenberg J, Maturi RA., et al. Detection of edema associated with myocardial ischemia by computerized tomography in isolated, arrested canine hearts. Circulation 1977; 55(1): 99–108.
8. Dodge HT, Sandler H, Baxley WA, Hawley RR. Usefulness and limitations of radiographic methods for determining left ventricular volume. Am J Cardiol. 1966; 18(1): 10–24.
9. Holliday D, Resnich R. Archimedes' Principle. In: Physics (Wiley, New York, 1966); 430.
10. Lipton MJ, Hayashi TT, Boyd DF, Carlsson E. Measurement of left ventricular cast volume by computerized tomography. Radiol. 1978; 127(2): 419–23.
11. Lipton MJ, Hayashi TT, Davis PL, Carlsson E. The effects of orientation on volume measurements of human left ventricular casts. Invest Radiol 1980; 15(6): 469–74.
12. Skioldebrand CG, Ovenfors CO, Mavroudis C, Lipton MJ. Assessment of ventricular wall thickness in vivo by computed transmission tomography. Circulation 1980; 61(5): 960–65.
13. Skioldebrand CG, Lipton MJ, Mavroudis C, Hayashi TT. Determination of left ventricular mass by computed tomography. Am J Cardiol 1982; 49(1): 63–70.
14. Berninger WH, Redington RW, Doherty P, Lipton MJ, Carlsson E. Gated cardiac scanning: canine studies. J Comput Assist Tomogr. 1979; 3(2): 155–63.
15. Godwin JD, Herfkens RJ, Skioldebrand CG, et al. Detection of intraventricular thrombi by computed tomography. Radiol. 1981; 138(3): 717–21.
16. Lackner K, Thurn P. Computed tomography of the heart: ECG-gated and continuous scans. Radiol. 1981; 140(2): 413–20.
17. Masuda Y, Yoshida H, Morooka N, et al. ECG synchronized computed tomography in clinical evaluation of total and regional cardiac motion: comparison of postmyocardial infarction to normal hearts by rapid sequential imaging. Am Heart J. 1982; 103(2): 230–8.
18. Mattrey RF, Slutsky RA, Long SA, Higgins CB. In vivo assessment of left ventricular wall and chamber dynamics during transient myocardial ischemia using prospectively ECG-gated computerized transmission tomography. Circulation 1983; 67(6): 1245–51.
19. Berninger WH, Redington RW, Leue W, et al. Technical aspects and clinical applications of CT/X, a dynamic CT scanner. J Comput Asst Tomogr 1981; 5: 206–15.
20. Carlsson E, Lipton MJ, Berninger WH, Doherty P, Redington RW. Selective left coronary myocardiography by computed tomography in living dogs. Invest Radiol 1977; 12(6): 559–62.
21. Doherty PW, Lipton MJ, Berninger WH, et al. The detection and quantitation of myocardial infarction in vivo using transmission computed tomography. Circulation 1981; 63(3): 597–606.
22. Newell JD, Higgins CB, Abraham JL, et al. Computerized tomographic appearance of evolving myocardial infarctions. Invest. Radiol. 1980; 15: 207–14.
23. Lipton MJ, Higgins CB. Evaluation of ischemic heart disease by computerized transmission tomography. Radiologic Clinics of NA 1980; 18(3): 557–76.
24. Siemers PT, Higgins CB, Schmidt W, Ashburn W, Hagan P. Detection, quantitation and contrast enhancement of myocardial infarction utilizing computerized axial tomography: comparison with histochemical staining and 99mTc-pyrophosphate imaging. Invest Radiol 1978; 13(2): 103–9.
25. Ringertz HG, Palmer RG, Lipton MJ, Carlsson E. CT attenuation ratio of myocardium and blood pool in the normal and infarcted canine heart. Acta Radiological [Diagn] 1983; 24(1): 11–16.
26. Gerber BL, Belge B, Legros GJ, et al. Characterization of acute and chronic myocardial infarcts by multidetector computed tomography: comparison with contrast-enhanced magnetic resonance. Circulation 2006; 113(6): 823–33.
27. Lardo AC, Cordeiro MA, Silva C, et al. Contrast-enhanced multidetector computed tomography viability imaging after myocardial infarction: characterization of myocyte death, microvascular obstruction, and chronic scar. Circulation 2006; 113(3): 394–404.
28. Kramer PH, Goldstein JA, Herkens RJ, Lipton MJ, Brundage BH. Imaging of acute myocardial infarction in man with contrast-enhanced computed transmission tomography. Am Heart J. 1984; 108(6): 1514–23.
29. Koyama Y, Matsuoka H, Mochizuki T, et al. Assessment of reperfused acute myocardial infarction with two-phase contrast-enhanced helical CT: prediction of left ventricular function and wall thickness. Radiology 2005; 235(3): 804–11.

30. Ritman EL. The DSR – a unique x-ray computed tomographic scanner for exploring the power of the dynamic spatial reconstruction. Am J Card Imaging 1994; 8(2): 161–7.

31. Ritman EL. Cardiac computed tomography imaging: a history and some future possibilities. Cardiol Clin. 2003; 21(4): 491–513.

32. Boyd DP. A proposed dynamic cardiac 3-D densitometer for early detection of and evaluation of heart disease. IEEE Trans Nucl Sci. 1979; 26: 2724.

33. Boyd DP, Couch JL, Napel SA, Peschmann KR, Rand RE. Ultrafast cine CT: Where have we been? What lies ahead? Am J Card Imaging, 1987; 1: 175.

34. Redington RW, Berninger WH, Lipton MJ, et al. Cardiac computed tomography. SPIE: Recent and future developments in medical imaging II. 1979; 206: 67–72.

35. Boyd DP. Instrumentation and Principles of CT, Chapter II. Cardiac PET and PET/CT Imaging. Di Carli M, Lipton MJ, eds, published by Springer (in press).

36. Kalender WA, Seissler W, Klotz E, Vock P. Spiral volumetric CT with single-breath-hold technique, continuous transport, and continuous scanner rotation. Radiology 1990; 176(1): 181–3.

37. Hubener KH, Lipton MJ. Digital radiography (scanning projection): Possibilities and perspective. In: Radiology Today, 2nd ed, FH Heuck and MW Donner, eds. Heidelberg (Springer-Verlag, 1983) 298–306.

38. Lipton MJ, Boyd DP. Contrast media in dynamic computed tomography of the heart and great vessels. Proceedings of the CT International Workshop, Berlin, Exerpta Medica 1981; 204–13.

39. Reiter SJ, Rumberger JA, Feiring AJ, Stanford W, Marcus ML. Precision of measurements of right and left ventricular volume by cine computed tomography. Circulation 1986; 74(4): 890–900.

40. Roig E, Chomka EV, Castaner A, et al. Exercise ultrafast computed tomography for the detection of coronary artery disease. J Am Coll Cardiol. 1989; 13(5): 1073–81.

41. Caputo, Gould R, Dery R., et al. Ultrafast CT evalauation of exercise induced ischemia: a feasibility study. Dynamic Cardiovascular Imaging 1989; 2(2): 110–19.

42. Lipton MJ, Rumberger JA. Exercise Ultrafast Computed Tomography: Preliminary findings on its role in diagnosis of Coronary Artery Disease. Editorial. JACC 1989; 13(5): 1082–84.

43. Lanzer P, Garrett J, Lipton MJ, et al. Quantitation of regional myocardial function by cine computed tomography: Pharmacologic changes in wall thickness. J Am Coll Cardiol 1986; 8(3): 682–92.

44. Smiseth OA, Refsum H, Junemann M, et al. Ventricular diastolic pressure-volume shifts during acute ischemic left ventricular failure in dogs. JACC 1984; 3(4): 956–77.

45. Smiseth OA, Frais MA, Junemann M, et al. Left and right ventricular diastolic function during acute pericardial tamponade. Clinical Physiology 1991; 11(1): 61–71.

46. Jaschke W, Gould RG, Assimakopoulos PA, Lipton MJ. Flow measurements with a high speed computed tomography scanner. Med Physics 1987; 14(2): 238–43.

47. Jaschke W, Cogan MG, Sievers R, Gould R, Lipton MJ. Measurement of renal blood flow by cine computed tomography. Kidney Intl 1987; 31(4): 1038–42.

48. Gould RG, Lipton MJ, McNamara MT, et al. Measurement of regional myocardial blood flow in dogs by ultrafast CT. Invest Radiol 1988; 23(5): 348–53.

49. Rumberger JA, Feiring AJ, Lipton MJ, et al. Use of ultrafast CT to quantitate regional myocardial perfusion: a preliminary report. JACC 1987; 9(1): 59–69.

50. Koyama Y, Mochizuki T, Higaki J. Computed tomography assessment of myocardial perfusion, viability, and function. J Magn Reson Imaging 2004; 19(6): 800–15.

51. Ringertz H, Jaschke W, Sievers RE, Lipton MJ. Relative carotid blood flow measurements in dogs by high-speed CT. Invest Radiol 1987; 22(12): 960–64.

52. Herfkens RJ, Axel L, Lipton MJ, et al. Measurement of cardiac output by computed transmission tomography. Invest Radiol 1982; 17(6): 550–3.

53. Garrett JS, Lanzer P, Jaschke W, et al. Measurement of cardiac output by cine computed tomography. Am J Cardiol 1985; 56(10): 657–61.

54. Brundage BH, Lipton MJ, Herfkens RJ, et al. Detection of patent coronary bypass grafts by computed tomography. A preliminary report. Circulation 1980; 61(4): 826–31.

55. Stanford W, Brundage BH, MacMillan R, et al. Sensitivity and specificity of assessing coronary bypass graft patency with ultrafast computed tomography: results of a multicenter study. JACC 1988; 12(1): 1–7.

56. Rumberger JA and Lipton MJ. Ultrafast cardiac CT scanning. Cardiology Clinics, Wolfe C. ed. (W. B. Saunders Company, Philadelphia, PA 1989), 7(3); 713–34.

57. Rumberger JA, Feiring AJ, Hiratzka, et al. Quantification of coronary artery bypass flow reserve in dogs using cine-computed tomography. Circ Res. 1987; 61(5 Pt 2): II, 117–23.

58. Garrett JS, Jaschke W, Aherne T, et al. Quantitation of intracardiac shunts by cine-CT. JCAT 1988; 12(1): 82–7.

59. Eldridge WJ, Diethelm NE, Lipton MJ. Ultrafast computed tomography in the diagnosis of congenital heart disease. In: Pediatric Cardiovascular Imaging. Tonkin ILD, Ed. (WB Saunders Company: Philadelphia, 1992) 177–201.

60. Di Carlo LA, Schiller NB, Herfkens RJ, Brundage BH, Lipton MJ. Noninvasive detection of proximal pulmonary artery thrombosis by two-dimensional echocardiography and computerized tomography. Am Heart J 1982; 104(4) Part 1: 879–81.

61. Kareiakis DJ, Herfkens RJ, Brundage BH, Gamsu G, Lipton MJ. Computerized tomography in chronic thromboembolic pulmonary hypertension. Am Heart J 1983; 106(6): 1432–36.

62. Himmelman RB, Abbott JA, Lipton MJ, Schiller NB. Cine computed tomography compared with echocardiography in the evaluation of cardiac function in emphysema. Am Jrnl of Cardiac Imaging 1988; 2(4): 283–91.

2

Physics of and Approaches to Cardiovascular Computed Tomography

Marc Kachelrieß

I INTRODUCTION

Cardiac computed tomography (CT) challenges the problem of imaging moving objects without showing motion artifacts. The aim is to provide high fidelity images that allow to perform coronary CT angiography, coronary calcification measurements, soft plaque detection and dynamic CT studies of the heart.

In general, CT requires at least 180° plus fan angle of projection data to perform image reconstruction. This implies that the intrinsic temporal resolution of a standard CT scan is in the order of $t_{rot}/2$ or worse, where t_{rot} is the time needed for a full rotation of the scanner and lies in the order of 0.33 s to 0.5 s, today. With modern cone-beam CT scanners it is possible to achieve $t_{rot}/2 = 165$ ms which is not sufficient to perfectly image the anatomical details of the moving human heart. Standard spiral CT image reconstruction further makes use of all the data contributing to a given voxel and therefore exhibits a temporal resolution of about t_{rot}/p where p is the spiral pitch value defined by the ratio of the table increment per rotation and the total collimation (number of slices times slice thickness). The value $1/p$ quantifies the number of rotations that contribute to a single point in the object. Typical pitch values lie in the range from 0.1 to 1.5.

Special reconstruction algorithms have been designed to allow reducing the data to a single 180° segment to always come close to $t_{rot}/2$. If the object is moving in a periodic fashion it is further possible to use dedicated cardiac reconstruction algorithms that divide the required 180° into one, two or more smaller segments and collect these smaller data segments from adjacent motion periods (e.g. heart cycles) and that ensure that the same motion phase always enters the image. Thereby, the temporal resolution can be improved proportionally to the number of segments used and 4D phase-correlated imaging of the heart is achieved. The alignment of these allowed data intervals (be it one or several segments) to a desired motion phase generates images where the object's motion is frozen in the desired motion state. These basic concepts of phase-correlated CT imaging were first proposed and evaluated in Kachelrieß and Kalender[1] and since then they are widely used in clinical CT.[2–12]

To further improve the temporal resolution, new scanner concepts that simultaneously utilize two x-ray sources and two detector arrays were introduced in 2005. These dual source CT (DSCT) scanners require only a 90° rotation to acquire sufficient data and hence exhibit a temporal resolution in the order of $t_{rot}/4$ or less. Thereby, 83 ms temporal resolution are routinely achieved which is sufficient to image patients with high heart rates and with arrhythmia throughout all motion cycles.

This chapter gives an introduction into the basics of cardiac CT as it is in use today. It focuses on physics, technology and image reconstruction. Dose issues and cardiac CT applications are addressed elsewhere in this book.

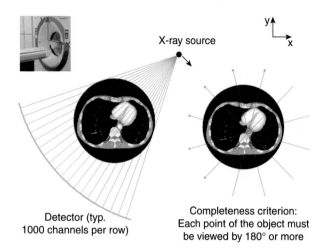

Figure 2.1 Clinical CT is the measurement of x-ray photon attenuation along straight lines. The in-plane scan geometry is the fan-beam geometry with one point-like source and many detector elements. During a rotation of the gantry many line integrals are measured – enough to perform image reconstruction.

2 CT BASICS

Clinical CT is the measurement of an object's x-ray absorption along straight lines. As long as each object point is probed by x-rays under an angular interval of 180° image reconstruction of that point is possible. Therefore, clinical CT scanners have an x-ray focal spot that rotates continuously around the patient. On the opposing side of the x-ray tube a cylindrical detector consisting of about 10^3 channels per slice is mounted (Figure 2.1). The plane of rotation is the x-y-plane.

The number of slices that are simultaneously acquired is denoted as M (Figure 2.2). In the longitudinal direction (perpendicular to the plane of rotation), the size of the detectors determines the thickness S of the slices that are acquired. During a full rotation approximately of 10^3 read-outs of the detector are performed. Altogether about 10^6 intensity measurements are taken per slice and rotation. The negative logarithm $p(L)$ of each intensity measurement I corresponds to the line integral along line L of the object's linear attenuation coefficient distribution $\mu(x, y, z)$:

$$p(L) = -\ln\frac{I(L)}{I_0} = \int_L dL\, \mu(x,y,z).$$

I_0 is the primary x-ray intensity and is needed for proper normalization.

The CT image $f(x, y, z)$ is a close approximation to the true distribution $\mu(x, y, z)$. The process of computing the CT image from the set of measured projection values $p(L)$ is called image reconstruction and is one of the key components of a CT scanner. For circle scans that perform measurements at a fixed z-position, image reconstruction is rather simple. It consists of a convolution of the projection data

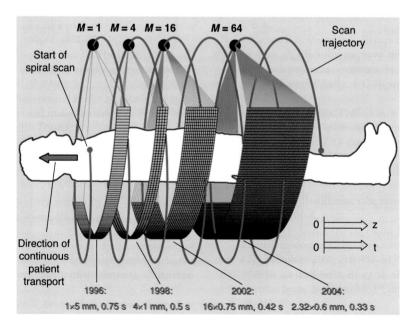

Figure 2.2   Spiral CT principle. Four scanner generations are shown: single-slice, 4-slice, 16-slice and 64-slice spiral CT scanners.

with the reconstruction kernel followed by a backprojection into image domain:

$$f(x,y) = \int_0^\pi d\vartheta\, p(\vartheta,\xi) * k(\xi)\Big|_{\xi = x\cos\vartheta + y\sin\vartheta}$$

where ϑ is the angle and ξ is the distance of the measured ray L that is defined as $x\cos\vartheta + y\sin\vartheta = \xi$. The algorithm is called the filtered backprojection (FBP) and is implemented in all clinical CT scanners. Several reconstruction kernels $k(\xi)$ are available to allow modifying image sharpness (spatial resolution) and image noise characteristics.

The reconstructed image $f(x, y, z)$ is expressed in CT values. They are defined as a linear function of the attenuation values. The linear relation is based on the demand that air (zero attenuation) has a CT value of -1000 HU (Hounsfield units) and water (attenuation μ_{water}) has a value of 0 HU. Thus, the CT value is given as a function of μ as follows:

$$CT = \frac{\mu - \mu_{water}}{\mu_{water}} 1000\,\text{HU}.$$

The CT values are often called the Hounsfield values. They have been introduced by Hounsfield to replace the handling with the rather inconvenient μ values by an integer-valued quantity. Since the CT value is directly related to the attenuation values, which are proportional to the density of the material, we can interpret the CT value of a pixel or voxel as being the (approximate) density of the object at the respective location. It should be noted here that CT, in contrast to other imaging modalities such as magnetic resonance imaging or ultrasound imaging, is highly quantitative regarding the accuracy of the reconstructed values. The reconstructed attenuation map can therefore serve for quantitative diagnosis such as the quantification of coronary calcifications.

3 SPIRAL CT

In the late 1980s, just when continuously rotating scanners became available, a new scan mode was introduced by Willi A. Kalender.[9,13,14] In spiral CT data acquisition is performed continuously while the patient moves at constant speed through the gantry. Viewed from the patient the scan trajectory is a spiral. Although not obvious spiral scans turned out to yield better image quality than conventional scans. This, however, requires the addition of z-interpolation as an additional image reconstruction step.[9]

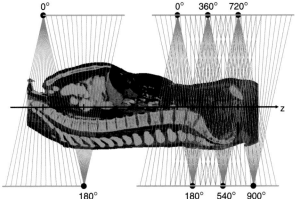

Maximum table increment: $p \approx 1.5$ Overlapping data acquisition: $p < 1.5$

Maximum increment: angular range = 180° (completeness)
Overlapping scan: angular range > 180° (completeness + redundancy)

Figure 2.3 The pitch value's upper limit is determined by the completeness criterion (c.f. Figure 2.1). Smaller pitch values mean that redundant data are acquired. Cardiac CT makes use of the data redundancy to select only interesting data intervals, i.e. those that are in the desired phase of cardiac motion.

A new scan parameter has been introduced in spiral CT: the table increment d is the distance the table travels during one rotation of the gantry. In conventional CT (circle scans) this value has typically been equal to the collimated thickness (adjacent but non-overlapping images). In spiral CT we can choose d smaller or greater than $M \cdot S$. One uses the so-called pitch value to relativize the definition of the table increment [15]:

$$p = \frac{d}{W_{tot}}.$$

W_{tot} is the total collimation and usually equal to the product of the number of slices × nominal slice thickness, i.e. $W_{tot} = M \cdot S$. Small pitch values yield overlapping data and the redundancy can be used to decrease image noise (more quanta contribute to one z-position), to reduce artifacts or, in case of cardiac CT, to improve temporal resolution (Figure 2.3). Large pitch values increase the scan speed and complete anatomical ranges can be covered very fast. Typical values lie between 0.1 and 1.5 and spatial resolution is not a function of the pitch value. However, for some scanners pitch values up to 2 are allowed and the longitudinal spatial resolution (z-resolution) decreases whenever the pitch exceeds the value 1.5.

The inverse pitch $1/p$ measures how many rotations contribute to each z-position. For example with $p = 1$ we find that a given z-position is covered by exactly one rotation and for $p = 0.5$ two rotations contribute to the z-position, i.e. a 720° angular interval.

4 CARDIAC CT

The aim of cardiac CT is to provide images of the heart that are free of motion artifacts and that correspond to a specified motion phase. Only then can applications such as coronary CT angiography or coronary calcification quantification be carried out reliably and guarantee reproducible results.

To achieve this goal one must be able to synchronize data acquisition and/or image reconstruction with the cardiac motion and one must achieve a fairly high temporal resolution. Synchronization is typically done using the patient ECG signal that is recorded simultaneously with CT data acquisition (Figure 2.4). Alternative approaches that derive the motion signal directly from the patient raw data or from a set of reconstructed images are in use, too.[16, 17]

Typical heart rates lie in the range from 40 bpm to 120 bpm and correspond to a duration of the heart cycle between 0.5 s and 1.5 s. To avoid blurring due to heart motion it is desired to have no more than 10% of the motion cycle show up in the reconstructed images and the temporal resolution should be in the order of 50 ms to 150 ms, depending on the heart rate. Since this cannot always be achieved, high heart rates (above 70 bpm) are frequently avoided by using premedication with beta blockers. CT imaging requires projection data from at least 180° plus fan angle. Using this minimal data interval guarantees

a temporal resolution of slightly above $t_{rot}/2$ where t_{rot} is the time needed for one scanner rotation. An example that shows the differences between a standard reconstruction that uses all available data and a phase-correlated reconstruction that only shows the minimal data required is given in Figure 2.5.

4.1 Prospective triggering

One way to obtain phase-correlated CT images of the heart is to use the ECG to trigger the scan (x-ray and data acquisition on). This prospective technique is typically used in combination with circle scans. The scanner is continuously rotating, the patient table is at rest and the x-rays and data acquisition are switched on whenever the ECG signal is about to arrive at the desired motion phase. X-rays and data acquisition and are switched off after 180° plus fan angle of data have been acquired. After one acquisition the table is advanced by a certain amount (that typically corresponds to the total collimation) and the procedure is repeated until the complete heart is covered. The temporal resolution lies in the order of $t_{rot}/2$ and image reconstruction is a simple partial scan reconstruction (filtered backprojection of 180° plus fan angle).

Since prospective gating is nothing but a sequential CT scan (step-and-shoot scan, multiple circle scan) triggered by an external signal it does not benefit from the higher image quality that can be achieved with spiral CT. For example data inconsistencies due to patient motion between different table positions may show up in the

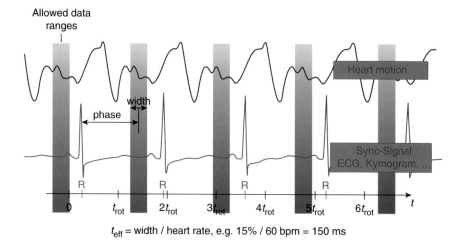

t_{eff} = width / heart rate, e.g. 15% / 60 bpm = 150 ms

Figure 2.4 In cardiac CT only data corresponding to a certain motion phase shall contribute to the images. In prospective gating techniques this phase is fixed, for retrospective gating one can vary the phase from reconstruction to reconstruction. The width of the data intervals determines the temporal resolution.

Standard   Phase-correlated

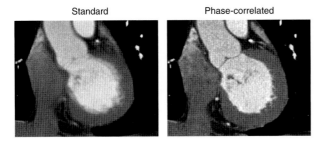

Figure 2.5 Example images of the heart using a standard reconstruction (left) and a phase-correlated reconstruction (right). Due to the low temporal resolution the standard image is a superposition of all cardiac phases and hence all structures are significantly blurred. This is not the case for the phase-correlated image. $C = 150$ HU, $W = 700$ HU.

reconstructed images and volumetric displays of the data may not be of state-of-the-art quality.

4.2 Retrospective gating

One of the most prominent special CT applications today is retrospectively gated CT of the heart. It combines the advantages of spiral CT with phase-correlated imaging and thereby guarantees highest image quality, isotropic spatial resolution, fast scanning and high temporal resolution. Cardiac spiral CT started with the introduction of dedicated

phase-correlated reconstruction algorithms for single-slice spiral CT in 1997[1] and since then they have been extended to multi-slice and cone-beam CT and are widely used in clinical routine.[2–12]

The underlying principle of phase-correlated spiral CT is to acquire highly overlapping spiral data using a small pitch value. In this case the acquired data are highly redundant and a given voxel or z-position is covered by far more than the 180° actually needed. Dedicated image reconstruction algorithms make use of this data redundancy by selecting a small 180° interval from the large and redundant data range (Figure 2.6).

Freely selecting such a data interval within the cardiac motion cycle implies that the time t_{rot}/p the scanner covers a given z-position (or a given voxel) is longer than the duration $1/f_H$ of one heart cycle: Whenever the spiral pitch, the patient heart rate and the scanner rotation time fulfill the requirement

$$P < f_H \cdot t_{rot}$$

it is possible to retrospectively select a 180° interval at any desired cardiac motion phase. Only then can one reconstruct the complete heart as a function of time.

As an example, consider a patient with a heart rate of 60 bpm and assume the scanner rotation is 0.33 s. Choosing a pitch value of 0.2 or 0.3 would be adequate in this case, a pitch value of 0.4 would be too high to allow for

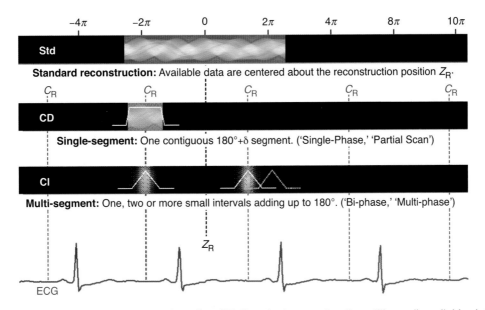

Figure 2.6 Principle of retrospectively gated cardiac CT. Standard reconstruction utilizes all available data, i.e. $1/p$ full rotations. Cardiac reconstruction combines one or more data segments to yield a complete 180° data range with maximum temporal resolution.

phase correlation. Note that lower heart rates require lower pitch values and thus imply slower scanning.

With this so-called partial scan, single-segment or single-phase approach one achieves a temporal resolution of $t_{rot}/2$. In case of a 0.33 s rotation these are 165 ms. However, one can further increase the temporal resolution by splitting up the required 180° into two or more data segments that are collected from adjacent heart beats (Figure 2.6). These so-called multi-segment or multi-phase approaches have the advantage of increasing the temporal resolution by up to a factor two or three, respectively. Of course, the scan speed must be decreased to allow for two or three heart beats during the coverage of a given z-position and the relation $P < f_H \cdot t_{rot}$ must be replaced by $P < f_H \cdot t_{rot}/2$ or $P < f_H \cdot t_{rot}/3$, respectively. In practice, the algorithms are adaptive and automatically choose the appropriate data segments as a function of the scan pitch, the rotation time and the patient heart rate[1]: low heart rates typically imply single-segment reconstruction, high heart rates are handled with multi-segment approaches, in case of varying heart frequency the algorithms may adaptively switch between single- and multi-segment mode.

However, the technique to collect data from multiple heart cycles suffers from the fact that a lower pitch value is required and that their benefit is dependent on the heart rate. In a case where the heart rate is in resonance with the scanner rotation, e.g. when the patient has 60 bpm and the scanner rotates with 0.5 s, the multi-phase approaches exhibit the same temporal resolution as the single-phase approaches because after one heart beat the scanner 'sees' exactly the same view angles as have been acquired already during the first heart cycle. Therefore, the temporal resolution exhibits a rather complex behavior (top curve in Figure 2.7) and in case of resonances the multi-segment algorithms exhibit the same low temporal resolution as the single-segment reconstruction.[5–18]

4.3 Dual-source CT

From Figure 2.1 we have learned that a 180° data interval is required to perform image reconstruction. Typically, this requirement limits the temporal resolution to 50% of the scanner rotation time. However, when more than one x-ray tube and more than one detector, i.e. more than one spiral thread, are built into the same gantry one can acquire the 180° data range with less than 180° rotation (Figure 2.8). With multi-source CT scanners the achievable temporal resolution increases proportionally with the

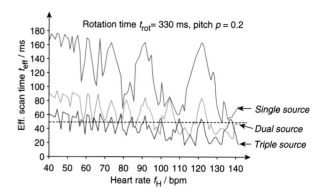

Figure 2.7 Temporal resolution in phase-correlated cardiac spiral CT as a function of heart rate for scanners with one, two and three source-detector systems. The temporal resolution of multi-phase approaches is always equal to or better than the temporal resolution of a single phase or partial scan algorithm.[5,18]

number of sources used. For multi-segment phase-correlated image reconstruction the heart rate dependency turns out to far smaller with multi-source CT scanners than with single source CT scanners (Figure 2.7, bottom two curves).[18]

Regarding the literature the first multi-source CT systems that were realized attempted achieving fully four-dimensional imaging by completely sampling large object regions in the spatial and temporal domain with high spatial

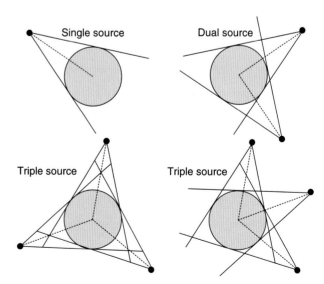

Figure 2.8 CT systems with two or three x-ray sources require only a 90° or 60° acquisition interval to obtain complete data. Hence, their temporal resolution is increased by a factor of two and three, respectively, compared to single source CT scanners.

and temporal resolution.[19–21] Cost and image quality issues did not allow to commercialize this system. Liu et al.[22] also proposed a multi-threaded CT scanner to improve temporal resolution but no system was realized. Neither of these systems considered phase-correlated image reconstruction, no design optimizations regarding temporal resolution were carried out and no reconstructions of clinical cardiac CT data were provided.

Recently, the first clinical dual source dual detector CT system became available. It uses two threads, a z- and an α-flying focal spot (see Flohr et al.[23] and Kachelrieß[24] for details regarding the flying focal spot), and it reads out 32 detector rows per thread (Somatom Definition, Siemens Medical Solutions, Forchheim, Germany).[25] Each projection thus consists of 2·2·32 slices (Figure 2.9).

The Definition scanner rotates at 0.33 s and thereby achieves a temporal resolution of 83 ms for single-phase (partial scan) cardiac image reconstruction. This is high enough to obtain superb artifact-free images for a wide range of heart rates, even in cases of arrhythmia. For example Figure 2.10 shows a clear delineation of the coronary arteries even into the most distal segments. Even more, reconstructions can be performed at any cardiac phase with nearly equal image quality (Figure 2.11). Higher temporal resolution can be achieved with DSCT using multi-segment reconstruction techniques, just in the single-source case and may be of use for functional assessment of the heart. In any case, the DSCT experience gathered so far meets the expectations and proves a significant benefit over single-source CT systems.[26,27]

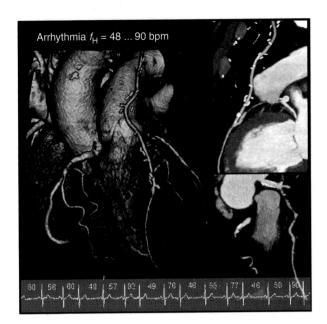

Figure 2.10 Heart rate independent cardiac imaging with dual source CT: arrhythmic patient, heart rate from 48 bpm to 90 bmp, 83 ms temporal resolution, 0.33 s rotation, 13 s for 137 mm. Data courtesy of University of Erlangen, Germany.

4.4 Kymogram-correlated cardiac CT

Typically, phase-correlated cardiac CT imaging uses the patient ECG signal for synchronization and for correlation. However, the ECG is an electric signal and does not exactly map to the mechanical motion of the heart. Signals that

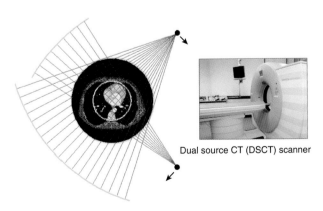

Dual source CT (DSCT) scanner

Figure 2.9 The DSCT scanner Somatom Definition (Siemens Medical Solutions, Forchheim, Germany) comprises two tube detector systems mounted at an angle of 90° and thereby requires only a quarter rotation to acquire a complete CT data set. With 0.33 s required for a full rotation its temporal resolution is 0.33 s/4 = 83 ms.

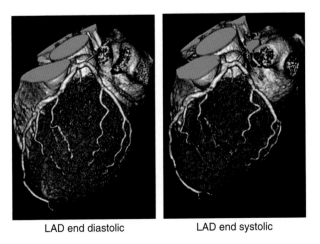

LAD end diastolic   LAD end systolic

Figure 2.11 Heart rate independent cardiac imaging with dual source CT throughout all cardiac phases: patient heart rate from 79 bpm to 86 bmp, 83 ms temporal resolution, 0.33 s rotation, 6 s for 120 mm. Data courtesy of University of Erlangen, Germany.

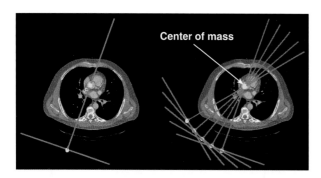

Figure 2.12 Kymogram principle. A few projections suffice to triangulate the center of mass of the heart. Since this COM moves as a function of time one can use the resulting kymogram as a synchronization signal for cardiac imaging.

directly reflect the cardiac motion, which is the source of motion artifacts, may be promising alternatives for synchronization. A raw data-based signal that fulfills this criterion is the so-called kymogram function.[16] It is based on the center of mass theorem that allows to deduce the object center of mass (COM) from the projection center of mass. All that is required are a number of adjacent CT projections. From these projections one can obtain the object center of mass by

simple triangulation (Figure 2.12). Due to the heart motion the so derived object COM moves as a function of time and this motion signal, the kymogram, can be used to synchronize image reconstruction.

A recent study shows that kymogram-based image reconstruction and ECG-based image reconstruction are of comparable quality with ECG-based imaging being slightly superior.[28] Even though this is true on average, in about 5% of the cases the kymogram provides diagnostic images while the ECG does not (Figure 2.13). Therefore one may regard the kymogram as a backup solution for those cases or for cases where the ECG is not available at all or where it is deficient.

4.5 Optimal reconstruction phase

Since the heart's contractile motion is a non-uniform quasi-periodic motion, not all phase intervals in the cardiac cycle are equally well suited with respect to the phase-correlated reconstruction algorithm. The systolic phase corresponds to the contraction of the heart and the myocardium shows a high velocity. After relaxation the heart is almost at rest which corresponds to the diastolic phase. The diastolic phase represents the optimal cardiac reconstruction phase

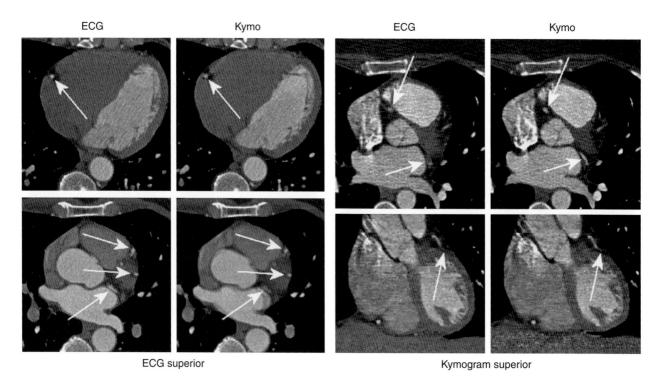

Figure 2.13 In most cases both synchronization approaches are comparable. For some patients the ECG performs better than the kymogram (left), for other patients the kymogram is superior (right). All four reconstructions show the optimal reconstruction phase (found by manual selection). $C = 150$ HU, $W = 700$ HU.

Maximal enhancement   Time to peak   Perfusion (maximum)

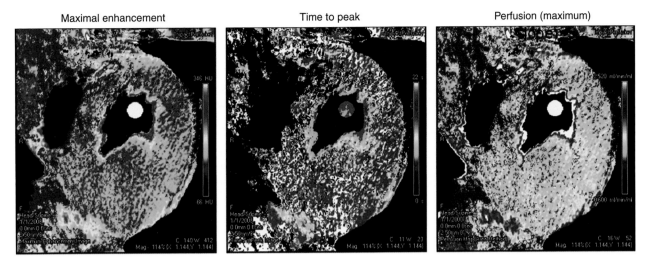

Figure 2.14   Assessment of cardiac function requires 5D imaging (spatial domain + cardiac motion phase + contrast bolus).[31,32]

for most cases,[29] since the temporal window for the data acquisition covers the period of rest. With increasing heart rate, the systolic phase more frequently provides optimal image quality. However, a general prediction of the optimal reconstruction phase showing a minimum of motion is not possible. On the one hand, the possibility of an optimal reconstruction in either the systolic or the diastolic phase (both is possible depending on the patient), prohibits this prediction. On the other hand, a slight patient-dependent variation of the typical ECG phases makes the prediction uncertain. Hence, it is common practice to approach the optimal image quality adaptively by image reconstruction at different phase points. To overcome these problems fully, automatic algorithms, among them the said raw data-based kymogram approach, have been proposed providing the optimal reconstruction phase.[17,30] Hereby, cardiac images with an optimal image quality can be achieved with a single image reconstruction process.

5 SUMMARY AND OUTLOOK

Motion artifact-free phase-correlated CT images of the heart require fast rotating scanners in combination with dedicated image reconstruction algorithms that are able to synchronize the cardiac motion with the raw data. In most cases the ECG signal is used for synchronization but alternative approaches, such as the raw data-based kymogram signal or the image-based motion map, are available, too.

Single-segment reconstruction algorithms obtain a temporal resolution of roughly half of the scanner rotation time. Multi-segment approaches that collect data from adjacent heart cycles may obtain a significantly higher temporal resolution, given that the heart beat is not in resonance with the scanner rotation and given a rather low pitch value. Temporal resolution can be further increased by using dual-source CT scanners and the first clinical studies show that this DSCT technology appears to keep its promises or even outperform them.

Today, the fastest scanners rotate at 0.33 s and one routinely achieves a temporal resolution of far below 100 ms. In combination with isotropic sub-millimeter spatial resolution the resulting CT images of the heart are of highest diagnostic value.

In the future, scanners are likely to improve in temporal and in spatial resolution. Better detector technology, faster rotation times and multiple source-detector arrangements will be required. Increasing the number of simultaneously acquired slices — today 64 slices is standard — will allow to scan the complete heart with just one circle trajectory. This opens the door to phase-correlated dynamic scans of the heart[31,32] (Figure 2.14).

REFERENCES

1. Kachelrieß M and Kalender WA. Electrocardiogram-correlated image reconstruction from subsecond spiral CT scans of the heart. Med Phys 1998; 25(12): 2417–31.

2. Flohr T, Stierstorfer K, Bruder H, and Kachelrieß M. A new cone-beam spiral CT reconstruction approach for 16 slice CT scanner with full dose utilization at arbitrary pitch. Radiology 2001; 221(P): 543.

3. Grass M, Manzke R, Nielsen T, et al. Helical cardiac cone-beam reconstruction using retrospective ECG gating. Phys Med Biol 2003; 48(18): 3069–84.

4. Flohr T, Ohnesorge B, Bruder H, et al. Image reconstruction and performance evaluating for ECG-gated spiral scanning with 16-slice CT system. Med Phys 2003; 30(10): 2650–62.

5. Kachelrieß M, Ulzheimer S, and Kalender WA. ECG-correlated image reconstruction from subsecond multi-slice spiral CT scans of the heart. Med Phys 2000; 27(8): 1881–1902.

6. Kachelrieß M, Ulzheimer S, and Kalender WA. ECG-correlated imaging of the heart with subsecond multi-slice spiral CT. IEEE Trans Med Imaging (Special issue) 2000; 19(9): 888–901.

7. Kachelrieß M, Fuchs T, Lapp R, et al. Image to volume weighting generalized ASSR for arbitrary pitch 3D and phase-correlated 4D spiral cone-beam CT reconstruction. In: Proc. of the 6th Int. Meeting on Fully 3D Image Reconstruction 2001: 179–82.

8. Kachelrieß M, Knaup M, and Kalender WA. Extended parallel backprojection for standard 3D and phase-correlated 4D axial and spiral cone-beam CT with arbitrary pitch and 100% dose usage. Med Phys 2004; 31(6): 1623–41.

9. Kalender WA. Computed Tomography. Fundamentals, System Technology, Image Quality, Applications. 2nd ed. Publicis Erlangen 2005.

10. Manzke R, Grass M, Nielsen T, Shechter G, and Hawkes D. Adaptive Temporal Resolution Optimization in Helical Cardiac Cone Beam CT Reconstruction. Med Phys 2003; 30(12): 3072–80.

11. Taguchi K and Anno H. High temporal resolution for multi-slice helical computed tomography. Med Phys 2000; 27(5): 861–72.

12. Achenbach S, et al. Noninvasive coronary angiography by retrospectively ECG-gated multislice spiral CT. Circulation 2000; 102(12): 2823–28.

13. Kalender WA, Seissler W, and Vock P. Single-breath-hold spiral volumetric CT by continuous patient translation and scanner rotation. Radiology 1989; 173(P): 414.

14. Kalender WA, Seissler W, Klotz E, and Vock P. Spiral volumetric CT with single-breathhold technique, continuous transport, and continuous scanner rotation. Radiology 1990; 176(1): 181–3.

15. IEC. International Electrotechnical Commission, 60601-2-44: Medical electrical equipment – Part 2-44: Particular requirements for the safety of X-ray equipment for computed tomography, Geneva, Switzerland, 1999.

16. Kachelrieß M, Sennst D-A, Maxlmoser W, and Kalender WA. Kymogram detection and kymogram-correlated image reconstruction from subsecond spiral computed tomography scans of the heart. Med Phys 2002; 29(7): 1489–503.

17. Manzke R, Köhler T, Nielsen T, Hawkes DJ, and Grass M. Automatic phase determination for retrospectively gated cardiac CT. Med Phys 2004; 31(12): 3345–62.

18. Kachelrieß M, Knaup M, and Kalender WA. Multi-threaded cardiac CT. Med Phys 2006; 33(7): 2435–47.

19. Boyd DP. Transmission computed tomography. In: Radiology of the skull and brain. Technical aspects of computed tomography. Vol. 5. T. Newton and D. Potts, Editors. C.V. Mosby Company, St. Louis, 1981: 4357–71.

20. Robb R and Ritman EL. High speed synchronous volume computed tomography of the heart. Radiology 1979; 133: 655–61.

21. Robb R, Hoffmann E, Sinak LJ, Harris LD, and Ritman EL. High-speed three-dimensional x-ray computed tomography: The dynamic spatial reconstructor. Proc. IEEE 1983; 71: 308–19.

22. Liu Y, Liu H, and Wang G. Half-scan cone-beam CT fluoroscopy with multiple X-ray sources. Med Phys 2001; 28(7): 1466–71.

23. Flohr T, Stierstorfer K, Ulzheimer S, et al. Image reconstruction and image quality evaluation for a 64-slice CT scanner with z-flying focal spot. Med Phys 2005; 32(8): 2536–47.

24. Kachelrieß M, Knaup M, Penßel C, and Kalender WA. Flying focal spot (FFS) in cone-beam CT. Trans Nuclear Science 2006; 53(3): 1238–47.

25. Flohr T, et al. First performance of a dual-source CT (DSCT) system. Eur Radiol 2006; 16: 256–68.

26. Achenbach S, et al. Contrast-enhanced coronary artery visualization by dual-source computed tomography – Initial experience. Eur J Radiol. 2006; 57(3): 331–5.

27. Johnson TRC, et al. Dual-source CT cardiac imaging: initial experience. Eur Radiol 2006; 16: 1409–15.

28. Ertel D, Pflederer T, Kachelrieß M, et al. Validation of a rawdata-based synchronization signal (kymogram) for a phase-correlated cardiac image reconstruction. IEEE Trans Med Imaging 2006; submitted.

29. Achenbach S, Ropers D, Holle J, et al. In-plane coronary arterial motion velocity: Measurement with electron-beam CT. Radiology 2000; 216(2): 457–63.

30. Ertel D, Kachelrieß M, Pflederer T, et al. Raw data-based detection of the optimal reconstruction phase in ECG-gated cardiac image reconstruction. 9th International Conference on Medical Image Computing and Computer Assisted Intervention. In: Proceedings MICCAI 2006. Springer Berlin Heidelberg: 348–55.

31. Kachelrieß M. Phase-correlated dynamic CT. In: Proc. of the IEEE International Symposium on Biomedical Imaging 2004: 616–19.

32. Ulzheimer S, Muresan L, Kachelrieß M, et al. Considerations on the assessment of myocardial perfusion with multislice spiral CT (MSCT) scanners. Radiology 2001; 221(P): 458.

3

Radiation Dose in Computed Tomography

Michael F. McNitt-Gray

The purpose of this chapter is to provide a discussion of radiation dose in X-ray computed tomography (CT), with specific application to CT of the cardiovascular system. Although CT represents a small percentage of radiological procedures performed, CT contributes a significant amount to the collective effective radiation dose from all radiological procedures.[1] Rapid advances in CT technology have increased both the utility and utilization of CT in many clinical diagnostic applications. Specifically, as tube rotation times climbed to the 0.5 second range and as the number of detector rows first reached 16 and then continued on to 64, the ability to perform CT scans for the coronary arteries has increased dramatically.[2–4] This has led to a significant increase in the number of patients being scanned for cardiovascular problems, both in a screening and diagnostic context.

This chapter will first describe some terms related to radiation dose and describe their methods of measurement. In the next section, the effects of some key CT technical factors on radiation dose will be described briefly. The following section will describe a few common uses of CT in cardiac imaging, providing estimates of radiation dose for each. Finally, a brief discussion will be provided for some additional advances in CT (e.g. Dual Source CT) as well as some radiation dose reduction technologies.

1 RADIATION DOSE BASICS

1.1 Radiation dose terms

1.1.1 Exposure

The term *exposure* is a term often used in the context of radiation dose discussions. It is defined as the ability of X-rays to ionize air and is measured in units of Roentgen or Coulomb/kg.[5] This term generally describes the concentration of radiation in air at a specific point. While it does describe how much ionization is created in air, it does not tell how much energy is absorbed by tissues, nor does it reflect the relative radiosensitivity of any particular tissue.

1.1.2 Radiation dose

The term *radiation dose* refers to the amount of energy absorbed per unit mass at a specific point.[5] This quantity is measured in Grays (SI unit, where 1 Gy = 1 Joule/kg) or rads (English unit, where 1 rad = 1 erg/gram), with the conversion between the two being 100 rads = 1 Gy. Radiation doses from CT in tissue are usually expressed in mGy (thousandths of a Gray) range. This quantity does describe how much energy is absorbed from ionizing radiation in a small volume centered at a specific point. However, it generally does not specifically describe where that radiation dose is absorbed or reflect the relative radiosensitivity or risk of detriment to tissues being irradiated.

1.1.3 Effective dose

The term *effective dose* is not a physically measurable quantity, but is rather a construct designed to take into account not only where the radiation dose is being absorbed, but the relative radiosensitivity of the various tissues being irradiated.[6,7] It attempts to reflect the equivalent whole-body dose that results in a stochastic risk that is equivalent to the stochastic risk from a non-uniform, partial-body irradiation such as a CT scan. Effective dose is calculated by estimating the individual organ dose to a specific set of radiosensitive organs, and then taking a weighted average of organ doses, as described in Equation (1):

$$E = \sum_T w_T w_R D_{T,R} \qquad (1)$$

where E is the effective dose, w_T is the tissue weighting factor, w_R is the radiation-weighting coefficient (1 for X-rays), and $D_{T,R}$ is the average absorbed dose to tissue, where the subscript T represents each radiosensitive tissue, and the subscript R represents each type of radiation (in CT, only X-rays are present). The relative weighting factors are estimated for each radiosensitive organ in Publication 60 of the International Commission on Radiological Protection (ICRP).[6] It should be noted that these factors are under review and that significantly different weighing factors have recently been proposed by the BEIR VII (Biological Effects of Ionizing Radiation) report that is expected to be released in 2007. Effective dose is measured in Sieverts (Sv) or rems. The conversion between Sieverts and rem is 100 rem = 1 Sv. Typical values of effective dose from CT scans range from < 1 to 10 mSv (.001 Sv to .01 Sv).

Although methods to calculate the effective dose have been established (ICRP Publications 60),[6] these methods depend heavily on the ability to estimate *the dose to the radiosensitive organs* from the CT procedure ($D_{T,R}$). However, estimating the radiation dose to these organs is problematic and direct measurement is not possible. Several methods to estimate organ radiation dose, especially from CT are outlined in McNitt-Gray.[8]

1.1.4. CTDI

While the above definitions are general for any form of radiation, specific definitions for radiation dose from CT were developed because of its unique geometry and usage. While most conventional imaging methods (e.g. radiography) involve the use of a source at a single stationary position, in CT the source rotates around the patient. In addition, multiple exposures are acquired along the length of the patient to cover the desired anatomic region(s). This kind of usage resulted in a rotationally symmetric radiation dose distribution that extends along some length of the patient.

To help characterize this unique geometry and usage, methods were developed to calculate the radiation dose in a set of standardized phantoms, referred to as the Computed Tomography Dose Index (CTDI). In the original definition, developed by investigators in the FDA,[9,10] CTDI was defined as the average dose in the center slice of a series of several contiguous slices, when measured in one of two cylindrical phantoms. The large phantom is 32 cm in diameter and is referred to as the 'body' phantom. The smaller phantom is 16 cm in diameter and is referred to as the 'head' phantom. Both are made of polymethylmethacrylate (PMMA or an acrylic) and extend 15 cm in length. They each also have 5 holes drilled along the length of them to obtain a standard set of measurements; one in the center of the phantom and one each at ordinal positions 1 cm from the surface of the phantom at the 12:00, 3:00, 6:00 and 9:00 positions around the periphery of the phantom. Typically, measurements were made in the center position as well as in at least one of the four peripheral positions. Figure 3.1 shows a schematic of the CTDI measurement in a phantom, along with an example of a single axial scan radiation dose profile measured in the center position of the phantom and the dose distribution along the longitudinal direction that results from a series of contiguous axial scans, measured at the center position in the phantom.

These investigators[9,10] showed that in order to get the average dose in the center slice of a series of several contiguous slices, one need only estimate the area under the radiation profile along the z-direction (longitudinal axis) of a single axial tube rotation, integrate over the number of slices, and divide by the total nominal beam collimation. Therefore, a method was developed that allowed the use of a long, integrating pencil ionization chamber placed at the center of a single axial scan, to first measure the exposure along the length of the phantom (at a specific measurement position) and then use that measurement to calculate the CTDI value at a specific position (e.g. center or 12:00).

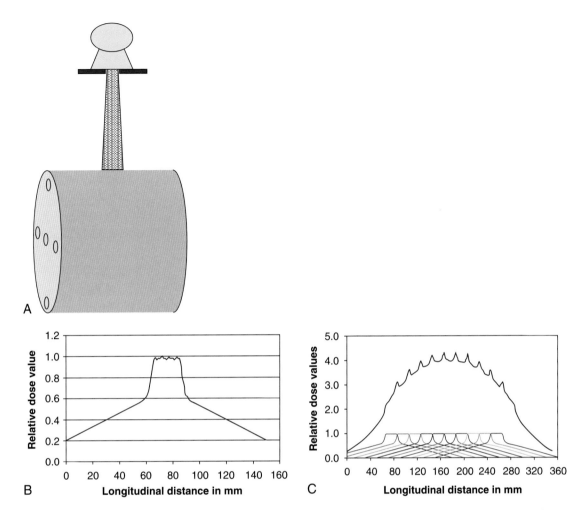

Figure 3.1   (a) Diagram illustrating the CTDI measurement geometry where a single axial scan is performed around one of two phantoms; (b) the radiation profile measured along the longitudinal axis of the phantom at the center position resulting from a single axial scan; and (c) graph of the radiation profile measured along the longitudinal axis of the phantom at the center position resulting from a series of contiguous axial scans, where the graph shows both profiles from the individual scans and the total that results from the summation of all of these scans.

Originally, this was specified for 14 contiguous slices and is often referred to as $CTDI_{FDA}$. So that:

$$CTDI_{FDA} = \frac{1}{NT}\int_{-7T}^{7T} D(z)dz$$

where N = the number of simultaneous slices produced in a single rotation, T = width of each slice (so that the product of NT yields the nominal width of the x-ray beam), and $D(z)$ is the measured radiation profile of a single axial tube rotation exposure using that nominal beam width NT.

Because the standard length of the measuring device (the pencil ionization chamber) is 100 mm, a slightly different CTDI index was developed.[11] In this metric, rather than specifying 14 slices at a specific beam width, it was recognized that the measurement was performed over 100 mm.

Therefore, the definition of $CTDI_{100}$ was developed that was very similar to that of $CTDI_{FDA}$, but with fixed measurement limits that extend from −50 mm to +50 mm:

$$CTDI_{100} = \frac{1}{NT}\int_{-50mm}^{50mm} D(z)dz$$

This $CTDI_{100}$ value is measured at the center and peripheral locations of each phantom.

Because the center and peripheral positions will result in different values (there is often a factor of two difference from center to periphery in a 32 cm phantom), a weighted average CTDI value was developed[11]:

$$CTDI_w = \left(\frac{1}{3}CTDI_{100,center}\right) + \left(\frac{2}{3}CTDI_{100,peripheral}\right)$$

Finally, with the introduction of helical scanning, a CTDI was developed to take into account the effects of the relative table speed using the pitch factor.[11] This is referred to as $CTDI_{vol}$ (vol stands for volume) and is defined as:

$$CTDI_{vol} = \frac{CTDI_w}{Pitch}$$

This definition reflects the fact that, with all other factors held constant, the radiation dose will be inversely proportional to pitch. That is, as pitch decreases, the dose will increase linearly by that same amount. This has significant implications for cardiac scanning.

In summary, a series of dose indices have been developed through the years that are unique to CT:

- $CTDI_{FDA}$ represents the measurement across 14 widths of the nominal beam width and hence the measured length varies with the nominal beam width;
- $CTDI_{100}$ represents values measured with a fixed length of the 100 mm pencil ionization chamber, regardless of the nominal beam width;
- $CTDI_w$ is a weighted average of $CTDI_{100}$ values measured at peripheral and central positions within the cylindrical phantom;
- $CTDI_{vol}$ represents the extension of $CTDI_w$ that takes into account the table feed or pitch of the actual scan acquisition.

Because it is measured in a cylindrical phantom that is similar to patients only in approximate diameter, these CTDI values are not intended to reflect the actual radiation dose to any specific patient; instead they are just relative indices of the radiation dose. While they may not be very useful for estimating, radiation dose to the breast for a specific CT exam, they are very useful in comparing the relative radiation dose of a scan with one set of technical parameters versus another. This is illustrated below.

2 KEY TECHNICAL FACTORS IN CT AND THEIR EFFECT ON RADIATION DOSE

In X-ray CT, there are several factors that have a strong effect on the radiation dose. These include the tube current-time product (mAs), beam energy (kilovolt peak or kVp), pitch (or relative table speed) and beam collimation among other factors. These factors and the magnitude of their effect on radiation dose will be described below.

2.1 Tube current-time product (mAs)

The tube current-time product is often referred to as the product of tube current (mA) and gantry rotation time (in seconds), or just simply 'mAs.' This term is meant to be proportional to the photon fluence, or total number of photons (regardless of the energy of the photons, which will be discussed in the next section), that are emitted by the x-ray tube.

There are several variations on the term 'mAs.' When the x-ray beam is on for the entire rotation around the patient, then the mAs value just equals the product of the tube current setting in mA and the gantry rotation time. However, as will be described below in section 3, there are times when the beam is not actually on for the entire rotation (such as when a partial scan is performed). In this case, the mAs value will be the product of the tube current setting in mA and the actual beam on time (and *not* the gantry rotation time). Another variation on this term is the term 'effective mAs' or 'mAs/slice'; these terms take into account the pitch value and will be described below in section 2.3.

Radiation dose is directly proportional to this mAs value as it represents the number of photons that are being emitted by the x-ray tube. Therefore, as one increases the mAs, the radiation dose will increase. Similarly, as one decreases the mAs, the radiation dose will decrease. This is illustrated in Table 3.1, in which some $CTDI_{vol}$ values (defined above) were measured while the mAs value was varied.

2.2 Beam energy – kVp

X-ray CT uses an X-ray beam that contains a spectrum of energies. Each spectrum is characterized by the peak

Table 3.1 Typical radiation dose values measured by $CTDI_{vol}$ (in mGy) for different mAs settings; all values based on measurements done in 32 cm diameter CTDI phantom for 120 kVp, 12 × 1.5 mm beam collimation, pitch 1.0

mAs	$CTDI_{vol}$
100	7.7 mGy
200	15.4 mGy
300	23.1 mGy
400	30.8 mGy
500	38.5 mGy
600	46.2 mGy

Table 3.2 Typical radiation dose values measured by CTDI$_{vol}$ (in mGy) for different kVp settings; all values based on measurements done in 32 cm diameter CTDI phantom for 300 mAs, 12 × 1.5 mm beam collimation, pitch 1.0

kVp	CTDI$_{vol}$
80	7.1 mGy
100	14.3 mGy
120	23.1 mGy
140	35.0 mGy

Table 3.3 Typical radiation dose values measured by CTDI$_{vol}$ (in mGy) for different pitch values; all values based on measurements done in 32 cm diameter CTDI phantom for 120 kVp, 300 mAs, 12 × 1.5 mm beam collimation.

Pitch	CTDI$_{vol}$
0.20	115.5 mGy
0.24	96.3 mGy
1.0	23.1 mGy
1.5	15.4 mGy
2.0	11.6 mGy

(or maximum) voltage (kVp) that is applied to the x-ray source. The influence of the kVP setting on radiation dose is illustrated in Table 3.2. This table shows CTDI$_{vol}$ values measured at different kVp settings. When all other factors (mAs, beam collimation, etc.) are held constant, changing the kVp from 120 to 140 kVp increases the radiation dose by approximately 50%.

2.3 Pitch

Pitch is defined for helical scanning as the table travel per rotation divided by the total nominal beam collimation and reflects the relative table speed:

$$\text{Pitch} = \frac{\text{Table Travel per Rotation}}{\text{Total Beam Collimation}}$$

A pitch value of 1.0 represents a contiguous acquisition where the table advances one beam collimation width every rotation. For example, in a 64 slice scanner where the nominal beam collimation might be 64 × 0.625, the total beam collimation would be 40 mm. If the table travel per rotation were 40 mm, then a pitch of 1.0 would result. If the table travel were faster, say 60 mm per rotation, then a pitch value of 1.5 would result. Often in cardiac scanning, a lower pitch value is used, such as 0.2; this means that the table would only move 8 mm per rotation for that 40 mm nominal beam collimation.

Pitch is accounted for in the CTDI$_{vol}$ definition. This definition demonstrates that, with all other factors held constant, radiation dose is *inversely* proportional to pitch. That is, the radiation dose for pitch = 2.0 is half of that resulting from using pitch 1.0. Similarly, the radiation dose resulting from using pitch 0.2 is *five times* that resulting from using pitch 1.0. This is shown in Table 3.3.

2.4 Beam collimation

In Multidetector row CT (MDCT) scanners, there are often several choices of total nominal beam collimation settings. Note that this refers to the total nominal width of the X-ray beam at the scanner isocenter and *not* the width of the reconstructed slices. A specific example would be for a 64 slice MDCT scanner that has options for beam collimation settings of 8 × 0.625 mm, 16 × 0.625 mm, 32 × 0.625 mm and 64 × 0.625 mm. Each of these would result in a different total nominal beam collimation width at the scanner's isocenter; however, each of these beam collimation settings would allow reconstruction of 0.625 and 1.25 mm thick slices (and perhaps even more slice thicknesses). For MCDT, the actual radiation beam width at isocenter is slightly larger than the nominal beam width; this ensures that all detectors see the same amount of radiation, even the detector rows at the extreme edges. This discrepancy between nominal and actual beam width can have implications on patient dose. Since we are interested in the radiation dose, the radiation dose profile can be measured in air at isocenter and this would describe how close the actual radiation beam width would be to the nominal beam width. Typically for MDCT, when the beam collimation is set to the largest possible width (e.g. 64 × 0.625 mm for a 64 detector row scanner), there is a relatively small difference between the measured beam width and the nominal beam width. However, when the narrowest beam collimation settings are used (e.g. 8 × 0.625 mm setting), the actual beam collimation can be significantly larger than the nominal. This 'overbeaming' can result in significant additional dose. Note that the setting with the least amount of overbeaming is not always the widest setting; for the particular scanner investigated for Table 3.4, the setting with the measured beam width closest to nominal was the 20 mm beam width, not the 40 mm beam width, though the difference

Table 3.4 Measured beam widths compared to nominal beam collimation settings for a 64 detector row scanner

Nominal beam collimation	Total nominal beam width	Measured beam width	% over nominal
8 × 0.625 mm	5 mm	7.3 mm	46.0%
16 × 0.625 mm	10 mm	11.4 mm	14.0%
32 × 0.625 mm	20 mm	20.3 mm	1.5%
64 × 0.625 mm	40 mm	42.4 mm	6.0%

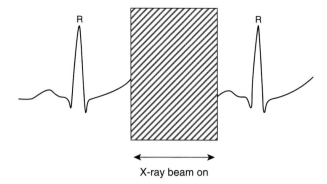

X-ray beam on

Figure 3.2. This figure illustrates that in prospective ECG gating, the x-ray beam is turned on only during the quietest phase of the heart cycle – typically starting at 40% of the R-R interval.

between these two is not large. These results are described in Table 3.4.

3 COMMON CARDIOVASCULAR CT EXAMS AND THEIR RADIATION DOSE

In other chapters within this book, many applications using CT for the cardiovascular system are described. While it is not possible here to describe the radiation dose implications for each one individually, this section will describe a few very common exams and describe the radiation dose that results from each one. The two most common exams of the coronary arteries are a scan for coronary artery calcium and a coronary artery computed tomography angiography (CTA) exam. These two exams are carried out in quite different ways and this has significant implications for radiation dose.

3.1 Prospective ECG-triggered CT – coronary artery calcium scanning

A coronary artery calcium study is often performed on asymptomatic patients and the aim is to assess (and quantify) the amount of calcium present in the coronary arteries. Therefore, this study acquires images just of the coronary arteries with as little motion as possible and, because these are often asymptomatic patients, using as little radiation dose as possible. This means that the examination is done without any intravenous contrast agent and is done using prospective ECG gating in a sequential axial acquisition, although helical scanning techniques are also sometimes used.

In prospective ECG (or cardiac) triggering, the x-ray source is turned on and off so that image projection data is collected only during certain predetermined R-R intervals of the ECG wave (a typical value would be 40% of the

R-R interval, but this has been varied in some studies). In fact, the x-ray source is essentially being triggered (turned on and off) by the ECG wave. This is done so that all of the required projections are acquired during the quietest phases of the ECG cycle to minimize cardiac motion in the resulting image. This is illustrated in Figure 3.2. Note that the arteries are therefore only imaged at one phase of the cardiac cycle, because that is all that is required to quantify the amount of calcium present.

In this exam, the x-ray beam will only be on long enough to create what is known as a 'partial scan.' This means that the x-ray beam is on just long enough to collect the minimum amount of data necessary to reconstruct an image; this minimum is 180° of rotation plus the fan angle which typically equals approximately 240° (or 2/3 of a full rotation). For a scanner that can perform a full rotation in 0.5 second, this partial scan time is approximately 0.33 second. For a scanner that can perform a full rotation in 0.33 second, the partial scan time reduces to 0.22 second. Obviously, the shorter the scan acquisition time, the less likely there will be motion while imaging the coronary arteries.

After each exposure, the table will be incremented by the nominal beam width as in conventional contiguous axial (or sequential) scanning. In MDCT scanners, multiple detector rows are used simultaneously to acquire multiple axial images. For example in a 12 × 1.5 mm scan acquisition mode, the nominal beam width is 12 × 1.5 mm, or 9 mm, and the table feed would also be 9 mm to create the contiguous axial scans. In this case, there are 12 separate images, each having 1.5 mm thickness; note that the projection data can also be combined to create six 3 mm thick images (because quantification of coronary artery calcium is typically done on 3 mm thick images). For a 64 detector row scanner, the scan acquisition might be done as a 64 × 0.625 mm scan acquisition with

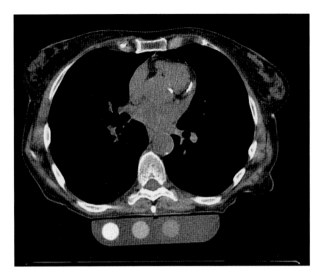

Figure 3.3 Image of a CT scan to assess coronary artery calcium; this image shows a calcified plaque in the left anterior descending coronary artery.

number (and higher k-edge, creating more photoelectric absorption and hence, higher x-ray attenuation).

The radiation dose for these exams is relatively low. This is because they use prospective ECG gating, partial scans, contiguous axial scans and they are performed at low mA settings. Table 3.5 shows some typical technical parameter settings and CTDI$_{vol}$ values for this kind of exam. These values can be compared to those in previously published works[12–14] for coronary artery exams. These previous estimates of CTDI$_{vol}$ ranged from 2.2 to 5 mGy and effective dose estimates ranged from 0.6 to 1.6 mSv. These will be compared with other types of exams described in subsequent sections within this chapter.

3.2 Retrospective gated CT – coronary angiography scanning

The aim of this examination is to assess whether there is narrowing in any of the coronary arteries. This study is typically performed on patients with symptoms of coronary artery disease and is performed with high resolution imaging in all planes (including thin slices) so that multiplanar reformations and 3D reconstructions can be performed and covering several, if not all, of the phases of the heart cycle, both systole and diastole.

To meet these requirements, and in contrast to the prospective gating done to assess coronary artery calcium, the coronary CT angiogram (CTA) is performed using

a 40 mm table feed and images reconstructed with 2.5 mm thickness. Because these scans are done with contiguous axial scans, this results in the equivalent of a pitch of 1.0.

CT scans to quantify coronary artery calcium are typically done at low mA settings. This is possible because of the higher attenuation values (Hounsfield Units or HU) observed where there is significant calcium in the coronary arteries (Figure 3.3), which are primarily due to calcium's higher atomic

Table 3.5 Radiation dose values estimated from a prospective ECG gated, contiguous axial CT scan typically performed for coronary artery calcium assessment. Note that CTDI$_{vol}$ values are based on measurement data and that the effective dose and organ doses that follow are based on estimates obtained from the ImPACT CT Dose calculator version 0.99 × [15]

Gating used	Prospective ECG	Prospective ECG	Prospective ECG
Number of detector rows	4	16	64
Beam energy in kVp	120	120	120
Beam collimation	4 × 2.5 mm	16 × 1.25 mm	64 × 0.625 mm
Total nominal beam width	10 mm	20 mm	40 mm
Table feed	10 mm	20 mm	40 mm
Rotation time	0.5 sec	0.5 sec	0.33 sec
Partial scan time (Actual beam on time)	0.33 sec	0.33 sec	0.24 sec
mA	190	190	264
mAs	63 mAs	63 mAs	63 mAs
CTDI$_{vol}$ (mGy)	6.4	6.2	5.9
Effective dose (mSv)	1.5	1.5	1.3
Breast dose (mGy)	7.1	6.7	6.0
Esophagus dose (mGy)	3.2	3.3	2.9
Thyroid dose (mGy)	0.12	0.12	0.12
Lung dose (mGy)	5.5	5.2	5.0

an injection of an intravenous contrast agent, retrospective ECG gating (described below), and a helical scan with a pitch much less than 1.0. This results in radiation doses that are much higher than in the previous section.

In retrospective ECG gating, the X-ray source is kept on so that image projection data is collected continuously during the helical scan. To ensure that sufficient image projections are acquired for each location at all phases of the ECG wave, the table movement is slowed down significantly by using a low pitch value – typically 0.2 to 0.3. This is done so images can be reconstructed for any phase of the cardiac cycle.

To be able to accurately assess the coronary arteries in any plane, thin slice (≤ 2 mm) acquisitions are performed. With the advent of 16 and 64 slice scanners, these acquisitions are typically done with submillimeter (≤ 1 mm) slice thicknesses. However, when these thinner slices are used, the image noise increases.

These CTA scans are typically done at much higher mA settings than the scans to assess coronary artery calcium. This is true primarily because thin slice images require a higher mA to keep image noise to an acceptable level where the diagnosis can be made with confidence.

Therefore, the radiation dose for CTA exams is higher than for coronary artery calcium scans. This is primarily because this exam uses: (a) retrospective ECG gating which requires low pitch values and (b) thin sections and relatively low image noise, which requires high mAs. Table 3.6 shows some typical technical parameter settings and CTDI$_{vol}$ values

for this kind of exam. These values can be compared with the values found in references,[12–14] which estimated CTDI$_{vol}$ to range from 36–55 mGy and effective dose to range from 7–13 mSv for retrospectively gated coronary CTA exams. Please note that these values are significantly higher than the values encountered for the coronary artery calcium scans described in the previous section.

4 RECENT ADVANCES IN CT

As multidetector row CT (MDCT) has advanced rapidly in the last several years, there have also been significant developments related to the reduction of radiation dose from MDCT as well.[16] These are discussed in this section along with their strengths and weaknesses in terms of their ability to reduce radiation dose in clinical practice.

4.1 Tube current modulation (automatic exposure control for CT)

The purpose of automatic tube current modulation is to maintain constant image quality regardless of patient attenuation characteristics, thus allowing radiation dose to patients to be reduced.[17] That is, rather than using the same tube current through both thick and thin parts of the patient

Table 3.6 Radiation dose values estimated from a retrospective ECG gated, helical scan with low pitch values performed for coronary artery CT angiography. Note that CTDI$_{vol}$ values are based on measurement data and that the effective dose and organ doses that follow are based on estimates obtained from the ImPACT CT Dose calculator version 0.99 x [15]

Gating used	Retrospective ECG	Retrospective ECG	Retrospective ECG
Number of detector rows	4	16	64
Beam energy in kVp	120	120	120
Beam collimation	4 × 2.5 mm	16 × 1.25 mm	64 × 0.625 mm
Reconstructed slice width	2.5 mm	1.25	0.625 mm
Total nominal beam width	10 mm	20 mm	40 mm
Table feed per rotation	2 mm	4.8 mm	9.6 mm
Pitch	0.2	0.24	0.24
Rotation time	0.5 sec	0.5 sec	0.33 sec
mA	250	300	450
mAs	125 mAs	150 mAs	150 mAs
Effective mAs (= mAs/pitch)	625	625	625
CTDI$_{vol}$(mGy)	63.2	61.9	57.5
Effective dose (mSv)	15	15	13
Breast dose (mGy)	71	67	59
Esophagus dose (mGy)	32	32	29
Thyroid dose (mGy)	1.2	1.2	1.2
Lung dose (mGy)	55	52	49

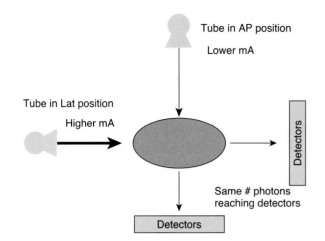

Figure 3.4 This figure illustrates that for the typical non-circularly shaped patient, the tube current can be varied as the x-ray tube is moved around the patient, resulting in the same number of photons reaching the detectors for each projection angle, which produces a constant noise level while reducing radiation dose.

(such as when the tube moves from an AP position to a lateral position around the patient), the tube current could be reduced when the thinner, less attenuating part of the patient is encountered. This would save radiation dose to the patient and, even though fewer x-ray photons came out of the tube at that position, there would be approximately the same number of photons reaching the detectors because there would be less attenuation through that portion of the body; yielding the same image quality as when a higher number of photons were used in a thicker portion of the body. Thus image quality is maintained, but radiation dose is lowered for that projection through the less attenuating part of the patient. This is illustrated in Figure 3.4.

4.1.1 Conventional tube current modulation methods

There are several kinds of tube current modulation, all of which share this same basic idea.[17–21] The first kind is an angular tube current modulation, where the tube current is only varied with the angle of the x-ray tube current around the patient. This is the kind of tube current modulation referred to in Figure 3.4. In angular (x- and y-axis) tube current modulation, the tube current is varied to equalize the photon flux to the detector as the x-ray tube rotates about the patient (e.g. from the anterior-posterior direction to the lateral direction). Thus, an initial tube current value (or tube current-time product value) is chosen and then the tube

current is modulated (typically, decreased) from that initial value within one gantry rotation. The resulting tube current values might be as shown in Figure 3.4.

The next tube current modulation scheme varies the tube current along the longitudinal (or z-axis) of the patient. In this scheme, the tube current is varied to yield approximately the same image quality across different anatomic regions (e.g. shoulders vs. lung, or abdomen vs. pelvis) despite there being large differences in attenuation. Therefore, the tube current is higher through the more dense/attenuating regions (e.g. shoulders) and then reduced for the lower attenuating regions (e.g. lung). This is illustrated very well in McCollough et al.[17] This can result in substantial dose reduction compared to a constant tube current scheme.

The last of the conventional tube current modulation schemes is a combination where the tube current is modulated in both the angular and longitudinal directions (x, y and z) of the patient, as illustrated in Figure 3.5. This involves variation of the tube current both during gantry rotation and along the z-axis of the patient (i.e., from the anteroposterior direction to the lateral direction, *and* from the shoulders to the abdomen). This comprehensive scheme provides the advantages of both methods above and therefore the dose is adjusted according to the patient-specific attenuation in all three directions.

4.1.2 ECG-gated tube current modulation

In ECG-gated tube current modulation,[22] the tube current is raised and lowered in relation to the ECG wave, rather than based on patient attenuation characteristics as described above. These schemes keep the tube current value high during the portion of the heart cycle where motion is reduced (e.g. diastole) and then reduce the tube current when motion is expected to be high (e.g. systole); this is illustrated in Figure 3.6. In this way, radiation dose can be reduced without incurring much of an image quality penalty as the projections acquired with low mA would typically have significant motion and would not be used. Jakobs et al,[22] reported a mean dose reduction of nearly 50% when this scheme was used.

4.2 Dual source CT

In 2006, a dual source CT was introduced by Siemens (Definition, Siemens Medical Solutions, Forcheim, Germany).[23] This unique scanner placed two x-ray

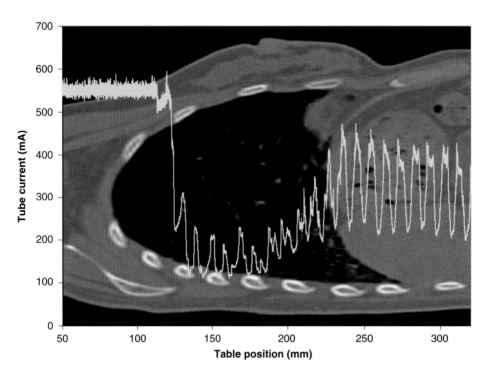

Figure 3.5   Graph of the tube current (mA) shown with reference to a sagittal plane image of an adult female patient. In this tube current modulation scheme, the tube current is varied both as the tube rotates around the patient (causing the rapid changes in tube current value) and as the tube moves along the longitudinal position of the patient.

sources on the same gantry in the same imaging plane, but offset by 90°; two separate sets of detectors (similar to that used in the Siemens Sensation 64) are also placed in the same imaging plane, opposite each x-ray source. The primary purpose of this distinctive arrangement was to improve temporal resolution for cardiac imaging. In their article describing system performance,[23] the authors describe a temporal resolution of 83 ms. That is, a complete set of projection data necessary to reconstruct an image was acquired within 83 msec, using single segment reconstruction (temporal resolution improves to an average of 60 msec down to a minmum of 42 msec when dual segment reconstruction methods are used). In addition, because so many projections are acquired simultaneously, this

temporal resolution is maintained for heart rates ranging from 40 bpm all the way up to 120 bpm. This has allowed coronary CT angiogram studies to be performed on patients with a much wider range of heart rates and still yield a successful study with a minimum of cardiac motion in the image.

4.2.2 Dose reduction technologies utilized

While at first glance the notion of two x-ray tubes would suggest a doubling of the radiation dose to the patient for a cardiac CT exam, there have been several dose reduction technologies employed for this scanner. The first is the

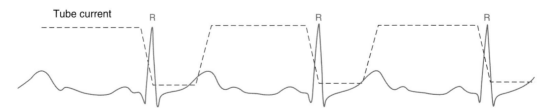

Figure 3.6   ECG-controlled tube current modulation. The tube current is lowered during phases of ECG wave where cardiac motion is expected to be high, and restored to higher values where cardiac motion is expected to be low.

ECG gated tube current modulation described above. For this scanner, because the amount of time that the x-ray actually has to be on is shorter, the tube current can be reduced for more of the cardiac cycle, thus allowing more dose reduction than in 16 or 64 slice scanners. Another dose reduction technology employed is that, as the heart rate *increases*, the pitch is allowed to increase as well. Therefore, rather than employing a fixed pitch value (typically 0.20 to 0.24) regardless of heart rate, this scanner allows pitch values to range from 0.20 (for heart rates as low as 40 bpm) to 0.40 (for heart rates up to 120 bpm). Thus, not only does this scanner allow imaging at these faster heart rates, the radiation dose is actually decreased at those faster heart rates. While there are other methods employed as well, these two are the primary radiation dose reduction technologies used in this scanner to help keep the radiation dose to levels comparable to previous technologies used for cardiac scanning.

5 SUMMARY

CT is being used for a wide variety of cardiac imaging applications, ranging from exams to assess coronary artery calcium to detailed coronary CTA studies of the arteries. In this section, the elements of radiation dose were defined as well as the technical factors that influence dose. The magnitude of radiation dose from several types of CT exams was described as well as some technologies for radiation dose reduction.

As CT technology continues to develop the ability to cover more of the patient with better spatial and temporal resolution, especially if this continues to develop in a cost-effective manner, then its utilization will also increase. Because CT does use ionizing radiation, it is prudent to continue to understand issues related to radiation dose and to encourage methods that will reduce the radiation dose necessary to accomplish the clinical objectives of the imaging study.

REFERENCES

1. Stern SH, Kaczmarek RV, Spelic DC, Suleiman OH. Nationwide Evaluation of X-ray Trends (NEXT) 2000–2001 survey of patient radiation exposure from computed tomographic (CT) examinations in the United States (abstr). Radiology 2001; 221(P): 161.
2. Mollet NR, Cademartiri F, Krestin GP, et al. Improved diagnostic accuracy with 16-row multi-slice computed tomography coronary angiography. J Am Coll Cardiol. 2005; 45(1): 128–32.
3. Meijboom WB, Mollet NR, van Mieghem CA, et al. 64-slice Computed Tomography Coronary Angiography in Patients with Non-ST Elevation Acute Coronary Syndrome. Heart 2007 (in press).
4. Herzog C, Zangos S, Zwerner P, et al. CT of coronary artery disease. J Thorac Imaging 2007 Feb; 22(1): 40–8.
5. Bushberg JT, Seibert JA, Leidholdt EM, Boone JM. The essential physics of medical imaging. 2nd ed. Philadelphia, Pa: Lippincott Williams & Wilkins, 2001.
6. International Council on Radiation Protection. 1990 recommendations of the International Commission on Radiological Protection. Publication 60, Annals of the ICRP 1991; 21. Oxford, England: Pergamon, 1991.
7. McCollough CM, Schueler BA. Calculation of effective dose. Med Phys 2000; 27: 838–44.
8. McNitt-Gray MF. AAPM/RSNA Physics Tutorial for Residents: Topics in CT. Radiation dose in CT. Radiographics. 2002 Nov–Dec; 22(6): 1541–53.
9. Shope TB, Gagne RM, Johnson GC. A method for describing the doses delivered by transmission x-ray computed tomography. Med Phys 1991; 8: 488–95.
10. Department of Health and Human Services, Food and Drug Administration. 21 CFR Part 1020: Diagnostic x-ray systems and their major components; amendments to performance standard; Final rule. Federal Register 1984, 49, 171.
11. European Guidelines on Quality Criteria for Computed Tomography (EUR 16262 EN, May 1999). Available at: www.drs.dk/guidelines/ct/quality/index.htm. Accessed March 2007.
12. Gerber TC, Kuzo RS, Morin RL. Techniques and parameters for estimating radiation exposure and dose in cardiac computed tomography. Int J Cardiovasc Imaging 2005 Feb; 21(1): 165–76.
13. Bae KT, Hong C, Whiting BR. Radiation dose in multidetector row computed tomography cardiac imaging. J Magn Reson Imaging 2004 Jun; 19(6): 859–63.
14. Morin RL, Gerber TC, McCollough CH. Radiation dose in computed tomography of the heart. Circulation 2003 107(6): 917–22.
15. Imaging Performance Assessment of CT (ImPACT) CT Patient Dosimetry Calculator, version 0.99x. Created 1/20/06. Available at: http://www.impactscan.org/ctdosimetry.htm.
16. Linton OW, Mettler FA Jr. National Council on Radiation Protection and Measurements. National conference on dose reduction in CT, with an emphasis on pediatric patients. Am J Roentgenol. 2003 Aug; 181(2): 321–9.
17. McCollough CH, Bruesewitz MR, Kofler JM Jr. CT dose reduction and dose management tools: overview of available options. Radiographics 2006; 26(2): 503–12.
18. Haaga JR, Miraldi F, MacIntyre W, et al. The effect of mAs variation upon computed tomography image quality as evaluated by in vivo and in vitro studies. Radiology 1981; 138: 449–54.
19. Kalra MK, Maher MM, Toth TL, et al. Techniques and applications of automatic tube current modulation for CT. Radiology 2004 Dec; 233(3): 649–57.
20. Gies M, Kalender WA, Wolf H, Suess C. Dose reduction in CT by anatomically adapted tube current modulation. I. Simulation studies. Med Phys 1999; 26: 2235–47.

21. Kalender WA, Wolf H, Suess C. Dose reduction in CT by anatomically adapted tube current modulation. II. Phantom measurements. Med Phys 1999; 26: 2248–53.

22. Jakobs TF, Becker CR, Ohnesorge B, et al. Multislice helical CT of the heart with retrospective ECG gating: reduction of radiation exposure by ECG-controlled tube current modulation. Eur Radiol 2002; 12: 1081–86.

23. Flohr TG, McCollough CH, Bruder H, et al. First performance evaluation of a dual-source CT (DSCT) system. Eur Radiol. 2006 Feb; 16(2): 256–68.

4

Cardiovascular Computed Tomography: A Clinical Perspective

Mario J. Garcia

1 INTRODUCTION

Coronary artery disease (CAD) is one of the leading causes of death and disability in the industrialized world. Invasive coronary angiography is considered the diagnostic standard for establishing the presence and severity of significant CAD. However, interventional treatment is generally performed in no more than 50% of diagnostic procedures. As invasive procedures have an associated mortality (0.15%) and morbidity (1.5%),[1] attention has been turned to finding accurate noninvasive diagnostic tests. Noninvasive imaging testing for the detection of CAD has evolved significantly over the last 50 years. From resting ECG, to stress ECG, and stress echocardiography and nuclear imaging tests, we have gradually improved our ability to detect CAD. Stress testing is useful to establish prognosis in patients with suspected coronary artery disease but has limited diagnostic utility.[2] In the best circumstances, the accuracy of stress imaging tests is <85% for the detection of obstructive disease and negligible for the detection of non-obstructive CAD.

Recent technological advances have led to a substantial increase in spatial and temporal resolution, as well as shortening of the image acquisition time, making it possible to visualize the beating heart with electron-beam (EBCT) and multi-detector computed tomography (MDCT). The first clinical applications were focused on the evaluation of cardiac volumes and function, the pericardium and the great vessels. More recently, cardiac MDCT has gained popularity for the detection and quantification of coronary artery disease.[3,4,5] The evolution of MDCT technology has occurred much faster than EBCT over the last decade. The number of uninterpretable MDCT coronary studies has gradually decreased from 20–40% using 4-slice, to 15–25% with 16-slice and is now as low as 3–10% with 64-slice systems. Cardiac MDCT is the fastest growing noninvasive diagnostic cardiac imaging modality in the US, with dedicated cardiovascular systems available now in most large hospital and outpatient cardiology practices. In addition to coronary angiography, MDCT is commonly utilized for 3-dimensional planning of electrophysiological and surgical procedures, such as radiofrequency ablation, redo-myocardial revascularization and aortic aneurysm and dissection repair.

In this chapter we will review the current and developing clinical applications of the rapidly evolving field of cardiac MDCT.

2 PATIENT SELECTION

2.1 Technical considerations

The physical principles and instrumentation of cardiac MDCT have been discussed at length in previous chapters. However, it is important to revise the technical considerations that are pertinent to patient selection. Cardiac imaging demands a very high temporal resolution, as the heart is in almost constant, rapid phasic motion, which involves short axis and long axis deformation as well as torsion. Current generation MDCT systems require the acquisition of 6–10 cardiac cycles in order to visualize the complete cardiac volume. In order to obtain a high quality cardiac study the following conditions need to be met: (1) the heart rate and/or the temporal resolution of the scanner are sufficiently low to complete a phase acquisition during either iso-volumic relaxation or diastasis; (2) the heart rate variability is minimal, therefore the temporal registration coincides for all or most of the acquired cardiac cycles; and (3) the time of acquisition is short, therefore respiratory motion is avoided and contrast delivery is optimized. Accordingly, cardiac MDCT may not be suitable for patients with fast or irregular heart rhythms or those with severe pulmonary disease. In addition, image quality has been shown to be decreased in morbidly obese patients. These considerations apply primarily for MDCT coronary angiography since motion artifacts are rarely severe enough to impair the visualization of larger structures such as the left atrium, pulmonary veins, cardiac masses or the aorta.

2.2 Radiation dose and patient safety

Cardiac MDCT, like invasive angiography involves radiation exposure. The 'effective dose,' expressed in milli-Sieverts (mSv), depends on multiple factors, including volume of acquisition required, duration of the scan, and radiation energy level used. The volume of acquisition is typically 12–16 cm for coronary angiography and 18–25 cm for angiography for coronary bypass conduits. The radiation energy level required to obtain adequate image quality will depend on the width of the patient's chest, the type of study and desired spatial resolution. Current MDCT systems with 64 detectors provide a typical dose range in the order of 8 to 20 mSv for coronary angiography. This compares to 2–6 mSv for invasive angiography, and 10–30 mSv for nuclear myocardial perfusion imaging. Strategies to minimize effective dose in MDCT include dose modulation, which, depending on heart rate, may reduce total radiation exposure up to 50%. It is estimated that the risk of cancer may increase by 1:2000 in MDCT coronary studies, depending on the age of the patient. Because of these concerns, the wide application of MDCT as a screening test is not justified until more outcome data becomes available.

The relative risk of contrast nephropathy needs to be considered when ordering a contrast-enhanced cardiac

MDCT study. In patients who are determined to be at higher risk, the risk/utility of MDCT needs to be compared with that of alternative diagnostic tests. An invasive diagnostic coronary angiogram may be performed in many cases using a lower amount of contrast (30–50 ml), and thus may be a preferred option for patients with renal insufficiency.

3 CLINICAL APPLICATIONS

3.1 Calcium scoring

The volume of calcified atherosclerotic plaque burden in the coronary arteries may be measured based around a radiographic density-weighted volume of plaques with pixel numbers of a least 130 HU. The prognostic value of the calcium is well established.[6] The presence of coronary calcification is a predictor of adverse cardiovascular events. The risk increases above a calcium score > 100 (RR = 1.9), although several studies indicate that the predictive value is higher when adjusted for gender and age. Although the utility of screening asymptomatic individuals remains controversial, several studies support that the calcium score provides prognostic information independent of conventional risk factors, particularly for individuals at intermediate and high risk. In a recent study published by Greenland et al., a calcium score >300 was associated with a significant increase in CHD event risk compared with that determined by clinical score alone.[7] In patients with Framingham risk scores of 10–15, patients with a calcium score >300 had a 7% cardiac event rate compared to 4% in those with a calcium score of <100. In those with Framingham risk scores of 15–20, a calcium score >300 was twice as high as in those with a score <100 (Figure 4.1). Patients determined at low risk by clinical

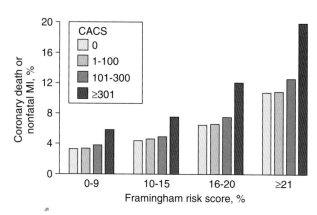

Figure 4.1 Risk of cardiac events according to Framingham risk and calcium score (From Greenland et al.)[7]

criteria, however, appear to derive minimal additional prognostic benefit from calcium scoring. Some experts even suggest that a calcium score may in aggregate have a detrimental effect on the quality of life of screening populations.[8]

3.2 MDCT coronary angiography

The use of contrast-enhanced ECG gated CT for visualization of the coronary arterial lumen and vessel wall became available first with EBCT, but has gained popularity with the introduction of 16–64-slice MDCT scanners. Guidelines for training have been recently issued by the American College of Cardiology and American Heart Association.[9]

Figures 4.2–4.4 are examples of atherosclerotic coronary arteries as seen by MDCT and invasive coronary angiography. From these images it is easy to appreciate that MDCT and conventional coronary angiography provide different information and, therefore, one should not expect a perfect agreement in their quantitative determination of luminal stenosis. Unlike conventional angiography, MDCT provides visualization of the atherosclerotic plaque. In some cases, calcified plaque volume may be overestimated by MDCT due to partial volume and blooming artifacts, leading to overestimation of stenosis severity. In other instances, stenosis severity may be underestimated by conventional angiography. Typically, only 2 or 3 projections are obtained in a conventional angiogram for each vessel. In contrast, MDCT is a 3-dimensional imaging technique, and thus provides an infinite number of projections.

Several studies[10,11,12,13,14,15,16,17,18,19,20] have compared the results of 16-slice MDCT coronary angiography for the detection of coronary artery stenosis with conventional angiography in patients with known or suspected CAD referred. In most studies, analysis of MDCT data was performed by investigators blinded to the results of invasive angiography and, in all but two, was limited to coronary segments of more than 1.5 or 2 mm in diameter. In most cases, significant coronary artery stenosis was defined as a $\geq 50\%$ lesion. The prevalence of significant CAD in patients enrolled in these studies ranged from 42–83%, since most included patients with high probability of CAD clinically referred for cardiac catheterization. It should be also noted that about 5–30% of all analyzable segments were excluded from analysis due to motion, severe calcified plaques and other imaging artifacts. These single center studies have reported sensitivities and specificities for the detection of obstructive coronary lesions using 16-row MDCT scanners ranging between 30–95% and 86–98%, respectively. A few 16-slice MDCT studies have reported accuracy using each patient as the unit of analysis. The sensitivity for detecting obstructive CAD per patient has been reported between 85–100%, and the specificity between 78 and 86%.

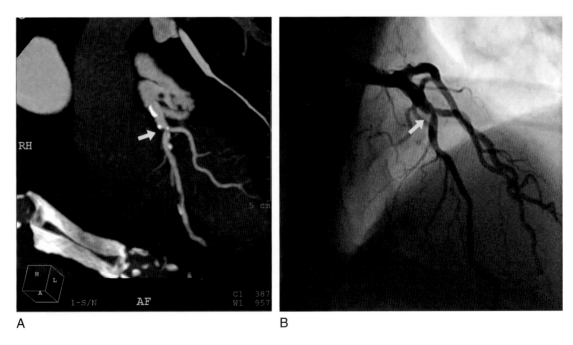

A   B

Figure 4.2   A. This MDCT oblique coronal image obtained from a patient with anginal symptoms demonstrates a moderately severe stenosis at the bifurcation of the left anterior descending coronary artery and the first diagonal branch. B. The coronary angiogram confirms moderately severe stenosis of the vessel.

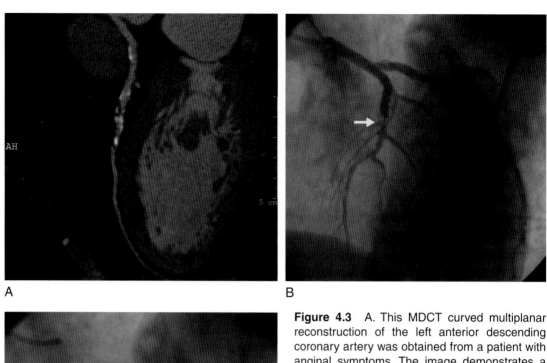

A

B

C

Figure 4.3 A. This MDCT curved multiplanar reconstruction of the left anterior descending coronary artery was obtained from a patient with anginal symptoms. The image demonstrates a severe stenosis in the mid segment of the vessel caused by an ulcerated plaque. B. The coronary angiogram confirms severe stenosis in the middle left anterior descending coronary artery (arrow). C. The delayed frame from the angiogram demonstrates residual contrast in the ulcerated plaque area.

Positive predictive values have ranged between 72 and 90% per segment and 81–97% per patient, and negative predictive values between 97–99% and 82–100%, respectively. As expected, sensitivity has been higher in those studies that excluded small vessel segments. However, most experts agree that the ability of detecting obstructive coronary disease in smaller caliber vessels is less important, since myocardial revascularization is often not required or unable to be performed. The accuracy of MDCT coronary angiography appears to be also reduced when performed in patients with morbid obesity. Clinical data show that standard currently available temporal resolution is not sufficient to cover the normal range of resting heart rates. This deficiency is corrected with beta-blocker-induced heart rate reduction, which prolongs diastole and extends the phases of low cardiac and subsequent coronary motion to allow artifact-free imaging. Two strategies have emerged to increase temporal resolution. One is based on faster gantry rotation. The reconstruction of one MDCT frame depends on a 180° turn of the gantry; thus temporal resolution increases linearly with shortening of the gantry rotation.[21] The second strategy is based on shortening the reconstruction window within a single heart cycle by segmenting image data acquisition over multiple heart beats.[22] An adaptive multi-cycle reconstruction approach combines data from consecutive cardiac cycles and enhances temporal resolution to an average of 140 ms.[23]

We recently completed a multicenter trial that studied the accuracy of MDCT coronary angiography performed with 16-slice scanners.[24] In this study, we enrolled

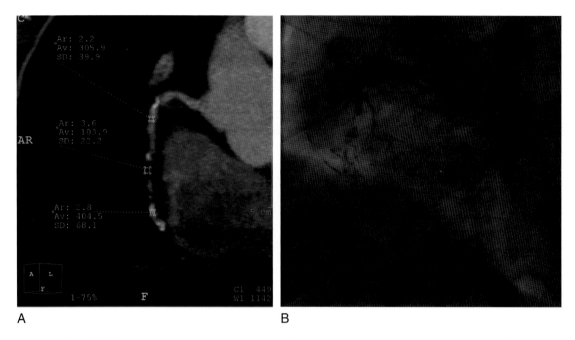

A   B

Figure 4.4   A. This MDCT oblique sagittal image obtained from a patient with history of myocardial infarction demonstrates a totally occluded right coronary artery with retrograde collateral filling. The mid portion of the artery is filled by thrombus/non-calcified plaque (105 Hounsfield units). B. The coronary angiogram confirms complete occlusion of the vessel.

238 patients with high or intermediate risk who were clinically referred for diagnostic angiography. Patients first underwent a calcium score scan followed by MDCT angiography prior to invasive angiography if the Agatston calcium score was <600. Coronary angiography and MDCT data sets were quantitatively and analyzed by blinded independent core laboratories. In the 187 patients who underwent MDCT, there were 89 segments (5.5%) in 59 patients (32%) with stenosis >50% by conventional angiography. Of 1629 segments >2 mm in diameter, 71% were evaluable on MDCT. All nonevaluable segments were censored as 'positive,' since in clinical practice they would also lead to performance of angiography. Using this approach, the sensitivity, specificity, positive and negative predictive values for detecting >50% luminal stenoses were 89%, 65%, 13% and 99%. In a patient-based analysis, the sensitivity, specificity, positive and negative predictive values for detecting subjects with at least one 'positive' segment were 98%, 54%, 50% and 99%. The high number of non-evaluable and false-positive segments in this study indicates that 16-slice MDCT may lead to an excessive number of catheterizations or additional functional testing if applied indiscriminately. Nevertheless, given its high sensitivity and negative predictive value, 16-row MDCT may be very useful excluding coronary disease in selected patients in whom a false-positive or inconclusive stress test result is suspected.

It is anticipated that the lower number of nonevaluable segments seen with 64-slice scanners will likely result in higher specificity and positive predictive values, allowing wider implementation of this test.

An important advantage of the new generation 32, 40 and 64-channel MDCT systems is their greater craniocaudal coverage per rotation, which allows shorter breath-holds and consequently higher contrast injection rates, smaller contrast injection volumes, and fewer artifacts related to patient breath-hold compliance and heart rate variability.[25,26,27] Studies have shown that the superior performance characteristics of 64-slice MDCT in terms of spatial and temporal resolution lead to measurable improvement in image quality.[28] The sensitivities and specificities for the detection of coronary artery stenosis studies have been reported between 92–95% and 95–99%, respectively, using 64-slice scanners. The number of nonevaluable segments excluded has been reduced below 10% in most studies, also representing a significant improvement when compared with previous generation scanners. One of the most recent analyses of 64-slice MDCT with state-of-the-art scanning and analysis of all segments identified 19 of 21 severe lesions requiring revascularization at subsequent catheterization.

Evaluating coronary artery stenosis in patients with extensive coronary artery calcifications may be difficult. Reconstructions involving calcified structures tend to overestimate the volume set representing calcium ('blooming') because of the 'partial volume averaging,' by which much of the coronary lumen is apparently occupied by calcified plaque, and because of 'beam hardening,' where the calcium shields the true lumen. A recent study has analyzed the performance of MDCT after excluding patients with very high calcium score.[28] In their series the respective sensitivity and specificity were 77 and 97% for all patients (n = 60) vs. 98 and 98% when only those patients with a score <1000 were included (n = 46). Since symptomatic patients with very high calcium score have a very high probability of having obstructive coronary artery disease, it is reasonable to avoid MDCT angiography and proceed directly to invasive catheterization in these patients.

The assessment of previously stented coronary vessels remains an important limitation to MDCT coronary angiography.[29] A study using 16-slice MDCT reported evaluable images in only 126 of 232 stented segments (64%).[30] In a recent study performed with 64-slice MDCT, 2 of 2 stents with severe stenosis were accurately identified, 2 of 2 stents with moderate stenosis were missed by MDCT, and 4 of 9 stents with no angiographic restenosis were determined as stenotic by MDCT. The ability to evaluate the lumen of stented vessels depends on the type and the diameter of the stent. Practical delineation of in-stent stenosis remains difficult in lumens smaller than 3 mm diameter, as the internal luminal diameter is often underestimated due to partial volume and blooming artifacts. Improved visualization may be obtained in some cases, however, using sharp reconstruction filters.[31]

MDCT coronary angiography is very useful in assessing the origin and course of congenitally anomalous coronary arteries.[32,33] Compared to conventional angiography, MDCT can easily determine the 3-dimensional relationship of anomalous coronary arteries with the aorta and pulmonary arterial trunk. In addition, MDCT can also detect arteriovenous fistulae, myocardial bridges and aneurysmal dilatation of the coronary vessels.

3.3 Evaluation of atherosclerotic plaque volume and morphology

Figures 4.5 and 4.6 show representative examples of calcified and noncalcified coronary atherosclerotic plaques. Acute rupture of vulnerable plaques has been shown to play a significant role in the development of acute coronary syndromes.[34] Until recently, intravascular ultrasound (IVUS) was the only diagnostic tool capable of detecting the

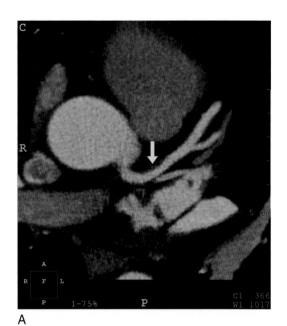

A

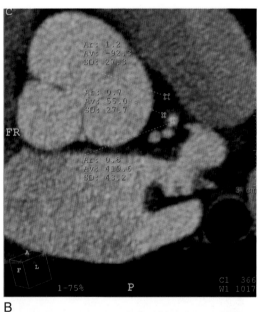

B

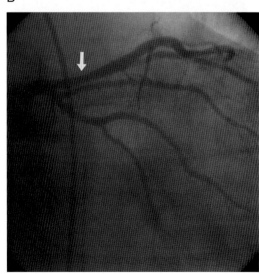

C

Figure 4.5 A. This MDCT axial image demonstrates mild narrowing of the proximal left anterior descending coronary artery caused by a non-calcified plaque. B. The zoomed cross-sectional view demonstrates the noncalcified plaque (55 Hounsfield units) causing mild narrowing of the coronary lumen (419 Hounsfield units). C. The coronary angiogram demonstrates mild narrowing of the proximal segment of the left anterior descending coronary artery (arrow).

presence, extent and composition of these plaques in the coronary arteries in-vivo.[35,36,37] Unfortunately, the wide application of IVUS as a screening tool for risk assessment is impractical due to the need for and high cost of invasive catheterization. In contrast to invasive coronary angiography, MDCT angiography is also capable of imaging the vessel wall. Recent studies have documented the ability of MDCT visualizing atherosclerotic coronary plaques[38,39,40] and differentiating calcified from non-calcified lesions based on Hounsfield unit values. In a series of 22 patients clinically referred for IVUS, MDCT correctly identified the presence of coronary atherosclerotic plaques in 41 of 50 affected segments.[41] The sensitivity of MDCT is greater for calcified (94%) than for mixed (78%) or soft (53%) plaques, and is limited for small caliber vessels. Plaque volume tends to be systematically underestimated by MDCT compared to IVUS, and luminal calcified plaque tends to be overestimated. In a recent study, there was reasonable correlation between mean plaque area defined by IVUS and 64-slice MDCT (r = 0.73), but sensitivity for detection for stenosis >75% was only 80%.

In addition to quantifying plaque volume, MDCT may be capable of characterizing, to some extent, plaque composition. We recently compared the IVUS and MDCT results of 40 patients with previously documented coronary artery disease.[42] Cross-sectional images obtained at 10 mm increments were assessed for percent luminal area reduction. Atherosclerotic plaques were classified by IVUS as soft, fibrous and calcified. In the matched MDCT images, regions of interest of 1–3 mm in diameter were placed inside each plaque, and tissue contrast was measured in Hounsfield Units (HU). From a total of 276 plaques examined by IVUS and MDCT, there were 188 (68.2%) soft, 45 (16.2%) fibrous and 43 (15.5%) calcified plaques. The MDCT attenuation values of soft, fibrous and calcified plaques were 71.5 ± 32.1, 116.3 ± 35.7 and 383.3 ± 186.1, p <0.001, respectively (Figure 4.7). Using a cutoff value of 185 HU, 273 of 276 (99%) plaques were correctly

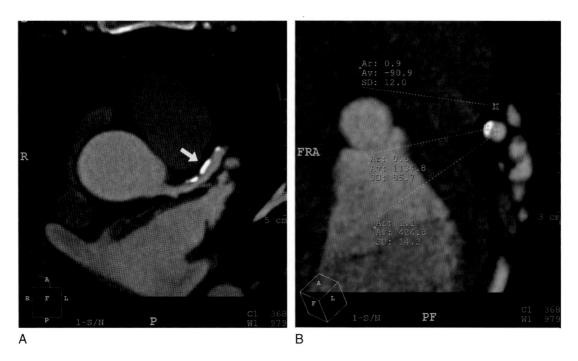

A   B

Figure 4.6 A. This MDCT oblique axial image obtained from a patient with atypical chest pain demonstrates eccentric calcified plaques (arrow) with mild stenosis of the proximal left anterior descending coronary artery. B. The zoomed cross-sectional view of the vessel demonstrates the eccentric calcified plaque (1134 Hounsfield units) causing mild narrowing of the coronary lumen (424 Hounsfield units).

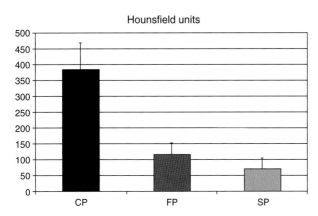

Figure 4.7 MDCT tissue contrast of calcified (CP), fibrous (FP) and soft plaques (SP) measured in Hounsfield Units (HU). (From Carrascosa et al.)[42]

classified as calcified or noncalcified. Using a cutoff value of 88 HU, 192 of 233 (82%) noncalcified plaques were correctly classified as fibrous or soft. Whether MDCT could be used in the clinical practice as a screening test remains to be proven, but in selected patients at low-intermediate risk, it could potentially help to justify life-long aggressive preventive intervention. MDCT plaque characterization could also potentially serve to device optimal revascularization strategies.

3.4 Evaluation of coronary artery bypass grafts

Several studies using 16-slice MDCT have investigated the accuracy in identifying stenosis in coronary bypass conduits. The reported sensitivity, specificity, positive and negative predictive values for detecting total graft occlusion have been reported at 96%, 95%, 81%, and 99%, respectively.[43] Imaging of the distal anastomosis site is feasible in almost 75% of patients (Figure 4.8). Although determining total vein graft occlusion is quite straightforward, quantifying moderate stenoses may be difficult. Motion artifacts and interference by surgical clips often limit the assessment of vessel anastomosis. Although graft position is easily visualized in patients following coronary artery bypass surgery (CABG), analysis of the native vessels is often more difficult in these patients, due to poor run-off, more extensive calcification and smaller lumen size. This can potentially limit the diagnostic utility of MDCT angiography in this setting. MDCT angiography may also help characterize the 3-dimensional location of preexisting coronary grafts in relationship to each other and to the chest wall in patients undergoing repeat sternotomy.

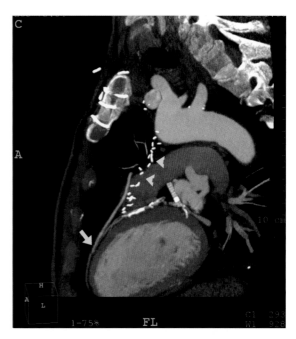

Figure 4.8 This MDCT oblique sagittal view was obtained from a patient with coronary artery disease and previous bypass surgery. The arrow demonstrates the distal anastomosis of an aorto-coronary bypass graft to the left anterior descending coronary artery. A previous internal thoracic artery graft to the same vessel is totally occluded and the metallic clips are visualized (arrowheads).

Stents/surgical clips artifacts remain a significant obstacle to image quality with MDCT. Metal artifacts may limit the assessment of the distal anastomosis of internal thoracic grafts, where the vessel lumen becomes essentially uninterpretable at that point.

3.5 Evaluation of myocardial function and perfusion

In patients with ischemic heart disease or cardiomyopathies, MDCT has the ability to combine retrospectively gated phases of the cardiac cycle allowing for accurate quantification of LV mass, volumes, and EF.[44] These methods create a 17-segment model, perform favorably in comparison to invasive ventriculography and may be used to quantify regional LV dysfunction. The data are acquired at the time of the coronary study and require no additional contrast or radiation.

Previous studies performed with electron beam computed tomography[45,46] have demonstrated hypodense areas in the left ventricular myocardium representing reduced iodine contrast appearance in the presence of flow-limiting coronary obstruction. More recently, similar findings have

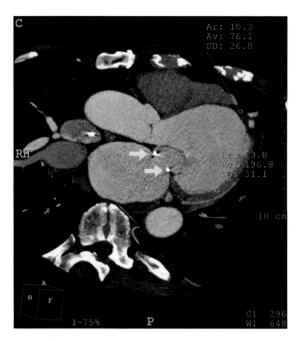

Figure 4.9 This MDCT oblique axial image was obtained in a patient with heart failure symptoms. There is thinning and reduced contrast enhancement of the anteroseptal and apical segments (76 Hounsfield units), consistent with a previous myocardial infarction. There is a mitral annuloplasty ring present (arrows).

been reported by MDCT in patients with acute myocardial infarction[47] (Figure 4.9).

3.6 Evaluation of intracardiac masses

MDCT is a useful imaging modality to determine the anatomical extent and the tissue characteristics of intracardiac masses.[48] MDCT offers certain potential advantages over echocardiography and MRI. First, MDCT may be performed much faster in patients who are hemodynamically unstable. Second, MDCT may be performed in patients with pacemakers or other implanted metallic devices in which MRI is contraindicated. Third, MDCT provides a more detailed evaluation of the lungs and mediastinal structures. Fourth, MDCT provides true 3D and 4D imaging in complex pathologies, quantifies calcification, vascularity and relationship to other mediastinal structures. However, it is important to recognize that MDCT may miss or incompletely characterize small mobile masses such as valvular vegetations due to its lower temporal resolution, it cannot visualize flow through intracardiac shunts or valvular regurgitation and it requires radiation exposure and the use

of intravenous contrast. Thus, in many cases, the information derived from MRI and MDCT is complementary.

MDCT has high sensitivity for the detection of left atrial appendage thrombi, but reduced specificity, as it is often difficult to differentiate reduced opacification due to slow flow vs. actual presence of a thrombus. Figure 4.10 demonstrates a left atrial appendage thrombus in the 2-chamber view in a patient undergoing cardiac MDCT prior to radiofrequency ablation of atrial fibrillation. There is lower attenuation in the LA appendage than in the body of the LA. The sharp transition from the LA thrombus and the non-thrombosed LA supports the presence of thrombus rather than flow stagnation (sludge).[49,50]

Most intracardiac tumors are benign in origin. Cardiac myxomas are the most common cardiac tumors. They originate from primitive mesenchymal cells that may differentiate into several cell types, including endothelial and lipidic cells. The tumor is benign but it may cause serious sequelae due to the high rate of embolization.[51] Figure 4.11 demonstrates an intramyocardial lipoma found in a patient with atypical chest pain undergoing MDCT coronary angiography. The low attenuation value is consistent with fat. Lipomas are rare and have no age or gender predisposition. Most are incidentally found in the interatrial septum or in the sub-endocardium or subpericardium of the free atrial or ventricular walls. About 25% of these tumors are intramuscular.[52]

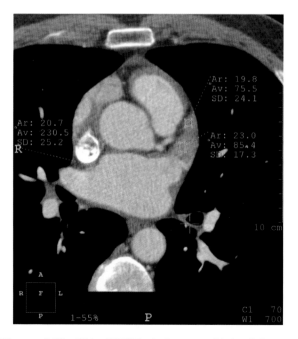

Figure 4.10 This MDCT study was obtained from a patient undergoing evaluation prior to radiofrequency ablation of atrial fibrillation. The axial image shows a thrombus in the left atrial appendage (75–87 Hounsfield units).

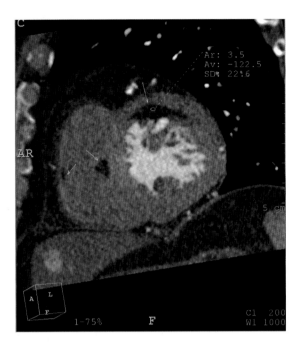

Figure 4.11 This cross-sectional view of the left and right ventricle was obtained from a patient undergoing evaluation of anginal symptoms. Multiple intramyocardial lipomas are incidentally noted (-122 Hounsfield units).

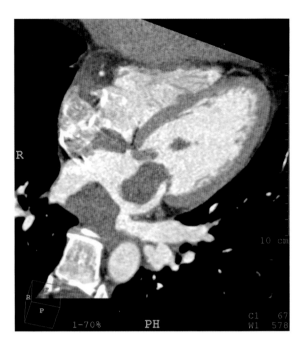

Figure 4.12 The MDCT axial image demonstrates multiple masses invading the left atrium, intraatrial septum, right atrium and encasing the right coronary artery. Biopsy demonstrated an angiosarcoma.

Fibromas are benign tumors that appear more frequently in children and adolescents. They often require resection due to their continuous growth and penetration into the pericardium causing hemorrhagic pericarditis and tamponade. MDCT typically demonstrates a calcified center, although delayed-enhancement MRI is better at demonstrating the surrounding fibrotic tissue.

Malignant cardiac tumors are often recognized by their irregular borders, invasion into the pericardium and mediastinal structures and heterogenous attenuation caused by areas of central necrosis, vascularity and calcification. Figure 4.12 demonstrates multiple large masses with attenuation similar to that of the LV myocardium, due to the rich vascularity and, therefore, contrast enhancement. Histological diagnosis was consistent with angiosarcoma. These tumors originate more commonly in the right atrium and may have intracavitary, polypoid or diffuse infiltrative appearance. Symptoms vary according to anatomical location. Obstruction of the superior and inferior vena cava and invasion of the pericardium are common. Most sarcomas are fatal within 4–24 months, regardless of treatment.

3.7 Evaluation of the pericardium

The pericardium is well visualized by MDCT and is usually surrounded by clearly delineated fat. MDCT may accurately

determine pericardial thickness and tissue characteristics in patients with pericardial disease. Pericardial effusions can be distinguished by their typical low attenuation values and calcification by the high attenuation (Figure 4.13). Primary pericardial tumors such as mesothelioma are rare, but it is a

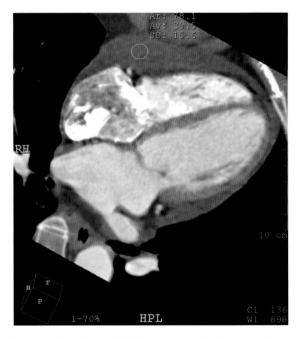

Figure 4.13 The MDCT oblique axial image demonstrates a pericardial effusion with an attenuation of 39.5 Hounsfield units.

frequent site of late metastasis from other sites, often accompanied by bloody effusions. Thickening (>2 mm) and calcification of the pericardium can suggest constriction, but MDCT is limited to establish the presence of constrictive physiology, thus echocardiography and MRI are superior in this regard. In the postoperative patient, MDCT is a robust tool to identify and localize pericardial fluid, hemorrhage and thrombus, and the Hounsfield score can be used to help differentiate thrombus from free fluid.

3.8 Cardiac MDCT in electrophysiology

Radiofrequency ablation of atrial fibrillation and cardiac resynchronization therapy in heart failure patients have become standard procedures in electrophysiology. Pulmonary vein isolation is effective in preventing recurrence of atrial fibrillation but may be associated with potentially serious complications such as esophageal perforation and pulmonary vein stenosis. The incidence of pulmonary vein stenosis varies according to the experience of the operator and the technique, but can be as high as 20%,[53] as detected by MDCT. The pulmonary veins have a complex anatomy, differing from patient to patient, and up to 20% of patients have less or more than 4 separate pulmonary vein ostia. MDCT provides excellent 3-dimensional visualization of the left atrium, pulmonary veins, and their relationship with surrounding structures. MDCT images can be registered with the catheter system to provide virtual 3-dimensional navigation during the procedure.[54]

MDCT may be used to evaluate the anatomy of the coronary sinus and its tributaries prior to implantation of biventricular pacing leads for cardiac resynchronization therapy, and allows the electrophysiologist to plan a two-stage procedure with epicardial lead implantation where the coronary sinus anatomy is unfavorable.[55]

4 FUTURE DIRECTIONS

Although there is considerable enthusiasm, many doubts remain about the appropriate clinical indications of cardiac MDCT studies. It is likely that outcome data will become available over time, with its increased clinical utilization. In the meantime, the high negative predictive value of MDCT coronary angiography makes this test ideal for establishing or excluding coronary artery disease in patients with low-intermediate probability. A normal MDCT study virtually excludes the presence of coronary artery disease. MDCT studies that demonstrate the presence of atherosclerotic plaque without significant luminal stenosis may establish the need for preventive interventions. In most cases, stress testing should follow MDCT studies that show moderate-severe stenosis, given the high prevalence of false-positive MDCT results. On the other hand, in those patients who have nondiagnostic, equivocal or unexpected functional stress test results, MDCT may also be useful as a confirmatory test, therefore reducing the need for diagnostic coronary angiography.

Future generations of MDCT systems will seek to improve temporal and spatial resolution and reduce radiation exposure. Alternative designs using multiple X-ray tubes and detector arrays or extra-wide detector coverage are currently been implemented. It is likely that temporal resolution will increase soon, but improvement in spatial resolution will come at the expense of increased radiation exposure. Until radiation exposure is significantly reduced, the wide application of MDCT as a screening test is not justifiable.

REFERENCES

1. Kennedy JW. Complications associated with cardiac catheterization and angiography. Cath Cardiovasc Diagn 1982; 8: 5–11.
2. Gibbons RJ, Abrams J, Chatterjee K, et al. ACC/AHA 2002 guideline update for the management of patients with chronic stable angina. J Am Coll Cardiol 2003; 41(1): 159–68.
3. Garcia MJ. Noninvasive coronary angiography: hype or new paradigm? JAMA 2005; 293: 2531–3.
4. Schoenhagen P, Stillman AE, Halliburton SS, et al. Non-invasive coronary angiography with multi-detector computed tomography: comparison to conventional X-ray angiography. Int J Cardiovasc Imaging 2005; 21: 63–72.
5. Hoffmann MHK, Shi H, Manzke R, et al. Noninvasive coronary angiography with 16-detector row CT: effect of heart rate. Radiology 2005; 234: 86–97.
6. Keelan PC, Bielak LF, Ashai K, et al. Long-term prognostic value of coronary calcification detected by electron-beam computed tomography in patients undergoing coronary angiography. Circulation 2001; 104: 412–7.
7. Greenland P, LaBree L, Azen SP, et al. Coronary artery calcium score combined with Framingham score for risk prediction in asymptomatic individuals. JAMA 2004; 291: 210–15.
8. O'Malley PG, Greenberg BA, Taylor AJ. Cost-effectiveness of using electron beam computed tomography to identify patients at risk for clinical coronary artery disease. Am Heart J. 2004; 148: 106–13.
9. Budoff MJ, Cohen MC, Garcia MJ, et al. ACCF/AHA clinical competence statement on cardiac imaging with computed tomography and magnetic resonance. Circulation 2005; 112: 598–617.

10. Nieman K, Cademartiri F, Lemos PA, et al. Reliable noninvasive coronary angiography with fast submillimeter multislice spiral computed tomography. Circulation 2002; 106: 2051–4.

11. Ropers D, Baum U, Pohle K, et al. Detection of coronary artery stenoses with thin-slice multi-detector row spiral computed tomography and multiplanar reconstruction. Circulation 2003; 107: 664–6.

12. Kuettner A, Beck T, Drosch T, et al. Diagnostic accuracy of noninvasive coronary imaging using 16-detector slice spiral computed tomography with 188 ms temporal resolution. J Am Coll Cardiol 2005; 45: 123–7.

13. Dewey M, Laule M, Krug L, et al. Multisegment and halfscan reconstruction of 16-slice computed tomography for detection of coronary artery stenoses. Invest Radiol 2004; 39: 223–9.

14. Kuettner A, Trabold T, Schroeder S, et al. Noninvasive detection of coronary lesions using 16-detector multislice spiral computed tomography technology-initial clinical results. J Am Coll Cardiol 2004; 44: 1230–7.

15. Mollet NR, Cademartiri F, Krestin GP, et al. Improved diagnostic accuracy with 16-row multi-slice computed tomography coronary angiography. J Am Coll Cardiol 2005; 45: 128–32.

16. Mollet NR, Cademartiri F, Nieman K, et al. Multislice spiral computed tomography coronary angiography in patients with stable angina pectoris. J Am Coll Cardiol 2004; 43: 2265–70.

17. Martuscelli E, Romagnoli A, D'Eliseo A, et al. Accuracy of thin-slice computed tomography in the detection of coronary stenoses. Eur Heart J 2004; 25: 1043–8.

18. Hoffmann MH, Shi H, Schmitz BL, et al. Noninvasive coronary angiography with multislice computed tomography. JAMA 2005; 293: 2471–8.

19. Kaiser C, Bremerich J, Haller S. Limited diagnostic yield of non-invasive coronary angiography by 16-slice multi-detector spiral computed tomography in routine patients referred for evaluation of coronary artery disease. Eur Heart J 2005; 26: 1987–92.

20. Kuettner A, Beck T, Drosch T. Image quality and diagnostic accuracy of non-invasive coronary imaging with 16 detector slice spiral computed tomography with 188 ms temporal resolution. Heart 2005; 91: 938–41.

21. Flohr T, Ohnesorge B. Heart rate adaptive optimization of spatial and temporal resolution for electrocardiogram-gated multislice spiral CT of the heart. J Comput Assist Tomogr 2001; 25(6): 907–23.

22. Grass M, Manzke R, Nielsen T, et al. Helical cardiac cone beam reconstruction using retrospective ECG gating. Phys Med Biol. 2003; 48(18): 3069–84.

23. Manzke R, Grass M, Nielsen T, et al. Adaptive temporal resolution optimization in helical cardiac cone beam CT reconstruction. Med Phys. 2003; 30(12): 3072–80.

24. Garcia MJ, Lessick J, Hoffmann MHK. Accuracy of 16-Row Multidetector Computed Tomography for the Assessment of Coronary Artery Stenosis. JAMA 2006; 296: 404–11.

25. Raff GL, Gallagher MJ, O'Neill WW, et al. Diagnostic Accuracy of Noninvasive Coronary Angiography Using 64-Slice Spiral Computed Tomography. J Am Coll Cardiol 2005; 46: 552–7.

26. Leber AW, Knez A, von Ziegler F, et al. Quantification of Obstructive and Nonobstructive Coronary Lesions by 64-Slice Computed Tomography: A Comparative Study With Quantitative Coronary Angiography and Intravascular Ultrasound. J Am Coll Cardiol 2005; 46: 147–54.

27. Mollet NR, Cademartiri F, van Mieghan CA, et al. High-Resolution Spiral Computed Tomography Coronary Angiography in Patients Referred for Diagnostic Conventional Coronary Angiography. Circulation 2005; 112: 2318–23.

28. Rius T, Goyenechea M, Poon M. Combined cardiac congenital anomalies assessed by multi-slice spiral computed tomography. Eur Heart J 2006; 27(6): 637.

29. Gilard M, Cornily JC, Rioufol G, et al. Noninvasive assessment of left main coronary stent patency with 16-slice computed tomography. Am J Cardiol. 2005; 95: 110–12.

30. Hong C, Chrysant GS, Woodard PK, et al. Coronary artery stent patency assessed with in-stent contrast enhancement measured at multi-detector row CT angiography: initial experience. Radiology 2004; 233: 286–91.

31. Seifarth H, Raupach R, Schaller S, et al. Assessment of coronary artery stents using 16-slice MDCT angiography: evaluation of a dedicated reconstruction kernel and a noise reduction filter. Eur Radiol. 2005; 15: 721–6.

32. Taylor AJ, Byers JP, Cheitlin MD, et al. Anomalous right or left coronary artery from the contralateral coronary sinus: "high-risk" abnormalities in the initial coronary artery course and heterogeneous clinical outcomes. Am Heart J. 1997; 133: 428–35.

33. Shi H, Aschoff AJ, Brambs HJ, et al. Multislice CT imaging of anomalous coronary arteries. Eur Radiol 2004; 14: 2172–81.

34. Burke AP, Farb A, Malcom GT, et al. Coronary risk factors and plaque morphology in men with coronary disease who died suddenly. N Engl J Med 1997; 336: 1276–82.

35. Nissen SE, Grinses CL, Gurley JC, et al. Application of a new phased-away ultrasound imaging catheter in the assessment of vascular dimensions: in vivo comparison to cine angiography. Circulation 1980; 81: 660–6.

36. Vince D, Dixon K, Cothern R, et al. Comparison of texture analysis methods for the characterization of coronary plaques in intravascular ultrasound images. Comput Med Imag Graph 2000; 24(4): 221–9.

37. Kostamaa H, Donoran J, Kasaoka E, et al. Calcified plaque cross-sectional area in human arteries: correlation between intravascular ultrasound and undercalcified histology. Am Heart J 1999; (3): 482–8.

38. Kopp A, Schoroeder S, Baumbach A, et al. Non-invasive characterization lesion morphology and composition by Multislice: Just results in comparison with intracoronary ultrasound. Euro Radiol 2001; 11(9): 1607–11.

39. Tobis JM., Mallery JA., Gessert J., et al. Intravascular ultrasound cross-sectional arterial imaging before and after ballon angioplasty in vitro. Circulation 1989; 70: 873–82.

40. Schoenhagen P, Tuzcu EM, Stillman AE, et al. Non-invasive assessment of plaque morphology and remodeling in mildly stenotic coronary segments: comparison of 16-slice computed tomography and intravascular ultrasound. Coron Artery Dis. 2003; 14: 459–62.

41. Achenbach S, Moselewski F, Ropers D, et al. Detection of calcified and noncalcified coronary atherosclerotic plaque by contrast-enhanced, submillimeter multidetector spiral computed tomography. A segment-based comparison with intravascular ultrasound. Circulation 2004; 109: 14–17.

42. Carrascosa PM, Capunay CM, Garcia-Merletti P, et al. Characterization of coronary atherosclerotic plaques by

multidetector computed tomography. Am J Cardiol 2006; 97(5): 598–602.

43. Schlosser T, Konorza T, Hunold P, et al. Noninvasive Visualization of Coronary Artery Bypass Grafts Using 16-Detector Row Computed Tomography. J Am Coll Cardiol 2004; 44: 1224–9.

44. Hundt W, Siebert K, Wintersperger BJ, et al. Assessment of global left ventricular function: comparison of cardiac multidetector-row computed tomography with angiocardiography. J Comput Assist Tomogr 2005; 29: 373–81.

45. Bell MR, Lerman LO, Rumberger JA. Validation of minimally invasive measurement of myocardial perfusion using electron beam computed tomography and application in human volunteers. Heart 1999; 81(6): 628–35.

46. Schmermund A, Bell MR, Lerman LO, Ritman EL, Rumberger JA. Quantitative evaluation of regional myocardial perfusion using fast X-ray computed tomography. Herz 1997; 22: 29–39.

47. Paul JF, Dambrin G, Caussin C, Lancelin B, Angel C. Sixteen-slice computed tomography after acute myocardial infarction: From perfusion defect to the culprit lesion. Circulation 2003; 108: 373–4.

48. Restrepo CS, Largoza A, Lemos DF, et al. CT and MR imaging findings of malignant cardiac tumors. Curr Probl Diagn Radiol 2005; 34: 1–11.

49. Jaber WA, White RD, Kuzmiak SA, et al. Comparison of ability to identify left atrial thrombus by three-dimensional tomography versus transesophageal echocardiography in patients with atrial fibrillation. Am J Cardiol 2004; 93(4): 486–9.

50. Tatli S, Lipton MJ. CT for intracardiac thrombi and tumors. Int J Cardiovasc Imaging 2005; 21(1): 115–31.

51. Grebenc ML, Rosado-de-Christenson ML, Green CE, et al. Cardiac myxoma: imaging features in 83 patients. Radiographics 2002; 22(3): 673–89.

52. Schvartzman PR, White RD. Imaging of cardiac and paracardiac masses. J Thorac Imaging 2000; 15(4): 265–73.

53. Saad EB, Rossillo A, Saad C, et al. Pulmonary vein stenosis after radiofrequency ablation of atrial fibrillation: functional characterization, evolution, and influence of the ablation strategy. Circulation 2003; 108(25): 3102–7.

54 Verma A, Marrouche N, Natale A. Novel method to integrate three-dimensional computed tomographic images of the left atrium with real-time electroanatomic mapping. Journal of Cardiovascular Electrophysiology Aug 2004; 15(8): 968.

55 Shinbane JS, Girsky MJ, Mao S, Budoff MJ. Thebesian valve imaging with electron beam CT angiography: implications for resynchronization therapy. Pacing Clin Electrophysiol 2004; 27: 1566–7.

5

Computed Tomographic Anatomy of the Heart

Amgad N. Makaryus and Lawrence M. Boxt

1 INTRODUCTION

Computed tomography (CT) of the heart provides significant morphologic and functional information needed for the diagnosis and management of patients with acquired and congenital heart disease. The clinical utility of cardiac CT is derived from its convenience, safety, and diagnostic accuracy. CT examinations are acquired in high contrast and spatial resolution, producing robust data sets from which detailed maps of x-ray attenuation may be produced. Contemporary workstations apply fast software for the production of 2-, 3-, and 4-dimensional imagery. Students of clinical medicine are increasingly confronted by anatomic 3-D displays (renderings) reconstructed from CT images. These images display the organs of the chest and abdomen in anatomical orientation allowing the student of anatomy to visualize the appearance of the organ, as well as the spatial relations of the adjacent organs. The dramatic improvement in temporal resolution achieved with ECG-gated multi-detector CT scanning set the stage for its implementation into the daily practice of cardiology. A particular characteristic of cardiac CT scanning is acquisition of image data in the axial body plane. This orientation of image data is unfamiliar to the cardiac imager because the heart lies obliquely in the chest, and the axial body section therefore displays cardiac structure oblique to the intrinsic cardiac axes. Image data obtained in this format, however, provides a wealth of anatomic information. The purpose of this chapter is to describe the normal anatomy of the heart as obtained in ECG-gated contrast-enhanced thin-section axial tomographic acquisitions. These images will be supplemented with oblique tomograms and 3-D volume rendered reconstructions obtained by processing the axial data from contrast-enhanced multi-slice 64-detector CT scans of the heart. Our description will follow the flow of blood into and out of the heart. Each particular anatomic structure will be described in terms of its intrinsic morphologic structure, place in the heart, and anatomic relationships. The reader is encouraged to treat the figures as slides in a discussion of a particular part of cardiac anatomy. Correlating axial acquisition images with oblique tomographic reconstructions and surface-rendered 3-dimensional figures will reinforce the overall organization and structure of the heart. Part of this discussion has been presented in a previous article.[1]

2 SUPERIOR VENA CAVA

The superior vena cava (SVC) is formed by the confluence of the innominate veins (Figure 5.1). It passes to the right and slightly posterior to the ascending aorta, draining into the right atrium (RA) just posterior to the orifice of the right atrial appendage (RAA). The posterior wall of the SVC as it enters the RA forms the sinus venosus portion of the interatrial septum (Figures 5.2–5.10, 5.27, 5.56, 5.58, 5.63).

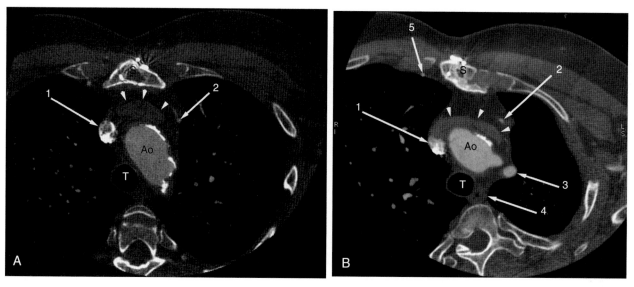

Figure 5.1 (a) Axial image obtained from a CT examination of a 66-year-old man presenting with chest discomfort and a history of previous coronary artery bypass graft surgery, through the moderately calcified aortic arch (Ao). The left-sided aortic arch displaces the trachea (T) toward the right. Contrast was injected via the right upper extremity; the right innominate vein (arrow 1) is highly opacified. Unopacified blood from the left innominate vein (arrowheads) is seen passing anterior to the Ao, immediately behind the sternum (S). The left internal mammary artery (arrow 2) has been dissected away from the anterior chest wall. (b) Oblique axial reconstruction 1.5 cm inferior to figure 1a. The left innominate vein (arrowheads) is just joining the opacified right innominate vein (arrow 1). The left internal mammary (arrow 2) and proximal left subclavian (arrow 3) arteries are opacified. Air is seen within the collapsed esophageal lumen (arrow 4), immediately posterior and toward the left of the trachea (T). The right internal mammary artery (arrow 5) is labeled.

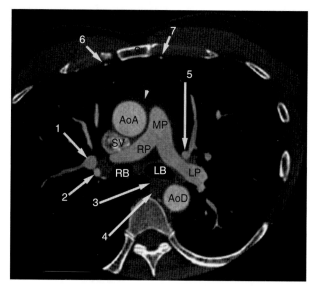

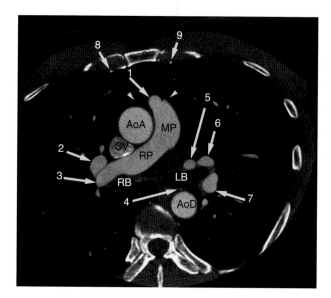

Figure 5.2 Axial acquisition image through the main pulmonary artery (MP) and left (LP) and right (RP) pulmonary arteries. The RP lies anterior to the right bronchus (RB); the LP has crossed over the left bronchus (LB). The superior vena cava (SV) lies behind the ascending aorta (AoA) and RP. The confluence of the branches of the right upper lobe pulmonary vein (arrow 1) lies immediately anterior to the right upper lobe pulmonary artery (arrow 2). The left upper lobe pulmonary vein (arrow 5) lies anterior to the LP. The collapsed esophagus (arrow 3) lies behind the LB, and anterior to the azygos vein (arrow 4) and descending aorta (AoD). The parietal pericardium (arrowhead) reflects over the ascending aorta (AoA) and MP. The right (arrow 6) and left (arrow 7) internal mammary arteries lie to the right and left of the sternum (S), respectively.

Figure 5.3 Axial acquisition image obtained just inferior to Figure 5.2. The anterior pulmonary artery sinus of Valsalva (arrow 1) is contained within the parietal pericardium (arrowheads). The confluent right upper lobe pulmonary vein (arrow 2) lies immediately anterior to the hilar right pulmonary artery (RP), which lies anterior to the right bronchus (RB). The segmental left upper lobe pulmonary veins (arrows 5 and 6) have not yet joined. The left pulmonary artery (arrow 7) has crossed, and is now posterior to the left bronchus (LB). A tiny bronchial artery (arrow 4) is viewed in cross section. The right (arrow 8) and left (arrow 9) internal mammary arteries lie to the right and left of the sternum (S), respectively.

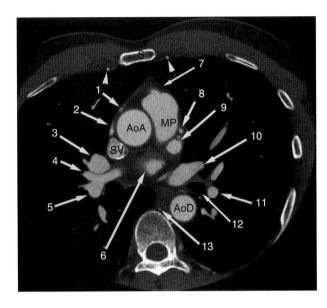

Figure 5.4 Axial acquisition image obtained just inferior to Figure 5.3, through the roof of the left atrium (arrow 6). The main pulmonary artery (MP) is enveloped by the parietal pericardium (arrow 7). The superior aspect of the right atrial appendage (arrows 1 and 2) lies anterior to the ascending aorta (AoA). At this level, the confluence of the right upper lobe pulmonary vein (arrow 3) is anterior to the right upper lobe pulmonary artery (arrow 4) as is splits off from the right lower lobe pulmonary artery (arrow 5). Portions of the cavity of the left atrial appendage (arrows 8 and 9) are separated from each other by the interposed pectinate muscles. Posterior to the left atrial appendage, the left upper lobe pulmonary vein (arrow 10) is seen draining into the posterior aspect of the left atrium. The left lower lobe pulmonary artery (arrow 11) lies to the left of the left lower lobe bronchus (arrow 12). An intercostal artery (arrow 13) is seen in cross section to the right of the descending aorta (AoD).

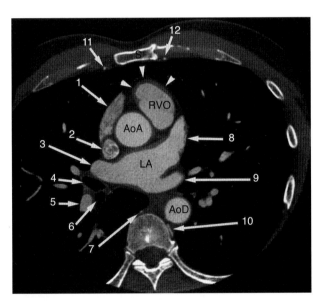

Figure 5.5 Axial acquisition image obtained through the bodies of the right (arrow 1) and left (arrow 8) atrial appendages. The left upper lobe pulmonary vein (arrow 9) is now seen draining into the body of the left atrium (LA). The LA lies between the ascending (AoA) and descending (AoD) aorta. A right-sided intercostals artery (arrow 7) is seen in cross section; a left-sided intercostal artery (arrow 10) is viewed in longitudinal section as it passes from the descending aorta (AoD) toward the underside of a left rib. Intracavitary filling defects characterize the pectinate muscles of the right atrial appendage (arrow 1). At this level, the superior vena cava (arrow 2) has not yet been incorporated into the right atrium. The right upper lobe pulmonary vein (arrow 3), right lower lobe pulmonary artery (arrow 5) and right upper (arrow 4) and lower (arrow 6) lobe bronchi comprise the right pulmonary hilum. At this level, below the level of the pulmonary valve, we view the myocardium (arrowheads) of the right ventricular outflow tract (RVO). The right (arrow 11) and left (arrow 12) internal mammary arteries lie to the right and left of the sternum (S), respectively.

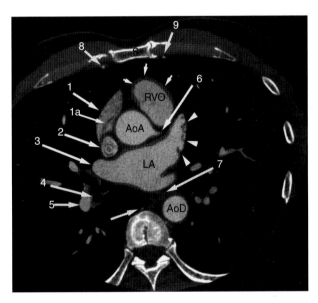

Figure 5.6 Axial acquisition image obtained through the ascending aorta (AoA) at the level of the origin of the left main coronary artery (arrow 6). The myocardium (arrowheads) of the right ventricular outflow tract (RVO) is visualized. A tubular filling defect (arrow 1a) within the right atrial appendage (arrow 1) represents a large pectinate muscle. Similarly, pectinate muscles of the left atrial appendage appear as short filling defects (arrowheads) along the lateral appendage wall. The superior vena cava (arrow 2) has not yet been assimilated into the right atrium. Immediately posterior to the superior vena cava, the right upper lobe pulmonary vein (arrow 3) has entered the left atrium (LA). The right lower lobe pulmonary artery (arrow 5) and bronchus (arrow 4) are viewed in cross section. Circular lucencies represent air within the nearly collapsed esophagus (arrow 7) sandwiched between the entrance of the left upper lobe pulmonary vein into the LA and the descending aorta (AoD). The right (arrow 8) and left (arrow 9) internal mammary arteries lie to the right and left of the sternum (S), respectively.

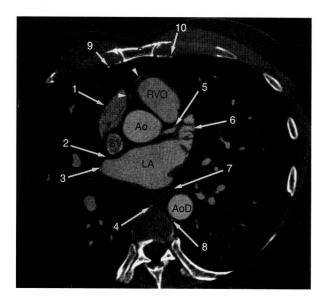

Figure 5.7 Axial acquisition image obtained through the aortic root (Ao) just after the origin of the left main coronary artery (arrow 5). The right atrial appendage (arrow 1) is anterior to the Ao. The low attenuation (fatty infiltrated) sinus venosus atrial septum (arrow 2) separates the posterior wall of the superior vena cava (SV) from the cavity of the left atrium (LA) adjacent to the entry of the right upper lobe pulmonary vein (arrow 3). The collapsed esophagus (arrow 7) is interposed between the LA and the descending aorta (AoD). A right-sided (arrow 4) and left-sided (arrow 8) intercostal artery is seen in cross section against the volume averaged vertebral body (VB). At this level, portions of the highest marginal branch (arrowheads) of the right coronary artery (the 'conus artery') can be seen passing anterior to the right ventricular outflow (RVO). The right (arrow 9) and left (arrow 10) internal mammary arteries lie to the right and left of the sternum (S), respectively.

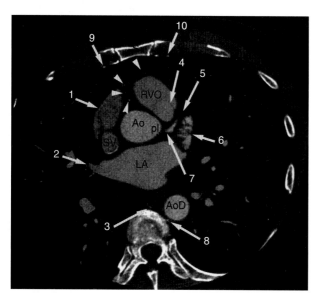

Figure 5.8 Axial acquisition image obtained through the aortic root (Ao) and posterior left (pl) aortic sinus of Valsalva. The distal left main coronary artery (arrow 7) has not yet dipped beneath the left atrial appendage (arrow 6) to become the circumflex artery. The proximal left anterior descending artery is seen passing along the superior aspect of the interventricular septum, posterior to the pulmonary artery sinuses of Valsalva (arrow 4) and right ventricular outflow (RVO). An isolated right middle lobe pulmonary vein (arrow 2) is seen entering the left atrium (LA). More proximal segments of the conus branch of the right coronary artery (arrowheads) are seen embedded in the fat between the right atrial appendage (arrow 1) and RVO. Adjacent to the vertebral body, a segment of a right (arrow 3) and left (arrow 8) intercostal artery is seen in cross section. The right (arrow 9) and left (arrow 10) internal mammary arteries lie to the right and left of the sternum (S), respectively. The superior vena cava (SV) and descending aorta (AoD) are labeled.

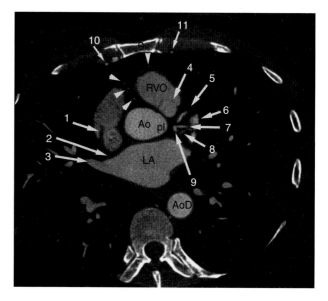

Figure 5.9 Axial acquisition image obtained through the aortic root (Ao) and posterior left (pl) aortic sinus of Valsalva. The proximal left anterior descending (arrow 5), proximal circumflex (arrow 9), and a ramus medianus branch are identified embedded in fat. Curving away from the ramus branch (arrow 7), the distal portion of the anterior interventricular vein (arrow 8) is passing toward the posterior atrioventricular ring. Segments of the conius artery (arrowheads) are embedded in the fat of the anterior atrioventricular ring, and along the epicardium of the right ventricular outflow (RVO) myocardium. At this level, the inferior aspect of a cusp of the pulmonary valve (arrow 4) is seen. The extension of the crista terminalis (arrow 1) appears as a thick, curving filling defect in the body of the right atrial appendage. The sinus venosus interatrial septum (arrow 2) is embedded in low attenuation fat. The inferior aspect of an isolated right middle lobe pulmonary vein (arrow 3) is seen entering the left atrium (LA). The right (arrow 10) and left (arrow 11) internal mammary arteries lie to the right and left of the sternum (S), respectively. The descending aorta (AoD) is labeled.

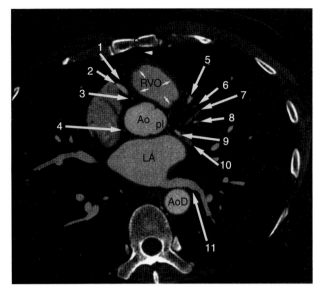

Figure 5.10 Axial acquisition image obtained through the aortic root (Ao) and posterior left (pl) aortic sinus of Valsalva. The anterior junction line (arrowhead) is formed by the visceral and parietal pleura meeting at the midline. The circumferential myocardium of the right ventricular infundibulum (small arrows) is also midline, residing behind the sternum (S). The proximal right coronary artery (arrow 2) and segments of the conus artery (arrows 1 and 3) are embedded within the fat of the anterior atrioventricular ring. A portion of the sinoatrial node branch of the right coronary artery (arrow 4) is seen behind the Ao passing toward the junction of the superior vena cava and atrial septum. A diagonal branch (arrow 6) of the anterior descending coronary artery (arrow 5) is seen in the epicardial fat above the interventricular septum. The ramus branch (arrow 8) has just passed beneath the anterior interventricular vein (arrow 7) on its path toward the posterior atrioventricular ring. Within the ring itself, the circumflex coronary artery (arrow 9) and great cardiac vein (arrow 10) are seen. The left lower lobe pulmonary vein (arrow 11) characteristically passes immediately in front of the descending aorta (AoD) before entering the left atrium (LA).

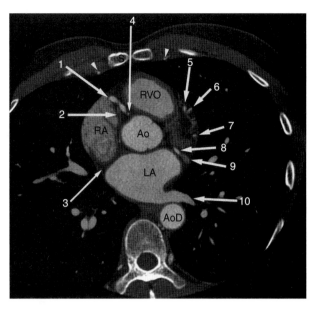

Figure 5.11 Axial acquisition image obtained through the aortic root (Ao) and posterior left (pl) aortic sinus of Valsalva immediately inferior to Figure 5.10. The origin of the conus artery (arrow 3) from the very proximal right coronary artery (arrow 2) is seen. Notice the course of the sinoatrial node branch (arrow 2) as it passes behind the right atrium (RA) toward the interatrial septum (arrow 3). Passing the right ventricular outflow (RVO), the mid-anterior descending coronary artery (arrow 5) and a diagonal branch (arrow 6) continue along the top of the interventricular septum and anterolateral wall of the left ventricle, respectively. The ramus branch (arrow 7) is seen passing along the anterolateral left ventricular wall. Within the posterior atrioventricular ring, the circumflex artery (arrow 8) and great cardiac vein (arrow 9) are intertwined. The left lower lobe pulmonary vein (arrow 10) passes anterior to the descending aorta (AoD) to enter the left atrium (LA). The right and left internal mammary arteries (arrowheads) lie to the right and left of the sternum (S), respectively.

3 THE CARDIAC VEINS

The venous drainage of the heart is carried by three very different sets of veins; the coronary sinus and its tributaries, the anterior cardiac veins, and the thebesian veins. Venous return from the left ventricular myocardium is through the anterior interventricular, the middle (or marginal) cardiac, and the posterior cardiac veins (Figures 5.9–5.20, 5.28–5.37, 5.39–5.53, 5.61, 5.62). The anterior interventricular (or anterior cardiac) vein ascends in the anterior interventricular sulcus, parallel with the anterior descending coronary artery, and passes over the base of the heart toward the posterior atrioventricular ring, to enter the great cardiac vein.

The great cardiac vein (GCV) extends from the confluence of the anterior interventricular vein in the posterior atrioventricular ring. It receives the middle ventricular and posterior cardiac veins, and then passes beneath the LA to the diaphragmatic surface of the heart. The coronary sinus is the confluence of the large cardiac veins. Before draining into the right atrium, the roof of the coronary sinus forms a portion of the floor of the left atrium. The coronary sinus (CS) drains into the right atrium medial, and slightly superior to the entry of the inferior vena cava. The eustachian valve separates these two structures.

The anatomy of the major cardiac veins varies considerably among individuals. The great cardiac vein spirals with the circumflex coronary artery in the posterior atrioventricular ring, receives the marginal and posterior cardiac veins,

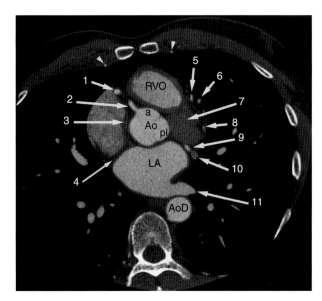

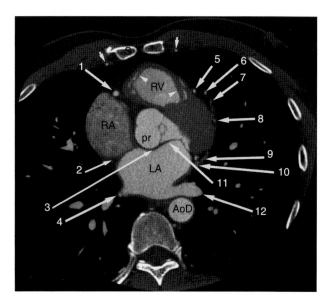

Figure 5.12 Axial acquisition image obtained through the aortic root (Ao) immediately inferior to Figure 5.11. The right coronary artery (arrow 2) arises from the anterior aortic sinus of Valsalva (a). The inferior aspect of the posterior left sinus (pl) is labeled. A segment of the proximal right coronary artery has looped superiorly (out of plane) and then inferiorly (arrow 1) to begin descent in the anterior atrioventricular ring. A portion of the sinoatrial node artery (arrow 3) is viewed passing toward the interatrial septum (arrow 4). The anterior descending artery (arrow 5), a diagonal branch of the anterior descending artery (arrow 6), and the ramus branch (arrow 8) have passed beyond the top of the myocardium of the anterior left ventricular wall (arrow 7). The circumflex artery (arrow 9) and great cardiac vein (arrow 10) are again seen intertwined in the posterior atrioventricular ring. The left lower lobe pulmonary vein (arrow 11) passes anterior to the descending aorta (AoD) to enter the left atrium (LA). The right and left internal mammary arteries (arrowheads) lie to the right and left of the sternum (S), respectively.

Figure 5.13 Axial acquisition image obtained through the posterior right aortic sinus of Valsalva (pr). The right coronary artery is viewed in cross section within the anterior atrioventricular ring. Muscle bundles (arrowheads) are seen within the sinus of the right ventricle (RV) passing between the interventricular septum and the RV free wall. Embedded within fat in the anterior interventricular groove, the anterior descending coronary artery (arrow 5) and a diagonal branch (arrow 6) are viewed in cross section. Similarly, along the anterior aspect of the left ventricle, the anterior interventricular vein (arrow 7) and ramus branch (8) are viewed in cross section. The pr abuts the right (RA) and left (LA) atrium, and the interatrial septum (arrow 2). Notice continuity between the anterior mitral leaflet (arrow 11) and the aortic annulus (arrow 3) supporting the pr. Within the posterior atrioventricular ring, the middle ventricular vein (arrow 9) is seen draining into the great cardiac vein (arrow 10). The right (arrow 4) and left (arrow 12) lower lobe pulmonary veins are seen draining into the LA. The right and left internal mammary arteries (small arrows) lie to the right and left of the sternum (S), respectively.

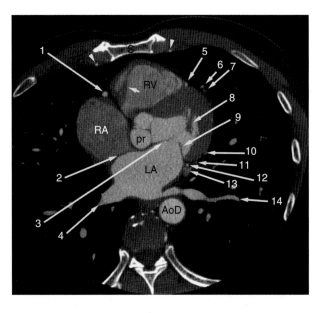

Figure 5.14 Axial acquisition image obtained through the posterior right aortic sinus of Valsalva (pr), inferior to Figure 5.13. The right coronary artery (arrow 1) is viewed in cross section. The pr is the inferior-most aortic sinus, lying between the right (RA) and left (LA) atrium. Note how thin the interatrial septum (arrow 2) is here. The anterior mitral leaflet (arrow 3) is in continuity with the aortic annulus beneath the pr. The posterior mitral leaflet (arrow 9) is attached on the posterior atrioventricular ring, which contains the great cardiac vein (arrow 13) and circumflex artery (arrow 12) and segments (arrows 10 and 11) of a marginal branch of the circumflex artery. A myocardial muscle bundle characteristically crosses the sinus of the right ventricle (RV) (short arrow); a left ventricular papillary muscle (arrow 8) protrudes from the lateral wall into the ventricular cavity. The right (arrow 4) and left (arrow 14) lower lobe pulmonary veins drain into the LA. The right and left internal mammary arteries (arrowheads) lie to the right and left of the sternum (S), respectively.

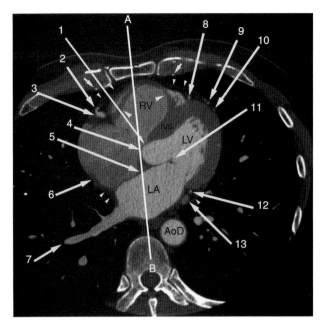

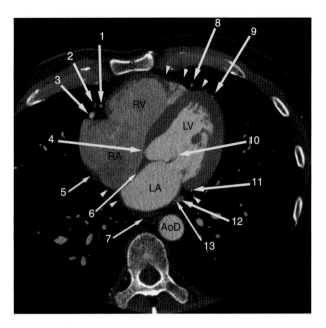

Figure 5.15 Axial acquisition image obtained through the inferior aspect of the posterior right aortic sinus of Valsalva (pr), inferior to Figure 5.14. Line AB 'divides' the heart into 'right' and 'left.' Notice how the inflow to the right ventricle (RV) lies to the right with respect to the inflow of the left ventricle (LV). The membranous (arrow 1) and atrioventricular (arrow 4) portions of the interventricular septum lie posterior and to the right of the muscular interventricular septum (ivs). The primum interatrial septum (arrow 5) and anterior mitral leaflet (arrow 11) are continuous with each other as well as the aortic annulus and primum atrial septum and atrioventricular and membranous interventricular septum. The origin of a marginal branch (arrow 2) of the right coronary artery (arrow 3) passes within the epicardial fat, beneath the pericardium (small arrowheads about the perimeter of the heart). Muscular trabeculations within the (RV) chamber pass from the septum to the free wall. Within the fat in the anterior interventricular groove, the anterior descending (arrow 8) and two diagonal branches (arrows 9 and 10) are viewed in cross section. The circumflex artery (arrow 12) and great cardiac vein (arrow 13) are viewed in cross section within the fat of the posterior atrioventricular ring. The descending aorta (AoD) is labeled. The right and left internal mammary arteries (small arrows) lie to the right and left of the sternum (S), respectively.

Figure 5.16 Axial acquisition image obtained through the atrioventricular septum, inferior to Figure 5.15. The atrioventricular septum (arrow 4), primum atrial septum (arrow 6) and anterior mitral leaflet (arrow 10) all share fibrous continuity. Viewed in cross section embedded in the fat of the anterior atrioventroicular ring are the right coronary artery (arrow 3), a marginal branch of the right coronary artery (arrow 1), and the anterior cardiac vein (arrow 2). The anterior descending artery (arrow 8) is viewed in cross section in the fat of the anterior interventricular groove. A diagonal branch of the anterior descending artery (arrow 9) passes over the left ventricular myocardium. A marginal branch of the circumflex artery (arrow 11) and the great cardiac vein (arrow 12) are seen in cross section in the posterior atrioventricular ring. The distal circumflex artery (arrow 13) continues in the distal atrioventricular ring as a very small vessel. Notice the intimate relationship between the air-filled esophagus (arrow 7) and the left atrium (LA). Portions of pericardium (arrowheads) are identified about the periphery of the heart.

Figure 5.17 Axial acquisition image obtained about 2 cm inferior to Figure 5.16. A marginal branch of the right coronary artery (arrow 1) passes along the free wall of the right ventricle (RV). The right coronary artery (arrow 2) is viewed in cross section within the fat of the anterior atrioventricular ring. The anterior descending coronary artery (arrow 5) is viewed in cross section. A marginal branch of the circumflex coronary artery (arrow 6) is viewed in longitudinal section along the posterior left ventricular (LV) wall. The moderator band, a muscular trabeculation (arrowhead) that extends from the interventricular septum to the right ventricular (RV) free wall is seen. The distal great cardiac vein disappears beneath the left atrium (LA), and emerges medially as the coronary sinus (arrow 4) to enter the right atrium (RA). The crista terminalis (arrow 3) is labeled.

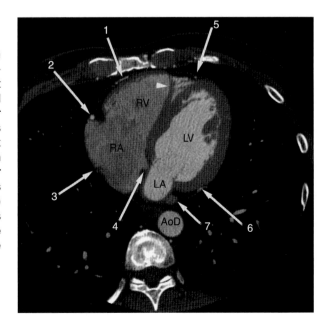

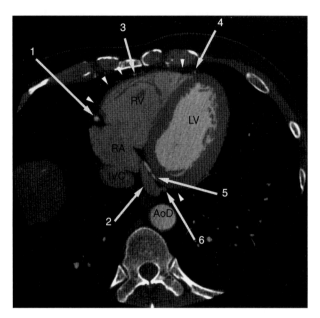

Figure 5.18 Axial acquisition image obtained through the dome of the right diaphragm (D), 1 cm inferior to Figure 5.17. The distal right coronary artery (arrow 1) is viewed in cross section. A marginal branch of the right coronary artery (arrow 3) passes along the right ventricular (RV) free wall. The distal anterior descending coronary artery (arrow 4) is seen near the cardiac apex. The coronary sinus (arrow 2) receives the middle (or marginal) cardiac vein (arrow 6). Running parallel to the coronary sinus (arrow 2) in the inferior aspect of the posterior atrioventricular ring is the posterior left ventricular branch (arrow 5) of the distal right coronary artery. At this level, the suprahepatic inferior vena cava (IVC) is just entering the right atrium (RA). Portions of pericardium (small arrowheads) are identified about the periphery of the heart.

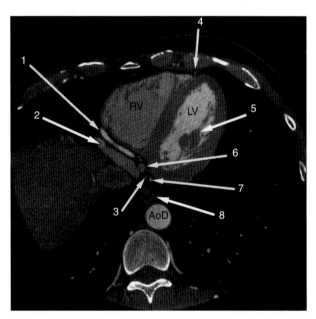

Figure 5.19 Axial acquisition image obtained through the liver (Li) and the inferior aspect of the anterior atrioventricular ring, 1 cm inferior to Figure 5.18. The distal right coronary artery (arrow 1) is viewed in longitudinal section, embedded within the fat of the atrioventricular ring, between the inferior aspect of the right atrium (arrow 2) and the cavity of the right ventricle (RV). At this level, the inferior interventricular vein (arrow 6) has not yet become confluent with the coronary sinus. The posterior left ventricular branch of the distal right coronary artery (arrow 7) and a tributary of the marginal cardiac vein (arrow 3) are viewed in cross section in the fat of the posterior atrioventricular ring. The distal anterior descending coronary artery (arrow 4) is viewed in cross section within the anterior interventricular groove. The posterior papillary muscle (arrow 5) of the left ventricle (LV) appears as a lobulated intracavitary filling defect. The esophagus is labeled.

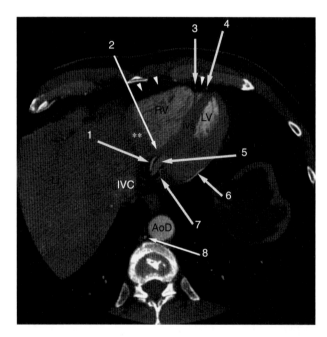

Figure 5.20 Axial acquisition image obtained through the liver (Li), the intrahepatic inferior vena cava (IVC), and the cardiac crux (arrow 2), the intersection of the interventricular septum (ivs) and the anterior (**) and posterior atrioventricular rings. The posterior descending coronary artery (arrow 1) runs with the posterior cardiac vein (arrow 5). Posterior to the vein, embedded in the fat of the inferior aspect of the posterior atrioventricular ring, a posterior left ventricular branch of the distal right coronary artery (arrow 7) runs along the inferior wall of the left ventricle (LV). This distal marginal branch is the posterior extension of this dominant right coronary artery. The distal anterior descending artery (arrow 4), and a tributary of an anterior cardiac vein (arrow 3) lie in the epicardial fat between the right (RV) and left (LV) ventricles. The descending aorta (AoD) and an intercostal artery in cross section (arrow 8) are labeled.

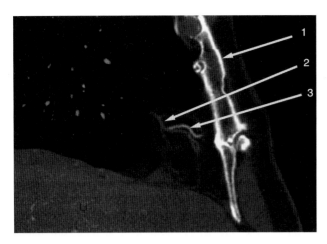

Figure 5.21 Right anterior oblique (RAO) reconstruction obtained through the body of the sternum (arrow 1) and liver (Li). A marginal branch of the right coronary artery (arrow 3) passes along the free wall of the right ventricle, crossing a tributary of the anterior cardiac vein (arrow 2).

and drains into the right atrium as the coronary sinus. The marginal cardiac veins originate from the posterior or lateral aspects of the left ventricle and drain into the great cardiac vein. Not uncommonly, they drain directly into the coronary sinus.

Venous drainage from the right ventricular free wall is via the anterior cardiac veins (Figures 5.16, 5.21–5.25, 5.50, 5.59, 5.63). These veins travel along the anterior aspect of the

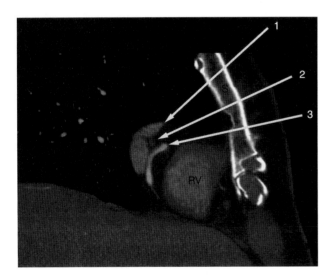

Figure 5.22 Right anterior oblique (RAO) reconstruction obtained through the sternum (S) and the anterior atrioventricular ring. The mid right coronary artery (arrow 3) runs within the low attenuation fat of the ring. The anterior cardiac vein (arrow 2) is viewed in cross section as it passes beneath the right atrial appendage (arrow 1) to drain into the right atrium.

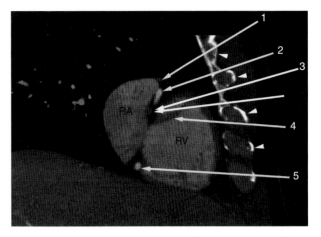

Figure 5.23 Right anterior oblique (RAO) reconstruction obtained to the left of Figure 5.22, through calcified right costal cartilages (arrowheads) and the anterior atrioventricular ring. Proximal (arrow 2) and distal (arrow 4) right coronary segments are viewed within the fat of the atrioventricular ring. The right atrial appendage (arrow 1) has a broad opening into the right atrium (RA). The cavity of the right ventricle (RV) is slightly inferior to the RA. Intracavitary filling defects within the RV (arrow 3) are muscle bundles extending from the interventricular septum to the free wall.

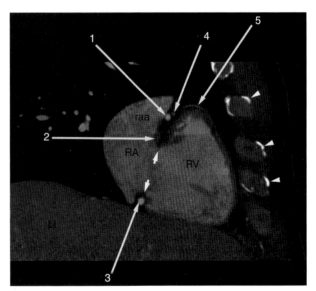

Figure 5.24 Right anterior oblique (RAO) reconstruction obtained to the left of Figure 5.23, through calcified right costal cartilages (arrowheads) and the anterior atrioventricular ring. In the fat of the superior aspect of the ring, the right coronary artery (arrow 1), and a proximal (arrow 4) and more distal segment (arrow 5) of the first marginal, or conus artery crosses the right ventricular (RV) infundibulum. The distal right coronary artery (arrow 3) passes immediately beneath the tricuspid annulus (short arrows). The anterior cardiac vein, viewed in cross section, has not yet drained into the right atrium (RA).

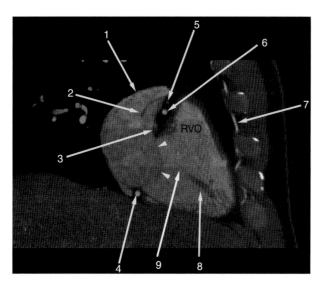

Figure 5.25 Right anterior oblique (RAO) reconstruction obtained to the left of Figure 5.24, through the left internal mammary artery (arrow 7), the tricuspid valve (arrowheads), and the proximal (arrow 6) and distal (arrow 4) right coronary artery. A right ventricular papillary muscle (arrow 8) appears as a large filling defect. The chordal attachment to the valve leaflet (arrow 9) is finer, and less apparent. The right atrial appendage (arrow 1) contains tubular filling defects (arrow 2) which are the pectinate muscles, similar in appearance to muscle bundles seen in the right ventricle. A more proximal segment of the conus artery is viewed in cross section cephalad to the proximal right coronary artery (arrow 6). The anterior cardiac vein is just breaking the wall of the right atrium. The myocardium of the infundibulum surrounds (and forms) the right ventricular outflow tract (RVO).

heart, cross the anterior atrioventricular ring, and enter the right atrium, either directly or through a small right atrial cardiac vein. The thebesian veins are very small vessels which drain myocardial blood directly back to the cardiac chambers.[1]

4 RIGHT ATRIUM

The right atrium is generally round in shape, and forms the right lower border of the heart (Figures 5.11–5.18, 5.23–5.31, 5.49–5.55, 5.58, 5.59, 5.63). The lateral RA wall is very thin; the distance between the cavity of the RA and the outer lateral border of the heart should be no greater than 3 mm. The cavity of the RA is segregated into an anterior trabeculated portion, and posterior smooth-walled portion, by the crista terminalis, the remnant of the vein of the sinus venosus (Figures 5.9, 5.15–5.17).

The interatrial septum usually bows toward the RA with normal thinning seen in the region of the foramen

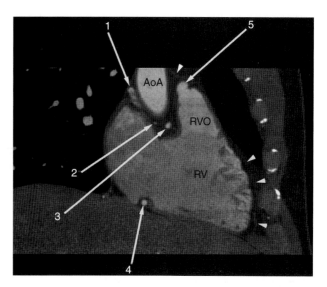

Figure 5.26 Right anterior oblique (RAO) reconstruction obtained to the left of Figure 5.25, through the posterior aspect of the right atrial appendage (arrow 1). The proximal (arrow 3) and distal (arrow 4) right coronary artery is viewed in cross section as it enters and passes under the anterior atrioventricular ring, respectively. The sinoatrial node artery (arrow 2) is viewed in cross section, as it passes posteriorly and superiorly toward the superior vena cava (out of the plane of this figure). Just above the right ventricular outflow (RVO), a sinus of Valsalva of the main pulmonary artery (arrow 5) is now seen. Portions of pericardium (small arrowheads) are identified about the periphery of the heart.

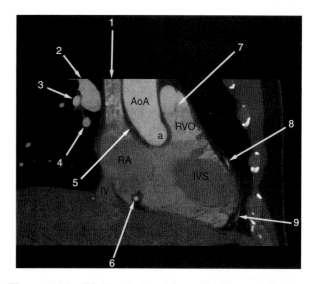

Figure 5.27 Right anterior oblique (RAO) reconstruction obtained to the left of Figure 5.26, through the anterior aortic sinus of Valsalva (a) and the muscular interventricular septum (IVS). The superior vena cava (arrow 1) passes to the right of the ascending aorta (AoA) to drain into the right atrium (RA). Anterior, and to the left of the AoA, the right ventricular outflow tract (RVO) is seen immediately inferior to leaflet tissue of the pulmonary valve (arrow 7). The sinoatrial node artery (arrow 5) and distal right coronary artery (arrow 6) are both viewed in cross section. Portions of the distal anterior descending artery (arrows 8 and 9) are viewed in longitudinal section as they pass along the superior aspect of the IVS.

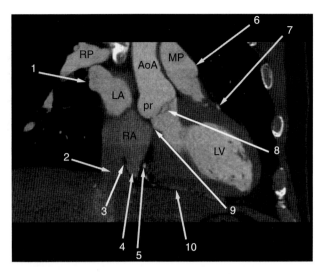

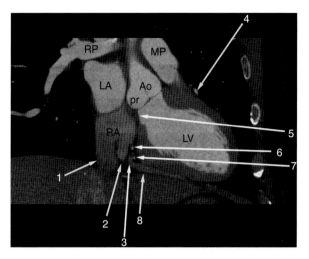

Figure 5.28   Right anterior oblique (RAO) reconstruction obtained to the left of Figure 5.27, immediately posterior to the interventricular septum, within the atrioventricular septum (arrow 9) and the left ventricle (LV). The right upper lobe pulmonary vein (arrow 1) drains into the left atrium (LA) after it passes beneath the right pulmonary artery (RP). Notice the relationship between the posterior right aortic sinus of Valsalva (pr) and the right (RA) and left (LA) atrium. The coronary sinus (arrow 4) entry into the RA is separated from the inferior vena cava (arrow 2) by the eustacian valve (arrow 3). Medial, and anterior to the coronary sinus, the distal right coronary artery (arrow 5) is becoming the posterior left ventricular branch, passing toward the posterior atrioventricular ring. The posterior interventricular vein (arrow 10) is viewed longitudinally along the inferior aspect of the interventricular septum. A segment of the left anterior descending artery (arrow 7) is viewed after passage behind the right ventricular outflow. The main pulmonary artery (MP) lies to the left of the ascending aorta (AoA). The pulmonary artery sinus of Valsalva (arrow 6) lies superior and to the left of the aortic valve.

Figure 5.29   Right anterior oblique (RAO) reconstruction obtained to the left of Figure 5.28, through the atrioventricular septum (arrow 5) and posterior right aortic sinus of Valsalva (pr). The left atrium (LA) lies superior and medial to the right atrium (RA), inferior to the transverse right pulmonary artery (RP), and posterior to the aortic root (Ao). Notice the right-to-left and inferior-to-superior relationship of the Ao and the main pulmonary artery (MP). A portion of the mid anterior descending coronary artery (arrow 4) is seen as it passes from behind the right ventricular outflow along the superior aspect of the anterior interventricular groove. The posterior interventricular vein (arrow 8) and great cardiac vein (arrow 3) become confluent with the coronary sinus (arrow 2) prior to drainage into the RA, medial, and slightly superior to drainage of the suprahepatic inferior vena cava (arrow 1).

ovale (Figures 5.11–5.14, 5.16, 5.54). The mid-portion of the interatrial septum is called the secundum septum, and it comprises the bulk of the interatrial septum. The right atrium usually appears nearly the same size as the left atrium. Measurement of right atrial size is less difficult than estimation of RA volume. Nevertheless, RA enlargement is associated with clockwise cardiac rotation.

The right atrial appendage is a broad-based, triangular structure, contained within the pericardium, which extends from about the middle of the heart obliquely around the ascending aorta (Figures 5.4–5.9, 5.22–5.25, 5.50–5.55, 5.58–5.61, 5.63). Pectinate muscles are characteristically seen in the RA anterior to the crista terminalis, appearing as intracavitary filling defects, analogous to myocardial bundles in the right ventricle (Figures 5.13–5.15, 5.17, 5.23).

The tricuspid valve is contained within the anterior atrioventricular ring. Its septal and anterior leaflets appear as long filling defects attached to the AV ring. Very fine chordae and papillary muscles of varying size are connected to the RV free wall and septum (Figures 5.24, 5.25).

5 RIGHT VENTRICLE

The right ventricle resides immediately posterior to the sternum, more or less in the midline (Figures 5.13–5.20, 5.20–5.24, 5.44–5.47, 5.59). Unless hypertrophied, the right ventricular free wall myocardium is only about 2 to 3 mm in thickness, and at end diastole may be difficult to visualize. The shape of the RV can be surmised by visualizing the ventricle as the sum of the axial sections obtained during CT examination. From the level of the pulmonary valve, moving caudad, the shape of the ventricle changes. The right ventricular outflow tract is round in shape (Figures 5.5–5.12, 5.25–5.27, 5.49, 5.60, 5.61, 5.63), surrounded

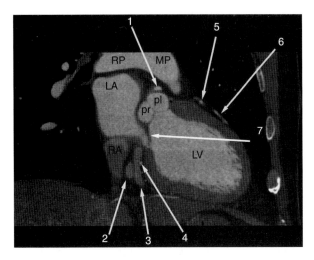

Figure 5.30   Right anterior oblique (RAO) reconstruction obtained to the left of Figure 5.29, through the posterior right (pr) and left (pl) aortic sinuses of Valsalva. The left main coronary artery (arrow 1) has just exited the pl. After passing behind the right ventricular outflow and main pulmonary artery (MP) the anterior descending artery (arrows 5 and 6) is seen in longitudinal section within the anterior interventricular groove along the superior aspect of the interventricular septum. The left atrium (LA) lies high and posterior, beneath the transverse right pulmonary artery (RP) and superior to the right atrium (RA). The anterior-most portion of the anterior mitral leaflet (arrow 7) is seen in continuity with the inferior aspect of the pr. At this level, the great cardiac vein (arrow 3) is viewed longitudinally within the posterior atrioventricular ring, slightly anterior, and not yet confluent with the coronary sinus (arrow 2). The posterior left ventricular branch of the distal right coronary artery (arrow 4) is viewed in cross section anterior to the great cardiac vein in the posterior atrioventricular ring.

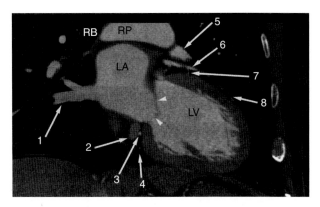

Figure 5.31   Right anterior oblique (RAO) reconstruction obtained to the left of Figure 5.30, posterior to the aortic root. The left atrium is posterior and superior to the left ventricle (LV), and inferior to the transverse right pulmonary artery (RP). The mitral valve (arrowheads) separates the LA from LV. The RP lies anterior to the right bronchus (RB). The right lower lobe pulmonary vein (arrow 1) is seen entering the LA. The anterior descending coronary artery (arrow 6) passes beneath the anterior-most extension of the left atrial appendage (arrow 5), and is seen giving a septal perforating branch (arrow 7) into the superior aspect of the interventricular septum. Farther down the anterolateral wall of the LV, a diagonal branch of the anterior descending artery (arrow 8) is seen. The great cardiac vein (arrow 2) and posterior left ventricular branch of the distal right coronary artery (arrow 3) lie side-by-side in the fat of the posterior atrioventricular ring. A distal branch of the posterior left ventricular branch of the right coronary artery (arrow 4) is viewed in cross section as it heads toward the posterior wall of the LV.

by the ventricular infundibulum, and lies to the patient's left. Moving in a caudad direction, the chamber increases in size, assuming a triangular shape (Figures 5.14–5.20, 5.24–5.26, 5.43–5.48, 5.58–5.61, 5.63); the base formed by the AV ring, and the apex at the intersection of the free wall and interventricular septum.[1]

The tricuspid valve is separated from the pulmonary valve by the infundibulum. The right ventricular surface of the interventricular septum is irregular. Although the septomarginal trabeculation may not always be identified, papillary muscles extending from it to the tricuspid valve leaflets are commonplace (Figures 5.15, 5.17, 5.46, 5.47). Numerous muscle bundles extend from the interventricular septum across the RV chamber to the free wall. The inferior-most of these is the moderator band, which carries the conducting system right bundle fibers.

The interventricular septum appears as intermediate attenuation muscle. The bulk of the septum appears relatively thick (never greater than 1.5 times the thickness of the free wall), and normally bows toward the right ventricle (Figures 5.15–5.20, 5.27, 5.40–5.48). The posterior superior aspect of the septum is embryologically derived from the endocardial cushions; this is the membranous and atrioventricular septum. It appears as a thin (not uncommonly fatty infiltrated, low attenuation) structure, which has a characteristic anatomic relationship with the aortic valve, primum interatrial septum, and anterior mitral and septal tricuspid leaflets (Figures 5.15, 5.16, 5.28, 5.29, 5.49).[2]

6 PULMONARY ARTERIES

The pulmonary valve lies slightly out of the axial plane, so may appear elongated in conventional axial acquisition (Figures 5.3, 5.9, 5.26–5.28, 5.49, 5.58–5.61). The caliber of the main pulmonary artery should be about the caliber of the ascending aorta at this anatomic level. The left pulmonary artery is the extension of the main PA over the top

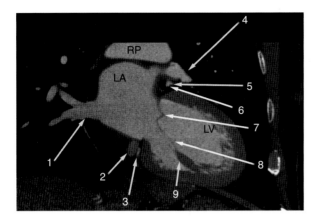

Figure 5.32 Right anterior oblique (RAO) reconstruction obtained to the left of Figure 5.31, through the anterior mitral leaflet (arrow 7). A left ventricular (LV) papillary muscle (arrow 9) and chordae tendineae (arrow 8) are seen connecting to the leaflet. The left atrial appendage (arrow 4) is seen draining into the left atrium (LA). Beneath the proximal portion of the left atrial appendage, the anterior descending (arrow 5) and circumflex (arrow 6) coronary arteries separate from the left main artery. The great cardiac vein (arrow 2) and posterior left ventricular branch of the distal right coronary artery (arrow 3) are seen within the posterior atrioventricular ring. The segmental veins of the right lower lobe (arrow 1) drain to the LA. The transverse portion of the right pulmonary artery (RP) passes along the superior aspect of the LA.

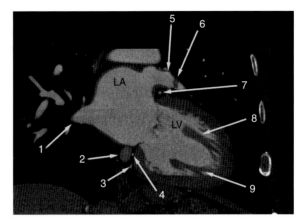

Figure 5.33 Right anterior oblique (RAO) reconstruction obtained to the left of Figure 5.32, through the posterior aspect of the left ventricle (LV). The superior (arrow 8) and inferior (arrow 9) papillary muscles lie nearly parallel to each other in this section. The entrance of the right lower lobe pulmonary vein (arrow 1) into the left atrium (LA) and left atrial appendage (arrow 5) are viewed in longitudinal section. Notice the filling defect of a pectinate muscle bundle (arrow 6) within the left atrial appendage. The circumflex coronary artery (arrow 7) passes beneath the left atrial appendage, to enter the posterior atrioventricular ring. Beneath the LA within the inferior aspect of the posterior atrioventricular ring, the great cardiac vein (arrow 2), and distal left ventricular branches (arrows 3 and 4) are viewed in cross section. The transverse portion of the right pulmonary artery (RP) passes along the superior aspect of the LA.

of the left atrium. When the PA crosses the left bronchus, it becomes the left PA (Figures 5.2, 5.3, 5.56, 5.58, 5.61). The right PA originates from the underside of the main PA, passes along the roof of the left atrium, posterior to the ascending aorta and superior vena cava, to enter the right hilum (Figures 5.2–5.4, 5.28–5.33, 5.54–5.58, 5.61). The pericardium is reflected over the top of the main PA.[3]

7 PULMONARY VEINS

The upper lobe pulmonary veins lie anterior to their respective pulmonary arteries (Figures 5.2–5.9, 5.27, 5.28, 5.35–5.37, 5.55–5.57, 5.58–5.63). As the left upper lobe vein courses inferiorly, it passes in front of the left PA, and enters the left atrium immediately posterior to the orifice of the left atrial appendage. The right upper lobe vein lies anterior to the right pulmonary artery. It passes from anterior to posterior and inferiorly to enter the left atrium immediately posterior to the entrance of the superior vena cava into the right atrium. The left lower lobe pulmonary vein always courses in a caudad direction directly anterior to the descending thoracic aorta before entering the posterior left

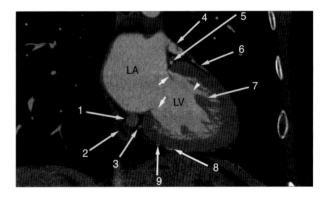

Figure 5.34 Right anterior oblique (RAO) reconstruction obtained to the left of Figure 5.33, through posterior aspects of the mitral leaflets (short arrows). The superior papillary muscle (arrow 7) and a chordae tendineae (arrowhead) are seen. The circumflex artery (arrow 5) is viewed in cross section within the fat of the posterior atrioventricular ring, inferior to the posterior aspect of the left atrial appendage (arrow 4). A diagonal branch of the anterior descending artery (arrow 6) is viewed in longitudinal section, as it passes over the anterolateral wall of the LV. The great cardiac vein (arrow 1) is viewed in cross section beneath the LA. A segment of a low marginal cardiac vein (arrow 3) is viewed prior to its confluence with the great cardiac vein. Segments of a distal posterior left ventricular branch of the distal right coronary artery (arrows 8 and 9) are viewed along the inferolateral LV wall. A segment of the air-filled esophagus (arrow 2) is seen.

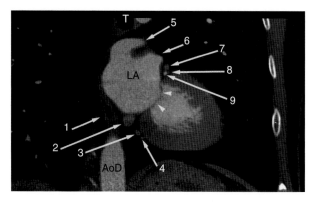

Figure 5.35 Right anterior oblique (RAO) reconstruction obtained to the left of Figure 5.34, through the distal trachea (T), esophagus (arrow 1) and descending aorta (AoD). The left upper lobe pulmonary vein (arrow 5) drains into the left atrium (LA) posterior and superior to the orifice of the left atrial appendage (arrow 6). A high marginal cardiac vein (arrow 8) has not yet drained into the proximal aspect of the great cardiac vein (arrow 7). The circumflex coronary artery (arrow 9) is viewed in cross section in the superior aspect of the posterior atrioventricular ring. A more proximal portion of a low marginal cardiac vein (arrow 3) and a posterior left ventricular branch of the distal right coronary artery (arrow 4) are viewed in the inferior aspect of the posterior atrioventricular ring, along with the great cardiac vein (arrow 2).

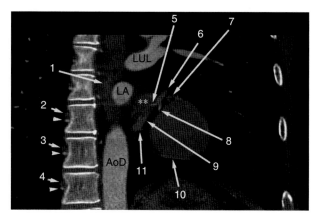

Figure 5.37 Right anterior oblique (RAO) reconstruction obtained to the left of Figure 5.36, through the thoracic spine, mid esophagus (arrow 1) and descending aorta (AoD). The posterior-most aspect of the left atrium (LA), myocardium of the posterior LA wall (**), and distal left upper lobe pulmonary vein (LUL) prior to its drainage into the LA are visualized. The proximal portion of a high marginal cardiac vein (arrow 7) is just about to drain into the great cardiac vein (arrow 6) cephalad to a segment of the circumflex artery (arrow 8). A low marginal cardiac vein along the posterior left ventricular wall (arrow 10) drains (arrow 11) into the distal great cardiac vein (arrow 9). Intercostal arteries (arrowheads) and veins (short arrows) lie adjacent to the thoracic vertebral bodies.

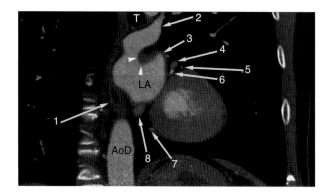

Figure 5.36 Right anterior oblique (RAO) reconstruction obtained to the left of Figure 5.35, through the trachea (T), esophagus (arrow 1), descending aorta (AoD) and posterior aspect of the posterior atrioventricular ring. The proximal (arrow 4) and distal (arrow 8) parts of the great cardiac vein and trunk circumflex artery (arrow 6) are viewed. The left upper lobe pulmonary vein (arrow 2) drains from upper left medially to enter the left atrium (LA) behind the orifice of the left atrial appendage (arrow 3). Note the apparent thickened endothelium between the upper lobe vein drainage and atrial appendage ostium (arrowheads). A proximal segment of a low marginal cardiac vein (arrow 7) passing along the posterior LV wall has not yet entered the great cardiac vein.

aspect of the left atrium (Figures 5.10–5.15, 5.31–5.33, 5.54–5.57, 5.60–5.62). The right lower lobe vein drains to the right posterior inferior aspect of the left atrium.[3]

8 LEFT ATRIUM

The left atrium lies posterior, superior, and toward the left with respect to the right atrium (Figures 5.14–5.17, 5.28–5.37, 5.51–5.57, 5.62). The two atria share the interatrial septum, which forms an oblique surface between the two. The interatrial septum normally thins in the region of the foramen ovale. The left atrium is just about the same size as the right atrium. The inner surface of the LA is bald smooth. The confluence of the left upper lobe pulmonary vein and orifice of the left atrial appendage is a redundant endothelium, which may appear to be thickened in its medial-most aspect (Figure 5.36). The left atrial appendage is long and finger-like (Figures 5.4–5.9, 5.31–5.36, 5.49–5.53). Analogous to the right atrial appendage, it contains pectinate muscles. However, these myocardial trabeculations are always smaller in caliber than those of the RAA, and almost never cross from one face of the appendage to the other. The LAA runs from caudad to cephalad, around the left aspect of the heart, below the level of the pulmonary valve.

The mitral valve lies within the posterior atrioventricular ring, immediately subjacent to the circumflex coronary artery (Figures 5.13–5.16, 5.30–5.35, 5.49, 5.50). Fibrous continuity between the anterior mitral leaflet and the aortic annulus is characteristically found in morphologic left ventricles (Figures 5.13–5.16, 5.30). Ordinarily, the chordae tendineae of the anterior and posterior mitral leaflets are not visualized on CT examination. However, introduction of ECG-gated 16 and 64-detector systems has improved the spatial and temporal resolution to a point where these structures are now commonly identified[1,2] (Figures 5.32, 5.34).

9 LEFT VENTRICLE

The left ventricle is generally in the shape of a prolate-ellipse. It is symmetrical, with a long axis and two orthogonal shorter axes. The left ventricular papillary muscles are always seen as filling defects in the LV cavity (Figures 5.14, 5.19, 5.32–5.34, 5.44–5.46). Analogous to visualization of the chordeae, attachment of the papillary muscles to the chordeae is frequently visualized on the newer scanners.

The posterior AV ring also contains the great cardiac vein. This vein lies anterior to the circumflex artery, and passes around the ring between the LA and LV, to run beneath the LA prior to its drainage into the RA. Before entering the RA, is receives other venous tributaries, which run along the epicardial surface of the heart.

The left ventricle lies posterior and to the left with respect to the right ventricle (Figure 5.15). The left ventricular myocardium is nearly uniform in thickness (1 cm at end diastole). However, in axial acquisition, the poster LV wall may appear thicker than the septal or apical myocardium, because it has been cut obliquely with respect to its internal axis (Figures 5.18–5.20). Although some trabecular myocardial filling defects may be identified within the ventricular cavity, the LV is characterized by its smooth walls and two large papillary muscles. These always originate from the posterior wall of the ventricle. The plane of the interventricular septum is directed anterior to the coronal plane, and inferiorly toward the left hip. It normally bows toward the RV (Figures 5.16–5.19, 5.27, 5.41–5.48). The aortic valve shares the fibrous trigone of the heart and is, as previously described, in continuity with the anterior mitral leaflet.[3]

10 AORTIC ROOT

The aortic valve has three sinuses of Valsalva, the right (anterior), the left (posterior), and the non-coronary (right posterior) (Figures 5.8–5.14, 5.27–5.30, 5.49–5.53). The right coronary artery (RCA) originates from the right sinus. The left main coronary artery (LMCA) arises from the left sinus. The non-coronary sinus is the most inferior sinus, and provides no coronary artery; it abuts the right and left atria.

11 CORONARY ARTERIES

The right coronary artery (Figures 5.7–5.36, 5.44–5.54, 5.58–5.61, 5.63) originates from the right aortic sinus of Valsalva. It takes a short right turn to enter the fat within the anterior atrioventricular ring, and passes around to the intersection of the A-V ring and the interventricular septum, the so-called crux of the heart. The RCA originates more caudally from the aorta than the LMCA.

The distal RCA usually gives the posterior descending artery (PDA) to perfuse the inferior interventricular septum. In 85% of individuals, the PDA arises from the distal right coronary artery; this is called a right dominant circulation. The PDA may also derive from the left circumflex artery (LCX), forming a left dominant circulation or there may be 'co-dominance' with derivation of the PDA from the RCA and LCX.

The sinoatrial node artery arises from the proximal RCA, and passes behind the superior vena cava to the top of the interatrial septum. Marginal branches from the RCA arise at a right angle from the plane of the AV ring, and then course within the epicardial fat across the right ventricular free wall. The highest marginal branch from the RCA is the conus artery. In right dominant circulations, the distal RCA continues in the posterior A-V ring as the posterior left ventricular branches.[4]

The LMCA arises from the left aortic sinus of Valsalva (Figures 5.6–5.8, 5.30. 5.32, 5.52, 5.53). The artery continues posteriorly, and passes beneath the left atrial appendage, to enter the posterior AV ring. It continues within the ring as the circumflex artery (Figures 5.9–5.17, 5.32–5.38, 5.50–52, 5.60–5.62). Marginal branches arise from the posterior AV ring, and pass along the posterior LV wall. In 15% of individuals, the circumflex artery continues around the posterior AV ring, and the PDA arises from the distal LCX, or is its continuation. This is called left dominant circulation.

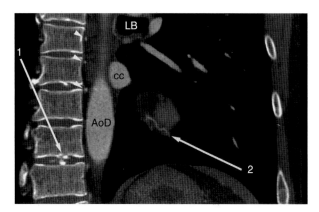

Figure 5.38   Right anterior oblique (RAO) reconstruction obtained to the left of Figure 5.39, through the thoracic spine, left bronchus (LB), confluence (cc) of the left lower lobe pulmonary veins prior to entering the left atrium, and descending aorta (AoD). Intercostal arteries (arrowheads) are viewed in cross section. A marginal branch of the circumflex coronary artery (arrow 2) is viewed in longitudinal section along the posterior aspect of the left ventricular myocardium. Note the calcified thoracic vertebral disc (arrow 1).

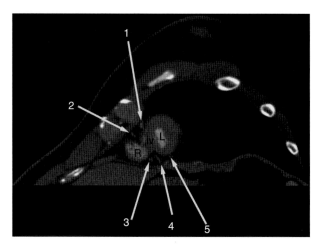

Figure 5.40   Short axis reconstruction obtained to the right of Figure 5.39, through the right ventricular apex (R). The anterior descending artery is seen just before (arrow 1) and after (arrow 4) it passes about the cardiac apex between the right (R) and left (L) ventricles. A branch from the distal anterior descending artery (arrow 5) passes toward the lateral wall. Reaching toward the cardiac apex, the distal posterior cardiac vein, beneath the interventricular septum (iv).

Before the left main artery passes beneath the LAA, the anterior descending artery arises along the top of the interventricular septum (Figures 5.7–5.20, 5.26–5.32, 5.39–5.51, 5.58–5.63). Within the epicardial fat, it passes along the top of the septum in the anterior interventricular groove to the cardiac apex. As the RCA defines the right margin of the RV, the LAD defines the left border, and thus the position of the RV, an indicator of RV size. Diagonal branches of the LAD pass along the anterolateral aspect of the ventricle.[4,5]

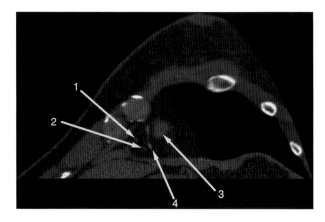

Figure 5.39   Short axis reconstruction obtained through the myocardium of the left ventricular apex (arrow 3). The distal anterior descending coronary artery (arrow 4) passes in the fat of the interventricular sulcus toward the underside of the apical interventricular septum. Running with the artery are segments of the anterior cardiac vein (arrows 1 and 2).

12 PERICARDIUM

The heart is contained within the middle mediastinum by the pericardium. The visceral pericardium is adherent to the ventricular myocardium, and cannot be visually separated from the epicardial fat. The parietal pericardium may be identified as a paper-thin high signal intensity surface surrounding the heart and great arteries (Figures 5.2, 5.3, 5.15, 5.16, 5.18, 5.20, 5.41–5.54). On the left side of the heart, it attaches over the top of the main pulmonary artery. The ascending aorta is enveloped up to about the level of the azygos vein. Recesses (potential spaces) in the pericardium are typically found anterior to the ascending aorta and medial to the main pulmonary artery (the anterior aortic recess), between the ascending aorta and transverse right pulmonary artery (the superior pericardial recess), and around the entry of the pulmonary veins to the left atrium. Visualization of the parietal pericardium depends upon the presence and extent of low-density fatty deposition in the pericardial fat pad and middle mediastinum.[1,2]

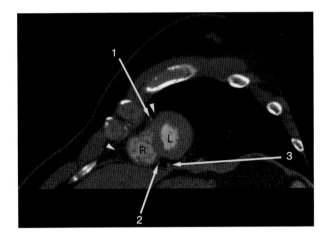

Figure 5.41 Short axis reconstruction obtained to the right of Figure 5.40. The anterior descending coronary artery is viewed in cross section along the distal anterior interventricular groove (arrow 1), and the inferior aspect of the distal interventricular septum (arrow 2). A branch from the distal anterior descending artery (arrow 3) passes toward the lateral wall. Portions of pericardium (small arrowheads) are identified about the periphery of the heart.

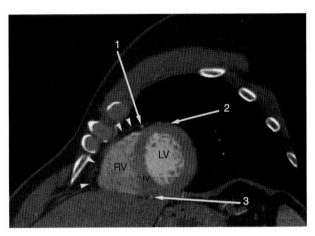

Figure 5.43 Short axis reconstruction obtained to the right of Figure 5.42. The anterior descending coronary artery (arrow 1) passes beneath the pericardium (arrowheads) along the anterior interventricular groove. The distal posterior cardiac vein (arrow 3) is viewed in cross section passing along the inferior aspect of the interventricular septum (iv) between the right (RV) and left (LV) ventricles. A high diagonal branch of the anterior descending artery (arrow 2) is viewed in cross section along the anterior wall.

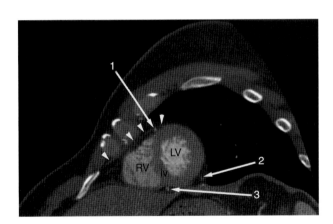

Figure 5.42 Short axis reconstruction obtained to the right of Figure 5.41. The anterior descending coronary artery (arrow 1) passes beneath the pericardium (arrowheads) along the anterior interventricular groove. The distal posterior cardiac vein (arrow 3) is viewed in cross section passing along the inferior aspect of the interventricular septum (iv) between the right (RV) and left (LV) ventricles. A branch from a distal posterior left ventricular branch of the distal right coronary artery (arrow 2) passes along the LV lateral wall.

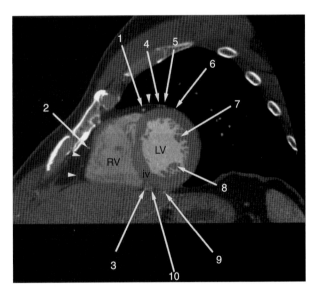

Figure 5.44 Short axis reconstruction obtained to the right of Figure 5.43. The anterior descending artery (arrow 1) and a diagonal branch (arrow 5) of the anterior descending artery are viewed in cross section. Between the two arteries, the anterior interventricular vein (arrow 4) is seen in cross section. A more distal diagonal branch (arrow 6) is within the anterior epicardium. Along the inferior aspect of the interventricular septum (iv), the posterior descending coronary artery (arrow 3) and the inferior interventricular vein (arrow 10) are viewed in cross section. A distal posterior left ventricular branch of the distal right coronary artery (arrow 9) is found along the inferior left ventricular (LV) wall. At this anatomic level, the papillary muscles of the LV (arrows 7 and 8) are seen as large intracavitary filling defects. A marginal branch of the right coronary artery (arrow 2) is seen in cross section, embedded in the epicardial fat of the right ventricular (RV) free wall. Portions of pericardium (small arrowheads) are identified about the periphery of the heart.

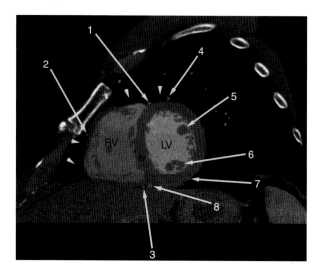

Figure 5.45   Short axis reconstruction obtained to the right of Figure 5.44. The anterior descending artery (arrow 1) is viewed in cross section along the superior aspect of the interventricular septum (iv). The posterior descending artery (arrow 3) and inferior interventricular vein (arrow 8) are viewed in cross section along the inferior aspect of the iv. A diagonal branch of the anterior descending artery (arrow 4) and a posterolateral branch of the distal right coronary artery (arrow 7) are viewed along the anterior and posterolateral walls, respectively. The papillary muscles of the LV (arrows 5 and 6) are seen as large intracavitary filling defects within the left ventricle (LV). A marginal branch of the right coronary artery (arrow 2) is viewed in the right ventricular (RV) free wall epicardium. Portions of pericardium (small arrowheads) are identified about the periphery of the heart.

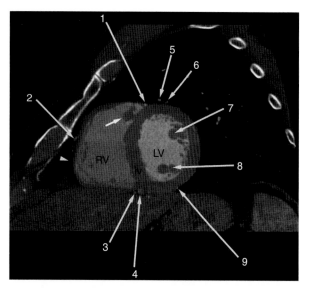

Figure 5.46   Short axis reconstruction obtained to the right of Figure 5.45. The anterior descending artery (arrow 1) and a diagonal branch of the anterior descending coronary artery (arrow 5) are viewed in cross section within the fat of the anterior left ventricular (LV) wall. In addition, a tributary of the anterior interventricular vein (arrow 6) is found within the fat, as well. The posterior descending artery (arrow 3) and the inferior interventricular vein (arrow 4) are viewed in cross section along the inferior aspect of the interventricular septum (iv). A posterolateral branch of the distal right coronary artery (arrow 9) is seen along the posterolateral LV wall. The papillary muscles of the LV (arrows 7 and 8) appear as filling defects toward the posterior aspect of the LV cavity. In this section, the parietal band of the crista supraventricularis (small arrow) appears as a filling defect in the superior portion of the right ventricle (RV). Portions of pericardium (small arrowheads) are identified about the periphery of the heart.

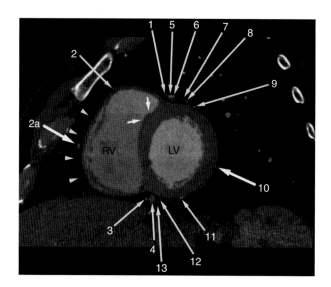

Figure 5.47   Short axis reconstruction obtained to the right of Figure 5.46. This section is proximal to the papillary muscles of the left ventricle (LV). The anterior descending coronary artery (arrow 5), a septal perforating branch (arrow 1) and a diagonal branch (arrow 6) are all viewed in cross section within the epicardial fat of the anterior wall of the LV. In addition, tributaries of the anterior interventricular vein (arrows 7 and 8) are found within the fat, as well. A proximal marginal branch of the circumflex coronary artery (arrow 9) is viewed in cross section. The posterior descending coronary artery (arrow 3), the inferior interventricular vein (arrow 4), and portions of the posterior left ventricular branch of the distal right coronary artery (arrows 11, 12, 13, and 14) are viewed in cross section beneath the interventricular septum (iv) and inferior LV wall. A distal marginal branch of the circumflex artery is viewed in cross section along the posterolateral LV wall (arrow 10). The conus artery (arrow 2) is viewed in cross section along the right ventricular (RV) outflow myocardium. A marginal branch of the mid right coronary artery is viewed in cross section (arrow 2a) within the epicardial fat of the RV free wall. Portions of pericardium (small arrowheads) are identified about the periphery of the heart.

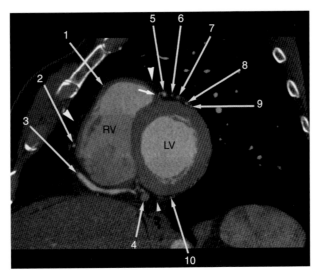

Figure 5.48 Short axis reconstruction obtained to the right of Figure 5.47, through the distal right coronary artery (arrow 3), passing within the inferior aspect of the anterior atrioventricular ring. The anterior descending coronary artery (arrow 5) and a diagonal branch of the anterior descending artery (arrow 6) are viewed in cross section within the epicardial fat of the anterior wall of left ventricle (LV). A small septal perforating branch (small arrow) is seen arising from the anterior descending artery. The anterior interventricular vein (arrow 7) is viewed in cross section as it passes toward the posterior atrioventricular ring. Both rami of a bifurcating marginal branch of the circumflex coronary artery (arrows 8 and 9) are viewed in cross section along the anterior LV wall. The inferior interventricular vein (arrow 4) is seen in cross section along the inferior aspect of the interventricular septum. A posterolateral branch of the distal right coronary artery (arrow 10) is seen along the inferior LV wall. The conus artery (arrow 1) and a marginal branch of the right coronary artery (arrow 2) are viewed in cross section along the free wall of the right ventricle (RV). Portions of pericardium (small arrowheads) are identified about the periphery of the heart.

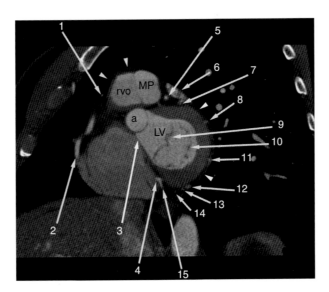

Figure 5.49 Short axis reconstruction obtained to the right of Figure 5.48, through the anterior aortic sinus of Valsalva (a). The mid right coronary artery (arrow 2) weaves through the fat of the anterior atrioventricular ring. A portion of the conus artery (arrow 1) is seen in cross section within the epicardial fat of the right ventricular outflow (rvo). The anterior descending artery (arrow 5) passes behind the main pulmonary artery (MP) and beneath the left atrial appendage (arrow 6) within the epicardial fat of the anterior left ventricular (LV) wall. The anterior interventricular vein (arrow 7) passes posteriorly, separating from the anterior descending artery as it enters the posterior atrioventricular ring. A tributary of the middle cardiac vein (arrow 8) and a segment of a marginal branch of the circumflex artery (arrow 11) are viewed in the epicardium of the posterior LV wall. Large (arrow 12) and small (arrow 14) tributaries of the posterior cardiac vein are viewed in cross section. The distal right coronary artery (arrow 4) and the origin of a posterior LV branch are viewed within the fat of the inferior aspect of the posterior atrioventricular ring. The anterior (arrow 9) and posterior (arrow 10) mitral valve leaflets are seen as redundant sheet-like filling defects within the LV cavity. The atrioventricular septum (arrow 3) lies along the posterolateral aspect of the anterior aortic sinus (a). Portions of pericardium (small arrowheads) are identified about the periphery of the heart.

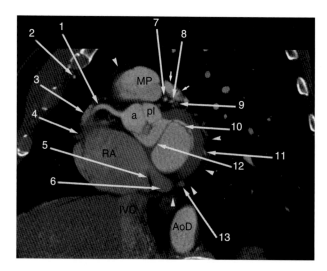

Figure 5.50   Short axis reconstruction obtained to the right of Figure 5.49, through the anterior (a) and posterior left (pl) aortic sinuses of Valsalva (a) and proximal right coronary artery (arrow 1). Immediately after it enters the fat of the anterior atrioventricular ring, the right coronary artery descends within the ring behind the right atrial appendage (arrow 3). The anterior cardiac vein (arrow 4) drains the right ventricle, and is seen passing toward the junction of the right atrial body (RA) and appendage (arrow 3). The anterior interventricular vein (arrow 9) has not yet drained into the great cardiac vein (not visualized). A low posterior cardiac vein (arrow 13) is about to drain into the great cardiac vein (arrow 6) and RA. The eustachian valve (arrow 5) segregates coronary sinus from inferior vena cava (IVC) blood flow. The very proximal most left anterior descending artery (arrow 7) is viewed in cross section. Notice the nonobstructive eccentric low attenuation fatty plaque. A high marginal branch is seen passing beneath the left atrial appendage (small arrows). Immediately adjacent, the anterior interventricular vein is passing toward the posterior atrioventricular ring. The anterior (arrow 12) and posterior (arrow 10) mitral leaflets are thin and well-defined. A segment of a marginal branch of the circumflex artery (arrow 11) is viewed in the epicardial fat of the posterior LV wall. Portions of pericardium (small arrowheads) are identified about the periphery of the heart.

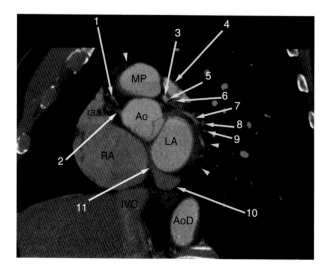

Figure 5.51   Short axis reconstruction obtained to the right of Figure 5.50, on the left atrial (LA) side of the posterior atrioventricular ring. The sinoatrial node artery (arrow 1) ascends in the epicardial fat beneath the right atrial appendage (raa) after originating from the proximal right coronary artery (arrow 2). The great cardiac vein (arrow 10) is confluent with the coronary sinus (arrow 11) prior to drainage into the right atrium (RA). The left anterior descending coronary artery (arrow 3), a marginal branch of the circumflex artery (arrow 5) and the circumflex artery itself (arrow 7) are in the fat posterior to the aortic root (Ao), beneath the left atrial appendage (arrow 4). The anterior interventricular vein (arrow 6) and a middle cardiac vein (arrow 8) have not yet drained into the great cardiac vein. A more distal marginal branch of the circumflex artery (arrow 9) is viewed in cross section after origin from the trunk circumflex artery (arrow 7). Portions of pericardium (small arrowheads) are identified about the periphery of the heart. The intrahepatic inferior vena cava (IVC) and descending aorta (AoD) are labeled.

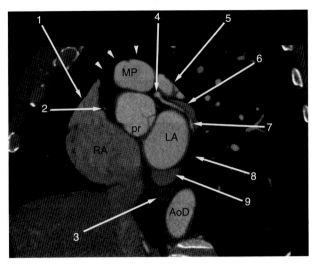

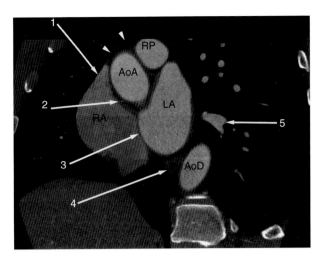

Figure 5.52 Short axis reconstruction obtained to the right of Figure 5.51, through the right atrial appendage (arrow 1), posterior right aortic sinus of Valsalva (pr), and the origin and proximal course of the circumflex coronary artery (arrow 7) from the left main coronary artery (arrow 4). The sinoatrial node artery is viewed in cross section (arrow 2) beneath the right atrial appendage. After originating from the left main artery, the circumflex artery (arrow 7) passes beneath the left atrial appendage (arrow 5) and runs with the great cardiac vein (arrow 6) in the fat of the posterior atrioventricular ring. A branch of a marginal cardiac vein (arrow 8) has not yet drained into the distal great cardiac vein (arrow 9), running along the floor of the left atrium (LA). The esophagus (arrow 3) and descending aorta (AoD) are labeled. Portions of pericardium (small arrowheads) are identified about the periphery of the heart.

Figure 5.54 Short axis reconstruction obtained to the right of Figure 5.53, through the cavities of the right (RA) and left (LA) atrium, ascending aorta (AoA) and proximal right pulmonary artery (RP). The sinoatrial node coronary artery (arrow 2) is viewed in cross section beneath the right atrial appendage (arrow 3). The interatrial septum (arrow 3) bows toward the RA as expected. A portion of the left lower lobe pulmonary vein (arrow 5) has not yet drained to the LA. The esophagus (arrow 4) and descending aorta (AoD) are labeled. Portions of pericardium (small arrowheads) are identified about the periphery of the heart.

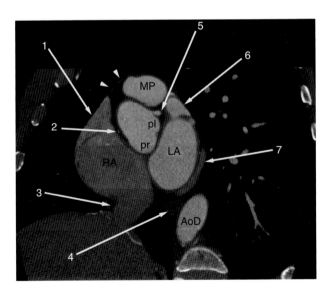

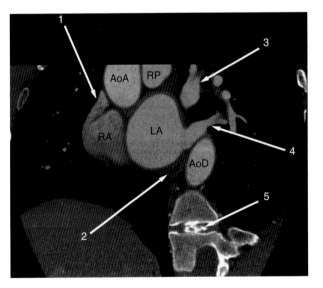

Figure 5.53 Short axis reconstruction obtained to the right of Figure 5.52, through the main pulmonary artery (MP), the posterior right aortic sinus of Valalva (pr), and the great cardiac vein (arrow 7) in the posterior atrioventricular ring. The sinoatrial branch of the right coronary artery (arrow 2) is seen beneath the right atrial appendage (arrow 1). The left atrial appendage (arrow 6) is not quite confluent with the left atrium (LA). The origin of the left main coronary artery from the posterior left aortic sinus of Valsalva (pl) is seen. Portions of pericardium (small arrowheads) are identified about the periphery of the heart. The suprahepatic inferior vena cava (arrow 3), esophagus (arrow 4) and descending aorta (AoD) are labeled.

Figure 5.55 Short axis reconstruction obtained to the right of Figure 5.54, through the cavities of the right (RA) and left (LA) atrium, ascending aorta (AoA) and proximal right pulmonary artery (RP). The right atrial appendage (arrow 1) lies anterior to the AoA. The left upper lobe pulmonary veins are about to drain into the LA; the left lower lobe veins (arrow 4) have entered the LA. The esophagus (arrow 2) and descending aorta (AoD) are labeled. Note the calcified lower thoracic intervertebral disc (arrow 5).

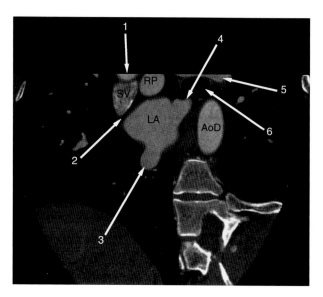

Figure 5.56 Short axis reconstruction obtained to the right of Figure 5.55, through the sinus venosus interatrial septum (arrow 2), the distal superior vena cava (SV), proximal right pulmonary artery, and lateral aspect of the left atrium (LA). The lateral aspect of the acending aorta (arrow 1) is on the periphery of the image. The left upper lobe (arrow 4) and right lower lobe (arrow 3) pulmonary venous drainage to the LA is labeled. In this plane, the left pulmonary artery (arrow 5) has just crossed over the top of the left bronchus (arrow 6). The descending aorta is labeled.

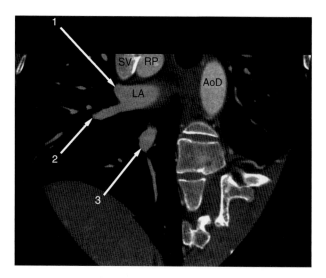

Figure 5.57 Short axis reconstruction obtained to the right of Figure 5.56, through the inferolateral aspect of the left atrium (LA), at the entry of a segmental right middle lobe pulmonary vein (arrow 2). The entry of the right upper lobe pulmonary vein (arrow 1) into the LA is noted. Note that the superior vena cava (SV) lies anterior and toward the right of the right pulmonary artery (RP). The descending aorta (AoD) is labeled.

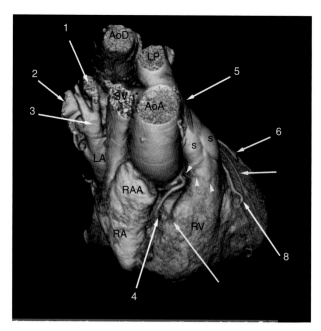

Figure 5.58 Surface rendered 3-dimensional reconstruction of the heart viewed from above and the right (i.e., caudally angulated right anterior oblique view). The proximal right coronary artery (RCA) (arrow 4) travels embedded in the (invisible) fat of the anterior atrioventricular (AV) ring. Marginal branches of the RCA cross the ring and course along the RV free wall. The ring is bordered along its right aspect by the right atrial appendage (RAA), and body of the right atrium (RA). The medial aspect of the right ventricle (RV) forms the leftward aspect of the atrioventricular ring. The superior vena cava (SV) lies to the right of the ascending aorta (AoA), and passes posteriorly and toward the right to enter the RA immediately anterior to the left atrium (LA). The pulmonary artery sinuses of Valsalva (s) characterize the proximal most portion of the pulmonary arteries. The pulmonary valve (at the base of the sinuses) is separated from the tricuspid valve (within the atrioventricular ring) by the RV infundibulum. The conus artery (arrowheads) is the highest marginal branch of the RCA. It travels along the surface of the infundibular free wall myocardium. The main pulmonary artery (arrow 5) passes to the left of the AoA, and continues as the left pulmonary artery (LP). The right pulmonary artery (*) is obscured by the AoA, SV, and right upper lobe pulmonary vein (arrow 3). The right upper lobe pulmonary artery (arrow 1) and hilar right pulmonary artery (arrow 2) both lie posterior to the right upper lobe pulmonary veins. The left anterior descending coronary artery (LAD) (arrow 8) passes in the anterior interventricular groove, demarking the leftward border of the RV. Further along the lateral wall of the left ventricle, a diagonal branch of the LAD is seen. Between the two arteries is the anterior interventricular cardiac vein (arrow 7). The descending aorta (AoD) is labeled.

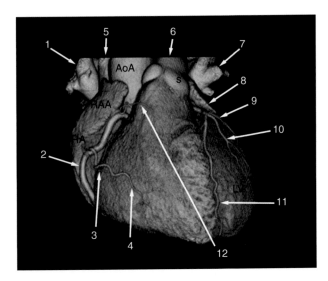

Figure 5.59 Surface rendered 3-dimensional reconstruction of the heart viewed from the front. The right ventricle (RV) is an anterior structure, bounded on the right by the right coronary artery (arrow 2) in the anterior atrioventricular ring and the left anterior descending coronary artery (arrow 11) in the anterior interventricular groove; the pulmonary artery (arrow 6) sinuses of Valsalva (s) define the superior-most aspect of the RV. The conus artery (arrow 12) runs along the high RV free wall; a marginal branch of the right coronary artery (arrow 4) runs along the mid RV free wall. The anterior cardiac vein (arrow 3) runs with the marginal branch, crossing the anterior atrioventricular ring to drain into the right atrium (RA). The anterior interventricular vein (arrow 9) and diagonal branch of the anterior descending artery (arrow 10) are seen passing from beneath the underside of the left atrial appendage (arrow 8) onto the anterolateral wall of the left ventricle (LV). The right (arrow 1) and left (arrow 7) upper lobe pulmonary veins, superior vena cava (arrow 5), and ascending aorta (AoA) are labeled.

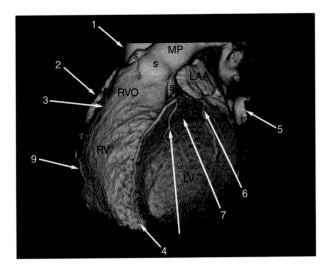

Figure 5.60 Surface rendered 3-dimensional reconstruction of the heart rotated toward the patient's right, viewed in left anterior oblique. The anterior descending coronary artery (arrow 9) divides the right ventricular cavity from the left (LV). A diagonal branch of the anterior descending artery (arrow 8) and a marginal branch of the circumflex artery (arrow 6) are seen passing over the anterolateral LV wall. The anterior interventricular vein (arrow 7) is viewed draining toward the posterior atrioventricular ring. The conus artery (arrow 3) is seen passing over the free wall of the right ventricular outflow (RVO); a marginal branch of the right coronary artery is viewed passing over the free wall of the right ventricular (RV) sinus. The pulmonary artery (MP) sinuses of Valsalva (s) define the top of the RVO. Portions of the ascending aorta (arrow 1), right (arrow 2) and left (LAA) atrial appendage and left lower lobe pulmonary veins (arrow 5) are labeled.

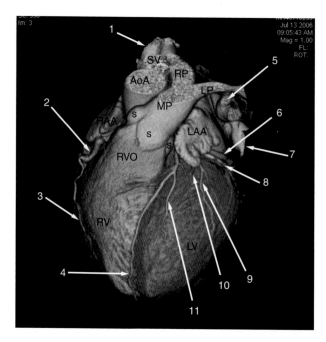

Figure 5.61 Surface rendered 3-dimensional reconstruction of the heart rotated toward the patient right, with the cardiac apex tipped inferiorly, displayed in cranialized left anterior oblique view. The anterior descending artery (arrow 4) gives a diagonal branch (arrow 11) after it emerges from beneath the left atrial appendage (LAA). The anterior interventricular vein (arrow 10) and a marginal branch of the circumflex artery (arrow 9) are viewed just distal to the LAA. The circumflex artery (arrow 8) and great cardiac vein (arrow 6) run together in the posterior atrioventricular ring. The proximal right coronary artery (arrow 2) is seen in the anterior atrioventricular ring. A marginal branch of the right coronary artery (arrow 3) passes around the free wall of the RV. The right upper lobe pulmonary veins (arrow 1), the left upper (arrow 5) and lower (arrow 7) pulmonary veins, the ascending aorta (AoA) and superior vena cava (SV) are labeled. The pulmonary artery sinuses of Valsalva (s), and bifurcation of the main pulmonary artery (MP) into left (LP) and right (RP) pulmonary arteries is displayed.

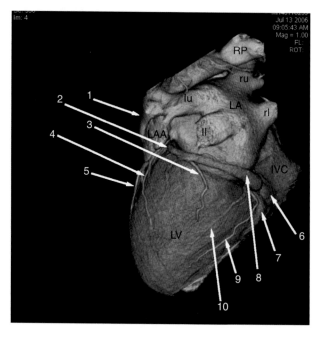

Figure 5.62 Surface rendered 3-dimensional reconstruction of the heart viewed from the posterior atrioventricular ring. The anterior descending coronary artery (arrow 5) runs down the anterior interventricular sulcus. A diagonal branch of the anterior descending artery (arrow 4) and a marginal branch of the circumflex artery (arrow 3) pass along the anterolateral and posterolateral left ventricular (LV) wall, respectively. The anterior interventricular vein (arrow 2) is joined by marginal cardiac vein (arrow 10) and the inferior interventricular vein (arrow 7) to form the great cardiac vein (arrow 8) which drains via the coronary sinus (arrow 6) into the right atrium, medial to the drainage of the inferior vena cava (IVC). The left upper (lu), right upper (ru), and left lower (ll) and right lower (rl) lobe pulmonary veins are seen draining to the posterior left atrium (LA). The left atrial appendage (LAA) and right pulmonary artery (RP) are labeled.

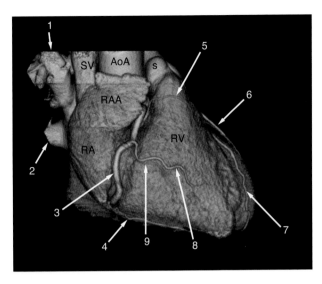

Figure 5.63 Surface rendered 3-dimensional reconstruction of the heart rotated toward the patient's left, displayed in right anterior oblique view. The right coronary artery passes from superior-to-inferior within the fat of the anterior atrioventricular ring. As the artery passes inferiorly, it provides the conus artery (arrow 5) which perfuses the right ventricular (RV) outflow, and a marginal branch (arrow 8) which perfuses the RV free wall. The posterior descending artery (arrow 4) arises from the distal right coronary artery, along the inferior aspect of the interventricular septum. The anterior cardiac vein (arrow 9) crosses the RV free wall and anterior atrioventricular ring to drain into the right atrium (RA). Toward the left, the anterior descending coronary artery (arrow 7) runs in the anterior interventricular groove; a diagonal branch of the anterior descending artery (arrow 6) is seen on the anterolateral wall. The right upper (arrow 1) and lower (arrow 2) lobe pulmonary veins, superior vena cava (SV), ascending aorta (AoA) and a pulmonary artery sinus of Valsalva (s) are labeled.

13 CONCLUSION

When carefully performed, contrast-enhanced ECG-gated computed tomography provides robust image data sets, from which a great deal of anatomic and physiologic information can be readily extracted. Recognition of the abnormal is based upon appreciation of its variance from normal. When carefully interpreted, CT examinations clarify difficult areas of cardiac morphology, characterize the severity of a particular lesion, and reflect the pathophysiologic sequelae of the underlying disease.

REFERENCES

1. Boxt LM. CT anatomy of the heart. Int J Cardiovasc Imaging 2005 Feb; 21(1): 13–27.
2. Guthaner DF, Wexler L, Harell G. CT demonstration of cardiac structures. AJR Am J Roentgenol. 1979 Jul; 133(1): 75–81.
3. Anderson RH, Razavi R, Taylor AM. Cardiac anatomy revisited. J Anat. 2004 Sep; 205(3): 159–77.
4. Rabin DN, Rabin S, Mintzer RA. A pictorial review of coronary artery anatomy on spiral CT. Chest 2000 Aug; 118(2): 488–91.
5. Lembcke A, Hein PA, Dohmen PM, et al. Pictorial review: electron beam computed tomography and multislice spiral computed tomography for cardiac imaging. Eur J Radiol. 2006 Mar; 57(3): 356–67.

6

Pathology of Coronary Artery Atherosclerosis: Aspects Relevant to Cardiac Imaging

Dylan V. Miller

Recent years have seen exponential improvements in rapidity and resolution of tomographic cardiac imaging, such that it seems the once science-fiction notion of externally 'scanning' near-microscopic details of living patients is becoming a reality. While histopathology remains the standard for definitively characterizing coronary plaques (as the oft-repeated pathology joke punchline goes) the answer comes a week too late. Consequently, there has been a cooperative striving among several disciplines for an accurate noninvasive means of assessing coronary disease and predicting which patients will develop acute coronary syndrome, and when. An exciting opportunity has arisen to connect the knowledge and experience from decades of histopathologic studies of autopsy and explanted hearts with the emerging ability to radiographically resolve fine details of plaque morphology. This chapter will attempt to realize that opportunity.

1 ATHEROSCLEROSIS

1.1 Definitions

Atherosclerosis is a term derived from the Greek 'athera-' meaning porridge and '-scleros' meaning hard. Coronary artery atherosclerosis is an intimal disease (though associated changes are seen in the media and adventitia) affecting the epicardial muscular arteries. It is characterized by both hardening of the artery wall and deposition of a soft material in the intimal layer. It follows a chronic progressive course from an initial 'fatty streak' to diffuse stenotic disease. This progression is thought to proceed via punctuated quantum evolution with periods of accelerated growth followed by recovery, stabilization, and return to quiescence. Atherosclerosis is thought to occur in three phases: (1) **initiation** or formation of the nascent lesion, (2) **progression** through the dynamic interplay of continued plaque growth and vessel adaptation, and (3) **complication** or clinical manifestation of disease.[1] Atherosclerosis should be distinguished from arteriosclerosis, a term which refers to a related processes of hypertrophy and/or calcification with intimal fibrosis but without plaque formation.

1.2 Distribution and macroscopic morphology

Plaques are not distributed randomly throughout the coronary circulation. There is a propensity for development in the proximal halves of the left anterior descending (LAD) and left circumflex (LCX) arteries, with the right coronary artery (RCA) showing a more even distribution throughout its course.[2,3] Plaques appear to develop at predisposed sites,

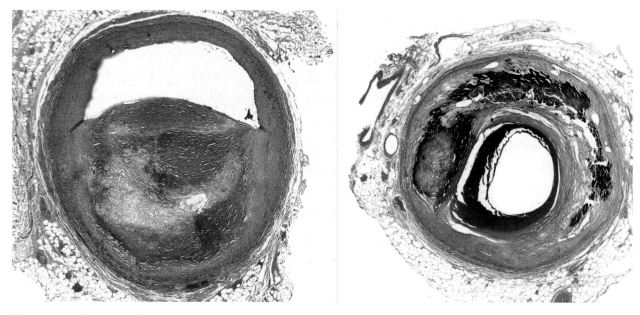

Figure 6.1   Eccentric (left) and concentric (right) lumen morphology. Because of asymmetric plaque distribution and growth, the majority (70%) of plaques result in eccentric luminal distortion. (H&E 12.5X)

such as arterial branchpoints and areas of flow turbulence.[4] Statistically, when a high grade stenosis of the LAD is present there is usually significant disease in all three vessels.[5] In autopsy studies, single vessel lesions of the left main and LAD are most frequent compared to angiographic studies where RCA and LCX disease predominates.[5]

Seventy percent of lesions show eccentric plaque formation when cut on cross section, with the remainder showing concentric lesions (Figure 6.1).[6] As stenosis becomes severe, the lumen is compressed and becomes ellipsoid, semilunar, or polymorphic in shape. In the setting of vasospasm, these factors become clinically significant as some configurations are more susceptible to flow reduction (Figure 6.2).

1.3 The atheroma

The fundamental unit of atherosclerosis is the atheroma or fibrofatty plaque. The pathogenesis of plaque formation is multifactorial and not entirely understood. The established theories regarding the initial inciting event(s) triggering plaque formation all focus on the intima and include: (1) A monoclonal expansion of cells (from a single smooth muscle myocyte) forms the initial lesion as a result of genetic 'transformation' due to viral infection or another (perhaps random) mutation event. The context of hyperlipidemia makes it more likely for these early lesions to propagate and enlarge.[7] (2) Endothelial injury, resulting from hemodynamic shear forces, toxic or oxidative damage (smoking or oxidized LDL), or infection, denudes the intima and exposes the basement membrane matrix. In the healing process, cells are recruited that initiate early plaque formation.[8–10] (3) As a response to non-lethal injury, including flow turbulence without traumatic shear forces, endothelial cells elaborate growth factors and cytokines that cause the intima to become permeable to monocytes as well as acting on medial smooth muscle cells, inducing early plaque formation.[11]

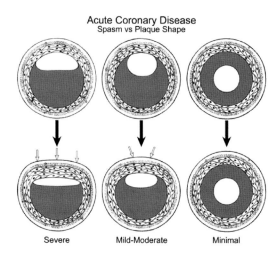

Acute Coronary Disease
Spasm vs Plaque Shape

Severe   Mild-Moderate   Minimal

Extent of Acute Luminal Obstruction

Figure 6.2   Compound effect of vasospasm on lumen morphology. Eccentricity and elongation of lumens narrowed by plaque are variably effected by vasospasm. The fibrous cap and distensible core of a plaque buffer the effects of medial constriction.

Though across race and gender, plaque histomorphology is remarkably constant, there is considerable variation from patient to patient and even from centimeter to centimeter within the same coronary artery. With age, there is also a general shift in plaque morphology to more frequent fibrotic and calcified plaques.[12] The composition of each plaque affects its appearance and physical properties. Lipid and necrotic debris-rich plaques are soft and compliant compared to collagen and calcium-rich plaques that are firm and rigid. Several components contribute to these properties of a plaque, and a brief discussion of each follows.

1.3.1 Lipid

For more than a century it has been known that serum lipids play a central role in atherogenesis. Early studies showed exclusive egg yolk and other lipid-rich diets fed to animals induce atherosclerosis. Genetic hyperlipidemia syndromes are also associated with severe and premature atherosclerosis.[13] More recent and sophisticated investigations have implicated modified LDL particles as the primary agents of plaque formation and propagation.[14] Lipids are predominantly in the esterified form and complexed within lipoprotein particles. The lipid particles gain entry to the vessels wall through endothelial cell receptor mediated endocytosis.

1.3.2 'Foam' cells

These conspicuous cells within plaques display cytoplasmic distention by numerous lipid vesicles microscopically resembling coalesced bubbles or foam. These cells are thought to derive from native vascular smooth muscle cells[15] as well as circulating monocytes that ingest the modified LDL particles.[16] These cells also elaborate cytokines and growth factors important in cell recruitment and plaque progression.

1.3.3 Blood and its breakdown products

Whether by incorporation of silent superficial thrombus resulting from microscopic endothelial injury or due to rupture of the plaque microvasculature, red blood cells and products of heme iron metabolism (hemosiderin laden cells, and extracellular iron) are frequently found in plaques.

1.3.4 Necrotic debris

As the intima thickens and expands and the distance from lumen to plaque core increases, the atheroma begins to outgrow its blood supply. Without sufficient oxygen tension, the smooth muscle and other cells in the plaque undergo cell death, emptying their contents into the plaque substance.

1.3.5 Cholesterol crystals

Lipids released during cell necrosis are rich in cholesterol which, no longer bound to protein, precipitates as large needle-like crystals. These crystals often incite a foreign-body giant cell reaction within the plaque.

1.3.6 Smooth muscle cells

The presence of these cells inside atheromas is well established although their origin and function is not. They may derive from endothelial cells, circulating stem cells, and/or the vascular media.[17] Smooth muscle cells also have been shown to phagocytose lipid and LDL particles, similar to a monocyte/macrophage.[15] Some evidence suggests a transformation from contractile phenotype to a synthetic phenotype occurs.[18,19] These cells also produce inhibitors of proteolytic enzymes, including matrix metalloproteinases.

1.3.7 Leukocytes

Foci of predominantly lymphocytic and monocytic inflammation are variably seen in plaques and are considered a feature of remodeling. They can also be associated with areas of collagen destruction in the fibrous cap and consequent plaque vulnerability. The presence of inflammation in both plaque remodeling and instability suggests this may have a central role and that these may be inter-related processes. These cells are the likely source of proteolytic enzymes active in the remodeling process.[20]

1.3.8 Microvasculature

Likely stimulated by low oxygen concentration in the plaque core, new growth of capillaries (neovascularization) extending inward from the adventitial vasa vasorum can be demonstrated in more established plaques.[21] These young vessels (part of so-called 'granulation tissue') are fragile and prone to leak or rupture, leading to accumulation of blood and iron deposits in the plaque as well.

1.3.9 Calcium

Calcification, associated both with the necrotic core and elsewhere in the fibrous parts of the plaque, are commonly seen. The composition is hydroxyapatite-like and contains phosphorus and carbonate as well. The mechanism of deposition is thought to be influenced by pH changes within the plaque[22] and it is thought that membrane-bound vesicles and cytoplasmic organelles of necrotic cells serve as the initial nidus for precipitation.[23] Enzymes reported to have primary function in bone metabolism, such as osteopontin,[24] have been reported to have a role in this process[25] and it is not uncommon to see true ossification of plaque calcium including the presence of lacunar cells and bone marrow elements.

Calcium deposition is typically a good indicator of overall plaque burden, but does not correlate highly with the degree of obstruction either at the site of calcification or elsewhere in a vessel. This is particulary true in older patients, as there is a general transition to rigid and calcified plaques with age.[12]

1.3.10 Collagen (fibrosis)

Like a scar forming at any other injury site in the body, dense fibrillary collagen formation is universal part of plaque structure. It is typically formed around the periphery of a plaque including a 'cap' separating the core material from the endothelium and vessel lumen. The thickness of this core if thought to be proportional to the protection it provides from plaque rupture and vessel thrombosis. Pharmacotherapy with angiotensin converting enzyme inhibitors and 'statin' agents is thought to promote and stabilize this fibrous cap.[26]

1.3.11 Fibrin and platelets (thrombus)

Activation of the coagulation cascade, together with platelet aggregation, occurs either when the core contents are exposed to luminal blood or when the delicate microvasculature is disrupted and blood (and serum) are spilled inside the plaque. Intraplaque fibrin material and platelet aggregates are not uncommonly seen and are highly associated with plaque vulnerability.

It should be borne in mind, however that these constituents exist in a dynamic and constantly changing state, such that one must resist the temptation to think of the plaque strata like rings of a tree trunk, marking a succession of thanksgiving feasts past or a retrospective chronicling of various dietary indiscretions. This constant turnover helps account for the apparent randomness of plaque instability (discussed later), but also suggests a mechanism for regression and plaque shrinkage.

1.4 Adventitia and vasa vasorum

In addition to the intimal changes detailed above, it is also becoming clear that the adventitia – particularly the vasa vasorum – plays an important role in plaque biology.[27] The adventitia underlying a plaque frequently shows a collar of dense mononuclear inflammation. There is also a significant expansion of the vasa vasorum network at these sites. Through detailed studies of vasculitis, it is evident that adventitial inflammatory cells, particularly dendritic cells, modulate the influx of cytotoxic cells through the vasa vasorum and into the media and intima.[28] It is possible that a similar phenomenon occurs in atherosclerosis and that intra-plaque inflammation associated with 'instability' can be tied to signaling from adventitial dendritic cells.[29]

2 VASCULAR REMODELING

As a coronary plaque enlarges, compensatory changes in the media occur in an attempt to maintain constant luminal area and thus flow.[30] (Figure 6.3) The media subjacent to the plaque becomes distended and atrophied. The media of the wall opposite the plaque often hypertrophies, possibly

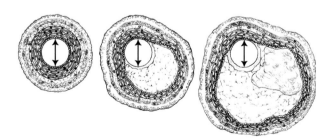

Figure 6.3 Vascular remodeling. As a plaque progresses in size, compensatory changes occur in the vessel wall resulting in dilatation and preservation of the original luminal diameter. The media underlying a plaque undergoes atrophy and the smooth muscle of the plaque-free wall hypertrophies.

becoming more prone to spasm. Both processes involve the combined effects of cell migration, proliferation, apoptosis and extracellular matrix metabolism.[31] Accommodation by the vascular wall is generally successful in preserving unimpeded flow until the plaque area approximates the luminal area, though an accelerated rate of plaque growth may outstrip the artery's ability to adapt appropriately and in time. These remodeling processes are also dynamic and can have the opposite effects in other segments of the artery or at later points in time, resulting in a reduction in wall thickness and luminal diameter when flow velocity is reduced.

The phenomenon of coronary remodeling has been recognized as a significant contributor to the occasional discordance between angiographic and histopathologic assessments of stenosis. Angiography and other methods of 'lumenography' are known to underestimate severity because in their percent occlusion equation, the denominator represents the least diseased adjacent segment of artery which may (either due to remodeling or simply diffuse disease) actually contain significant underlying plaque (Figure 6.4). This is especially true in the proximal LAD. Units of measure must also be reconciled as lumenography measures in a single linear dimension (mm) and cross sectional assessments are 2 dimensional (mm²); such that a 50% reduction in diameter corresponds roughly to a 75% area reduction and 70% stenosis angiographically equates to a 90% occlusion by cross sectional analysis. These mathematical calculations, however, are based on the assumption that the lumen remains circular, which often is not the case (hence the need for multiple orthogonal planes of imaging during cardiac catheterization). By lumenography concentric plaques typically show an hourglass type deformation and eccentric plaques are more wide-mouthed. It should also be kept in mind that coronary blood flow does not depend only on percent stenosis, but is also influenced by the length of a lesion, the shape of the lumen, the blood pressure reaching the coronaries, and extrinsic factors such as myocyte hypertrophy or an intramyocardial course of an artery.

3 ACUTE CORONARY SYNDROME AND VULNERABLE PLAQUE

The acute coronary syndrome (ACS) encompasses myocardial infarction, unstable angina and sudden cardiac death. It almost uniformly occurs in patients with coronary artery disease[32] and is due to acute thrombosis of usually a single coronary artery. Curiously, this phenomenon of thrombosis superimposed on atherosclerosis is as likely to involve non-critical plaques as it is areas of high grade stenosis.[33,34] Consequently, the occurrence of ACS is difficult to predict by any current imaging modality. It is also of interest to note that a partially obstructing thrombus may still cause symptoms and damage myocardium, though these more frequently lead to subendocardial rather than transmural infarction. Arterial spasm may also mimic ACS clinically, without any significant residual evidence obstruction.

The plaques associated with ACS-causing thromboses demonstrate consistent histomorphologic features (Figure 6.5).

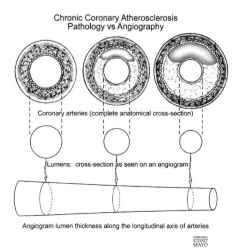

Figure 6.4 Effect of vessel remodeling on discrepancies between pathology and angiography.

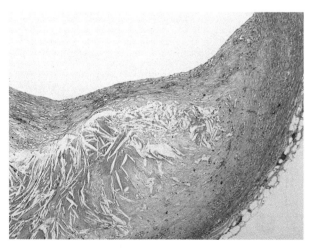

Figure 6.5 Histopathologic features of unstable plaque. Features of plaque instability are found in both critical and non-critical stenosing lesions and include abundant soft necrotic core material, a thin fibrous cap and active inflammation within the fibrous cap. Inflammation can also be seen in the adventitia (not pictured here). (H&E 50X)

They are typically lipid-rich with prominent soft necrotic cores, have a thinned fibrous 'cap,' and inflammatory foci within the cap, plaque substance, and/or adventitia.[26] Intraplaque hemorrhage and/or fibrin is also frequently seen.[35] In many cases, a breach of the fibrous cap can be found with exposure of the thrombogenic plaque contents to luminal blood. Using medical 'archeology' the sequence of events can be reconstructed based on the pathologic findings (Figure 6.6). The fibrous cap overlying a soft and pliable plaque is eroded by proteolytic enzymes produced from the inflammatory cells (representing an imbalance of degradation in the extracellular matrix metabolism). Pressure inside the plaque rises due to intraplaque hemorrhage, or else there is an endothelial injury (perhaps due to hypertensive reaction to emotional stress or some other 'trigger') causing disruption of the plaque. The coagulation cascade is activated by tissue factor and other thrombogenic plaque contents (plus platelet activation and aggregation) and thrombosis ensues.

A number of fates await a newly formed coronary artery thrombus. It may almost immediately begin to dissolve via intrinsic thrombolytic pathways. It, or portions of it, may dislodge and embolize to distal arteries and arterioles. It may remain stable and, if not removed by an interventional procedure, begin to organize and ultimately recanalize, typically with multiple luminal channels (Figure 6.7). The clinical manifestations of these events span a spectrum from completely silent partial obstructions that resorb (resulting in stepwise plaque progression) to sudden cardiac death and from myocardial infarction with cardiogenic shock to subtle changes in ejection fraction, eventually progressing to congestive heart failure or ischemic cardiomyopathy.

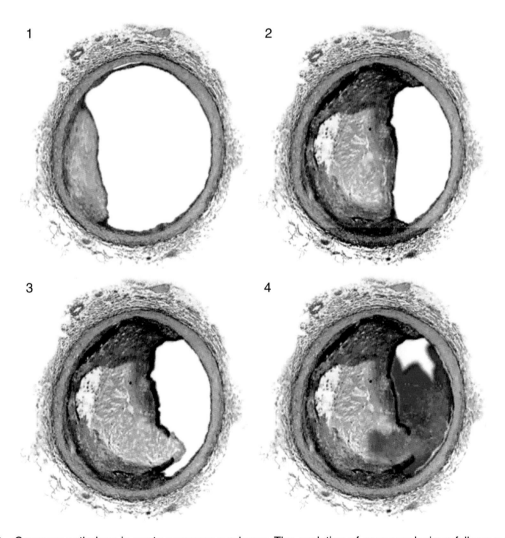

Figure 6.6 Coronary pathology in acute coronary syndrome. The evolution of coronary lesions follows a progression from (1) initial plaque formation, (2) plaque growth, (3) plaque vulnerability and rupture, and (4) thrombosis.

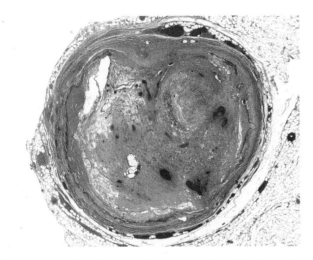

Figure 6.7   Organizing occlusive thrombus. The lumen is completely obliterated by organizing thrombus. Early recanalization is evident with multiple small vascular channels. (HE 12.5X)

4 CHRONIC CORONARY OBSTRUCTION AND RELATED CLINICAL SYNDROMES

Chronic flow-limiting obstructions of coronary arteries without superimposed thrombosis manifests clinically as stable, exertional angina. These typically correlate with diffuse disease that is slowly progressive and does not show features of plaque instability.

Chronic compromise of coronary blood flow may also occur in the absence of significant coronary obstruction. This can be due to coronary ostial stenosis, due to calcific aortic atherosclerosis (more often affecting the right coronary ostium), aortitis, or aortic dissection. Anomalous origins of the coronary arteries are also relatively rare causes of chronic intermittent flow obstruction.

Coronary disease in diabetes warrants special consideration as there is some evidence to suggest it differs from usual atherosclerosis in non-diabetic patients. These differences include greater calcification occurring in diabetic patients dying suddenly compared to non-diabetic sudden death

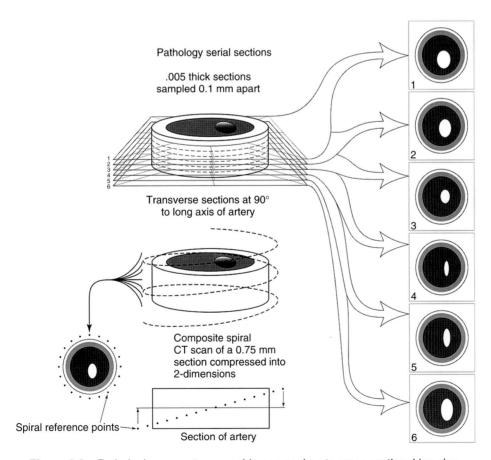

Figure 6.8   Pathologic versus tomographic approaches to cross sectional imaging.

controls, an increase in cell-rich areas and necrotic core content, as well as generally earlier and more diffuse lesions in comparison to a non-diabetic cohort.[36]

5 TOMOGRAPHIC IMAGING – HISTOLOGY CORRELATION

Potentially erroneous assumptions can be made when comparing histologic and tomographic visualizations of coronary arteries and this warrants some discussion. Images rendered from tomography are actually a 2-dimensional flattening of a complex 3-dimensional helical 'section' through the artery. As such they represent a summed average of the actual cross sectional morphologies from level to level throughout a given thickness of artery (e.g. approx. 0.75 mm or 750 microns using current CT scanners). Histologic sections, on the other hand, are 3-dimensional with a defined thickness of typically 5–10 microns and show the actual composition at a single microscopic level. This means that 1 CT slice can contain 100–150 histology slices, making a direct comparison of one CT slice with one histology slice difficult. However, due to technical aspects of microtomy using paraffin embedded tissue blocks (including 'facing in' to obtain a flat cutting surface as well as step sectioning to obtain sections at different levels through the block), by necessity, a significant number of sections end up on the cutting room floor. Fortunately, for both modalities, the variability in plaque morphology from millimeter to millimeter is negligible and when thrombi form they tend to propogate over distances of several milimeters, so these two approaches are reasonable approximations of each other when comparing percent stenosis, and lumen morphology (Figure 6.8).

BIBLIOGRAPHY

1. Gotlieb AI, Silver MD. Atherosclerosis: Pathology and Pathogenesis. In: Silver MD, Gotlieb AI, Schoen FJ, eds. Cardiovascular Pathology. Philadelphia: Churchill Livingstone; 2001: 68–106.
2. Jost S, Deckers JW, Nikutta P et al. Progression of coronary artery disease is dependent on anatomic location and diameter. The INTACT investigators. J Am Coll Cardiol. May 1993; 21(6): 1339–46.
3. Hochman JS, Phillips WJ, Ruggieri D et al. The distribution of atherosclerotic lesions in the coronary arterial tree: relation to cardiac risk factors. Am Heart J. Nov 1988; 116(5 Pt 1): 1217–22.
4. Gotlieb AI, Langille BL. Role of rheology in atherosclerotic coronary artery disease. In: Fuster V, Ross R, Topol EJ, eds. Atherosclerosis and Coronary Artery Disease. Philadelphia: Lippincott-Raven; 1996: 595–606.
5. Edwards WD. Pathology of Myocardial Infarction and Reperfusion. In: Gersch BJ, Rahimtoola SH, eds. Acute Myocardial Infarction. 2nd ed. New York: Chapman & Hall; 1997: 16–50.
6. Waller BF. The eccentric coronary atherosclerotic plaque: morphologic observations and clinical relevance. Clin Cardiol. Jan 1989; 12(1): 14–20.
7. Murry CE, Gipaya CT, Bartosek T et al. Monoclonality of smooth muscle cells in human atherosclerosis. Am J Pathol. Sep 1997; 151(3): 697–705.
8. Ross R, Glomset JA. The pathogenesis of atherosclerosis (second of two parts). N Engl J Med. Aug 19 1976; 295(8): 420–5.
9. Ross R, Glomset JA. The pathogenesis of atherosclerosis (first of two parts). N Engl J Med. Aug 12 1976; 295(7): 369–77.
10. Ross R. Atherosclerosis – an inflammatory disease. N Engl J Med. Jan 14 1999; 340(2): 115–26.
11. Dai G, Kaazempur-Mofrad MR, Natarajan S et al. Distinct endothelial phenotypes evoked by arterial waveforms derived from atherosclerosis-susceptible and -resistant regions of human vasculature. Proc Natl Acad Sci USA Oct 12 2004; 101(41): 14871–6.
12. Kragel AH, Reddy SG, Wittes JT et al. Morphometric analysis of the composition of atherosclerotic plaques in the four major epicardial coronary arteries in acute myocardial infarction and in sudden coronary death. Circulation Dec 1989; 80(6): 1747–56.
13. Fye WB. A historical perspective on atherosclerosis and coronary artery disease. In: Fuster V, Topol EJ, Nabel EG, eds. Atherothrombosis and Coronary Atery Disease. 2nd ed. Philadelphia: Lippincott William and Wilkins, 2004: 1–14.
14. Carmena R, Duriez P, Fruchart JC. Atherogenic lipoprotein particles in atherosclerosis. Circulation Jun 15 2004; 109(23 Suppl 1): III2–7.
15. Haust MD. The morphogenesis and fate of potential and early atherosclerotic lesions in man. Hum Pathol. Mar 1971; 2(1): 1–29.
16. Shashkin P, Dragulev B, Ley K. Macrophage differentiation to foam cells. Curr Pharm Des. 2005; 11(23): 3061–72.
17. Simper D, Wang S, Deb A, et al. Endothelial progenitor cells are decreased in blood of cardiac allograft patients with vasculopathy and endothelial cells of noncardiac origin are enriched in transplant atherosclerosis. Circulation Jul 15 2003; 108(2): 143–9.
18. Halayko AJ, Solway J. Molecular mechanisms of phenotypic plasticity in smooth muscle cells. J Appl Physiol. Jan 2001; 90(1): 358–68.
19. Birkedal-Hansen H. Proteolytic remodeling of extracellular matrix. Curr Opin Cell Biol. Oct 1995; 7(5): 728–35.
20. Libby P. Molecular bases of the acute coronary syndromes. Circulation Jun 1 1995; 91(11): 2844–50.
21. Moreno PR, Purushothaman KR, Sirol M et al. Neovascularization in human atherosclerosis. Circulation May 9 2006; 113(18): 2245–52.
22. Glimcher MJ. Mechanism of calcification: role of collagen fibrils and collagen-phosphoprotein complexes in vitro and in vivo. Anat Rec. Jun 1989; 224(2): 139–53.
23. Tanimura A, McGregor DH, Anderson HC. Calcification in atherosclerosis. I. Human studies. J Exp Pathol. Summer 1986; 2(4): 261–73.
24. Fitzpatrick LA, Severson A, Edwards WD et al. Diffuse calcification in human coronary arteries. Association of osteopontin with atherosclerosis. J Clin Invest. Oct 1994; 94(4): 1597–604.

25. Giachelli CM, Bae N, Almeida M et al. Osteopontin is elevated during neointima formation in rat arteries and is a novel component of human atherosclerotic plaques. J Clin Invest. Oct 1993; 92(4): 1686–96.

26. Kullo IJ, Edwards WD, Schwartz RS. Vulnerable plaque: pathobiology and clinical implications. Ann Intern Med. Dec 15 1998; 129(12): 1050–60.

27. Gossl M, Versari D, Mannheim D et al. Increased spatial vasa vasorum density in the proximal LAD in hypercholesterolemia – Implications for vulnerable plaque-development. Atherosclerosis Aug 17 2006.

28. Weyand CM, Ma-Krupa W, Pryshchep O et al. Vascular dendritic cells in giant cell arteritis. Ann N Y Acad Sci. Dec 2005; 1062: 195–208.

29. Erbel C, Sato K, Meyer FB et al. Functional profile of activated dendritic cells in unstable atherosclerotic plaque. Basic Res Cardiol. Mar 2007; 102(2): 123–32.

30. Glagov S, Weisenberg E, Zarins CK et al. Compensatory enlargement of human atherosclerotic coronary arteries. N Engl J Med. May 28 1987; 316(22): 1371–5.

31. Schoenhagen P, Nissen SE, Tuzcu EM. Coronary arterial remodeling: from bench to bedside. Curr Atheroscler Rep. Mar 2003; 5(2): 150–4.

32. Buja LM, Willerson JT. The role of coronary artery lesions in ischemic heart disease: Insights from recent clinicopathologic, coronary artiographic and experimental studies. Major Probl Pathol. 1991; 23: 42–60.

33. Brown BG, Gallery CA, Badger RS et al. Incomplete lysis of thrombus in the moderate underlying a therosclerotic lesion during intracoronary infusion of streptokinase for acute myocardial infarction: quantitative angiographic observations. Circulation Apr 1986; 73(4): 653–61.

34. Little WC, Constantinescu M, Applegate RJ et al. Can coronary angiography predict the site of a subsequent myocardial infarction in patients with mild-to-moderate coronary artery disease? Circulation Nov 1988; 78(5 Pt 1): 1157–66.

35. Davies MJ, Thomas AC. Plaque fissuring – the cause of acute myocardial infarction, sudden ischaemic death, and crescendo angina. Br Heart J. Apr 1985; 53(4): 363–73.

36. Schoenhagen P, Nissen SE. Coronary atherosclerosis in diabetic subjects: clinical significance, anatomic characteristics, and identification with in vivo imaging. Cardiol Clin. Nov 2004; 22(4): 527–40, vi.

7

Complementary Roles of Computed Tomography and Myocardial Perfusion Single Photon Emission Computed Tomography

Daniel S. Berman, Leslee J. Shaw, and Alan Rozanski

This book has been dedicated to the application of cardiac computed tomography (CT). However, a critical link to its effective implementation is the development of patient management strategies that integrate CT with conventional cardiac imaging. The focus of this chapter is on the complementary roles of CT and stress ischemia testing with myocardial perfusion single photon emission computed tomography (SPECT, SPECT MPI).

For several decades, stress-rest SPECT myocardial perfusion imaging (MPI) has been a mainstay for the noninvasive assessment of patients with suspected and known CAD. This test is effective both for the diagnostic assessment of patients with an intermediate pretest likelihood of CAD, and as a means for risk stratifying patients with either an intermediate-to-high likelihood of CAD or those with known CAD. Due to its proven effectiveness, SPECT MPI studies are now performed in more than 7 million Americans each year. Recently, cardiac CT has emerged as another means of assessing patients with suspected CAD. Cardiac CT provides high-resolution anatomic assessment of coronary artery calcification (CAC) in noncontrast studies and angiographic disease extent and severity using coronary CT angiography (CCTA). Potentially, SPECT MPI and cardiac CT may provide complementary information regarding physiology and anatomy. Herein, we first briefly review the current applications of SPECT MPI, followed by our review of the emerging role of cardiac CT,

including its potential complementary use to SPECT MPI for the clinical management of patients with suspected or known CAD.

1 CLINICAL ASSESSMENT WITH MPI

1.1 Stress-induced ischemia on SPECT MPI

Within the ischemic cascade, perfusion abnormalities develop prior to evidence of ST-segment changes on the surface electrocardiography or the onset of anginal symptoms. Thus, MPI provides a more sensitive diagnostic marker for obstructive CAD than clinical or stress ECG testing. The underlying mechanism for stress-induced ischemia is complex and both involves anatomic obstruction to coronary blood flow and dynamic physiological factors which may serve to cause reduced coronary blood supply with exercise (e.g., paradoxical vasoconstriction due to coronary endothelial dysfunction). Generally, coronary stenoses induce alterations in peak-stress myocardial blood flow if there is a moderate to severely obstructed lesion (>70% diameter narrowing), a degree of stenosis accepted by interventionalists as warranting revascularization. Stenoses of 50–70% frequently show no stress-induced perfusion defect by

SPECT MPI. By comparison, changes in resting myocardial blood flow are principally seen only in the setting of a critical stenosis (i.e., >90%).[1,2] However, it has recently been shown that a large proportion of acute coronary events occur in regions with only mild to moderate stenosis prior to the event. It is now considered likely that the dynamic component of unstable plaques may explain the high sensitivity of SPECT MPI for detecting patients at risk for cardiac events.

The need for stress SPECT MPI is for *diagnosis* determined by first assessing patients' pretest likelihood of CAD, as assessed from the Bayesian analyses of patient age, sex, risk factors, and symptoms, as initially developed by Diamond and Forrester.[3] Patients with an intermediate likelihood of CAD following the analyses of the above factors (generally in the range of 15–85% CAD likelihood) are considered the best candidates for stress testing (with or without imaging). Patients re-classified as "low likelihood" patients following stress testing will still generally require modification of coronary risk factors. Patients who are re-classified as having a high likelihood of CAD following stress testing may become appropriate referrals for cardiac catheterization, depending on the magnitude of inducible ischemia on stress testing. This diagnostic application has resulted in class I indications in the recent ACC/AHA/ASNC guidelines.[4]

Patients with an initially high likelihood of CAD prior to stress testing are unique in that the question regarding them is not diagnosis but rather *prognosis* – are they of sufficient risk to merit aggressive intervention? As a consequence, such high likelihood of CAD patients also commonly benefit from SPECT MPI as the next step in their clinical evaluation, because a normal SPECT MPI study identifies them as low-risk patients relative to future cardiac events (<1%).[5,6] When found to have normal SPECT MPI studies, these patients are at low risk of prognosis, and usually can be followed using medical management. Of note, approximately 60% of high likelihood of CAD patients have been found to have normal SPECT MPI examinations, allowing for consideration of a conservative management plan. Conversely, the more abnormal the SPECT MPI study is, the greater the likelihood that a patient would benefit from revascularization (e.g., PCI, CABG).[7] This approach is embodied in multiple ACC/AHA guidelines in which stress testing, with or without stress imaging, is considered a class I indication in many patients with an intermediate likelihood of CAD but class IIb indication for diagnostic testing in patients with either high or low pretest probability of CAD.[4,8–10]

1.2 Current evidence on risk stratification with SPECT MPI

Risk stratification, along with diagnostic testing, is the other common indicator for the use of SPECT MPI. A synthesis of available prognostic evidence with SPECT MPI reveals two key factors. First, a normal SPECT MPI is associated with a very low risk of major adverse cardiovascular events over the near term of follow-up (i.e., 1–3 years).[11,12] In general, longer term follow-up data estimating cardiac risk beyond 2–3 years is not currently available. A recent meta-analysis on the annualized cardiac death or myocardial infarction (MI) rates for a normal SPECT MPI are 0.3% for women and 0.8% for men.[13] A similar low rate of cardiac events has been reported when using all 3 available radioisotopes.[14] A synopsis of available risk stratification evidence is detailed in Table 7.1.[12,13,15] Second, risk of cardiac death or nonfatal MI is proportional to the extent and severity of stress SPECT MPI abnormalities, as summarized by various investigators.[4,12,16,17] The risk of cardiac events is slightly elevated with mild SPECT MPI abnormalities but can increase up to 10-fold for patients with moderate to severe SPECT MPI findings.[11] It is this strong relationship between major adverse cardiovascular events and SPECT MPI, as well as the numerous large registries and controlled clinical trials, that support numerous Class I indications for its use within guidelines from the ACC.[4]

Today, the preferred interpretive technique is based on semiquantitative perfusion assessment, utilizing a 17-segment myocardial model to define the extent of defects across the myocardium as well as the severity of defects within each region. Each segment is scored using a 5-point scoring system ranging from 0 = normal perfusion to 4 = absent perfusion. This score is applied to both the rest and stress images and summed to calculate a summed rest and stress score. The difference between the summed stress and rest score widely utilized index is of the amount of inducible ischemia (i.e., summed difference score).

More recently, we have advocated a new semiquantitative method for expressing the amount of myocardium at risk according to SPECT MPI.[7] This method divides the observed summed difference score in a given patient by 68 (maximum score possible) when using a 17-segment model. With this approach, the percent of the myocardium that is affected by reduced perfusion at stress or at rest can be reported. Using the latter scoring technique, a moderate to severely abnormal study is one encompassing ≥5% to ≥10% of the myocardium.[18] These thresholds were devised using validated prognostic models across diverse,

Table 7.1 Meta-analyses on the annual rates of cardiovascular death or myocardial infarction by low to high risk SPECT MPI

	Low risk or normal stress perfusion	High risk or severely moderate abnormal stress perfusion
Underwood	0.8%	5.2%
Shaw	0.6%	–
Tl-201, Tc-99m S*, & Tc-99m M*		
Shaw	0.85% (0.6%–1.2%)	5.9% (4.6%–8.5%)
Metz	1.2% (0.9%–1.5%)	–
Patient subsets		
Metz	0.4% (0.3%–0.5%)	–
Women		
Men		
Gender	1.4% (0.8%–2.1%)	6.3%
Women	0.7%	5.3%
Men	0.7%	
Diabetes		
Diabetics	1.9%	9.6%
Non-Diabetics	0.6%	5.8%
Diabetics		
Women	2.7%	10.9%
Men	1.3%	6.5%
Type of stress	0.7%	
Exercise	1.2%	5.6%
Pharmacologic stress		8.3%

Shaw report includes median event rates (25th, 75th percentile). For low risk, top values are in reports that highlighted only low risk studies and bottom included low- to high-risk subsets. *S = Sestamibi, M = Myoview.

large patient registries.[18,19] The benefit to using measures that identify the percent of the myocardium affected is that they are more easily understood by referring physicians.

In prior work from our group, when more than 10% of the myocardium is involved, such high risk patients were found to receive an improved outcome following coronary revascularization, based on observational data.[7,20] For symptomatic patients with high risk findings, such as >10% of ischemic myocardium, their risk of major adverse cardiovascular events exceeded 5% per year.[7] A recent meta-analysis revealed that the annual rates of cardiac death or nonfatal MI averaged 5.9% (25th percentile = 4.6% to 75th percentile = 8.5%) for a high risk MPI.[12] Of note, comorbidity will accentuate this risk, such that patients with a heavy risk factor burden may have annual event rates approaching 10% per year is the setting of a high risk study. These event rates are consistent with those observed in patients having a severe stenosis or multivessel coronary disease by angiographic procedures. As such, it has been recommended that this risk is sufficiently high to warrant referral to coronary angiography in patients who manifest these findings.[21]

A list of high-risk SPECT MPI findings is detailed in Table 7.2. These include large areas of reduced perfusion defects and multivessel perfusion abnormalities of moderate size. Patients with small perfusion defects can also be considered at sufficiently high risk to consider revascularization if there are ancillary markers suggesting high risk including transient ischemic dilation (TID) of the left ventricle[22] new wall motion abnormalities after stress (post-stress stunning),[23,24] increased lung uptake of radioactivity (associated with increased pulmonary capillary wedge pressure),[25] and unusually prominent right ventricular visualization,

Table 7.2 Examples of high-risk markers from stress SPECT MPI

1. Large anterior perfusion (fixed or reversible) defect
2. Multiple perfusion (fixed or reversible) defects of at least moderate size
3. Moderate perfusion defect in the left anterior descending vascular territory
4. Two or more defects with marked reduction in perfusion
5. ≥5% ischemic myocardium
6. Stress defects in ≥5% myocardium
7. Increased lung uptake
8. Transient ischemic dilation

reduced LVEF, and large end-systolic volumes. While both reversible (ischemic) and fixed ("infarct") defects confer risk, only the magnitude of the ischemic defect appears to be predictive of improvement in mortality risk after revascularization. Hachamovitch et al.[20] have recently shown that the predictive value of ischemia regarding survival benefit with revascularization extends across the range of ejection fractions as measured after stress with gated SPECT MPI. Finally, recent work from our institution has indicated the importance of assessing other clinical components in determining the need to consider invasive management, including factors such as age, symptoms (chest pain or shortness of breath),[26] exercise duration, heart rate at rest and percent heart rate response achieved, and inability to exercise.

2 CLINICAL ASSESSMENT WITH CAC SCANNING

2.1 Pathophysiology of coronary artery calcification

The occurrence of macroscopic CAC, the amounts required to be visualized by CT, is part of the atherosclerotic disease process.[27] Initially detected using fluoroscopic technique(s),[28] CAC in the current era is more frequently assessed utilizing electron beam (EBT) or multislice CT techniques[27,29] as discussed in Chapter 10. Teleologically, it is postulated that calcification of atherosclerotic plaque occurs in the body's effort to contain an 'active,' inflamed, or vulnerable coronary plaque.[29] Thus, the identification of a calcified region within a coronary artery is thought to reflect a more advanced stage of atherosclerotic plaque development, and it may have little relationship with disease activity. Coronary calcification can frequently occur with positive "remodeling" of the coronary artery with no resultant effect on the coronary lumen, a process known as the Glagov phenomenon.[30] Thus, a given CAC lesion is not site specific for an underlying obstructive coronary stenosis.

However, whereas CAC does not predict obstructive disease, it is strongly associated with the presence of ≥20% stenoses and thus provides a strong link to the overall burden of atherosclerosis. It is the accumulation of mild disease (i.e., ≥20% stenosis) that reflects the degree of atherosclerosis within the arterial wall.[31] Other data note a strong correlation between histopathologic evidence of coronary plaque and the extent of calcified and non-calcified plaque noted on CT (r >0.90).[32] Thus, the strength

of CT-determined CAC is that it is a measure of the global atherosclerotic disease burden.

2.2 Measurement of CAC

CAC is frequently measured using a scoring system initially devised by Agatston and colleagues.[33] Using this score, the extent and density of CAC is combined into one measure. The score is calculated using a semi-automatic computer-based program that is calculated as the product of calcified plaque area and the coefficient of its density, as expressed in peak Hounsfield units (HU). Coefficients are scored as 1 for 131–199 HU, 2 for 200–299 HU, 3 for 300–399 HU, and 4 for ≥400 HU, respectively. A CAC score is calculated for each coronary artery with a HU density ≥130. The score is summed for each coronary artery to obtain the commonly used total CAC score. Results are often assessed according to CAC ranges of 0, 1–10, 11–100, 101–399, 400–999, and ≥1,000 in clinical studies. Most investigators consider a prognostically relevant CAC score as ≥100 and a high risk score as ≥400. Another score, preferred for serial testing to evaluating disease progression, is the calcium volume score.[34,35]

2.3 Prevalence of CAC

CAC is common in adults with its prevalence increasing with age.[27] Nearly half of middle-age adults within the general population have some detectable CAC, but only 5% have a high risk score.[36] The prevalence of a high risk CAC increases with the number of clinical risk factors or the degree of comorbidity and is higher in patients with an intermediate- or high-risk Framingham risk score than in those with low risk scores. In contrast, nearly half of elderly patients have high-risk CAC score(s). Similar to CAD prevalence rates, the overall rates for women lag behind those of men by approximately 10–15 years.[37] Age and gender percentile scores are available that provide rough guides as to normative standards of CAC scores based on large datasets.[36,38]

2.4 Current evidence on risk stratification with CACS

Within the last few years, the results from a number of large observational registries have been published. These indicate a strong relationship between the extent of coronary calcium and major adverse cardiovascular events, including death or nonfatal MI.[29,31,39–46] The direct relationship between coronary artery calcium and hard cardiac events is most generally explained by the aforementioned strong relationship between the amount of calcified plaque and the overall plaque burden.[29] Thus, patients with extensive coronary calcium are also likely to manifest extensive noncalcified plaque, a plaque type more commonly associated with acute cardiac event(s).

A number of reports have been published on the relationship between CACS and all-cause mortality.[42,43,47,48] The largest of these was recently published by Budoff et al.[43] In this latter report, the authors pooled the data from two large observational registries including 35,364 asymptomatic patients clinically referred for EBT scanning and followed for 5–12 years.[43] Figure 7.1 plots the 5-year and 12-year all-cause mortality rates within a range of CACS. These results reveal a potent exponential relationship between CACS and death.[49]

Two recent consensus statements have summarized data indicating a strong, direct relationship between CACS and coronary heart disease (CHD) death and nonfatal MI.[29,31] A meta-analysis was included in the American College of Cardiology (ACC) expert consensus statement on CACS

synthesizing prognostic findings in 27,622 patients from 6 published reports.[29] Annual CHD death or MI rates ranged from 0.1% for a 0 CACS to 2.2% for high-risk CACS >1,000 (p < 0.00001).[29] Restricting outcome analyses to only those with an intermediate Framingham risk score, annual cardiac event rates (CHD death or annual nonfatal MI) were 0.4%, 1.3%, and 2.4% for CACS of 0–99, 100–399, and ≥400, respectively. This graded relationship between CHD events and mortality risk has been used to define a threshold for the utility of subsequent myocardial ischemia testing, as will be discussed further on.

2.5 Current evidence on the utility of stress SPECT MPI in patients with high risk CACS

SPECT MPI is generally applied for diagnostic purposes to patients with chest pain symptoms (or anginal equivalents) and asymptomatic patients with multiple CAD risk factors. The current increasing application of CAC scanning means that asymptomatic patients with even few or no CAD risk factors are now also being referred at times for SPECT MPI if they have evidence of substantial CAC. Emerging data

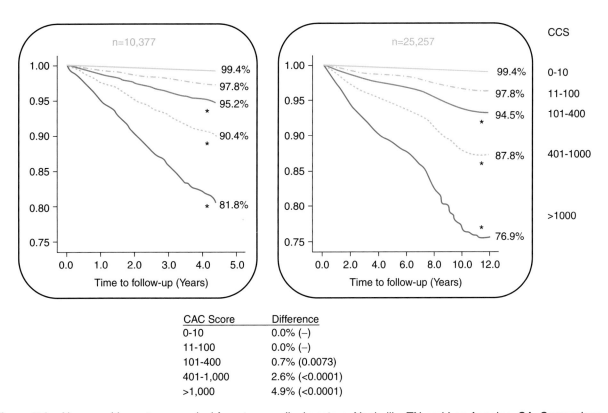

CAC Score	Difference
0-10	0.0% (–)
11-100	0.0% (–)
101-400	0.7% (0.0073)
401-1,000	2.6% (<0.0001)
>1,000	4.9% (<0.0001)

Figure 7.1   Near- and long- term survival from two medical centers: Nashville, TN and Los Angeles, CA. Comparison of 5-year mortality rates in two different cohorts. The results are quite consistent across different study groups. *p<0.01 vs. CCS 0-10, $\chi2$ = 1503, p < 0.0001, interaction p < 0.0001. (Adapted with permission from J Am Coll Cardiol.[49])

suggest that the detection of high risk CACS asymptomatic subjects is clinically concerning, especially when combined with other CAD risk factors.[29] Due to their heightened risk of major adverse cardiovascular events (i.e., 2% or higher per year or CHD risk equivalent status), patients with a high risk CACS should be considered candidates for evaluating their silent ischemic burden. There are currently 7 published reports on the relationship between the extent of CACS and the frequency of abnormal SPECT MPI.[50–58] Current Appropriateness Criteria by the ACC support the use of SPECT MPI in asymptomatic patients with a high CACS.[59] The use of SPECT MPI in patients with high CAC scores is also supported by a recent information statement from the American Society of Nuclear Cardiology (ASNC) on the complementary role of SPECT MPI and CACS,[56] and by a recent report from Rozanski et al. (JACC 2007).[84]

He and colleagues[50] were the first to report on the relationship between the frequency of inducible ischemia by SPECT MPI and CACS. These authors noted that among 411 patients, nearly half of those with a high-risk CACS had significant myocardial ischemia during SPECT MPI. More recent reports have failed to replicate such a high rate of ischemic defects in patients with a high-risk CACS. However, all of the results consistently report threshold relationships whereby the frequency of inducible ischemia on SPECT MPI increases substantially around a CAC score >400. For instance, Berman et al.[52] reported in a series of 1,195 patients a rate of SPECT MPI ischemia that was

<5% for CAC scores <400. A synthesis of all published series reveals that when the CACS is 400 or higher, the rate of SPECT MPI ischemia is approximately 20% (Figure 7.2).[29,56]

Berman et al.[52] also noted that in patients with a normal SPECT MPI, a surprisingly high number of patients had elevated CACS. Specifically, for the 1,119 patients with a normal SPECT MPI, 25%, 20%, and 11% had CACS from 100–399, 400–999, and ≥1,000, respectively. The frequency of significant atherosclerosis in patients with normal stress SPECT MPI exposes the limitation to SPECT MPI and uncovers the burden of disease that is undetected with 'stand alone' SPECT imaging. More than half of patients with normal SPECT MPI had a CACS >100.

It has been known for some time that patients with a greater risk factor burden, more comorbidity, or known CAD had higher rates of cardiac events in the setting of a normal SPECT MPI.[12,37,60,61] A synthesis of evidence reveals that, although the expected rate of cardiac events is < 1% for all patients, the risk of events is increased by 50% for the elderly, diabetics, those with peripheral arterial disease, known CAD, or for those with greater degrees of comorbidity and extensive atherosclerosis.[12] Thus, on average, for patients with a low-risk or normal SPECT MPI, the expected annual rate of cardiac death or nonfatal MI is 0.85% per year.[12] However, this expected yearly rate ranges from 0.6% for the clinically low-risk patients with no risk factors to 1.2% for clinically high-risk patients (e.g., diabetes, known

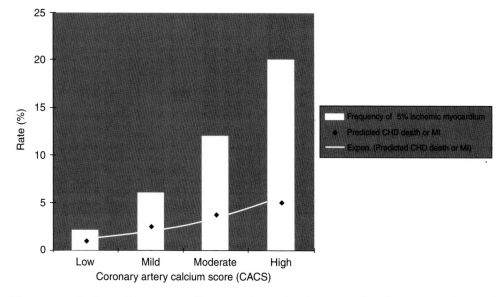

Figure 7.2 The expected relationship between the percent of ischemic myocardium from myocardial perfusion SPECT as compared with CT measurement of coronary artery calcification. Using published data, it is expected that the frequency of ≥5% ischemic myocardium is expected to increase from approximately 2% for patients with a low-risk coronary calcium score to nearly 20% for patients with high-risk coronary calcium score.

CAD, peripheral arterial disease, or extensive atherosclerosis).[12] However, visualizing high risk CACS for this subset of patients with normal SPECT MPI findings may provide a means to target patients requiring more intensive post-test management and, importantly, for excluding patients who do not require further testing or treatment.

In a recent report from Ramakrishna,[62] both the SPECT summed stress score (p = 0.009) and CACS (p = 0.005) were highly predictive of death or MI during very lengthy 10-year follow-up of 670 patients. These latter results reported a significant association of CACS and SPECT MPI findings in models estimating three outcomes: death from all causes; death or nonfatal MI; and the combination of death, nonfatal MI, or late revascularization. Furthermore, both CACS and SPECT MPI findings remained significant predictors of outcome in risk-adjusted or multivariable models controlling for diabetes, hypertension, and hypercholesterolemia. These results suggest that the combination of CACS and SPECT MPI measurements may provide a synergistic assessment of cardiac risk.

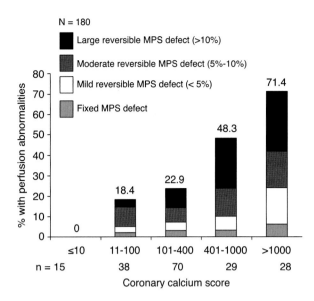

Figure 7.3 The frequency of an ischemic myocardial perfusion scan (MPS) by coronary artery calcium score measurements in type 2 diabetics.

2.6 Assessment of patients with diabetes, the metabolic syndrome, or a family history of premature CHD

With respect to the relationship between inducible ischemia and CAC scores, more recent evidence has identified selected patients in whom the likelihood for ischemia occurs at lower CAC thresholds. This includes patients who have diabetic, metabolic syndrome, or a family history of premature CHD.[51,53,55] This evidence yields a lower threshold upon which the rate of inducible ischemia increases. In such patients, the threshold for an increased rate of inducible ischemia is lower, with some suggesting that a threshold CAC ≥100 rather than a score ≥400 is a more appropriate threshold for ischemia in such patients. For instance, in a report by Wong and colleagues,[51] nearly 15% of patients with a CACS from 100–400 had inducible ischemia on SPECT MPI. This rate of ischemia was equivalent to that in patients with normal metabolic status and a CACS of 400 or higher.

Anand and colleagues[55] reported results from a controlled clinical trial of 510 asymptomatic, type-2 diabetics who underwent serial CT and SPECT MPI (Figure 7.3). SPECT MPI was peformed in all patients with a CACS >100 but also included imaging in a random sample of

53 patients with a CACS ≤ 100. In this series, diabetics with a CACS ≥100 had a nearly 4-fold higher odds of an abnormal SPECT MPI when compared to patients with lower CACS (p < 0.05). The odds of an abnormal SPECT MPI increased to ~11-fold for patients with a CACS >400 (p < 0.0001).

Two-year follow-up in this cohort of asymptomatic, type 2 diabetics revealed that both the CACS (p < 0.0001) and the percent of ischemic myocardium (p < 0.0001) were both highly predictive of major adverse cardiovascular events. In the cohort of 180 type-2 diabetics who underwent SPECT MPI, the relative risk of cardiac events was elevated 12.3-fold (95% CI = 3.4–43.7, p < 0.0001) for patients with ≥5% ischemic myocardium as compared to those with lesser or no inducible ischemia. Additionally, for those with a CACS ≥400, the relative risk for cardiovascular events was elevated up to 24-fold for patients with large reversible SPECT MPI exceeding 10% of the myocardium.

This latter report by Anand is intriguing given several prior series that attempted to establish a link between ischemic burden and diabetes through testing strategies that included initial SPECT MPI without CT.[63–65] In the observational series from Mayo Clinic, nearly 20% of asymptomatic diabetic patients had a high-risk SPECT MPI scan.[64] However, the most notable study was that of the Detection of Ischemia in Asymptomatic Diabetics (DIAD) study.[65] In this report, 1,124 patients were enrolled with 502 being randomized to undergo an adenosine Tc-99m sestamibi scan. Of the 502 asymptomatic diabetics, only 19% had provocative ischemia on SPECT MPI. These results reveal that employing direct imaging strategy that only utilize SPECT MPI will result in a lower yield in detecting at-risk patients when compared to serial imaging strategies that combine CT plus selective SPECT in patients with high-risk CACS findings. By comparison, by employing serial CT plus SPECT MPI, those with significant CACS, defined as a score >100, will have a much higher rate of ischemic abnormalities. This strategy of serial testing illustrates the principles of a multi-marker approach to risk assessment whereby risk increases additively as one examines patients with multiple risk markers (i.e., imaging abnormalities). Thus, the high frequency of silent ischemia in diabetics appears to be mediated by the extent of coronary atherosclerosis, which can be defined using CACS. Similar results have recently been published for patients with a family history of premature CHD.[53,66,67]

2.7 Serial testing paradigm with CT and SPECT MPI

Based on current evidence, Figure 7.4 details a potential clinical work-up strategy for the detection of inducible ischemia in patients undergoing CACS but also strategies targeted to selected high-risk patients including diabetics, those with metabolic syndrome, or those with a family history of premature CHD. A consensus of this evidence reveals that for all patients (excluding the high Framingham risk or other groups named above) with a CACS ≥400, subsequent stress SPECT MPI is effective at identifying at-risk patients. As mentioned earlier, approximately one-fifth of patients with a CACS ≥400 would be expected to have significant inducible ischemia. This testing strategy proposes a lower threshold of a CACS ≥100 in higher-risk patients that may include those

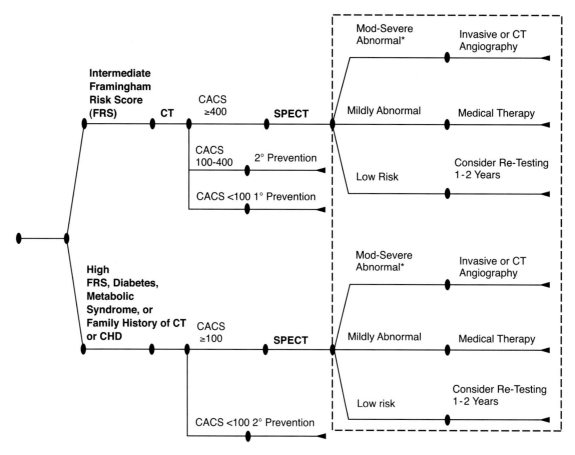

Figure 7.4 Clinical "work-up" algorithm for Intermediate Framingham Risk Score (FRS) patients as well as for high FRS, diabetics, those with the metabolic syndrome, or with a family history of premature Coronary Heart Disease (CHD). Dotted box includes patients who are candidates for treatment according to secondary prevention guidelines. (Adapted with permission from J Nucl Cardiol.[56])

with diabetes, metabolic syndrome, or patients with a family history of premature CHD. Prospective study is likely to define other potential risk factors or comorbid conditions that may alter the schema presented in this figure.

In summary, the current state of evidence for combined use of CT and SPECT MPI reveals strategies that support the use of CACS combined with serial application employing selective SPECT MPI for the detection of ischemic burden. Future strategies will allow for simultaneous assessment of combined CT-SPECT imaging. To date, current position statements from the ACC and ASNC support the use of SPECT MPI in patients with a CACS of 400 or higher. One would expect that clinically higher-risk patients with more frequent atherosclerosis have a higher rate of inducible ischemia, but do so at a significantly lower threshold of CAC.

3 DIAGNOSTIC TESTING WITH CORONARY CTA

The recent technologic advances in CT have led to a virtual explosion of interest in coronary CTA (CCTA), principally for detection and assessment of CAD. This application of CCTA provides an attractive alternative to stress testing and catheter-based coronary angiography. The principal breakthroughs in technology were increased speed of the x-ray tube rotation and increased numbers of detectors.

CCTA with multidetector CT first became feasible in 1998 when the 4 slice CT scanners were introduced. By 2005, there were 4 major manufacturers with commercially available 64-slice CT scanners with isotropic spatial resolution of ~0.4 mm. The greater coverage and speed provided by the 64-slice scanners has resulted in a reduction in the number of unevaluable segments than previously observed with scanners having fewer detectors.[31] In a recent meta-analysis by Schuijf and colleagues,[68] nearly 20% of segments were unevaluable using a 4- or 8-slice scanner as compared to <5% with more recent scanners. Additional advances in the 64-slice CT scanners include the ability to cover 20–40 mm with each rotation, thus requiring fewer heart beats for an image acquisition, in turn requiring less contrast and resulting in less heart rate increase during the procedure than with previous scanners. Total procedural time is ~10 minutes. Most centers generally also make a measurement of CAC prior to the contrast administration, as it is currently not reliably measured from contrast-enhanced images.

Over the last 5 years, numerous reports, several meta-analyses, and a position statement from the American Heart Association have addressed the correlation of CTA with x-ray angiography.[68-71] Generally, while the diagnostic accuracy of 16- as compared with 64-slice CT scanners is similar, there are fewer unevaluable segments with 64-slice scanners. Figure 7.5 details the pooled sensitivity (percent of positive studies with CAD) and specificity (percent of negative studies without CAD) from 8-, 16-, and 64-slice

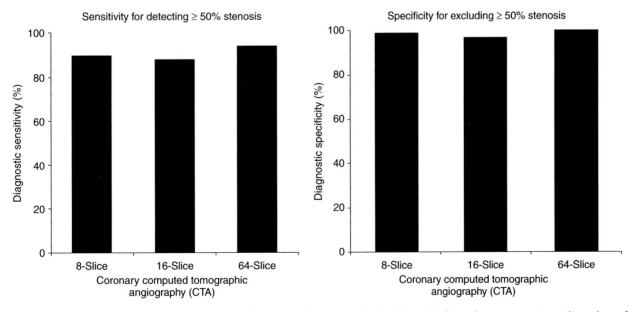

Figure 7.5 Diagnostic accuracy of Coronary Computed Tomographic Angiography based upon a systematic review of the evidence from 4-, 8-, 16-, and 64-Slice imaging. Data are presented based on a segment-based analysis. (Adapted with permission from Am J Med.[70])

CT scanners.[70] As a generalization, it appears that the sensitivity and specificity of 64-slice CT are approximately 95% and 90%, respectively. As technology improves, such as the recent introduction of the dual-source 64-slice CT scanner with temporal resolution of 83 msec, the frequency of artifacts is likely to decrease, resulting in a rise in specificity. In very small vessels (distal vessels, small branches), accuracy of CCTA declines, but such vessels are not candidates for revascularization and generally pose minimal prognostic risk (Table 7.3).[70] Thus, a relatively large and rapidly growing database supports a high degree of accuracy for detecting stenosis in all the major epicardial coronary vessels (Table 7.4),[70] and this accuracy appears to be higher than with any other noninvasive modality.

As mentioned above, current limitations for CTA include the ability to visualize the degree of coronary stenosis in segments with dense calcification. The size of the lumen as well as the distribution of calcium are major determinants as to whether an accurate estimate of coronary stenosis may be defined in a segment with dense calcification. Another limitation of imaging coronary stenosis with CCTA is the limited temporal resolution of most systems, such that there is improved image quality if resting heart rates are <65 beats/minute, minimizing coronary motion. Because of the problem of coronary motion with higher heart rates, beta-blockers are routinely given for patients with heart rates over 60 in most facilities. In general, CTA cannot be performed in patients with atrial fibrillation due

Table 7.4 Pooled diagnostic accuracy statistics of coronary computed tomographic angiography (CTA) by epicardial coronary arteries from blinded reports synthesized in the systematic review by Stein et al.

	Detection or exclusion of ≥50% stenosis	
	Sensitivity (number of reports)	Specificity (number of reports)
Left main artery		
16 slice	100% (8)	100% (6)
64 slice	100% (1)	100% (1)
Left anterior descending artery		
16 slice	90% (8)	84% (2)
64 slice	95% (1)	95% (1)
Left circumflex artery		
16 slice	82% (8)	89% (2)
64 slice	94% (1)	92% (1)
Right coronary artery		
16 slice	91% (8)	87% (2)
64 slice	93% (1)	96% (1)

to resultant beats/minute motion artifact. The speed of the recently released dual source CT system may make the scanning of these patients possible. In this regard, we have recently observed good image quality in several patients in atrial fibrillation and with varying heart rates when using the dual source CT (Figure 7.6).

Both CTA and SPECT MPI have a radiation burden associated with scanning. Even when dose modulation is performed to reduce radiation exposure during systole, CTA have similar exposures to SPECT MPI in the range of 10–20 mSev.[11] Several new developments in CTA are focused on reducing this exposure, and preliminary observations have suggested that if single phase imaging is used, greater dose modulation and/or lower KeV may result in an order of magnitude reduction in radiation exposure may already be achievable.

The estimation of the degree of coronary stenosis by CTA is not presently as highly correlated with segmental assessment by x-ray angiography as is the detection of stenosis *per se*. In general, the degree of coronary stenosis is overestimated by CTA. Raff and colleagues[72] recently reported that a 50% stenosis estimated by CTA can range from 25% to 75% by quantitative x-ray angiography. Practically, when 25% to 75% of lesions are the maximum observed by CCTA, additional testing is often recommended. In this latter case, SPECT or PET MPI, stress echocardiography, or stress MRI may be useful to define the functional significance of CTA-identified borderline stenoses.[11]

Table 7.3 Pooled diagnostic accuracy statistics evaluating the accuracy of coronary computed tomographic angiography (CTA) for detection and exclusion ≥50% stenosis for proximal, mid, and distal arterial segments from blinded reports synthesized in the systematic review by Stein et al.

	Detection or exclusion of ≥50% stenosis	
	Sensitivity (number of reports)	Specificity (number of reports)
Proximal segments (excluding left main stenosis)		
16 slice	90% (6)	95% (5)
64 slice	100% (1)	96% (1)
Mid segments		
16 slice	95% (5)	94% (4)
64 slice	94% (1)	90% (1)
Distal segments		
16 slice	83% (5)	97% (4)
64 slice	79% (1)	96% (1)

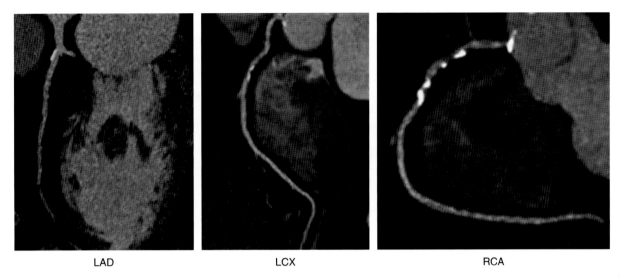

LAD   LCX   RCA

Figure 7.6 Dual-source coronary CT angiogram of a 62-year-old male with recent atrial fibrillation showing normal coronary arteries except calcified plaque with < 25% narrowing in mid and distal LAD. Left ventricular ejection fraction was 32%. Coronary calcium score was 237. The maximum heart rate during contrast injection was 88–133. Courtesy of Cedars-Sinai Medical Center.

A less-explored capability of CCTA is its ability to visualize the arterial wall and the potential to assess the burden of non-calcified plaque.[31] Currently, this assessment is a research tool, pending further development and clinical validation. The CT acquisition used for coronary CTA is also used to examine ventricular function, sizes of the cardiac chambers, LV mass, the pericardium, and cardiac valves. While some investigators are exploring the use of the single-contrast injection for assessment of coronary stenosis, pulmonary emboli, and aortic dissection (i.e., the "triple rule-out"), this approach is not currently in wide use since it compromises the quality of the examination for one of the organs involved.

3.1 CTA as the initial test

CTA is currently considered the test of choice for evaluation of coronary anomalies found or suspected at the time of cardiac catheterization. CTA may also become an effective initial test to discern ischemic from nonischemic cardiomyopathy. Given the high accuracy noted in the published literature for coronary CTA, it is not surprising that some "early adopters" have also proposed that CTA may become the initial test of choice for symptomatic patients with suspected CAD, potentially replacing SPECT MPI with this diagnostic application across the spectrum of pretest likelihood of CAD. Investigators in the field have proposed that coronary CTA may have its greatest advantage over stress testing as an initial test in patients with a low-intermediate likelihood of CAD. Thus far, the comparative accuracy of rest/stress SPECT MPI to coronary CTA has only been studied in one report including only 114 patients.[73] These investigators reported a high rate of normal SPECT MPI findings in patients with obstructive CAD noted on CTA and x-ray angiography (Figure 7.7). While some believe that this finding relates to the insensitivity of SPECT MPI, others suggest that these findings relate to an overestimation

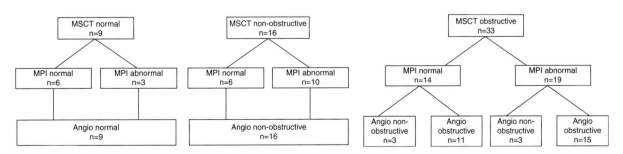

Figure 7.7 Relation between findings on multi-slice computed tomography (MSCT), myocardial perfusion imaging (MPI), and invasive coronary angiography (angio). (Adapted with permission from Am J Coll Cardiol.[73])

of stenosis severity by coronary CTA.[74] Further studies in larger patient series as well as prognostic data are needed to refine the comparative accuracy of CTA as compared to SPECT MPI. A large registry is currently underway which may provide additional data on this subject (SPARC).

3.2 Coronary CTA after SPECT MPI

A widely accepted indication of coronary CTA on clinical grounds is for a follow-up evaluation of patients with equivocal stress tests. While, in the past, some of these patients may have undergone an invasive coronary angiography in order to resolve diagnostic doubt, the very high negative predictive value of a coronary CTA allows this new procedure to be definitive in a large proportion of patients with equivocal stress tests. Quite possibly, data will emerge in which the same reasoning can be applied to patients with mild ischemia on SPECT MPI, as well as those with a positive stress electrocardiogram or exercise-induced chest pain in the setting of normal SPECT MPI, and those with persistent chest pain following a normal SPECT MPI (Figure 7.8). With regards to the latter, it is possible that in some patients SPECT MPI findings may even be normal but undetected due to diffuse subendocardial ischemia.[75] It has also been proposed that cardiovascular magnetic

resonance imaging may play a secondary role in testing patients with symptoms suggestive of myocardial ischemia yet normal SPECT MPI due to its ability to detect subendocardial ischemia.[76] Thus, it would appear that the relatively high frequency of normal invasive coronary angiography in patients after equivocal, mildly abnormal, or discordant stress test results may decline as CCTA becomes more widely used in these settings of clinical uncertainty. However, data supporting this application are limited.

3.3 Hybrid applications of SPECT-CT

Recent developments in instrumentation have combined both SPECT or PET MPI and CT into a single imaging device (e.g., SPECT/CT, PET/CT). These devices allow for combined assessment of myocardial perfusion, ventricular function, and CT defined CAC and CCTA. Hybrid PET/CT devices have become the standard for current PET machines. Almost all new PET systems available in the US are now combined with a high-resolution CT scan.

SPECT/CT systems are also now available from several manufacturers. The initial interest in the development of SPECT/CT was for attenuation correction, resulting in improved diagnostic specificity.[77–80] It is also possible on these newer systems to acquire a CAC scan, thus providing

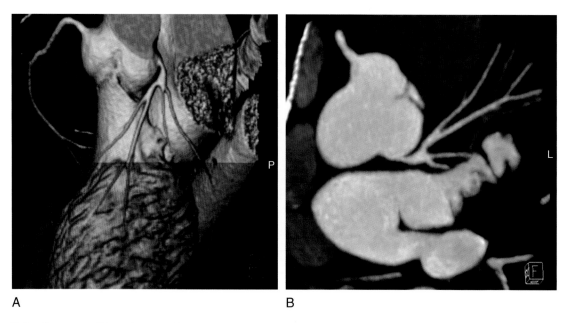

A   B

Figure 7.8   Coronary CT angiogram of a 53-year-old female with recent onset dyspnea and atypical chest pain showing >70% narrowing at ostial left main coronary artery, which subsequently revealed a 90% stenosis by conventional coronary angiography. Coronary calcium score was 0. The result of exercise SPECT myocardial perfusion imaging was borderline with ischemic stress ECG.

some anatomic information that can be combined with the myocardial perfusion findings. Recently, SPECT/CT systems with 64-slice CT have become available, allowing assessment of myocardial blood flow combined with coronary CTA findings. Although the use of coronary CT angiography may be a more precise measure than coronary calcium, its use in asymptomatic populations, given the radiation burden of combining CCTA with SPECT or PET MPI may be excessive for routine applications. Thus, the combination of the CACS as a marker for underlying disease with stress SPECT or PET MPI findings may prove to be an effective combination for improved disease detection and risk assessment.

There are presently only a small number of hybrid SPECT-CT systems in clinical use in the US. Current use is limited, in part, due to a current lack of evidence supporting the added value of anatomic CAC data with SPECT MPI findings. Based on current technology and data, the selective sequential imaging strategies, as discussed above, are likely to prevail over the use of the hybrid devices when both CCTA and MPI information is desired.

3.4 Clinical management strategies using MPI and CT

Optimal test strategies must be based on the specific clinical question being asked to be answered. In cardiology today, there are three core questions that clinicians need to ask regarding their approach to evaluating patients in clinical practice: (1) how to optimize early detection of atherosclerotic disease; (2) how to best diagnosis CAD in patients with possible cardiac symptoms? and (3) how to best assess the prognosis in patients with intermediate- to high-CAD likelihood?

3.5 Early detection of atherosclerosis

The issue of early detection of CAD should be differentiated from "screening" for CAD. Screening is currently accepted for certain select populations, such as the evaluation of individuals in high-risk occupations including pilots, firemen, or policemen, but there is unanimous agreement that widespread screening for CAD using stress testing is not advisable. Widespread testing for early disease detection using CAC scanning is also not widely practiced, but just such a

policy has recently been suggested[81] (Figure 7.9) for men >45 years and women >55 years, as a means of improving the estimation of individuals' long-term risk of cardiac death or nonfatal myocardial infarction.

When there is a clinical concern over a patient's cardiac risk factor burden, insurance companies appear increasingly supportive of an evaluation focusing on early detection of atherosclerotic disease. This would generally include patients with an intermediate Framingham risk score or those middle-aged adults with 2 or more cardiac risk factors. Other subsets, as discussed above, also include diabetics, those with metabolic syndrome, high-sensitivity C-reactive protein ≥ 3 mg/dl, or those patients with a family history of premature coronary heart disease. As discussed in Chapter 7, it is prudent for clinicians to not rely solely on a patient's Framingham risk score as a guide to testing, as it performs poorly in detecting risk in the young, women, and for those of diverse ethnicity (see chapter by Shaw). Thus, if a clinician believes other risk factors or co-morbidity is present, especially the presence of risk factors not included in the Framingham risk score, then testing for early detection of CAD may be warranted.

3.6 Diagnosis of CAD

Diagnostic testing using MPI is optimally applied in patients with an intermediate likelihood of CAD. In addition to defining the likely presence of a significant coronary lesion(s), such testing benefits clinical management by providing accurate estimation of patients' near term risk of major adverse cardiac events. For this latter question, the intensity of management is then based on the patient's risk estimate, with higher-risk patients receiving more intensive and early aggressive care. The chief management decision in the high risk patient is whether revascularization or medical therapy would be helpful in improving outcome. By comparison, lower risk patients require nothing more than a "watchful waiting" approach with follow-up limited to an evaluation for worsening symptoms at perhaps 1–2 years following the initial diagnostic test to re-assess patient risk.

Over the past few decades, both stress SPECT MPI and stress echocardiography have been the tests of choice for evaluation of the intermediate-risk patient. Future study will examine the relative use of CTA in such patients as well. Potentially, CTA could become the preferred first test in some defined diagnostic subgroups as proposed recently.[16,73] However, often, early evidence for any imaging modality is more selected and exhibits more favorable

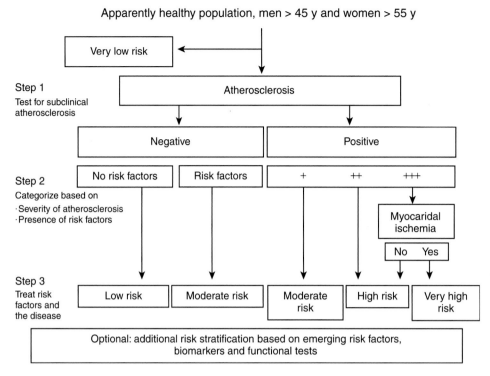

Figure 7.9   An approach to screening for atherosclerosis advocated by the Association for the Eradication of Heart Attacks (AHEA). Y = years. (Adapted with permission from Am J Cardiol.[81])

results. Validation of the early, favorable diagnostic accuracy data with coronary CTA in larger, diverse patient profiles will thus be important for continued development of this field. One can also envision a role for coronary CTA as a secondary test for patients with an equivocal SPECT MPI or echocardiogram, or in other cohorts of patients previously mentioned, including those with mildly abnormal test results or those with a normal SPECT MPI and abnormal stress electrocardiogram or those with other clinical reasons to suspect a false-negative SPECT study.

3.7 Risk stratification in patients with high CAD likelihood

High CAD likelihood patients are generally not candidates for diagnostic testing but may be referred for evaluation of their ischemic burden and for risk stratification purposes. Additionally, for medically treated patients, or for those with significant comorbidities, there may be a need to assess the extent and severity of SPECT MPI ischemia in order to more effectively guide medical decision making. There is evidence that these patients are excellent candidates for SPECT MPI with currently no support for the use of coronary CTA in

such patients. A recent study of over 1,000 patients with a high pre-scan likelihood of CAD from our group reported that initial testing with SPECT MPI was more cost effective than direct invasive coronary angiography.[5] Approximately 60% of these patients with normal MPI results associated with less than a 1% annual event rate as noted above. On the other hand, there has been no published data regarding the cost-effective application of CCTA in the general population of patients with a high pretest likelihood of CAD. Since CCTA is highly likely to be abnormal in their patients, CTA may not commonly result in a decision not to proceed to coronary angiography, while with SPECT, as noted above, this more frequently occurs.[82] As data regarding risk stratification by CCTA emerges over the next few years, CCTA could become useful in subgroups of these patients.

Using this paradigm of initial testing with SPECT MPI, selective invasive angiography would be reserved for patients with moderate to severe ischemia.[83] Of the remaining patients without inducible ischemia, their risk of major adverse cardiac events is low and medical management for control of symptoms and for risk factor modification has been shown to be most efficacious and clinically effective. Among patients with mild ischemia on SPECT MPI, a portion may benefit from additional risk stratification with CAC or with coronary CTA.

Table 7.5 American College of Cardiology / American Heart Association Criteria for pretest likelihood of CAD. Candidates for cardiac imaging are highlighted (in bold) as those with an intermediate pretest CAD likelihood. High-likelihood patients may also be candidates for stress MPS (and are italicized below).

Women				Men			
Age (y)	Typical angina	Atypical angina	Nonanginal chest pain	Age(y)	Typical angina	Atypical angina	Nonanginal chest pain
30–39	Intermediate	Low	Low	30–39	High	Intermediate	Low
40–49	Intermediate	Intermediate	Low	40–49	High	Intermediate	Low
50–59	Intermediate	Intermediate	Low	50–59	High	Intermediate	Intermediate
60–69	High	Intermediate	Intermediate	60–69	High	Intermediate	Intermediate
≥70	High	Intermediate	Intermediate	≥70	High	High	Intermediate

Reference: The ACC guidelines for stable angina

The latter decision would be based largely on their clinical risk, with higher-risk patients perhaps benefiting from a coronary CTA to eliminate high-risk angiographic disease.

While the dramatic improvements in CT have clearly caught the attention of clinical cardiologists for defining coronary anatomy, we believe the prominent role of the functional information provided by stress MPI in management of patients with CAD will not only continue but is likely to grow further over time, providing complementary information to CT.

REFERENCES

1. Gould KL, Lipscomb K. Effects of coronary stenoses on coronary flow reserve and resistance. Am J Cardiol. Jul 1974; 34(1): 48–55.
2. Aboul-Enein F, Hayes SW, Matsumoto N, et al. Rest Perfusion Defects in Patients with No History of Myocrdial Infarction Predict the Presence of a Critical Coronary Artery Stenosis. J Nucl Cardiol. 2003; 10: 656–62.
3. Diamond GA, Forrester JS. Analysis of probability as an aid in the clinical diagnosis of coronary-artery disease. N Engl J Med. 1979; 300(24): 1350–8.
4. Klocke FJ, Baird MG, Lorell BH, et al. ACC/AHA/ASNC Guidelines for the Clinical Use of Cardiac Radionuclide Imaging-Executive Summary. A Report of the American College of Cardiology/American Heart Association Task Force on Practice Guidelines (ACC/AHA/ASNC Committee to Revise the 1995 Guidelines for the Clinical Use of Cardiac Radionuclide Imaging). Circulation 2003; 108: 1404–18.
5. Hachamovitch R, Hayes SW, Friedman JD, Cohen I, Berman DS. Stress Myocardial Perfusion SPECT is Clinically Effective and Cost-effective in Risk-stratification of Patients with a High Likelihood of CAD but No Known CAD. J Am Coll Cardiol. 2004; 43: 200–8.
6. Poornima IG, Miller TD, Christian TF, et al. Utility of myocardial perfusion imaging in patients with low-risk treadmill scores. J Am Coll Cardiol. 2004; 43(2): 194–9.
7. Hachamovitch R, Hayes SW, Friedman JD, Cohen I, Berman DS. Comparison of the short-term survival benefit associated with revascularization compared with medical therapy in patients with no prior coronary artery disease undergoing stress myocardial perfusion single photon emission computed tomography. Circulation 2003; 107(23): 2900–7.
8. Gibbons RJ, Abrams J, Chatterjee K, et al. ACC/AHA 2002 guideline update for the management of patients with chronic stable angina—summary article: a report of the American College of Cardiology/ American Heart Association Task Force on Practice Guidelines (Committee on the Management of Patients With Chronic Stable Angina). Circulation 2003; 107(1): 149–58.
9. Gibbons RJ, Chatterjee K, Daley J, et al. ACC/AHA/ACP-ASIM guidelines for the management of patients with chronic stable angina: a report of the American College of Cardiology/American Heart Association Task Force on Practice Guidelines (Committee on Management of Patients With Chronic Stable Angina). J Am Coll Cardiol. Jun 1999; 33(7): 2092–97.
10. Gibbons RJ, Balady GJ, Bricker JT, et al. ACC/AHA 2002 guideline update for exercise testing: summary article: a report of the American College of Cardiology/American Heart Association Task Force on Practice Guidelines (Committee to Update the 1997 Exercise Testing Guidelines). Circulation 2002; 106(14): 1883–92.
11. Berman DS, Shaw LJ, Hachamovitch R, et al. Comparative use of radionuclide stress testing, coronary artery calcium scanning, and noninvasive coronary angiography for diagnostic and prognostic cardiac assessment. Semin Nucl Med. Jan 2007; 37(1): 2–16.
12. Shaw LJ, Iskandrian AE. Prognostic value of gated myocardial perfusion SPECT. J Nucl Cardiol. Mar–Apr 2004; 11(2): 171–85.
13. Metz LD, Beattie M, Hom R, et al. The prognostic value of normal exercise myocardial perfusion imaging and exercise echocardiography: a meta-analysis. J Am Coll Cardiol. Jan 16 2007; 49(2): 227–37.

14. Shaw LJ, Hendel RC, Borges-Neto S, et al. Prognsotic value of normal exercise and adenosine (99m)Tc-tetrofosmin SPECT imaging: results from the multicenter registry of 4,728 patients. J Nucl Med. 2003; 44(2): 134–9.

15. Underwood SR, Anagnostopoulos C, Cerqueira M, et al. Myocardial perfusion scintigraphy: the evidence. Eur J Nucl Med Mol Imaging. Feb 2004; 31(2): 261–91.

16. Berman DS, Hachamovitch R, Shaw LJ, et al. Roles of nuclear cardiology, cardiac computed tomography, and cardiac magnetic resonance: noninvasive risk stratification and a conceptual framework for the selection of noninvasive imaging tests in patients with known or suspected coronary artery disease. J Nucl Med. 2006; 47: 1107–18.

17. Underwood SR, Shaw LJ, Anagnostopoulos C, et al. Myocardial perfusion scintigraphy and cost effectiveness of diagnosis and management of coronary heart disease. Heart Aug 2004; 90 Suppl 5: v34–6.

18. Berman DS, Abidov A, Kang X, et al. Prognostic validation of a 17-segment score derived from a 20-segment score for myocardial perfusion SPECT interpretation. J Nucl Cardiol. 2004; 11: 414–23.

19. Shaw LJ, Berman DS, Hendel RC, et al. Cardiovascular disease risk stratification with stress single-photon emission computed tomography technetium-99m tetrofosmin imaging in patients with the metabolic syndrome and diabetes mellitus. Am J Cardiol. May 15 2006; 97(10): 1538–44.

20. Hachamovitch R, Rozanski A, Hayes SW, et al. Predicting therapeutic benefit from myocardial revascularization procedures: Are measurements of both resting left ventricular ejection fraction and stress-induced myocardial ischemia necessary? J Nucl Cardiol. 2006; 13: 768–78.

21. Mowatt G, Vale L, Brazzelli M, et al. Systematic review of the effectiveness and cost-effectiveness, and economic evaluation, of myocardial perfusion scintigraphy for the diagnosis and management of angina and myocardial infarction. Health Technol Assess. Jul 2004; 8(30): iii–iv, 1–207.

22. Abidov A, Bax JJ, Hayes SW, et al. Integration of automatically measured transient ischemic dilation ratio into interpretation of adenosine stress myocardial perfusion SPECT for detection of severe and extensive CAD. J Nuc Med. 2004; 45: 1999–2007.

23. Sharir T, Berman DS, Waechter PB, et al. Quantitative analysis of regional motion and thickening by gated myocardial perfusion SPECT: normal heterogeneity and criteria for abnormality. J Nucl Med. 2001; 42(11): 1630–38.

24. Johnson LL, Verdesca SA, Aude WY, et al. Postischemic stunning can affect left ventricular ejection fraction and regional wall motion on post-stress gated sestamibi tomograms [see comments]. J Am Coll Cardiol. 1997; 30(7): 1641–8.

25. Bacher-Stier C, Sharir T, Kavanagh PB, et al. Postexercise lung uptake of 99mTc-sestamibi determined by a new automatic technique: validation and application in detection of severe and extensive coronary artery disease and reduced left ventricular function. J Nucl Med. Jul 2000; 41(7): 1190–7.

26. Abidov A, Rozanski A, Hachamovitch R, et al. Complaints of dyspnea among patients referred for cardiac stress testing. New Eng J Med. 2005; 353: 1889–98.

27. O'Rourke RA, Brundage BH, Froelicher VF, et al. American College of Cardiology/American Heart Association Expert Consensus document on electron-beam computed tomography for the diagnosis and prognosis of coronary artery disease. Circulation Jul 4 2000; 102(1): 126–40.

28. Diamond GA, Forrester JS, Hirsch M, et al. Application of conditional probability analysis to the clinical diagnosis of coronary artery disease. J Clin Invest. 1980; 65(5): 1210–21.

29. Greenland P, Bonow RO, Brundage BH, et al. ACCF/AHA 2007 clinical expert consensus document on coronary artery calcium scoring by computed tomography in global cardiovascular risk assessment and in evaluation of patients with chest pain: a report of the American College of Cardiology Foundation Clinical Expert Consensus Task Force (ACCF/AHA Writing Committee to Update the 2000 Expert Consensus Document on Electron Beam Computed Tomography). Circulation 2007; 115(3): 402–26.

30. Glagov S, Weisenberg E, Zarins CK, Stankunavicius R, Kolettis GJ. Compensatory enlargement of human atherosclerotic coronary arteries. N Engl J Med. May 28 1987; 316(22): 1371–5.

31. Budoff MJ, Achenbach S, Blumenthal RS, et al. Assessment of coronary artery disease by cardiac computed tomography: a scientific statement from the American Heart Association Committee on Cardiovascular Imaging and Intervention, Council on Cardiovascular Radiology and Intervention, and Committee on Cardiac Imaging, Council on Clinical Cardiology. Circulation Oct 17 2006; 114(16): 1761–91.

32. Rumberger JA, Simons DB, Fitzpatrick LA, Sheedy PF, Schwartz RS. Coronary artery calcium area by electron-beam computed tomography and coronary atherosclerotic plaque area. A histopathologic correlative study. Circulation Oct 15 1995; 92(8): 2157–62.

33. Agatston AS, Janowitz WR, Hildner FJ, et al. Quantification of coronary artery calcium using ultrafast computed tomography. J Am Coll Cardiol. Mar 15 1990; 15(4): 827–32.

34. Callister TQ, Raggi P, Cooil B, Lippolis NJ, Russo DJ. Effect of HMG-CoA reductase inhibitors on coronary artery disease as assessed by electron-beam computed tomography. N Engl J Med. Dec 31 1998; 339(27): 1972–78.

35. Raggi P, Callister TQ, Shaw LJ. Progression of coronary artery calcium and risk of first myocardial infarction in patients receiving cholesterol-lowering therapy. Arterioscler Thromb Vasc Biol. Jul 2004; 24(7): 1272–77.

36. Hoff JA, Chomka EV, Krainik AJ, et al. Age and gender distributions of coronary artery calcium detected by electron beam tomography in 35,246 adults. Am J Cardiol. Jun 15 2001; 87(12): 1335–39.

37. Mieres JH, Shaw LJ, Arai A, et al. Role of noninvasive testing in the clinical evaluation of women with suspected coronary artery disease: consensus statement from the Cardiac Imaging Committee, Council on Clinical Cardiology, and the Cardiovascular Imaging and Intervention Committee, Council on Cardiovascular Radiology and Intervention, American Heart Association. Circulation Feb 8 2005; 111(5): 682–96.

38. Goff DC, Jr., Bertoni AG, Kramer H, et al. Dyslipidemia prevalence, treatment, and control in the Multi-Ethnic Study of Atherosclerosis (MESA): gender, ethnicity, and coronary artery calcium. Circulation Feb 7 2006; 113(5): 647–56.

39. Greenland P, LaBree L, Azen SP, Doherty TM, Detrano RC. Coronary artery calcium score combined with Framingham score for risk prediction in asymptomatic individuals. Jama Jan 14 2004; 291(2): 210–15.

40. Arad Y, Goodman KJ, Roth M, Newstein D, Guerci AD. Coronary calcification, coronary disease risk factors, C-reactive protein, and atherosclerotic disease events: the St. Francis Heart Study. J Am Coll Cardiol. 2005; 46: 158–65.

41. LaMonte MJ, FitzGerald SJ, Church TS, et al. Coronary artery calcium score and coronary heart disease events in a large cohort of asymptomatic men and women. Am J Epidemiol. Sep 1 2005; 162(5): 421–29.

42. Shaw LJ, Raggi P, Schisterman E, Berman DS, Callister TQ. Prognostic value of cardiac risk factors and coronary artery calcium screening for all-cause mortality. Radiology Sep 2003; 228(3): 826–33.

43. Budoff MJ, Achenbach S, Fayad Z, et al. Task Force 12: training in advanced cardiovascular imaging (computed tomography): endorsed by the American Society of Nuclear Cardiology, Society for Cardiovascular Angiography and Interventions, Society of Atherosclerosis Imaging and Prevention, and Society of Cardiovascular Computed Tomography. J Am Coll Cardiol. Feb 21 2006; 47(4): 915–20.

44. Vliegenthart R, Oudkerk M, Hofman A, et al. Coronary calcification improves cardiovascular risk prediction in the elderly. Circulation Jul 26 2005; 112(4): 572–7.

45. Taylor AJ, Bindeman J, Feuerstein I, et al. Coronary calcium independently predicts incident premature coronary heart disease over measured cardiovascular risk factors: mean 3-year outcomes in the prospective army coronary calcium project. J Am Coll Cardiol. 2005; 46: 807–14.

46. Kondos GT, Hoff JA, Sevrukov A, et al. Electron-beam tomography coronary artery calcium and cardiac events: a 37-month follow-up of 5635 initially asymptomatic low- to intermediate-risk adults. Circulation May 27 2003; 107(20): 2571–6.

47. Raggi P, Shaw LJ, Berman DS, Callister TQ. Prognostic value of coronary artery calcium screening in subjects with and without diabetes. J Am Coll Cardiol. May 5 2004; 43(9): 1663–9.

48. Raggi P, Shaw LJ, Berman DS, Callister TQ. Gender-based differences in the prognostic value of coronary calcification. J Womens Health (Larchmt). Apr 2004; 13(3): 273–83.

49. Budoff MJ, Shaw LJ, Liu ST. Long-term prognosis associated with coronary calcification: observations from a registry of 25,253 patients. J Am Coll Cardiol. 2007: In press.

50. He ZX, Hedrick TD, Pratt CM, et al. Severity of coronary artery calcification by electron beam computed tomography predicts silent myocardial ischemia. Circulation 2000; 101(3): 244–51.

51. Wong ND, Rozanski A, Gransar H, et al. Metabolic syndrome and diabetes are associated with an increased likelihood of inducible myocardial ischemia among patients with subclinical atherosclerosis. Diabetes Care 2005; 28: 1445–50.

52. Berman DS, Wong ND, Gransar H, et al. Relationship between stress-induced myocardial ischemia and atherosclerosis measured by coronary calcium tomography. J Am Coll Cardiol. 2004; 44: 923–30.

53. Blumenthal RS, Becker DM, Yanek LR, et al. Comparison of coronary calcium and stress myocardial perfusion imaging in apparently healthy siblings of individuals with premature coronary artery disease. Am J Cardiol. Feb 1 2006; 97(3): 328–33.

54. Moser KW, O'Keefe JH, Bateman TM, McGhie IA. Coronary calcium screening in asymptomatic patients as a guide to risk factor modification and stress myocardial perfusion imaging. J Nucl Cardiol. 2003; 10: 590–8.

55. Anand DV, Lim E, Hopkins D, et al. Risk stratification in uncomplicated type 2 diabetes: prospective evaluation of the combined use of coronary artery calcium imaging and selective myocardial perfusion scintigraphy. Eur Heart J. Mar 2006; 27(6): 713–21.

56. Shaw LJ, Berman DS, Bax JJ, et al. Computed tomographic imaging within nuclear cardiology. J Nucl Cardiol. 2005; 12: 131–42.

57. Ramakrishna G, Breen JF, Mulvagh SL, McCully RB, Pellikka PA. Relationship between coronary artery calcification detected by electron-beam computed tomography and abnormal stress echocardiography: association and prognostic implications. J Am Coll Cardiol. Nov 21 2006; 48(10): 2125–31.

58. Miller TD, Breen JF, Araoz PD, Hodge DO, Gibbons RJ. Relationship and Prognostic Value of Coronary Artery Calcification by Electron Beam Computed Tomography to Stress-induced Ischemia by Single Photon Emission Computed Tomography. Am Heart J. 2007: In press.

59. Hendel RC, Patel MR, Kramer CM, et al. ACCF/ACR/SCCT/SCMR/ASNC/NASCI/SCAI/SIR 2006 appropriateness criteria for cardiac computed tomography and cardiac magnetic resonance imaging: a report of the American College of Cardiology Foundation Quality Strategic Directions Committee Appropriateness Criteria Working Group, American College of Radiology, Society of Cardiovascular Computed Tomography, Society for Cardiovascular Magnetic Resonance, American Society of Nuclear Cardiology, North American Society for Cardiac Imaging, Society for Cardiovascular Angiography and Interventions, and Society of Interventional Radiology. J Am Coll Cardiol. Oct 3 2006; 48(7): 1475–97.

60. Hachamovitch R, Hayes S, Friedman JD, et al. Determinants of risk and its temporal variation in patients with normal stress myocardial perfusion scans: what is the warranty period of a normal scan? J Am Coll Cardiol. 2003; 41(8): 1329–40.

61. Kang X, Berman DS, Lewin HC, et al. Incremental prognostic value of myocardial perfusion single photon emission computed tomography in patients with diabetes mellitus. Am Heart J. Dec 1999; 138(6 Pt 1): 1025–32.

62. Ramakrishna G, Miller TD, Breen JF, et al. Relationship and Prognostic Value of Coronary Artery Calcification by Electron Beam Computed Tomography to Stress-induced Ischemia by Single Photon Emission Computed Tomography. Am Heart J. 2007: In press.

63. De Lorenzo A, Lima RS, Siqueira-Filho AG, Pantoja MR. Prevalence and prognostic value of perfusion defects detected by stress technetium-99m sestamibi myocardial perfusion single-photon emission computed tomography in asymptomatic patients with diabetes mellitus and no known coronary artery disease. Am J Cardiol. Oct 15 2002; 90(8): 827–32.

64. Miller TD, Rajagopalan N, Hodge DO, Frye RL, Gibbons RJ. Yield of stress single-photon emission computed tomography in asymptomatic patients with diabetes. Am Heart J. May 2004; 147(5): 890–6.

65. Wackers FJ, Young LH, Inzucchi SE, et al. Detection of silent myocardial ischemia in asymptomatic diabetic subjects: the DIAD study. Diabetes Care Aug 2004; 27(8): 1954–61.

66. Blumenthal RS, Becker DM, Moy TF, et al. Exercise thallium tomography predicts future clinically manifest coronary heart disease in a high-risk asymptomatic population. Circulation Mar 1 1996; 93(5): 915–23.

67. Blumenthal RS, Becker DM, Yanek LR, et al. Detecting occult coronary disease in a high-risk asymptomatic population. Circulation Feb 11 2003; 107(5): 702–7.

68. Schuijf JD, Bax JJ, Shaw LJ, et al. Meta-analysis of comparative diagnostic performance of magnetic resonance imaging

and multislice computed tomography for noninvasive coronary angiography. Am Heart J. Feb 2006; 151(2): 404–11.

69. Budoff MJ, Diamond GA, Raggi P, et al. Continuous probabilistic prediction of angiographically significant coronary artery disease using electron beam tomography. Circulation Apr 16 2002; 105(15): 1791–6.

70. Stein PD, Beemath A, Kayali F, et al. Multidetector computed tomography for the diagnosis of coronary artery disease: a systematic review. Am J Med. Mar 2006; 119(3): 203–16.

71. Achenbach S. Computed tomography coronary angiography. J Am Coll Cardiol. Nov 21 2006; 48(10): 1919–28.

72. Raff GL, Gallagher MJ, O'Neill WW, Goldstein JA. Diagnostic accuracy of noninvasive coronary angiography using 64-slice spiral computed tomography. J Am Coll Cardiol. Aug 2 2005; 46(3): 552–57.

73. Schuijf JD, Wijns W, Jukema JW, et al. Relationship between noninvasive coronary angiography with multi-slice computed tomography and myocardial perfusion imaging. J Am Coll Cardiol. Dec 19 2006; 48(12): 2508–14.

74. Dorbala S, Hachamovitch R, Di Carli MF. Myocardial perfusion imaging and multidetector computed tomographic coronary angiography: appropriate for all patients with suspected coronary artery disease? J Am Coll Cardiol. Dec 19 2006; 48(12): 2515–17.

75. Duvernoy CS, Ficaro EP, Karabajakian MZ, Rose PA, Corbett JR. Improved detection of left main coronary artery disease with attenuation-corrected SPECT. J Nucl Cardiol. Nov–Dec 2000; 7(6): 639–48.

76. Panting JR, Gatehouse PD, Yang GZ, et al. Abnormal subendocardial perfusion in cardiac syndrome X detected by cardiovascular magnetic resonance imaging. N Engl J Med. Jun 20 2002; 346(25): 1948–53.

77. Masood Y, Liu YH, Depuey G, et al. Clinical validation of SPECT attenuation correction using x-ray computed tomography-derived attenuation maps: multicenter clinical trial with angiographic correlation. J Nucl Cardiol. Nov–Dec 2005; 12(6): 676–86.

78. Fricke E, Fricke H, Weise R, et al. Attenuation correction of myocardial SPECT perfusion images with low-dose CT: evaluation of the method by comparison with perfusion PET. J Nucl Med. May 2005; 46(5): 736–44.

79. Dondi M, Fagioli G, Salgarello M, et al. Myocardial SPECT: what do we gain from attenuation correction (and when)? Q J Nucl Med Mol Imaging Sep 2004; 48(3): 181–7.

80. Duvall WL, Croft LB, Corriel JS, et al. SPECT myocardial perfusion imaging in morbidly obese patients: image quality, hemodynamic response to pharmacologic stress, and diagnostic and prognostic value. J Nucl Cardiol. Mar–Apr 2006; 13(2): 202–9.

81. Naghavi M, Falk E, Hecht HS, et al. From Vulnerable Plaque to Vulnerable Patient-Part III: Executive Summary of the Screening for Heart Attack Prevention and Education (SHAPE) Task Force Report. Am J Cardiol. 2006; 98: 2–15.

82. Hachamovitch R, Hayes SW, Friedman JD, et al. Is there a referral bias against revascularization of patients with reduced LV ejection fraction? Influence of ejection fraction and inducible ischemia on post-SPECT management of patients without history of CAD. J Am Coll Cardiol. 2003; 42: 1286–94.

83. Shaw LJ, Hachamovitch R, Berman DS, et al. The economic consequences of available diagnostic and prognostic strategies for the evaluation of stable angina patients: an observational assessment of the value of precatheterization ischemia. J Am Coll Cardiol. 1999; 33(3): 661–9.

84. Rozanski A, Gransar H, Wong ND, Shaw LJ, Miranda-Peats R, Polk D, Hayes SW, Friedman JD, Berman DS. Clinical Outcomes After Both Coronary Calcium Scanning and Exercise Myocardial Perfusion Scintigraphy. J Am Coll Cardiol 2007; 49: 1352–61.

8

Measurement of Coronary Artery Calcium by Computed Tomography

Thomas C. Gerber, Christoph R. Becker, and Birgit Kantor

The association between vascular calcification and vascular atherosclerosis has been known to anatomists and pathologists for centuries. The value of coronary artery calcification (CAC) for predicting the presence of coronary artery disease and the occurrence of future cardiac events is discussed in detail elsewhere in this book in chapters 9 (Knez A) and 10 (Shaw LJ et al.). In short, calcium is deposited in diseased coronary arteries in the form of hydroxyapatite, which contains 40% calcium by weight. The area of CAC is proportional to, but represents only approximately 20 percent of, the coronary artery plaque area on histological examination of excised coronary arteries.[1] CAC does not correlate well with the degree of coronary artery narrowing on a site-by-site basis,[2] and the relationship of CAC with coronary artery plaque that is prone to rupture is not well understood.[3] Nonetheless, if used in the appropriate clinical context, measurement of CAC can be useful in the diagnosis and prognostication of patients suspected of having coronary artery disease.[4]

This chapter will focus on the technical aspects of detecting and quantifying CAC, in particular diagnostic accuracy, reproducibility, agreement between imaging modalities, and algorithms used to quantify CAC from computed tomography (CT) images.

Most noninvasive X-ray-based imaging modalities can detect CAC. For example, the diagnostic and prognostic value of CAC detected by fluoroscopy has been examined in several studies.[5,6] However, the sensitivity of fluoroscopy

and chest X-ray for the detection of CAC is low compared with CT, and quantification is not possible.[7,8]

CT can detect the presence of CAC very sensitively. The performance of CT in the detection of CAC depends on many scanner- and patient-related factors. The ability to modify scanner-related features varies between the available CT modalities, which include conventional CT,[9,10] spiral [11] and multidetector-row CT (MDCT),[12] and electron beam CT (EBCT).[13] Investigators scanning for CAC with CT recognized early that, because of the rapid, constant motion of the coronary arteries throughout the cardiac cycle, temporal resolution is particularly important for the accuracy of CAC quantification by CT.[14] Among current CT scanners, MDCT and EBCT have the fastest temporal resolution (see also Chapter 2 [Kachelriess M]). Therefore, conventional and early spiral CT scanners no longer play a relevant role in coronary artery imaging or the quantification of CAC.

1 PERFORMING CARDIAC COMPUTED TOMOGRAPHY FOR CAC SCANNING

For imaging of CAC by CT, no patient preparation is required, and iodinated contrast medium is not administered. Depending on the type of scanner used, the scan duration is approximately 5–20 seconds. CT images of the heart can show calcium in locations other than the coronary arteries,

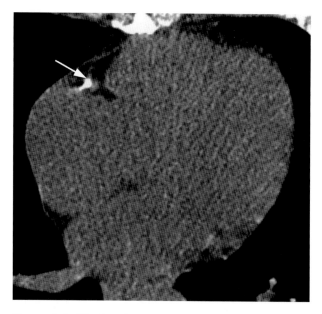

Figure 8.1. Electron beam computed tomography image of a calcification in the right coronary artery that is distorted by motion artfact in typical 'crescent shape' fashion (arrow). Reprinted with permission from Horiguchi et al.[15]

particularly the aorta, mitral annulus, papillary muscles, myocardium, and pericardium. Initial quantification of CAC is typically performed interactively on dedicated computer workstations by trained radiology technologists. The interaction with the computer software consists of highlighting which calcifications are part of the coronary artery walls and which are not. Physician review of the images should occur to ascertain that only coronary calcifications are scored. Aortic and coronary ostial calcifications are not included, and coronary calcifications distorted by cardiac motion artifact (Figure 8.1) are included as is without editing.

2 QUANTIFICATION OF CAC: AGATSTON SCORE

Imaging of CAC with EBCT was first described in 1989.[13] In 1990, Agatston et al. proposed a method for quantifying CAC with EBCT.[16] This algorithm, which is based on the X-ray attenuation expressed in Hounsfield units (HU) and the area of calcium deposits, is still widely used.

The original definition of the Agatston score is for a slice thickness of 3 mm and a temporal resolution of 100 msec, with image acquisition triggered at 80% of the RR-interval of the electrocardiogram. Any area of ≥ 1 mm^2 with a CT number of ≥ 130 HU is defined as 'calcification.' The requirement for a calcified area to have an area of least 1 mm^2 in order to be counted is meant to minimize the influence of 'noise' on CAC quantification in the form of single pixels with a CT density above the threshold of 130 HU.[17]

Table 8.1 Weighting factors for determination of Agatston score based on maximal CT number (HU) in calcified lesions

Maximal HU	Weighting factor
130–199	1
200–299	2
300–399	3
≥ 400	4

A weighting factor is assigned to each calcified area on each CT image based on the maximum CT number in that lesion, as listed in Table 8.1. A score is then calculated for each lesion by multiplying the area of calcification (expressed in mm^2) with the weighting factor. The total Agatston score (which has no units) is then calculated by summing up all lesion scores from all image slices. At the time when the Agatston score was first devised, EBCT scanners could only acquire 20 slices per scan which were typically arranged to cover the cranial portion of the heart, and with it the proximal and middle segments of the coronary arteries. This limitation was disadvantageous in those patients who have CAC only in the distal portions of the coronary arteries. Later generations of EBCT scanners could acquire enough slices to image the entire heart in 1 scan (typically 12 cm, or 40 contiguous, non-overlapping slices of 3 mm thickness, in craniocaudal direction of the z-axis), and the definition of the Agatston score was adapted to include the increased number of slices.

2.1 Variability of CAC quantification

For a reproducibility sufficient to be certain that patients undergoing CAC scanning are reliably classified into the appropriate risk categories, and to make serial scanning to detect changes of CAC over time (see also Chapter 11 [Schmermund A et al.]) meaningful, the variability of CAC quantification should be as low as possible. For example, based on the 3-sigma criterion, the variability between repeated measurements of CAC should be approximately $\leq 10\%$ to detect with confidence the 20–30% annual progression of CAC that occurs in asymptomatic patients or symptomatic patients on medical therapy. In early studies, the interobserver and intraobserver variability of the Agatston score was very low.[18] However, the variability (typically expressed as the difference divided by the mean) between two scans, performed minutes apart on the same patient with the same EBCT scanner (interscan variability), was as high as 50%.[17,19-22]

Table 8.2 Factors affecting the variability of CAC scoring. For details see text

Problem	Possible solution
Coronary motion artifact	• Use scanner with high temporal resolution • Careful selection of timepoint for trigger or gating
Partial volume averaging	Small slice thickness*
Misregistration	Overlapping slices*
Differences between scan protocols	Standardization of scanning protocols
• tube current and voltage	
• reconstruction algorithms (kernel)	
Patient size	Adaptation of tube current*
Attenuation dependence of Agastston score	Alternate quantification algorithms

*Will increase radiation dose to patient to maintain noise (slice thickness, patient size) or because of overlapping exposure to the X-ray beam (overlapping slices).

This variability had numerous sources (Table 8.2). As a simple mathematical matter, a given absolute difference between the CAC score from 2 CT scans results in a smaller relative variability (expressed in percent) in the presence of high than in the presence of low CAC scores. Because of the arbitrary HU-dependent weighting function of the Agatston score, the numerical value of the score is highly susceptible to factors that affect X-ray attenuation or image noise, both of which are the result of complex interactions between a number of patient- and scanner-related factors. Patient size and the settings of tube current affect the standard deviation of X-ray attenuation, i.e., image noise. As discussed in Section 2 of this chapter, image noise can affect the quantification of CAC if some of the noise has HUs ≥ 130 and is counted as calcium. The setting of tube voltage affects mean attenuation and hence, the HUs in calcified plaques seen on CT. Differences of tube voltage are of particular interest because they can result in different CAC scores even on the same scanner.

In addition, if images are acquired during a time point during the cardiac cycle where coronary motion velocity, particularly of the right coronary artery, is high, motion artifact may lead to 'smearing' of the calcified area that has random effects on the HU.[23] Motion artifacts are more prominent on scanners with low temporal resolution. The type of kernel used in filtered back-projection of the projection data (see Chapter 2 [Kachelriess M et al.]) does not significantly impact mean attenuation (HUs) of calcified plaques but will affect image noise, and hence the visibility of small calcifications in particular. As a result of partial volume averaging, calcifications that are small relative to the image slice thickness or a given voxel, but are high in density, can contribute disproportionately to the CAC score by making the entire voxel count toward calcification. As a

result of volume averaging, small calcifications that would have an HU near the definition threshold if a thinner slice thickness were used may go undetected depending on their position within the slice. If contiguous, non-overlapping slices are used (such as in the original Agatston protocol) registration artifacts due to patient motion or breathing can create gaps or unintended overlap between adjacent slices. In these cases, calcifications may be missed or counted doubly.

3 APPROACHES TO MAXIMIZING ACCURACY AND MINIMIZING VARIABILITY OF CAC QUANTIFICATION

The scanner- and patient-related factors that affect the accuracy and variability of CAC scoring can be addressed in various ways. Important concepts include appropriate choice of scanning equipment and of scanning and image reconstruction protocols.

3.1 Technical minimum requirements for CAC scanning

In a scientific statement from the American Heart Association published in 2006,[24] the writing group proposed the following minimum technical requirements be met in CAC scanning by CT (Table 8.3). These requirements are meant to ascertain that temporal and spatial resolution of the scanners used are sufficient, and that patient exposure to ionizing radiation is as low as possible.

Table 8.3 Minimum requirements for coronary artery calcium scanning by computed tomography.

1. Use of an electron beam scanner or a 4-slice (or greater) MDCT scanner
2. Cardiac gating
3. Prospective triggering for reducing radiation exposure
4. A gantry rotation of at least 500 ms
5. Reconstructed slice thickness of 2.5 to 3 mm to minimize radiation in asymptomatic persons (and to provide consistency with established results)
6. Early to mid-diastolic gating

MDCT, multidetector computed tomography.
Reprinted with permission from Budoff et al.[24]

3.2 Selection of slice thickness, overlap, and timepoint for trigger or gating

In one study, the use of 6 mm slice thickness on EBCT significantly reduced variability by one-half compared to protocols using 3 mm slice thickness, probably by reducing image noise and increasing volume averaging.[25] However, in such an approach, small calcifications may be missed because they no longer exceed the definition threshold of ≥130 HU as a result of volume averaging. Slice thicknesses >3 mm for CAC scoring have not been pursued in other studies.

With the prospective 'step and shoot' triggering used in EBCT, slice overlap can with most scanners be created only by choosing a table advance that is smaller than the slice thickness. The use of overlapping (3 mm thickness, 2.5 or 2 mm table advance), compared with contiguous slices on EBCT to reduce the likelihood of misregistration between image slices and make use of section averaging, lead to significantly lower interscan variability in one phantom study.[26] In MDCT, CAC can be imaged in 2 ways: with prospective triggering without slice overlap, and with retrospective gating of helical scans where continuous projection data acquisition always involves overlapping sampling at every anatomic level. The variability of CAC scores is lowest in scans performed with continuous projection data acquisition and reconstruction of overlapping slices, intermediate with non-overlapping slices reconstructed from continuous projection data acquisition, and highest for scans performed with prospective triggering.[15,27,28] An important disadvantage is that continuous projection data acquisition by helical scanning or overlapping slices in EBCT scanning is

associated with an increase in radiation dose to the patient (see Chapter 3 [McNitt-Gray M]).

Varying the timepoint for triggering image acquisition prospectively or reconstructing images by retrospective gating affects the variability of CAC scores. CT images for the quantification of CAC have typically been triggered or reconstructed in late diastole, at approximately 80% of the R-R interval of the electrocardiogram. However, the longest periods of the relatively lowest coronary motion velocity may occur at 40–50% of the R-R interval.[29,30] Triggering EBCT image acquisition at 40% instead of 80% of the R-R interval reduced interscan variability of EBCT from 17.4% to 11.5%[31] in one study, whereas it had no significant influence on variability in another.[32] Of note, in the latter study, the median variability was already low at 5.7%. The optimal trigger point associated with the least motion artifact may vary with patient's heart rate in that it more frequently occurs early in the cardiac cycle in patients with high heart rates.[33] With continuous projection data acquisition by MDCT, images can be reconstructed by retrospective gating at any time point during the cardiac cycle. The numeric value of the CAC score is dependent on the reconstruction window chosen. In one study using 16-slice MDCT, the minimal and maximal CAC scores were randomly distributed across the cardiac cycle when scores were systematically measured on images reconstructed every 10% of the R-R interval,[34] most likely because of blurring and distortion of calcified lesions by motion artifacts.[23] In a later study with 64-slice MDCT, the mean Agatston score was not significantly different among 5 image data sets per patient reconstructed between 50 and 70% of the R-R interval, and variability could be minimized by reconstructing overlapping slices.[35]

3.3 Standardization of scanning protocols

The effects of differences in X-ray attenuation can be addressed by using calibration phantoms to adjust attenuation values and calibrate calcium measurements (Figure 8.2). This approach can reduce the variability of serial measurements of CAC scores on the same scanner[36] and improve the agreement between CAC scores measured on different scanners or scanner types.[37,38]

The Physics Task Group of the International Consortium on Standardization on Cardiac CT has, based on phantom measurements, recently formulated a multiinstitutional, multimanufacturer international standard for quantification at cardiac CT that describes suggestions

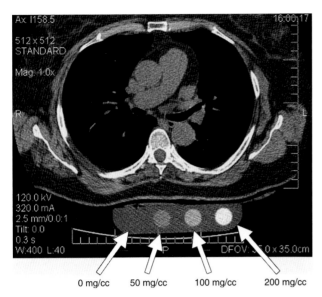

Figure 8.2. Electron beam computed tomography image of a patient's thorax and a calibration phantom placed under the thorax. The arrows point to the cross-sections of four calibration rods, which contain calcium hydroxyapatite at concentrations between 0 and 200 mg per cubic centimeter (cc). Reprinted with permission from Nelson et al.[38]

for scan acquisition and image reconstruction parameters, a technique for the adaption of tube current to patient size, and the measurement of calcium mass with the ultimate goal of minimizing the effect of patient- and scanner-related factors on CAC scoring variability.[37] These recommendations are listed in Table 8.4.

3.4 Alternate algorithms for CAC quantification

As a result of its definition, the Agatston score can vary considerably with minor changes of the maximal CT number of a calcified area. For example, the score of a calcified lesion with an area of 8 mm² increases from 16 to 24 (variability, 40%) if the maximal CT number changes by only 10 HU from 295 to 305. A number of approaches to CAC quantification have been suggested that are designed to reduce interscan variability.

3.4.1 Volume score

To reduce the influence of the arbitrary, HU-dependent multiplication factor used for calculation of the Agatston score on the variability of CAC measurements, volumetric scoring

methods for EBCT have been developed. In a simple approach, the 'calcified volume' is calculated by summing up all voxels with a CT number ≥130 HU, excluding extracoronary calcifications.

A refined version of this approach uses isotropic interpolation to create voxels with a size smaller than that of the voxels in the original 3-dimensional CT dataset.[39] By sampling the 3-dimensional dataset at cross-sections between the original tomographic slices, voxels with edges of equal length can be interpolated. For example, original voxel size in an EBCT scan with 3 mm thickness obtained with a field of view of 30 cm² is 0.586 mm × 0.586 mm × 3 mm = 1.03 mm³, whereas interpolated voxel size is 0.586 mm × 0.586 mm × 0.586 mm = 0.201 mm³. Based on the HU on the original tomogram, and the distance of the interpolated cross-section from the original tomogram, a numeric value is assigned to each of these smaller voxels. All interpolated voxels whose value exceeds 130 are counted toward the calcified volume. The immediate result is a volume estimated as a fraction of a cubic centimeter, but for the purpose of presenting an integer number and easier comparison with the Agatston score, the measured calcified volume is multiplied by 1,000.[39] In principle, the smaller size of interpolated voxels should allow a more precise volumetric reconstruction of coronary calcium, and make CAC quantification independent of slice thickness.

As an important disadvantage, the volume score, like the Agatston score, uses a fixed threshold of ≥130 HU to define calcification. This approach does not take into account the scanner- and patient-related factors that can influence attenuation, and hence HU values that are discussed above, and does not represent an actual physical measure. The volume score tends to overestimate the volume of coronary calcifications containing very high HU values and to underestimate the volume of coronary calcification with HUs near the definition threshold of CAC.[40] It is important to realize that the numerical values of the Agatston and volume scores strongly depend on the threshold used to define calcium. As an example, if the threshold for the definition of CAC is lowered, the numerical values of CAC scores increase.[41]

3.4.2 Calcium mass

The measurement of hydroxyapatite (calcium) mass automatically corrects for partial volume effects, does not use a fixed HU threshold for the definition of CAC, and is largely independent of scanner settings if the scanner is calibrated appropriately.[40]

Table 8.4 Recommended scan acquisition parameters for measurement of coronary artery calcium by computed tomography

Parameter	Imatron (electron-beam)	Light speed plus	MX8000	Volume zoom	Volume zoom	Volume zoom	Aquilion	Sensation 64
					Scanner			
Acquisition mode	Sequential	Sequential	Sequential	Sequential	Spiral		Sequential	Spiral
Electrocardiographic synchronization	Prospective	Prospective	Prospective	Prospective	Retrospective		Prospective	Retrospective
Peak voltage (kVp)	130	120	120	120	120		120	120
Rotation time (sec)	0.1 (scanning time)	0.5	0.5	0.5	0.5		0.5	0.33
Tube current-time product (mAs)*	63 (fixed)	25, 70, 145	10, 30, 65	20, 55, 135	20, 50, 115		20, 45, 90	20, 70, 145
Detector configuration (mm)	1×3	4×2.5	4×2.5	4×2.5	4×2.5		4×3	64×0.6
Section thickness (mm)	3	2.5	2.5	2.5	3		3	3
Table feed (millimeters per rotation)	3	10	10	10	3.75		12	3.84
Pitch	1	1	1	1	0.375		1	0.2
Reconstruction algorithm	Sharp	Standard	B	B35f	B35f		FC01	B35f
Effective dose (mSv)†	1.0	1.7	0.6	1.1	2.5		1.4	5.25

The Imatron scanner is manufactured by Imatron (South San Francisco, Calif); the LightSpeed Plus, by GE Healthcare; the MX8000, by Philips Medical Systems; the Aquilion, by Toshiba Medical Systems; and the Volume Zoom and Sensation 64, by Siemens Medical Solutions.

*For all scanners except the Imatron unit, the first milliampere-second value is for small patients; the second value, for medium-size patients; and the last value, for large patients.

†Calculated for medium-size patients by using ImPACT CT Patient Dosimetry Calculation, version 0.99W (*http://www.impactscan.org/ctdosimetry.htm*).

Reprinted with permission from McCollough et al.[37]

The calculation of calcium mass relies on the concept that the physical value of 'density' (ρ) of hydroxyapatite is proportional to the CT number on the reconstructed images. For a calcified volume, calcium mass equals the mean CT number, in that volume is multiplied by the volume expressed in mm^3 and a calibration constant. That calibration constant can be determined by scanning a phantom containing calcification with a known hydroxyapatite density, and then dividing this known hydroxyapatite density by the CT number determined from the images of the calcification phantom. Importantly, because the CT numbers of calcified lesions depend on the X-ray spectrum used, each scanning protocol and each scanner require individual calibration. As a result of its definition, the calcium mass determined from CT images will typically underestimate actual calcium mass somewhat.[40]

4 STUDIES COMPARING SCANNER TYPES AND QUANTIFICATION ALGORITHMS

The technical differences between EBCT and MDCT create concern that the CAC scores obtained with these two types of scanners might not be equivalent. This would make the use of CAC scores derived from MDCT scanners to risk-stratify patients based on prospective data obtained on EBCT scanners invalid. Because of ethical concerns related to the radiation exposure of scanning patients twice with different scanners, the equivalence of CAC scores derived from EBCT and MDCT scanners has been evaluated in a few studies only.

The results of comparing 4-slice MDCT to EBCT have varied from 17% variability between imaging modalities for the volume score[42] to 32% for the Agatston score,[12] both with very high correlation between the scores derived from both modalities. However, in another study from the same era,[41] the CAC scores obtained from EBCT and MDCT were significantly different from each other. Nonetheless, for clinical purposes CAC scores obtained with MDCT are now used interchangeably with those derived from EBCT, and interpreted in the context of the prognostic value determined in studies that used EBCT. Recognizing the potential differences between CAC quantification on the different scanner types, an Agatston score derived from MDCT is often referred to as an 'Agatston score equivalent.'

In a study using a variety of CT scanners available in the year 2000, EBCT and MDCT (Figure 8.3) had equivalent

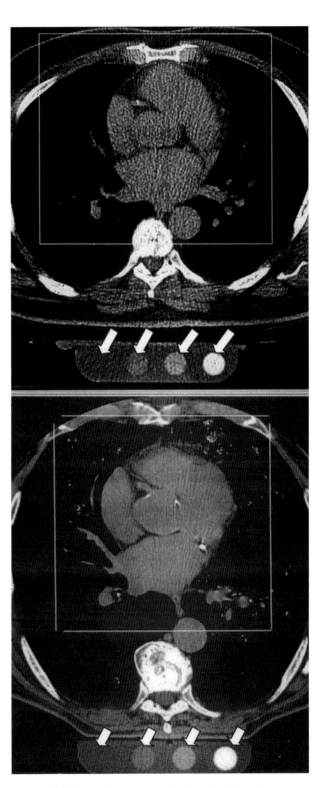

Figure 8.3. Typical images of the heart obtained by electron-beam computed tomography (top) and multi-detector row computed tomography (bottom). A calibration phantom is placed below thorax as in Figure 8.2. Reprinted with permission from Detrano et al.[43]

Threshold = 130 Hu
(103.2 mg/cm^3 CAHA)

Artery	Number of lesions (1)	Volume [mm^3] (3)	Equiv. mass [mg/cm^3 CAHA] (4)	Score (2)
LM	0	0.0	0.00	0.0
LAD	2	79.9	20.35	99.9
CX	0	0.0	0.00	0.0
RCA	0	0.0	0.00	0.0
Total	2	79.9	20.35	99.9

(1) Lesion is volume based
(2) Equivalent Agatston score
(3) Isotropic interpolated volume
(4) Calibration factor: 0.794

Figure 8.4. Example of coronary calcium scoring results listing Agatston score equivalent ('Score'), volume equivalent ('Volume'), and absolute mass of calcium ('Equiv. mass') in a patient with 2 calcified lesions in the left anterior descending artery (LAD).

reproducibility for measuring CAC.[43] The reproducibility of the volume score was not significantly lower than that of the Agatston score.[43] In another recent study examining a phantom on variety of scanners, the variability of the volume scores measured with the different scanners was higher than the variabilities of the Agatston score or calcium mass.[37] Use of a fixed hydroxyapatite threshold, as opposed to a fixed HU threshold, to define CAC reduced the variability between Agatston and calcium mass scores measured on different scanners.[37]

5 REPORTING CAC SCORES

CAC scores are typically reported for each major coronary artery (left main, left anterior descending, circumflex, right coronary artery) separately. However, for the purpose of risk stratification or measurement of CAC progression, the 'total' score that incorporates all regional scores is reported.

Given the fact that almost all information on the diagnostic and prognostic value is derived from studies that used the Agatston score, and because its numeric range is familiar to most physicians who refer patients for CAC scanning, this score is almost always reported at the current time despite its conceptual shortcomings. The volume score tends to be numerically similar to the Agatston score except at very high and very low scores. The numeric value of the calcium mass is typically much lower than that of the Agatston score (Figure 8.4). The evidence base for the prognostic value of these scores, in particular the calcium mass, is currently being developed.[44]

Because the increase in incidence and quantity of CAC with age can make interpretation of CAC scanning difficult, and because adverse cardiac events can occur at different quantities of CAC, CAC is often also reported as gender- and age-based percentile ranks based on asymptomatic cohorts [45,46] (Tables 8.5 and 8.6). In one study, where 22% of cardiac events occurred in patients with an Agatston score >400, although only 7% of the study population had a score that high, a percentile rank of >75 for age and gender was a better predictor of future cardiac events than the absolute Agatston score.[46] However, most studies examining the predictive value of CAC have used the absolute Agatson score to predict risk and a percentile rank >75 is not universally accepted as an indicator of high cardiovascular risk.[4]

6 SUMMARY AND RECOMMENDATIONS

CAC quantification can be performed with EBCT or MDCT without exposure of patients to iodinated contrast medium.

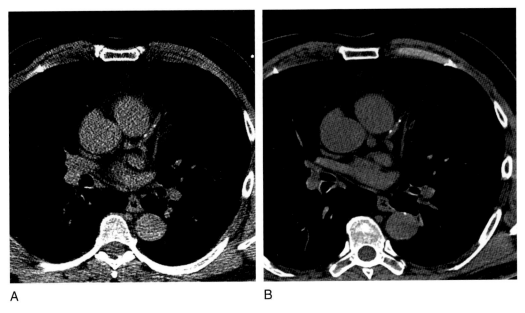

A   B

Figure 9.3 Determination of two calcified plaques in the proximal LAD with EBCT (a) and MDCT (b).

diagnostic accuracy of EBCT to diagnose possible CAD in symptomatic patients and to compare it with other non-invasive tests.[12] A total of 3,682 patients were enrolled in these studies. Inclusion criteria were the indication for coronary angiography, no prior history of CAD or prior cardiac transplantation, Definition of significant disease compromises >50%, ≥50%, ≥70% and ≥75% luminal diameter stenosis in any epicardial coronary artery, criteria for a pathologic scan were different, including any detectable calcium, score >0, score >1, score ≥5 and score >100. Individual study sensitivities ranged from 68% to 100% where as specificities ranged from 21% to 100%, predictive accuracy ranged from 49% to 51%. On average, significant coronary disease (≥50% or ≥70% stenosis by coronary angiography) was reported in 57% of the patients. Presence of calcium was reported on average in 65.8% of patients (defined as a score >0 in all but one report). With determination of any calcium (score >0) the summary odds were elevated 20 fold. Additional summary Ors were also calculated with various anatomic and calcium score cut points. For detection of minimal, >50%, and >70% angiographically documented stenosis, the summary odds increased from 6.8-fold to 50-fold, which means that odds of significant coronary disease increased when greater angiographic lesion thresholds were used for significant disease. Higher coronary calcium scores increased the likelihood of detecting significant disease. A threshold of detectable calcium or a score greater than 5 was associated with an odds of significant disease of 25.6-fold, but at the expense of a high percentage of false-negative results, which may lead to unnecessary additional investigation. Schmermund et al. used a different approach. They examined 291 patients with suspected CAD and a clinically indicated angiography who underwent risk factor determination as defined by the National Cholesterol Education Program (NCEP) and determination of coronary calcium with EBCT. On the basis of a simple noninvasive index = $\log_e$ [LAD score] + $\log_e$ [LCx score] + 2 [if diabetic] + 3 [if male] they could demonstrate sensitivities from 87–97% and specificities from 46–74% for separating patients with, versus without, angiographic three-vessel and/or left main CAD. A noninvasive index >14 increased the probability of angiographic 3-vessel and/or left main

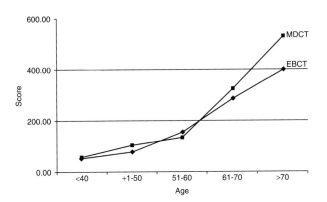

Figure 9.4 Comparison of the 75th percentile value of the volumetric calcium score derived from an EBCT study in a comparable patient population with the present study in men and women.

disease from 23% (pretest) to 65–100% (posttest), and noninvasive index <10 increased the probability of no three-vessel and/or left main CAD from 77% (pretest) to 95–100% (posttest).[13] Despite these encouraging results, no further study has ever applied this algorithm in a large prospective cohort. Further studies have tested the value of different absolute calcium thresholds for the prediction of significant disease. Guerci et al. found in a symptomatic patient population of 290 men and women that a coronary calcium score >80 was associated with an increased likelihood of any coronary disease, regardless of the number of risk factors and a coronary calcium score ≥170 was associated with an increased likelihood of obstructive coronary disease, regardless of the number of risk factors.[14] Kennedy et al. demonstrated in a multicenter trial with 368 patients that by multivariate analysis, only male sex and coronary calcification were predictive of angiographic disease.[15] An increase in the coronary calcium score from 10 to 100 more than doubles the probability of angiographic disease and an increase from 100 to 1,000 increases the probability by a factor of 12. Conversely, patients with low calcium scores (e.g. <75) have a low probability of disease (25%) and thus may not warrant coronary angiography. All three studies show that coronary calcification is a stronger independent predictor of angiographically obstructive CAD than are standard risk factors in symptomatic patients referred for angiography. Thus coronary calcification, when considered as a risk factor, was the most powerful of these for such patients.

In 2001, Haberl et al. correlated the EBCT derived calcium scores with the results of coronary angiography in 1,764 symptomatic patients (women = 539, age = 59 ± 12 years) in order to assess its value to predict or exclude significant coronary artery disease.[7] The strength of the study was that all patients were evaluated in a single center with the same technology. Due to the inclusion criteria, typical/atypical chest pain and/or signs of

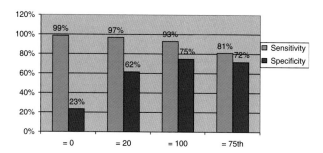

Figure 9.6   Accuracy of different cut off values to detect significant disease.

myocardial ischemia or noninvasive tests (bicycle stress test in most cases) all patients had a high pretest probability of coronary artery disease. Despite this high pretest probability, only 56% of men and 47% of women (Figure 9.5) revealed significant coronary artery disease (≥50% diameter stenosis).

The positive finding of coronary calcium (score >0) had the best sensitivity (99% in men and 100% in women) and the best negative predictive power (97% in men and 100% in women) to detect stenosis ≥50% and stenosis ≥75% in men and women. Conversely, the specificity was low, 23% in men and 40% in women. Higher calcium values (≥20, ≥100, ≥75th percentile) were associated with decreased sensitivity to detect significant CAD, but increased specificity (Figure 9.6).

Otherwise, the exclusion of coronary calcium was associated with extremely low probability of significant stenosis in men and women. No calcium was found in 128 (24%) of 540 men and in 116 (41%) of 284 women without significant disease. Figure 9.7 represents the sensitivity, specificity, positive and negative predictive value for a score of 0 for significant CAD (luminal diameter >70%).

Thus, exclusion of coronary calcification was associated with a low likelihood of significant stenosis in men and women. Only in five cases did coronary angiography

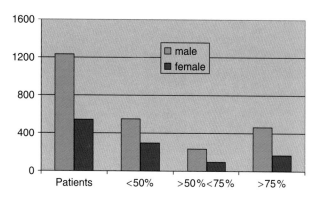

Figure 9.5   Distribution of the extent of coronary stenosis in 1,764 symptomatic patients.

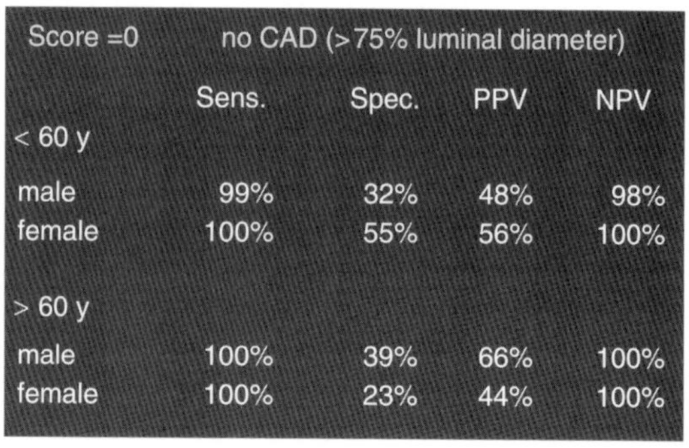

Score =0	no CAD (>75% luminal diameter)			
	Sens.	Spec.	PPV	NPV
< 60 y				
male	99%	32%	48%	98%
female	100%	55%	56%	100%
> 60 y				
male	100%	39%	66%	100%
female	100%	23%	44%	100%

Figure 9.7   Diagnostic accuracy of Score=0 for exclusion of obstructive disease in older (>60 years) and younger (<60 years) individuals; Sens. = Sensitivity, Spec. = Specificity, PPV = positive predictive value, NPV = negative predictive value.

reveal a significant stenosis despite a calcium score of zero. The results show that EBCT calcium screening can identify a subset of patients with a very low risk of significant CAD in whom diagnostic procedures may be omitted.

The study from Budoff et al. showed that 1,851 patients with suspected CAD applied a multivariate logistic prediction model to overcome verification bias as a consequence of the preferential referral of positive test responders to angiography and negative test responders away from angiography.[16] Study prediction models were designed to be continuous, adjusted for age and sex, corrected for verification bias, and independently validated in terms of their incremental diagnostic accuracy. The overall sensitivity was 95% and specificity was 66% for coronary calcium to predict obstructive disease (= 50% lumen diameter) on angiography. With calcium scores >20, >80 and >100, the sensitivity to predict stenosis decreased to 90%, 79% and 76% whereas the specificity increased to 58%, 72% and 75%, respectively. The logistic regression model exhibited excellent discrimination (receiver operating characteristic curve area of 0.84 ± 0.02) and calibration (chi-square goodness of fit of 8.95, p = 0.44). The study documents the clinical applicability of EBCT-derived calcium scores for the noninvasive diagnosis of CAD in two broad areas: for diagnosis, by the correlation of posterior probability with angiographic prevalence (Figure 9.8) and for evaluation, by the relation of posterior probability to the anatomic severity of disease.

As in other studies, the addition of calcium scores added independent and incremental information to predict obstructive disease over age and sex. Interestingly, those patients who exhibited the greatest change from pretest to posttest probability were those patients with pretest probability ranging from 20% to 70%, representing an intermediate pretest likelihood of CAD. This was consistent with many other cardiovascular tests, including exercise stress and thallium testing. As proposed by the authors the model

described can assist clinicians to develop post-test probability that will be useful for establishing a high (75% to 92%) as opposed to a low (<10%) probability of significant disease. In accordance with the study from Haberl et al. exclusion of coronary calcium defines a substantial subgroup of patients, albeit symptomatic with a low probability of significant stenosis. The high negative predictive value (96–100%) of exclusion of coronary calcium is highlighted in the AHA/ACC document on EBCT for the diagnosis and prognosis of CAD (Table 9.1).[12]

A complementary role for coronary calcium and MPS measurements was demonstrated by He et al., who noted a threshold phenomeon with almost no observable myocardial hypoperfusion among patients with CAC score <100 with a marked increase in the frequency of an abnormal MPS in patients with high CAC values (>100).[17] These findings were confirmed in a recent study of 1,195 patients who underwent CAC measurement and MPS assessment. The presence of coronary calcium was the most powerful predictor that a nuclear test would be positive for ischemia and <2% of all patients with a coronary calcium score <100 had positive EBCT studies.[18] Recent ACC/ASNC appropriateness criteria support that a low calcium score precludes the need for MPS assessment and a high score warrants further assessment.[19] These appropriateness criteria suggest nuclear testing may generally be inappropriate in patients with calcium scores <100, as the probability of obstruction or abnormal scan is very low. However, more recent evidence suggests that MPS may be indicated in patients with diabetes and those with a family history of CAD who have a calcium score <100.[20–21]

In summary, coronary calcium screening may be an effective filter before undertaking invasive diagnostic procedures, hospital admission or stress nuclear imaging, with more caution in younger patients, which has been shown in a large study of patients (n = 2215) with suspected CAD (mean

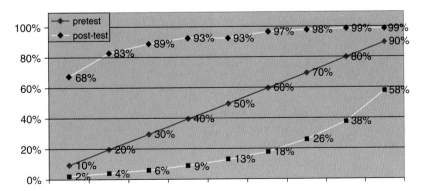

Figure 9.8 A 55-year-old man with a pretest probability of 53% has a posttest probability of 13% with a calcium score of 0 (■). The same 55-year-old man has with a score of 400 a posttest probability of 93% (◆).

Table 9.1 Interpretation and recommendation for coronary calcium scoring (adapted from ACC/AHA expert consensus document).[4]

- A negative test (score = 0) makes the presence of atherosclerotic plaque, including unstable or vulnerable plaque, highly unlikely
- A negative test (score = 0) makes the presence of significant luminal obstructive disease highly unlikely (negative predictive power by EBCT on the order of 95% to 99%)
- A negative test is consistent with a low risk (0.1% per year) of a cardiovascular event in the next 2 to 5 years
- A positive test (CAC > 0) confirms the presence of a coronary atherosclerotic plaque

age = 62 ± 19 years). A false negative result (score = 0) was observed in 7/8 patients with <45 years of age (Figure 9.9).[22]

In another study in 668 consecutive patients with chest pain syndrome, obstructive CAD was present in 9 patients (7%) despite a score = 0. Seven of the 9 patients were women and mean age was 50 years.[24] Therefore, most experts suggest in younger patients contrast with chest pain syndrome enhanced noninvasive coronary angiography to definitely rule out significant disease. Otherwise three studies have documented that coronary calcium screening is a rapid and efficient screening tool for patients admitted to the emergency department with chest pain and nonspecific electrocardiograms.[25–26] These small-scale studies (sample size 105 to 192) showed sensitivities of 98% to 100% for identifying patients with acute MI and very low subsequent event rates for persons with negative tests. The high sensitivity and high negative predictive value may allow early discharge of those patients

with nondiagnostic ECG and negative CAC scans (score = 0). Long term follow-up of one patient cohort demonstrated a very low risk of events in patients without demonstrated CAC at the time of emergency room visit. Therefore future studies in large patient cohorts are needed and should allow for adequate length of follow-up and assessment of larger numbers of hard endpoint events, especially all-cause mortality and myocardial infarction. The high sensitivity and negative predicitive value of a calcium score = 0 leads in patients with chest pain is implemented in the AHA/ACC recommendation. Patients with chest pain and equivocal or nomal ECGs and negative cardiac enzyme studies may be considered for CAC assessment (Class IIb, Level of Evidence: B).[4]

There is still no agreement for either what score cutpoint for determination of significant disease should be used in a clinical setting or if an age and gender related cut-off value (=75th percentile) is superior to an absolute threshold (>100, >400). It has been proposed that incorporation of age and gender distributions of coronary calcium should be used among younger patients and in women ≥60 years old which have lesser atherosclerotic plaque burden and would be overlooked otherwise.[22] Generally, scores <100 are typically associated with a low probability (<2%) of abnormal perfusion on nuclear stress test (28) and less than 3% probability of significant obstruction (>50% luminal diameter) on coronary angiography.[6–7] A person with an Agatston score >400 may benefit from functional testing to detect occult ischemia.

It is appropriate to compare CAC scoring with established diagnostic tests including stress electrocardiography, myocardial perfusion imaging and stress echocardiography. In direct comparison EBCT coronary calcium has been shown to be comparable to nuclear exercise testing in the

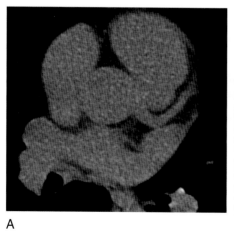
A

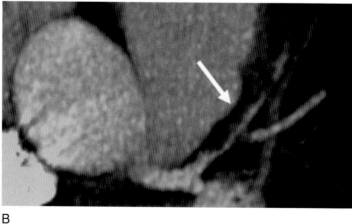
B

Figure 9.9 Absence of coronary calcium in the non-contrast scan despite the presence of high grade stenosis in the proximal left anterior descending artery (LAD) seen in the contrast enhanced scan in a 45-year-old woman (confirmed by angiography).

Table 9.2 Sensitivity and specificity of diagnostic tests for evaluation of CAD

	No. of patients	Sensitivity %	Specificity %
Stress treadmill[25]	2456	52	71
Exercise SPECT[26]	4480	87	73
Stress echocardiography[25]	2637	85	77
EBCT calcium[27]		85	75

detection of obstructive CAD (Table 9.2).[26–27] Opposite to these tests, EBCT is not limited by concurrent medication, the patient's ability to exercise, baseline ECG abnormalities, or existing wall motion abnormalities and can be easily performed by a technician, although more comparison work between modalities is clearly needed.

2 CORONARY CALCIUM MEASUREMENT IN SYMPTOMATIC PATIENTS WITH CARDIOMYOPATHY

The clinical manifestation of patients with ischemic cardiomyopathy are often distinguishable from those with primary dilated cardiomyopathy. One large study of 120 patients with heart failure of unknown etiology demonstrated that the presence of coronary calcium was associated with 99% sensitivity for ischemic cardiomyopathy.[28] Another study demonstrated this similarly high sensitivity using spiral CT to differentiate ischemic from nonischemic cardiomyopathy. Direct comparison studies have demonstrated this methodology to be more accurate than echocardiography and myocardial perfusion study techniques.[29–30] Additional comparative prognostic and diagnostic evidence is required to evaluate the role of CT as compared with conventional stress imaging techniques, as well as an assessment developing marginal cost-effectiveness models. CAC measurement in symptomatic patients to determine the etiology of cardiomyopathy is considered due to the AHA/ACC scientific statement a Class II B, level of evidence: B indication.[4]

3 CORONARY CALCIUM AND ACUTE CORONARY SYNDROME (ACS)

Coronary artery calcification is accepted as a marker of atherosclerosis. However, there is still controversy over what constitutes a vulnerable plaque. Some believe that calcification is an attempt by the body to protect weakened myocardium by strengthing the atherosclerotic plaque prone to rupture. However the stiffened calcified area can induce stress at the junction of calcified and noncalcified sections, a common site of plaque rupture.[31] On the other hand, others believe that a mildly or moderate stenotic plaque is more likely to rupture and lead to a coronary event.[33] The reasoning is that the presence of calcium implies the presence of unstable and vulnerable lipid-rich plaques. This correlates with Rumberger et al's finding that only 20% of plaque is calcified.[8] A useful histopathologic definition of unstable plaques has been provided by the AHA on the basis of work by Herbert Stary et al. (Figure 9.10).[33]

This classification describes the natural history of plaque initiation and development designated by lesions types I (earliest lesion) through VI (complicated lesion). Histopathologic studies have established plaque rupture (AHA lesion VIa) as the most common cause of acute coronary syndromes.[34–35] Otherwise, the pathology of acute coronary syndromes cannot be reduced to the analysis of a localized unstable plaque. In any given subject with coronary atherosclerosis, there is a spectrum of plaques at various stages of development. In addition, they can also be present in subjects without any history of CAD. This is pointed out in a study of apparently healthy individuals with traumatic death, that show plaque rupture ≤10% without any prior acute coronary event.[36] In respect to the complexity of the histopathology of atherosclerotic plaques and development of acute coronary syndrome is there any role for coronary calcium?

In a series of 50 patients with a mean age of 49 years, Farb et al. reported that calcium is a frequent feature of plaque rupture.[37] Calcium was associated less frequently with plaque erosion. Burke et al. classified culprit plaques in 108 victims of sudden cardiac death with a mean age of 50 years as stable (n = 20), erosion (n = 33), acute rupture (n = 37) and healed rupture (n = 18). The most frequently calcified plaques were healed ruptures.[38] There are also histopathologic reports suggesting that ruptured plaques are less likely to be calcified.[39]

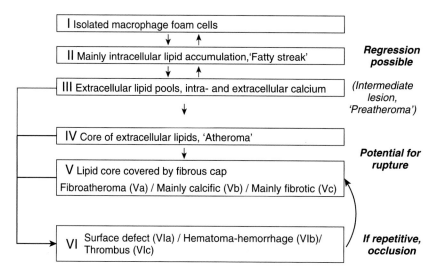

Figure 9.10   Histopathologic classification of coronary lesions adapted from the AHA.[33]

Schmermund et al. performed EBCT in 118 consecutive patients with previous myocardial infarction or unstable angina as the first manifestation of CAD. The vast majority of patients with at least moderate angiographic disease had measurable calcium by EBCT.[40] Those patients with a negative scan had minimal or no atherosclerotic plaque formation as confirmed by IVUS. Raggi et al. could demonstrate in 172 patients with a first acute myocardial infarction that in 87% the extent of coronary calcium was greater than would have been expected based on their age and sex.[41] These data suggest that, even in patients with an acute coronary syndrome as the first manifestation of CAD, coronary calcium is almost always present and usually exceeds the amount observed in asymptomatic subjects or patients with atypical symptoms. Acute coronary syndromes result from extensive coronary atherosclerosis.[32] Nevertheless, the extent of calcified plaques in patients with an acute coronary syndrome is significantly lower than in patients with stable angina demonstrated by Leber et al. (Figure 9.11).[42]

In summary, calcification frequently is observed in patients with acute coronary syndromes, although calcium cannot be used to identify unstable plaques. Because there is considerable overlap between all types of plaques, calcium is a marker for neither unstable nor stable plaques. Otherwise patients with a negative calcium test rarely have angiographic CAD, and multivessel CAD is almost never observed.[12,23,31]

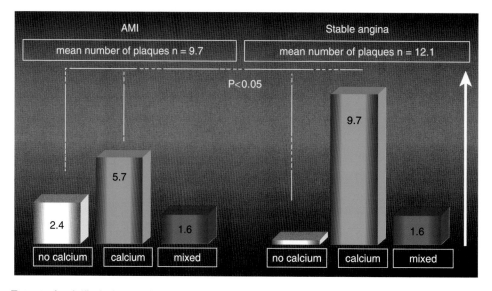

Figure 9.11   Extent of calcified plaques in patients with acute myocardial infarction (AMI) as compared to patients with stable angina.

REFERENCES

1. Raggi, P. Role of coronary calcium screening in preventive cardiology. Prev Cardiol 2000; 6: 214–16.

2. Taylor AJ, Feuerstein I, Wong H et al. Do conventional risk factors predict subclinical coronary artery disease? Results from the Prospective Army Coronary Calcium Project. Am H J 2001; 3: 463–8.

3. Greenland P, Bonow RO, Brundage BH et al. ACCF/AHA 2007 clinical expert consensus document on coronary artery calcium scoring by computed tomography in global cardiovascular risk assessment and in evaluation of patients with chest pain: a report of the American College of Cardiology Foundation Clinical Expert Consensus Task Force (ACCF/AHA Writing Committee to Update the 2000 Expert Consensus Document on Electron Beam Computed Tomography) developed in collaboration with the Society of Atherosclerosis Imaging and Prevention and the Society of Cardiovascular Computed Tomography. J Am Coll Cardiol 2006; 3: 378–402.

4. Budoff MJ, Achenbach S, Blumenthal RS et al. Assessment of coronary artery disease by cardiac computed tomography: a scientific statement from the American Heart Association Committee on Cardiovascular Imaging and Intervention, Council on Cardiovascular Radiology and Intervention, and Committee on Cardiac Imaging, Council on Clinical Cardiology. Circulation 2006; 16: 1761–91.

5. Budoff MJ, Georgiou D, Brody A et al. Ultrafast computed tomography as a diagnostic modality in the detection of coronary artery disease: a multicenter study. Circulation 1996; 93: 898–904.

6. Budoff MJ, Diamond GA, Raggi P et al. Continuous probabilistic prediction of angiographically significant coronary artery disease using electron beam tomography. Circulation 2002; 105: 1791–6.

7. Haberl R, Becker A, Leber A et al. Correlation of coronary calcification and angiographically documented stenoses in patients with suspected coronary artery disease: results of 1,764 patients. J Am Coll Cardiol 2001; 37: 451–7.

8. Rumberger JA, Simons DB, Fitzpatrick LA, Sheedy PF, Schwartz RS. Coronary artery calcium area by electron-beam computed tomography and coronary atherosclerotic plaque area. A histopathologic correlative study. Circulation 1995; 92: 2157–62.

9. Simons DB, Schwartz RS, Edwards WD et al. J Am Coll Cardiol 1992; 2: 1118–26.

10. Detrano R, Froelicher V, A logical approach for screening for coronary artery disease. Ann Intern Med 1986; 6: 846–52.

11. Agatston AS, Janowitz WR, Hildner FJ et al. Quantification of coronary artrey calcium using ultrafast computed tomography. Journal of the American College of Cardiology 1990; 15: 827–32.

12. O'Rourke RA, Brundage BH, Froelicher VF et al. American College of Cardiology/American Heart Association Expert Consensus Document on electron-beam computed tomography for the diagnosis and prognosis of coronary artery disease. J Am Coll Cardiol 2000; 36: 326–40.

13. Schmermund A, Bailey KR, Rumberger JA et al. An algorithm for noninvasive identification of angiographic three-vessel and/or left main coronary artery disease in symptomatic patients on the basis of cardiac risk and electron-beam computed tomographic calcium scores. J Am Coll Cardiol 1999; 33: 444–52.

14. Guerci AD, Spadaro LA, Goodman KJ et al. Comparison of electron beam computed tomography scanning and conventional risk factor assessment for the prediction of angiographic coronary artery disease. J Am Coll Cardiol 1998; 32: 673–9.

15. Kennedy J, Shavelle R, Wang S, Budoff M, Detrano RC. Coronary calcium and standard risk factors in symptomatic patients referred for coronary angiography. Am Heart J 1998; 4: 696–702.

16. Budoff MJ, Diamond GA, Raggi P et al. Continuous probabilistic prediction of angiographically significant coronary artery disease using electron beam tomography. Circulation 2002; 105: 1791–6.

17. He ZX, Hedrick TD, Pratt CM et al. Severity of coronary artery calcification by electron beam computed tomography predicts silent myocardial ischemia. Circulation 2000; 3: 244–51.

18. Berman DS, Wong ND, Gransar H et al. Relationship between stress-induced myocardial ischemia and atherosclerosis measured by coronary calcium tomography. J Am Coll Cardiol 2004; 44: 923–30.

19. Hendel RC, Patel MR, Kramer CM et al. ACCF/ACR/SCCT/SCMR/ASNC/NASCI/SCAI/SIR 2006 appropriateness criteria for cardiac computed tomography and cardiac magnetic resonance imaging: A Report of the American College of Cardiology Foundation Quality Strategic Directions Committee Appropriateness Criteria Working Group, American College of Radiology, Society of Cardiovascular Computed Tomography, Society for Cardiovascular Magnetic Resonance, American Society of Nuclear Cardiology, North American Society for Cardiac Imaging, Society for Cardiovascular Angiography and Interventions, and Society of Interventional Radiology. J Am Coll Cardiol 2006; 7: 1475–97.

20. Anand DV, Lim E, Hopkins D et al. Risk stratification in uncomplicated type 2 diabets: prospective evauation of the combined use of coronary artery calcium imaging and selective myocardial perfusion scintigraphy. Eur Heart J 2006; 27: 713–21.

21. Shaw L, Raggi P, Callister TQ, Bergman DS. Prognostic value of coronary calcium screening in asymptomatic smokers and nonsmokers. Eur Heart J 2006; 27: 968–75.

22. Knez A, Becker A, Leber A et al. Relation of coronary calcium scores using Electron Beam Tomography to obstructive disease in 2115 symptomatic patients. Am J Cardiol. 2004; 93(9): 1150–2.

23. Rubinshtein R, Gaspar T, Halon DA et al. Prevalence and extent of obstructive coronary artery disease in patients with zero or low calcium score undergoing 64-slice cardiac multidetector computed tomography for evaluation of a chest pain syndrome. Am J Cardiol 2007; 4: 472–5.

24. Laudon DA, Behrenbeck TR, Vukov LF, Breen JF. Coronary artery calcification scanning in patients presenting to the emergency department with chest pain: do we need a negative scan? Acad Emerg Med 2003; 10: 555.

25. Georgiou D, Budoff MJ, Kaufer E et al. Screening patients with chest pain in the emergency department using electron beam tomography: a follow-up study. J Am Coll Cardiol. 2001; 38: 105–10.

26. Schmermund A, Denkt AE, Rumberger JA et al. Independent and incremental value of coronary artery calcium for predicting the extent of angiographic coronary artery disease: comparison with cardiac risk factors and radionuclide perfusion imaging. J Am Coll Cardiol 1999; 34: 777–86.

27. Shavelle DM, Budoff MJ, Lamont DH et al. Exercise testing and electron beam computed tomography in the evaluation of coronary artery disease. J Am Coll Cardiol 2000; 36: 32–8.

28. Budoff MJ, Shavelle DM, Lamont DH et al. Usefulness of electron beam computed tomography scanning for distinguishing ischemic from nonischemic cardiomyopathy. J Am Coll Cardiol 1998; 32: 1173–78.

29. Le T, Ko JY, Kim HT, Akinwale P, Budoff MJ. Comparison of echocardiography and electron beam tomography in differentiating the etiology of heart failure: Clin Cardiol 2000; 23: 417–20.

30. Budoff MJ, Jacob B, Rasouli ML et al. Comparison of electron beam computed tomography and technetium stress testing in differentiating cause of dilated versus ischemic cardiomyopathy. J Comput Assist Tomogr 2005; 29: 699–703.

31. Wexler L, Brundage B, Crouse J et al. Coronary artery calcification: pathophysiology, epidemiology, imaging methods, and clinical implications. A statement for health professionals from the American Heart Association. Writing Group. Circulation 1996; 94: 1175–92.

32. Roberts WC, Kragel AH, Gertz SD et al. Coronary arteries in unstable angina pectoris; acute myocardial infarction, and sudden coronary death. Am Heart J 1994; 127: 1588–93.

33. Stary HC, Chandler AB, Dinsmore RE et al. A definition of advanced types of atherosclerotic lesions and a histological classification of atherosclerosis. A report from the Committee on Vascular Lesions of the Council on Arteriosclerosis, American Heart Association. Circulation 1995; 92: 1355–74.

34. Fuster V. Mechanism leading to myocardial infarction: insights from studies of vascular biology. Circulation 1994; 90: 2126–46.

35. Virmani R, Kolodgie FD, Burke AP et al. Lessions from sudden coronary death: a comprehensive morphological classification scheme for atherosclerotic lesion. Arteriosler Thromb Vas Biol 2000; 20: 1262–75.

36. Davies MJ, Thomas A. Thrombosis and acute coronary-artery lesions in sudden cardiac ischemic death. N Eng J Med 1984; 310: 1137–40.

37. Farb A, Burke AP, Tang AL et al. Coronary plaque erosion without rupture into a lipid core. A frequent cause of coronary thrombosis in sudden coronary death. Circulation 1996; 93: 1354–64.

38. Burke AP, Taylor A, Farb A et al. Coronary calcification: insight from sudden coronary death victims. Z Kardiol 2000, 89(suppl 2): 49–53.

39. Gertz SD, Roberts WC. Hemodynamic shear force in rupture of coronary arterial atherosclerotic plaques. Am J Cardiol 1990; 66: 1368–72.

40. Schmermund A, Baumgart D, Adamzik M et al. Comparison of electron-beam computed tomography and intracoronary ultrasound in detecting calcified and noncalcified plaques in patients with acute coronary syndromes and no or minimal to moderate angiographic coronary artery disease. Am J Cardiol. 1998; 81: 141–6.

41. Raggi P, Callister TQ, Cooil B et al. Identification of patients at increased risk of first unheralded acute myocardial infarction by electron-beam computed tomography. Circulation 2000; 101: 850–5.

42. Leber AW, Knez A, White CW et al. Composition of coronary atherosclerotic plaques in patients with acute myocardial infarction and stable angina pectoris determined by contrast-enhanced multislice computed tomography. Am J Cardiol. 2003; 91: 714–18.

10

Coronary Artery Calcification and Prediction of Major Adverse Cardiovascular Events

Leslee J. Shaw, Paolo Raggi, Matthew J. Budoff, and Daniel S. Berman

Initial developments in the field of computed tomography (CT) provided data on the diagnostic accuracy of coronary artery calcification (CAC). In the 2000 American College of Cardiology (ACC) expert consensus document on CAC, there were nearly 20 published reports on the diagnostic sensitivity and specificity of CAC.[1] Due to its ability to directly visualize arterial plaque, it was hoped that CT-determined CAC could more clearly define a patient's obstructive coronary artery disease burden, resulting in improved diagnostic classification when compared to ischemia tests, such as stress electrocardiography. However, the diagnostic evidence, largely derived from selected catheterized cohorts, revealed a markedly diminished specificity (~45%). That is, an elevated CAC score often did not accurately signify an associated coronary stenosis. This diminished specificity exposed both the limitations of CT-determined CAC as a diagnostic test but also re-oriented researchers toward a greater understanding of the strength of this modality. It was surmised that CAC with its strong association to the burden of atherosclerosis could be focused as a measure of a patient's global cardiac risk. Since this 2000 ACC document,[1] there has been an explosion of available prognostic evidence as to the accuracy of CAC to estimate major adverse cardiovascular events. This chapter will provide a theoretical perspective on how evidence of CAC can estimate cardiovascular outcomes as well as a synopsis of available data on this subject. Much of the discussion on the prognostic value of CAC will focus on the use of the Agatston score as the lion's share of outcomes data have been derived using this calculation.

1 CAC AND ITS THEORETICAL RELATIONSHIP WITH ACUTE CORONARY HEART DISEASE EVENTS

Atherosclerotic plaque progresses through stages, with calcification occurring in later phases of development.[1] The disease process is one of waxing and waning through periods of instability and including, at times, rupture followed by mechanisms acting as stabilizing forces. The homeostatic balance that occurs within the disease process includes the development of CAC as a mechanism to stabilize a damaged arterial bed. The disease process is not static and does not occur uniformly throughout the coronary arteries. As such, CAC can be documented within the milieu of noncalcified plaque that is in a flux of enhanced vulnerability. Additionally, CAC may be observed within the arterial wall as well as within a stenotic lesion and, therefore, may document both positive and negative remodeling. Positive remodeling is the process of plaque deposition (generally) occurring early in the disease process and represents outward expansion of the external elastic membrane and plaque deposition within the arterial wall. By comparison, later stages of the disease process include the development of atherosclerotic plaque encroaching within the lumen and therefore progressing toward ever increasing degrees of arterial stenosis (i.e., negative remodeling). As CAC can be documented within arterial wall as well as in stenotic lesions, the documentation of calcification cannot be site specific for a given stenotic lesion with the result being suboptimal diagnostic specificity. Furthermore, from the perspective of coronary event prediction, it cannot identify a given plaque that is prone to rupture and is, for practical purposes, suboptimal for localization of a vulnerable lesion.

As a result of this information, researchers have posited that, as CAC reflects stable atherosclerotic plaque, its association with cardiac event risk would be poor.[1] Yet, as we will discuss in this chapter, the observed data reveal a strong direct relationship between cardiac event risk and the extent of CAC. And, a key to understanding how this relationship works is to separate the poor site-specific detection of an obstructive lesion (i.e., diminished accuracy for detection of the vulnerable lesion) to its improved association with global risk and enhanced precision for identifying the vulnerable patient.[2]

Calcification occurs throughout areas of atherosclerotic plaque and has a strong association with histopathologic plaque area.[3] Therefore, the optimal clinical application for this marker may be as a surrogate for the extent of underlying atherosclerosis. And, as the extent of CAC is directly related to the extent of atherosclerosis, its strength lies in the detection of patient risk. A key to comprehending this reasoning is that the milieu of atherosclerotic plaque includes the coexistence of stable (i.e., calcified) as well as unstable plaque and that, the higher the CAC, patient risk is driven by the co-occurrence of and extent of vulnerable plaque. For the clinician not familiar with CT, an additional clinical analogy is that patients with high risk CAC scores (i.e., =400) have a greater frequency of obstructive coronary artery disease.[1] And that cardiac events occur more often in diseased than nondiseased patient populations. A caveat to this latter statement is that an extensive CAC *lesion* is not site-specific for a significant stenosis but a high risk CAC *score* is more often associated with a greater frequency of significant coronary artery disease.

As noncalcified plaque occurs with calcification, CAC has been defined as the 'tip of the iceberg' of patient risk. It is the determination of both arterial calcified and noncalcified plaque burden that would provide the ideal estimate of a patient's risk of acute coronary events. However, these prediction models are, as yet, unavailable.

2 WHY PROGNOSTICATE? – IMAGING AS MARKERS FOR RISK AND AS LINKS FOR TARGETING THERAPY

For tests that are able to accurately estimate important cardiovascular complications, patients with high risk imaging results may be more often aggressively treated when compared to those with lower risk test results. This reasoning represents an application of imaging markers as intermediate outcomes within therapeutic intervention strategies. Based on prognostic models, targeted treatment strategies may be devised to allocate more intensive care to those patients assigned to higher risk categories. Importantly, based on outcomes evidence, lower risk patients are treated less aggressively. From the 26th Bethesda Conference on secondary prevention, this type of management strategy was defined as changing the intensity of management based upon the patient's hazard or risk.[4] This concept of more aggressively treating high risk patients is an integral component of national guidelines for hypertension and hyperlipidemia.[5,6]

Given our CT data, prognostic evidence that assigns patients with more extensive CAC scores to a higher cardiac event risk may then be used to identify patients requiring more aggressive risk factor modification. The ensuing treatment is then based on clinical outcomes data and more precisely allocates resources to those in need (i.e., the high risk). Fundamental to this therapeutic reasoning is the premise that high risk patients receive a greater proportional risk reduction with treatment. In that, treatment will result in a more dramatic decline in patient risk for those whose baseline risk is high and that the proportional reduction in risk will be greater for high as compared to lower risk patients. Therefore, the identification of risk by CT-determined CAC and treatment initiation has the potential to result in optimal reduction in cardiovascular events. Although we will not discuss the treatment-based data that is available with CAC, understanding how the prognostic evidence may be applied in therapeutic management is key to affecting significant changes in patient outcome. As such, this chapter will focus on the available evidence on risk detection with CAC scoring. The reader may also wish to review the evidence on post-CAC treatment and ischemia testing that is highlighted in Chapter 7.

3 BASICS OF BAYESIAN THEORY – UNDERSTANDING PRETEST CLINICAL RISK

One additional preamble prior to our discussion on the available prognostic evidence is to introduce the concept of *prescan* clinical risk. This concept of clinical risk may be defined as a patient's baseline or underlying hazard for cardiac events that is largely driven by the extent and severity of risk factors as well as their degree of comorbidity. For patients with a greater clustering of cardiac risk factors, they have an accelerated risk of major adverse cardiovascular events. One method frequently used to estimate a patient's clinical risk of major CHD events is to calculate their Framingham risk score (FRS). This score assigns point values to a number of risk factors (smoking, hypertension, age, hyperlipidemia, and diabetes). The FRS then provides an estimate of the patient's 10-year risk of CHD death or nonfatal myocardial infarction (MI). Risk categories based on the FRS are low (i.e., CHD event rate <10% over 10 years), intermediate (i.e., CHD event rate from 10%–19.9% over 10 years), and high (i.e., CHD event rate = 20% over 10 years).

This latter high risk category is important as current guidelines recommend treatment to secondary prevention goals for patients with a high FRS.[5,6] Thus, as imaging or other novel risk markers detect more and more individuals whose risk is equivalent to a high FRS, then further improvements in our detection gap for atherosclerotic disease may be realized.[7]

One goal for the developing evidence base with CAC scanning is that it provides an equivalent, if not, superior ability to risk stratify patients over and above the FRS.[8] Practically speaking, if a CAC does not provide independent information, then it is hard to justify the expense of adding this test to a patient's clinical work-up. And, as we examine the prognostic evidence with CAC, we will review this data with an eye towards defining its predictive abilities in relation to the FRS.

As the FRS is the basis for current hypertension and hyperlipidemic treatment,[5,6] this initial calculation of risk also serves a 'gatekeeping' function for selecting optimal candidates for CAC scanning. The addition of a test within this strategy of hierarchical screening and selective CAC scanning requires some understanding of the potential for improved risk detection for patients whose FRS ranges from low to high risk. Thus, for this point, some understanding of Bayesian theory is needed. Bayesian theory states that the predictive accuracy of a given test is largely determined by a patient's *prescan* clinical risk. For imaging, a posttest assessment of risk will be used to modify their *prescan* risk calculation. Across the range of *prescan* FRS, the degree of change or shifting in *posttest* risk assessment varies. That is, for the patient with a low FRS, the addition of any test results in minimal shifting from *pre-* to *posttest* risk assessment; largely as a result of so few events occurring in this subset of patients. For the low FRS patient whose 10-year risk of CHD death or MI may be 0.6%, a high risk CAC may only shift their expected event risk to 1%, thus rendering them still within the same low risk category. A minimal shift from *pre-* to *posttest* risk is not ideal, with the result being a cost inefficient testing strategy. It is for this reasoning that the USPSTF[9] and more recently guidelines from the ACC[10] and American Heart Association (AHA)[11] do not recommend testing low risk patients.

By comparison, the goal of testing a patient with an intermediate FRS is that a sizeable proportion of these patients may then be shifted, given the results of a scan, to either a lower or higher risk group. In fact, the greatest shift from *pre-* to *post-scan* risk occurs for the intermediate FRS patient. In this category of patients, CAC screening will result in as many as 25% to 50% of patients reclassified to having a risk equivalent to those with a high FRS.[12,13]

'Risk equivalent' status, defined as having an expected event rate similar to patients with a high FRS, would mean that a patient's 10-year (or annual) risk of CHD death or MI would be 20% (or 2%) or higher. A number of other patient subsets have also been allocated to this risk equivalent status including diabetics and those functionally disabled, with peripheral arterial disease, or with chronic kidney disease.[5,14] Thus, should a high risk CAC score be able to identify patients whose cardiac event risk is equivalent to diabetics or to those with a high FRS, then this testing strategy could be easily integrated into accepted standards for risk detection that are now based on the use of global risk scores (e.g., FRS). All patients categorized as having a high FRS or those allocated to the risk equivalent group are then treated to more aggressive standards with secondary prevention goals for risk factor modification.[5,6]

4 LIMITATIONS OF THE FRS

The FRS is one example of a global risk score; others include the *Prospective Cardiovascular Münster* (PROCAM) score from Germany and the European Systemic Coronary Risk Evaluation (SCORE).[10] They are all similar in that they assign a point value to cardiac risk factors in order to estimate patient prognosis. As stated above, global risk scores, such as the FRS, form the basis for many guidelines including the National Cholesterol Education Program – Adult Treatment Panel III[5] and the National High Blood Pressure Education Program – Joint National Committee 7[6] where more intensive treatment is recommended to patients with a high FRS.

There are, however, notable limitations to the FRS that have implications for risk stratification. The prognostic weightings assigned to key patient subsets undervalue risk detection for women, younger patients, and for those patients living outside the US or for those of diverse ethnicity residing in the US.[12,15–17] There are also key risk factors currently excluded from the FRS that form a large proportion of patients referred for CHD risk assessment, including obese patients or those with a family history of premature CHD. Other novel risk factors also not contained within the FRS form an additional cohort of candidates who may be referred for screening, including patients with the metabolic syndrome or those with an elevated high sensitivity C-reactive protein (Hs-CRP), a generalized inflammatory marker.

Thus, although the FRS is an acceptable initial step for evaluating patient risk, clinicians should be aware of its limitations and inabilities to identify risk in several patient groups. In a recent report by Nasir et al., more than half of patients with a high risk CAC ≥400 were not classified as high risk by the FRS.[12] Shaw et al., in a related report, calculated that nearly half of low and high FRS patients could be reclassified based on CAC findings.[13] Thus, for a sizeable proportion of patients, CAC scanning may be helpful for risk stratification when the FRS assignment does not coincide with the physician's clinical impression of patient risk.

5 PROGNOSIS BY CAC MEASUREMENTS

There have been 3 critical time periods in the development of prognostic evidence with CAC. These time periods include early evidence reported through the 2000 ACC expert consensus document,[1] followed by additional evidence used in the US Preventive Services Taskforce[9,18] evaluation of CHD screening strategies, including publications through 2002, and, finally, more recent data published since 2003 with a number of large, prospectively-collected observational registries on the prognostic value of CAC.[19–24] Each time period is critical as they demarcate a juncture following which significant improvements in data quality were realized.

For example, early published reports were fraught with methodological challenge, as early evidence in any area

often is. They included the use of retrospective patient series, the inclusion of 'soft' end points (notably coronary revascularization as cardiac events), and were limited to smaller patient series followed for a short time period.[1] In the 2000 ACC expert consensus document, the prognostic evidence up to the year 2000 was criticized for being of modest quality, noting that the CAC score was not able to accurately risk stratify.[1] A second meta-analysis on the prognostic accuracy of CAC was performed by the USPSTF using additional data published through 2002.[18] The Pletcher meta-analysis[18] did a more rigorous and systematic review of the quality of the published literature and noted continuing deficiencies in the methods applied in defining the prognostic accuracy of CAC. Based on the Pletcher meta-analysis,[18] the USPSTF recommended against the use of CAC for routine CHD screening.[9] A synopsis of early prognostic data is plotted in Figure 10.1.[1,18]

During these early years, a number of investigators embarked on prospective registries, including several population-based cohort studies, examining long-term (i.e., 3–5 year) cardiac outcomes in asymptomatic individuals or consecutive patient series.[19–24] These studies, such as the Prospective Army Coronary Calcium Project[19] and the St. Francis Heart Study,[20] were initiated with the primary aim to evaluate the prognostic accuracy of CAC in asymptomatic individuals who had 1 or more pre-scan cardiac risk factors; thus, identifying patients at-risk for atherosclerotic disease. During this same time period, there were also a number of very large patient registries that examined death rates across the CAC scores.[25,26] We will start our discussion of prognosis by a review of evidence on the association of CAC to all-cause death.

6 CAC FOR RISK PREDICTIONS – MODEL # 1 – ESTIMATING ALL-CAUSE MORTALITY

Although the lion's share of evidence has focused on the estimation of cardiac events, there are several large observational, referred patient cohorts that have also been published on the relationship of the CAC score to estimating death from all causes.[13,25–29] In a middle-aged to elderly population, approximately 35% of deaths are the result of cardiovascular disease.[30] Thus, the estimation of death from all causes provides a reasonable approximation of a patient's cardiovascular risk. There is also one additional point and that has to do with the frequent imprecision with which cause of death is defined. In a sizeable proportion of patients, causation is frequently misclassified.[31] As such, models relying on death

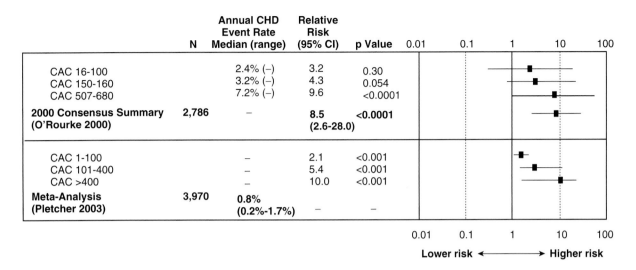

	N	Annual CHD Event Rate Median (range)	Relative Risk (95% CI)	p Value
CAC 16-100		2.4% (–)	3.2	0.30
CAC 150-160		3.2% (–)	4.3	0.054
CAC 507-680		7.2% (–)	9.6	<0.0001
2000 Consensus Summary (O'Rourke 2000)	2,786	–	**8.5** (2.6-28.0)	**<0.0001**
CAC 1-100		–	2.1	<0.001
CAC 101-400		–	5.4	<0.001
CAC >400		–	10.0	<0.001
Meta-Analysis (Pletcher 2003)	3,970	0.8% (0.2%-1.7%)	–	–

Figure 10.1   Early published reports on the prognostic value of coronary artery calcification (CAC) including analysis from the 2000 American College of Cardiology expert consensus statement and meta-analysis by Pletcher et al. of published reports through 2002.

from all causes do not suffer from the imprecision of incorrect classification of the cause of death.

Two groups have focused on developing mortality models with CT-determined CAC and include registries led by Drs. Tracy Callister[26] and Matt Budoff.[25] Both registries have enrolled large series of referred patients including sample sizes of 10,377 and 25,253 patients with average

follow-up from 5 to up to 12 years, respectively. Figure 10.2 provides a synopsis of prognostic evidence from these 2 registries.[25,26] Similar to what we will see with cardiac events, there appears to be a graded relationship between the extent of CAC, defined with the Agatston score, and mortality rates. Another way of defining this relationship is with the epidemiologic term, direct proportionality, where increases

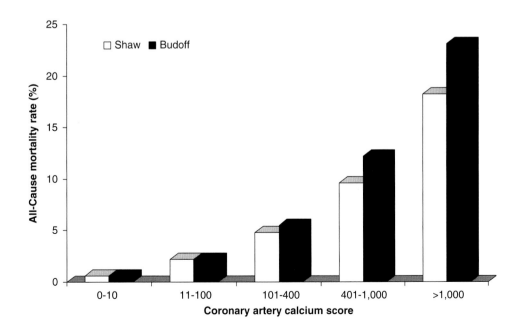

Figure 10.2   5- and 12-year all-cause mortality rates as reported from 2 large observational registries of 35,364 patients clinically referred for CT screening with coronary calcification.

in the CAC score are associated with higher mortality rates. For example, 5-year mortality rates ranged from 0.6% to 18.2% for CAC scores ranging from 0–10 to >1,000 (Figure 10.2).[26]

Longer term outcome data through 12 years of follow-up reveal the warranty period for a low risk CAC score. That is, for patients with a CAC score <100, their risk of death remains constantly low throughout nearly a decade of follow-up.[25] There appears to be no long-term detriment or clinical worsening beyond 5 years and through 12 years of observation. Specifically, a patient with a CAC score of 0–10 and 11–100 has a 12-year mortality risk that is 0.6% and 2.2%, revealing stability in their low mortality risk for an extended time period. However, for patients with higher CAC scores, clinical worsening is notable beyond 5 years as a result of accelerating disease progression. Mortality rates are approximately 15% to 30% higher for patients with CAC scores from 101–400 to >400; revealing the more active disease process in patients with more extensive atherosclerosis.

Other interesting findings based on all-cause mortality models have been published.[13,26–29] One recent report noted a higher mortality risk for women as compared to men for a given CAC score.[28] That is, for a woman with smaller arteries, a CAC score of 100 was associated with a higher mortality when compared with her male counterparts having the same score.[28] This is contradictory to conventional thought which states that women are generally at lower risk than men.[14] However, in many cases, women have a greater clustering of risk factors and it is likely that their greater degree of comorbidity drives this difference in all-cause mortality.[32] Additional validation of these findings is clearly necessary prior to supporting any gender-specific testing strategies.

Raggi and colleagues[27] also reported that the CAC score was able to risk stratify diabetics. Recalling that diabetics are routinely classified as CHD risk equivalents, these authors hypothesized that evidence on risk stratification may be beneficial in identifying lower to higher risk subsets within those diagnosed with diabetes. Five-year mortality rates for diabetics were substantially higher than those reported for non-diabetics with death rates from ~2% to 20% for those with CAC scores ranging from 0–10 to >1,000, rates nearly 50% higher than non-diabetics.[27] Although more precise data on the relationship of CAC risk to glycemic control, type of diabetes, and concomitant metabolic syndrome, as well as other factors could be helpful, this preliminary evidence does make us think about the fact that, perhaps, not all diabetics should be within this risk equivalent grouping. Hopefully, additional evidence will reveal that diabetics with a low risk CAC (or other cardiovascular imaging marker)

may be identified as having a risk <20% CHD death or MI risk or lower than their current risk equivalent status.

A more recent report examined the prognostic value of CAC in smokers as compared to nonsmokers.[29] These results were similar to those noted with diabetics with substantially higher mortality rates for smokers as compared to nonsmokers. This evidence is helpful given that smoking is one of the greatest risk factors for acute coronary thrombosis. One interesting finding from the Shaw et al.[29] report was the high mortality risk for young patients with high risk CAC scores >1,000. The relative risk for death was elevated nearly 9-fold for patients <40 years of age with a CAC score >1,000, resulting in an expected loss in life expectancy of ~5 years. This data is of clinical import given the observation that young smokers may be particularly prone to acute coronary thrombosis.[29] This data may be helpful to clinicians whereby CAC, due to its ability to directly visualize atherosclerotic plaque, may serve as a more effective motivator for smoking cessation where prior efforts have failed.

A final report by Shaw et al.[13] took a unique approach to risk assessment in that she rescored the FRS using age that was adjusted based on the CAC score. Although the prevalence and extent of CAC increases with age, it may be proposed that younger patients with higher risk CAC scores may have a disease extent that is equivalent to someone many years their senior. Thus, these authors used the CAC score to estimate a patient's predicted age, based on the CAC, deriving a new or CAC-adjusted FRS. By using this strategy of integrating the CAC with the FRS, decrements in years of life of lost with atherosclerosis were defined (Table 10.1).[13] Table 10.1 reports on the number of years added or lost with CAC subsets and age deciles.[13] Based on this CAC-adjusted age,

Table 10.1 This table depicts the results from a model that recalculates a patient's age based upon the extent of coronary artery calcification (CAC). For example, for a young patient <40 years of age, documentation of a CAC score >1,000 estimates their biologic age at approximately 70 years old.

Age (years)	<10	11-100	101-400	401-1,000	>1,000
>40	0.0	15	15	20	30
40–49	0.0	2.5	2.5	5	10
50–59	0.0	2.5	2.5	2.5	2.5
60–69	−2.5	−1	0	2.5	2.5
70–79	−10	−5	−1	5	5
80+	−10	1	1	5	10

Source: revised from Shaw et al.[13]

more than half of low to intermediate FRS patients were reclassified to a higher FRS group.

7 CAC FOR RISK PREDICTIONS – MODEL # 1 – ESTIMATING CHD DEATH OR NONFATAL MI

Recent evidence has also examined the prognostic accuracy of CAC scores as estimators of CHD death on MI.[19–24] A benefit to using models that estimate CHD events is that they may be more easily integrated with the FRS data and applied within our current prevention treatment strategies.[5,6] The more recent reports on the prognostic accuracy of CAC are notable due to their consistently high methodologic quality and the inclusion of substantially larger sample sizes of asymptomatic individuals or patients.[19–24] For example, the Rotterdam study is a population-based study of 1,795 subjects age ≥55 years prospectively enrolled and followed for the occurrence of major cardiovascular events.[23] Additionally, the Greenland et al. report,[21] from the South Bay Heart Watch study, included an asymptomatic community sample with risk factors (N = 1,461) who were followed for 7 years. Other series such as the Prospective Army Coronary Calcium Project, St. Francis Heart Study, or Cooper Clinic series were large registries enrolling >1,000 asymptomatic individuals.[19,20,22,24]

This data from 6 recent published reports was recently synthesized in an updated expert consensus statement from the ACC.[10] Within this meta-analysis, the prognostic evidence from 27,622 asymptomatic subjects (from population series) and patients (from clinical cohorts) was synthesized. The summary prognostic findings are plotted in Figure 10.3.[10] Following each subset of CAC scores from very low (i.e., 1–10) to very high (i.e., >1,000), the individual study results are reported as well as the summary relative risk ratios across a range of CAC scores from very low to very high risk. For the clinician, summary ratios are integrated measures of the weighted average relative risks. This data revealed that, for patients with minimal CAC, defined as a score from 1–10, summary relative risk ratios were nonsignificantly elevated (p = 0.18) revealing a trend toward higher CHD event risk. However, summary relative risk ratios were substantially increased for patients with higher risk CAC scores. That is, the summary relative risk ratios were increased 2.1- (p = 0.003), 4.1- (p<0.0001), 6.7- (p<0.0001), and 10.8- (p<0.0001) fold for CAC scores 11–100, 101–400, 401–1,000, and >1,000, respectively. Pooled CHD death or MI rates were 0.1% (n = 2,353), 0.4% (n = 4,832), 0.7% (n = 3,327), 1.6% (n = 2,560), and 2.2%

(n = 196) for CAC scores of 0–10, 11–100, 101–400, 401–1,000, and >1,000, respectively[10] (Figure 10.4). This gradient of accelerating risk is consistent with the prior data estimating all-cause mortality.

One of the challenges with the current evidence is that the groupings of the CAC scores have been inconsistent causing variability in the relative risk ratios across the studies, as seen in Figure 10.3. For example, from the Cooper Clinic series, higher risk CAC scores were reported as ≥113 for women and ≥250 for men.[24] Improved precision in our risk estimates would be expected, similar to that of the Shaw et al.[26] and Budoff et al.[25] series, if consistent groupings of CAC were utilized across studies. However, it remains possible that different risk thresholds may be optimal for specific gender, age, or ethnic minority patient subsets. Despite this, a synopsis of evidence reveals that a score of '0' is the lowest risk group with very low risk noted for scores in the range of 1–10. Increasing risk groups are mild, moderate, high, and very high for CAC scores of 11–100, 101–400, 401–1,000, and >1,000, respectively.

In unselected patient series, such as that presented above, it is notable that patients with a CAC score >1,000 have cardiac event rates equivalent to those of a high FRS patient. Additional subset analyses from the recent ACC expert consensus document[10] reveals that risk equivalent status (i.e., >2% annual CHD death or MI rate) should also be applied to patients with an intermediate FRS who have a higher risk CAC score ≥400 (Figure 10.5). When we place this evidence within our prior discussions on the aim of imaging to define patients with event rates equivalent to patients with a high FRS, it is notable that the evidence does support the inclusion of patients with an intermediate FRS and a high risk CAC score as within the risk equivalent groupings, along with other patient subsets, including diabetes and peripheral arterial disease. The manner in which risk is aggregated herein (i.e., intermediate risk + higher risk CAC scores = high FRS) has been defined as a multimarker approach whereby risk is compounded when multiple risk factors or markers are combined.

One final observation on the available data has to do with the comparative predictive accuracy of CAC to the FRS. Using the reasoning that improved accuracy is a necessary criterion for adding a test to a patient's clinical work-up, referral to CT is justified if the test provides substantive, independent prognostic information.[8] For each of the 6 recent reports, CAC measurements provided added statistical information within predictive models estimating CHD death or MI above and beyond cardiac risk factors or

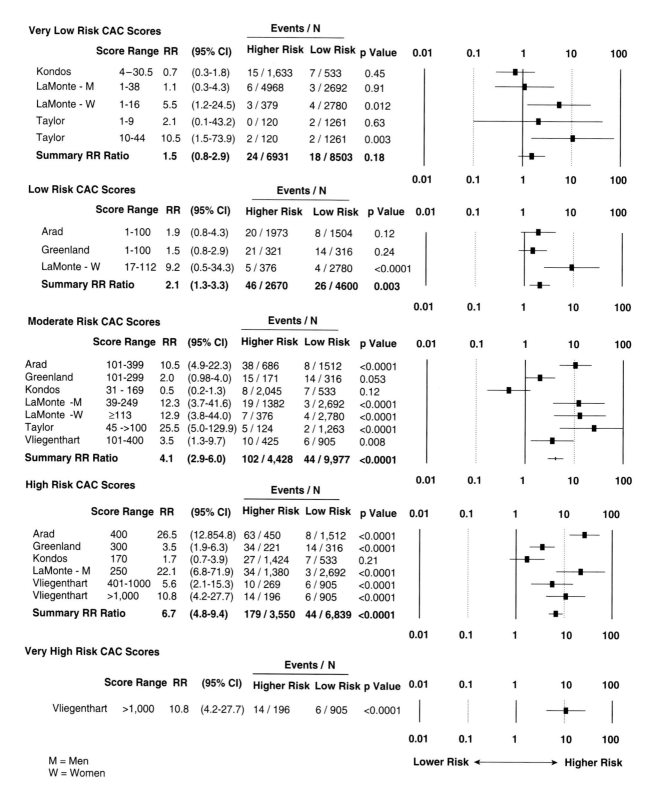

Figure 10.3 Meta-analysis on the prognostic value of CAC scores – relative risk (RR) ratios (95% confidence intervals [CI]).

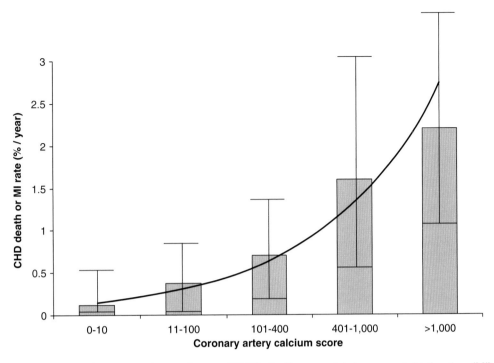

Figure 10.4   Annual rates of coronary heart disease (CHD) death or nonfatal myocardial infarction (MI) by coronary artery calcium score (in black solid line with 95% confidence intervals).

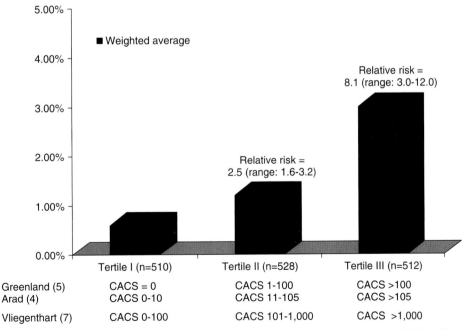

The weighted average calculation is weighted by the proportional sample size comprising the 1,550 sample. Relative risks were calculated using the Greenland, Arad, and Vliegenthart (4-5,7) series. However, the Vliegenthart series (7) used a Framingham risk score 20% as non-high risk in their elderly cohort.

Figure 10.5   Overall annual cardiac death or MI rate by tertiles of the Agatston score (n =1,550) in patients with an intermediate Framingham risk score.

the FRS. The CAC also provided improved risk prediction even when considering markers not currently within the FRS such as body mass index, Hs-CRP, and a family history of premature CHD.[19–23]

In fact, the CAC score provided independent predictive information not only above historical risk factor data but also when evaluating prognostication using measured laboratory measurements of cholesterol, blood pressure, body mass index, and Hs-CRP, a generalized inflammatory marker.[19,20,22–24] Clinicians should realize that continuous measures (e.g., LDL cholesterol) have improved delineation of risk when compared to categorical measures, such as hyperlipidemia (Yes or No). Thus, when the CAC provided independent prognostic information above and beyond many accepted cardiac risk factors such as blood pressure and cholesterol, this data was surprising to many observers. The strength of CAC as a strong prognosticator may lie within its ability to directly measure the extent of atherosclerosis as compared to indirect promoters of disease, such as cholesterol or blood pressure. In epidemiologic terms, CAC is more appropriately defined as a marker as compared to risk factors, such as blood pressure, and, as a marker, it would be expected to improve CHD event detection. Thus, although to many the improved estimation of risk noted with CAC in these 6 reports was surprising; to others its appropriate classification as a disease marker renders its superior accuracy understandable.

8 SCORING AND ESTIMATION OF CARDIOVASCULAR EVENTS

Although we have largely discussed the prognostic value of the Agatston score, age and gender percentile rankings are also commonly applied within clinical practice. The percentile rankings do have intuitive appeal due to ease of understanding for referring physician and patients. Limited prognostic data is available on the comparative accuracy of the Agatston score as compared to the percentile ranking data.[33] Clinically, limitations of the percentile ranking are that younger patients with relatively low CAC scores assigned to upper percentile groups will rarely have an event in the near term after testing. It is expected that their long term risk exceeds that of similarly-aged patients but, for event prediction in the 3–5 years, this young subset of patient's assigned rankings in the 75th to 90th percentiles will rarely have an event. Furthermore, elderly patients with CAC scores in the 100–400 range may be assigned middle (e.g., 50th) percentile ranks but have an

observed event rate that exceeds this classification. Thus, clinicians should be knowledgeable of how the percentile ranks may affect certain patient groups and qualify their use in a patient report within the context of the absolute CAC score.

9 COMPARATIVE DATA ON THE PROGNOSTIC VALUE OF THE EXERCISE ELECTROCARDIOGRAM AND OTHER IMAGING MODALITIES

In addition to the use of CAC, there are other tests that are also candidates for risk stratification. And, it would be helpful to know the predictive accuracy of CAC scoring in relation to other comparative modalities. Naghavi and colleagues[2] recently classified available cardiovascular imaging modalities as those residing within two categories: tests of (a) arterial structure and (b) arterial function. CAC is an example of a test of arterial structure similar to carotid intima-media thickness (C-IMT), or the evaluation of carotid plaque by magnetic resonance imaging. Tests of arterial function include those measuring endothelial function including brachial artery reactivity testing or vascular compliance using radial tonometry.

At least from the perspective of risk stratification, the data reported using CAC scanning are similar to the prognostic evidence in imaging for endothelial dysfunction with brachial artery reactivity and measurement of C-IMT made with high resolution B-mode ultrasound imaging.[34–35] Evidence of peripheral endothelial dysfunction, from a recent meta-analysis, was associated with a summary relative risk ratio that was 9.6-fold (95% CI = 7.1-12.8, $p<0.0001$) higher than for individuals with normal hyperemic brachial artery responsiveness.[34] The prognostic value of carotid IMT for future incident cardiovascular events has been demonstrated in multiple epidemiological studies to be graded and independent of other risk factors.[35–37] From the Atherosclerosis Risk in Communities Study (ARIC), enrolling 15,792 subjects aged 45 to 65 years between 1987–1989 from four regions of the United States,[35] the relative risk ratio comparing C-IMT measures >1 mm with >1 mm was elevated 5-fold for women and 1.9-fold for men.

Additional data is also available for use of ischemia testing for screening asymptomatic patients and subjects; although the majority of this data is dated when compared with CAC evidence.[38–41] For the clinician, the end point of an exercise test is the provocation of ST segment changes that result from an underlying obstructive coronary lesion. Thus, we can expect discordance between ischemic markers as compared to markers of arterial structure, such as the CACS, as a result of a greater extent of diffuse atherosclerosis (i.e., positive CACS) without significant coronary narrowing (i.e., positive remodeling). Furthermore, the occurrence of ST segment changes in an asymptomatic individual occurs infrequently and often fails to identify patients with more extensive atherosclerosis, such as with CAC scanning. In fact, abnormal test results are often classified as 'false-positive' results due to their lack of association with an obstructive coronary stenosis. Despite this, a review of evidence on the utility of screening with the exercise ECG was recently reported by the USPTF.[38] This evidence revealed that the median relative risk for CHD events was elevated 3.5-fold for those individuals with abnormal ST segment changes during exercise testing as compared to those with a normal peak exercise ECG.[38]

The data on ischemia testing also includes a few reports on the role of nuclear imaging in asymptomatics with hyperlipidemia or those with a family history of premature CHD.[39–41] Currently, the use of nuclear testing in asymptomatics is not recommended by current guidelines[42–43] as other tests with equivalent accuracy are more cost and clinically effective 'first line' test choices; such as CAC scanning.[44] A discussion of the role of nuclear imaging in asymptomatic individuals is detailed in Chapter 7.

10 PROGNOSTIC EVIDENCE AND TECHNOLOGY ASSESSMENT TOWARD GAINING REIMBURSEMENT

We have discussed heretofore a review of prognostic evidence with CAC and focused our discussion on the role of risk stratification in asymptomatic subjects. Ideally, the goal of developing this evidence would be that global screening strategies would ensue, similar to those used for breast or lung cancer screening. Although a number of clinicians are actively using CAC as a screening test, current guidelines do not support its utility.[9] For example, the recent USPSTF statement[9] recommends against the use of a CAC scan for risk stratification purposes because of the concern over 'false positive' test results. The authors concluded that 'false positive' test results would cause harm to patients and result in an abundance of unnecessary procedures and treatments as well as erode a

patient's quality of life due to mislabeling. The USPSTF concluded that the harms resulting from CAC scanning exceeded the benefits.[9] Although one can argue against statements that a patient with a high risk CAC score that fails to die or have an MI may be defined as 'false-positive,' it must be realized that our current state of evidence does in some ways fall short of accepted standards for screening; despite the strength of prognostic evidence. A major criterion utilized in guidelines or technology assessments has been that a screening test must have a high level of evidence on the effect of screening on health outcomes. This type of research details an improvement in either quantity or quality of life years as a result of the screening procedure. One example of where evidence is lacking lays with a lack of available evidence on a proven treatment for patients with a high risk CAC, resulting in a reduction in their observed event rates.

Although some have argued that direct evidence of an impact on clinical outcome is the only standard upon which new technology should be evaluated, others support the notion that unfolding a reasonable chain of logic regarding outcomes evidence with supporting links between testing, treatment, and outcome may be sufficient for clinical application of a new technology. Of course, the authors as well as most clinicians agree with the latter stance in large part, due to the extensive resources required to undertake a large randomized trial on CAC versus, for example, the FRS. This stance is also supported by the fact that much of the cardiac imaging literature has focused on devising standards for cardiovascular imaging that are based on the quality of their prognostic evidence. This standard of defining the relationship between imaging markers and CHD event risk has been effectively used to support resource utilization for echocardiography and nuclear imaging.[42,43,45] The rationale for the delineation of risk evidence in sufficiently powered patient samples allows for this data to be easily integrated with clinical trial data on therapeutic risk reduction.

In practice, there appears to be a two-stage process for risk stratification evidence: (1) testing to detect risk and (2) treatment to lower risk. Substantial evidence exists that treatment patterns do not always correlate with the extent of abnormalities noted on cardiovascular imaging.[46] It may be that the development of cardiovascular imaging evidence may be better guided by more stringent criteria on accuracy and longer term risk estimation beyond the current 3–5 years of follow-up noted by studies to date.

As a result, we are seeing a shift toward a greater acceptance of CAC as a tool that now has a growing evidence base with regard to its ability to differentiate risk in asymptomatic patients and subjects. It is for this reason that both statements from the ACC[10] and AHA[11] now are more supportive of CAC as an effective risk stratifier but recommendations will fall short of supporting routine screening of the adult population. Despite this, clinicians may be able to utilize the available prognostic evidence to revise local recommendations for screening strategies within targeted patient populations, such as those with an intermediate FRS or those not currently assigned risk within a global risk score (e.g., those with a family history of premature CHD).

11 LIMITATIONS OF THE PROGNOSTIC EVIDENCE WITH CAC SCANNING

Limitations of the current prognostic evidence base with CAC must also be acknowledged. It is important to note that not all patients with high risk CAC scores will die or have an acute MI during 3 to 5 years of follow-up. In fact, as we stated, only ~20% of patients with a CAC score >1,000 will be expected to have an event. This means that 80% will not have an event. Thus, the USPSTF[9] was correct that the majority of patients with high risk CAC results will not die or have an MI; they termed these patients as having 'false positive' test results. However, within the context of what we know about atherosclerosis, use of the term 'false positive' is a misnomer. A patient with a high-risk CAC score has atherosclerosis and the extensiveness of the disease process does not portend its degree of vulnerability per se; except as we discussed due to the co-occurrence of stable and vulnerable lesions. Clinicians should also understand that the assessment of absolute risk is relevant only within the context of knowing the degree of elevation in patient risk. Thus, although only 20% of those with a CAC score >1,000 will have an event, their risk is elevated more than 10-fold over patients with a low risk CAC score of 0–10. Physicians should understand at least the basics of population risk statistics to realize expected event rates as they relate to the general adult population.

A final limitation to the available CAC prognostic evidence is the lack of data in key subsets including those of diverse ethnicity. We await the results from the Multi-Ethnic Study of Atherosclerosis (MESA) to provide additional evidence on this subject.[47]

12 CONCLUSIONS

A review of the available evidence reveals that the extent of CAC is highly predictive of CHD or all-cause death as well

as acute MI. For this reason, it should be considered one of the few tests that may identify vulnerable patients with CAC scanning having the potential to serve as an effective screening test for CHD. Although guidelines are slow to adopt this concept, current statements from the ACC and AHA are more supportive of the role of CT-determined CAC as an effective prognosticator.[10–11] In particular, the data support the fact that patients with an intermediate FRS may be reclassified as being at CHD risk equivalent status. Upcoming data from the NIH-sponsored MESA study should provide needed data on the ability of CAC scoring to estimate risk in patients of diverse ethnicity.[47]

REFERENCES

1. O'Rourke RA, Brundage BH, Froelicher VF et al. American College of Cardiology/American Heart Association Expert Consensus Document on Electron Beam Computed Tomography for the Diagnosis of Coronary Artery Disease (Committee on Electron Beam Computed Tomography). J Am Coll Cardiol 2000; 36(1): 326–40.
2. Naghavi M, Falk E, Hecht H et al. for the SHAPE Task Force. From vulnerable plaque to vulnerable patient – Part III: Executive summery of the screening for heart attack and prevention and education (SHAPE) task force report. Am J Cardiol 2006 Jul 17; 98(2 Suppl 1): 2–15.
3. Rumberger JA, Simons DB, Fitzpatrick LA, Sheedy PF, Schwartz RS. Coronary artery calcium area by electron-beam computed tomography and coronary atherosclerotic plaque area. A histopathologic correlative study. Circulation 1995; 92: 2157–62.
4. Califf RM, Armstrong PW, Carver JR, D'Agostino RB, Strauss WE. Stratification of patients into high, medium, and low risk subgroups for purposes of risk factor management. J Am Coll Cardiol 1996; 27: 964–1047.
5. http://www.nhlbi.nih.gov/guidelines/cholesterol/index.htm., access date: August 29, 2006.
6. http://www.nhlbi.nih.gov/guidelines/hypertension/index.htm., access date: August 29, 2006.
7. Pasternak RC, Abrams J, Greenland P et al. 34th Bethesda Conference: Task force #1 – Identification of coronary heart disease risk: is there a detection gap? J Am Coll Cardiol 2003 Jun 4; 41(11): 1863–74.
8. Redberg RF, Vogel RA, Criqui MH et al. 34th Bethesda Conference: Task force #3 – What is the spectrum of current and emerging techniques for the noninvasive measurement of atherosclerosis? J Am Coll Cardiol 2003 Jun 4; 41(11): 1886–98.
9. http://www.ahcpr.gov/clinic/uspstf/uspsacad.htm, access date: September 28, 2004.
10. Greenland P, Bonow RO, Post WS et al. Coronary Artery Calcium Scoring By Ultrafast Computed Tomography: ACCF/AHA Writing Committee to Update the 2000 Clinical Expert Consensus Document on Electron-Beam Computed Tomography for the Diagnosis and Prognosis for Coronary Artery Disease. Circulation 2007; 115: 402–26.

11. Budoff MJ; Achenbach S, Blumenthal RS et al. Assessment of Coronary Artery Disease by Cardiac Computed Tomography: A Statement for Health Professionals From the American Heart Association. Circulation 2006; Oct 17; 114(16): 1761–91.

12. Nasir K, Michos ED, Blumenthal RS, Raggi R. Detection of High-Risk Young Adults and Women by Coronary Calcium and National Cholesterol Education Panel-III Guidelines. J Am Coll Cardiol 2005 Nov 15; 46(10): 1931–6.

13. Shaw LJ, Raggi P, Berman DS, Callister TQ. Coronary artery calcium as a measure of biologic age. Atherosclerosis 2006; 188: 112–19.

14. Mieres JH, Shaw LJ, Arai A et al. for the Cardiovascular Imaging Committee. American Heart Association – Cardiac Imaging Committee Consensus Statement: The role of cardiac imaging in the clinical evaluation of women with known or suspected coronary artery disease. Circulation 2005; 111: 682–96.

15. Brindle P, Emberson J, Lampe F et al. Predictive accuracy of the Framingham coronary risk score in British men: prospective cohort study. BMJ 2003 Nov 29; 327(7426): 1267.

16. Bertomeu A, Garcia-Vidal O, Farre X et al. Preclinical coronary atherosclerosis in a population with low incidence of myocardial infarction: cross sectional autopsy study. BMJ 2003 Sep 13; 327(7415): 591–2.

17. Grundy S. The changing face of cardiovascular risk. J Am Coll Cardiol 2005; 46(1): 173–5.

18. Pletcher MJ, Tice JA, Pignone M, Browner WS. Using the Coronary Artery Calcium Score to Predict Coronary Heart Disease Events. A Systematic Review and Meta-analysis. Arch Intern Med 2004; 164: 1285–92.

19. Taylor AJ, Bindeman J, Feurerstein I et al. The independent prognostic value of coronary calcium over measured cardiovascular risk factors in an asymptomatic male screening population: 6-year outcomes in the prospective army coronary calcium project. J Am Coll Cardiol 2005 Sep 6; 46(5): 807–14.

20. Arad Y, Goodman KJ, Roth M, Newstein D, Guerci AD. Coronary Calcification, Coronary Disease Risk Factors, C-Reactive Protein, and Atherosclerotic Cardiovascular Disease Events: The St. Francis Heart Study. J Am Coll Cardiol 2005; 46: 158–65.

21. Greenland P, LaBree L, Azen SP et al. Coronary artery calcium score combined with Framingham score for risk prediction in asymptomatic individuals. JAMA 2004; 291: 210–15.

22. Kondos GT, Hoff JA, Sevrukov A et al. Coronary Artery Calcium and Cardiac Events Electron-Beam Tomography Coronary Artery Calcium and Cardiac Events: A 37-Month Follow-Up of 5,635 Initially Asymptomatic Low to Intermediate Risk Adults. Circulation 2003; 107: 2571–76.

23. Vliegenthart R, Oudkerk M, Hofman A et al. Coronary calcification improves cardiovascular risk prediction in the elderly. Circulation 2005; Jul 26; 112(4): 572–7.

24. LaMonte MJ, FitzGerald SJ, Church TS et al. Coronary artery calcium score and coronary heart disease events in a large cohort of asymptomatic men and women. Am J Epidemiol 2005 Sep 1; 162(5): 421–9.

25. Budoff MJ, Shaw LJ, Liu ST et al. Long-term prognosis associated with coronary calcification: observation from a registry of 25,253 patients. J Am Coll Cardiol (in press).

26. Shaw LJ, Raggi P, Schisterman E, Berman DS, Callister TQ. Prognostic value of cardiac risk factors and coronary artery calcium screening for all-cause mortality. Radiol 2003; 228(3): 826–33.

27. Raggi P, Shaw LJ, Berman DS, Callister TQ. Prognostic value of coronary artery calcium screening in subjects with and without diabetes. J Am Coll Cardiol 2004; 43(9): 1663–9.

28. Raggi P, Shaw LJ, Berman DS, Callister TQ, Gender-based differences in the prognostic value of coronary calcification. J Women's Health 2004; 13(3): 273–82.

29. Shaw LJ, Raggi P, Callister TQ, Berman DS. Prognostic value of coronary artery calcium screening in asymptomatic smokers and non-smokers. Eur Heart J 2006 Apr; 27(8): 968–75.

30. Shaw LJ, Hendel RC, Cerquiera M et al. Ethnic differences in the prognostic value of stress tc-99m tetrofosmin gated spect myocardial perfusion imaging. J Am Coll Cardiol 2005; 45: 1494–1504.

31. Lauer MS, Blackstone EH, Young JB, Topol EJ. Cause of death in clinical research: time for a reassessment? J Am Coll Cardiol 1999; 34: 618–20.

32. Shaw LJ, Bairey Merz CN, Reis SE et al. for the WISE Investigators. Ischemic heart disease in women: Insights from the NHLBI-sponsored Women's Ischemia Syndrome Evaluation (WISE) study. Part I: Sex Differences in Traditional and Novel Risk Factors, Symptom Evaluation and Gender-Optimized Diagnostic Strategies. J Am Coll Cardiol 2006; 47: S4–S20.

33. Cooil B, Callister TQ. Use of electron beam tomography data to develop models for prediction of hard coronary events. Am Heart J 2001 Mar; 141(3): 375–82.

34. Bairey Merz CN, Shaw LJ, Reis SE et al. for the WISE Investigators. Ischemic heart disease in women: Insights from the NHLBI-sponsored Women's Ischemia Syndrome Evaluation (WISE) study. Part II: The Role of Micro- and Macro-vascular Disease Affecting Gender Differences in Presentation, Diagnosis, and Outcome. J Am Coll Cardiol 2006; 47: S21–S29.

35. Chambless LE, Folsom AR, Clegg LX et al. Carotid wall thickness is predictive of incident clinical stroke: the Atherosclerosis Risk in Communities (ARIC) study. Am J Epidemiol 2000; 151: 478–87.

36. O'Leary DH, Polak JF, Kronmal RA et al. Carotid-artery intima and media thickness as a risk factor for myocardial infarction and stroke in older adults. Cardiovascular Health Study. New Engl J Med 1999; 340: 14–22.

37. Bots ML, Hoes AW, Koudstaal PJ et al. Common carotid artery intima-media thickness and risk of stroke and myocardial infarction: the Rotterdam Study. Circulation 1997; 96: 1432–7.

38. Fowler-Brown A, Pignone M, Pletcher M et al. Exercise tolerance testing to screen for coronary heart disease: A systematic review for the U.S. Preventive Services Task Force. Ann Intern Med 2004; W-9-W-24.

39. Blumenthal RS, Becker DM, Moy TF et al. Exercise thallium tomography predicts future clinically manifest coronary heart disease in a high-risk asymptomatic population. Circulation 1996 Mar 1; 93(5): 915–23.

40. Blumenthal RS, Becker DM, Yanek LR et al. Detecting occult coronary disease in a high-risk asymptomatic population. Circulation 2003 Feb 11; 107(5): 702–7.

41. Gould KL, Ornish D, Scherwitz L et al. Changes in myocardial perfusion abnormalities by positron emission tomography after long-term, intense risk factor modification. JAMA 1995; 274(11): 894–901.

42. http://www.acc.org/qualityandscience/clinical/pdfs/SPECTMPIACPubFile.pdf2., access date: July 20, 2006.

43. Klocke FJ, Baird MG, Lorell BH et al. American College of Cardiology; American Heart Association; American Society for Nuclear Cardiology. ACC/AHA/ASNC guidelines for the clinical use of cardiac radionuclide imaging—executive summary: a report of the American College of Cardiology/American Heart Association Task Force on Practice Guidelines (ACC/AHA/ASNC Committee to Revise the 1995 Guidelines for the Clinical Use of Cardiac Radionuclide Imaging). J Am Coll Cardiol 2003 Oct 1; 42(7): 1318–33.

44. Anand DV, Lim E, Hopkins D et al. Risk Stratification in Uncomplicated Type 2 Diabetes: Prospective Evaluation of the Combined use of Coronary Artery Calcium Imaging and Selective Myocardial Perfusion Scintigraphy. Eur Heart J 2006 Mar; 27(6): 713–21.

45. Gibbons RJ, Abrams J, Chatterjee K et al. ACC/AHA 2002 guideline update for the management of patients with chronic stable angina – Summary article. J Am Coll Cardiol 2003; 41: 159–68.

46. Mowatt G, Brazzelli M, Gemmell H et al. Aberdeen Technology Assessment Group. Systematic review of the prognostic effectiveness of SPECT myocardial perfusion scintigraphy in patients with suspected or known coronary artery disease and following myocardial infarction. Nuc Med Comm 2005 Mar; 26(3): 217–29.

47. Bild DE, Detrano R, Peterson D et al. Ethnic differences in coronary calcification: the Multi-Ethnic Study of Atherosclerosis (MESA). Circulation 2005 Mar 15; 111(10): 1313–20.

11

Progression of Coronary Artery Calcium and its Pharmacologic Modification

Axel Schmermund and Raimund Erbel

1 BACKGROUND

Coronary artery calcium (CAC) is intimately associated with coronary atherosclerosis. As outlined in detail in chapters 8 to 10, CAC predicts the overall extent and severity of atherosclerotic plaque formation in the coronary arteries, whether measured at autopsy[1,2] or in the living patient by using invasive coronary angiography[3–6] or intravascular ultrasound.[7–8] It has also been demonstrated that patients with more advanced CAC have more frequent and severe stress-induced myocardial ischemia as determined by single-photon emission computed tomography.[9,10] Finally, patients with greater amounts of CAC have consistently been reported to carry an increased cardiovascular event risk.[11–13] All these relationships have been analyzed using CAC measurements in a cross-sectional manner. Much less is known about the progression of CAC over time.

CAC shares the same risk factor relationships established for the pathogenesis of coronary atherosclerosis and cardiovascular events. Age, male sex, smoking, high serum cholesterol levels, systemic hypertension, and diabetes have been consistently found to predict CAC scores.[14] Still, a substantial proportion of the interindividual variability in CAC scores remains unexplained. Against this background, it is only logical to ask about the natural history of CAC progression, the factors leading to greater or less CAC progression, the prognostic implications associated with it, and potential therapies to influence CAC progression in a beneficial manner. This has been an area of intense and continued research over the past few years. Despite these activities, some basic questions remain unanswered.

2 PROGRESSION OF CORONARY ATHEROSCLEROSIS

Coronary angiographic studies have established the prognostic importance of atherosclerosis progression.[15,16] Patients with increased progression of either the number of angiographic stenoses or worst stenosis degree have a several-fold increased risk of unstable angina and myocardial infarction. Importantly, it has been demonstrated that atherosclerosis progression does not occur in a graded, continuous fashion. Severe stenoses can appear in coronary segments showing no or minimal angiographic disease in the initial angiogram only weeks to months before the second examination, and lesions in the same patient do not necessarily develop in the same direction: some lesions progress whereas others remain stable or even regress.[17,18] Accordingly, it is usually impossible to predict the progression of coronary atherosclerosis in an individual patient.

Recent data suggest that the progression of coronary atherosclerosis shares a common underlying mechanism with the acute coronary syndromes (Figure 11.1).[19,20] In patients at risk, intra-arterial thrombosis occurs as a result of plaque rupture or plaque erosion (and, less frequently, calcified

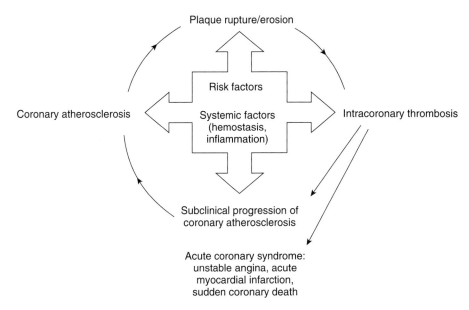

Figure 11.1 Simplified scheme of the relationship between coronary atherosclerosis progression and acute coronary syndromes. As explained in the text, similar mechanisms appear to be involved.

nodule formation). Depending on the extent of the thrombosis, myocardial ischemia ensues with the clinical manifestations of unstable angina, myocardial infarction, or sudden coronary death. In many cases, however, the intra-arterial thrombus formation remains clinically silent and only leads to rapid progression of atherosclerotic plaque formation, for example in the form of 'healed plaque rupture.'[20] Obviously, patients with such subclinical events are at a greatly increased risk of suffering a clinical event, explaining at least in part the above noted clinical observation that accelerated angiographic coronary lesion progression foretells an increased rate of clinical events. Indeed, on the basis of the clinical observations, Buchwald stated in 1992 that 'For an individual patient, changes in the severity of coronary atherosclerosis seen on sequential coronary arteriograms can serve as prognostic indicators for subsequent overall or atherosclerotic coronary heart disease mortality.'[21]

3 MEASURING THE PROGRESSION OF CORONARY ARTERY CALCIUM

Most of the studies examining CAC progression and its pharmacologic modification have been performed using electron-beam computed tomography (EBCT) (Figure 11.2). The median variability of the EBCT-derived CAC score (Agatston method or volumetric score) repeated in the same patient within a few minutes is in the order of 10% and thus

less than the annual rate of progression found in most patient groups.[22–24] Of note, the presence of CAC needs to be evaluated throughout the complete coronary arterial system and not only in the more proximal coronary segments to allow for a meaningful follow-up examination.

The original *Agatston score* has theoretic limitations with regard to reproducible measurements, because a density factor derived from the maximum CT density within the calcified lesion is used. The area of the lesion is then multiplied

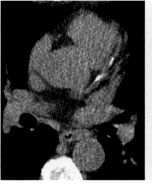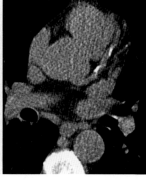

Figure 11.2 Serial examination of coronary artery calcium using electron-beam computed tomography. Sections at the level of the anterior descending coronary artery (LAD) are shown at baseline (left panel) and after an inter-scan interval of 14 months (right panel). Importantly, for serial coronary artery calcium studies, the complete coronary arterial system needs to be examined and not just portions of it. In this specific patient, the total Agatston coronary artery calcium score (comprising the complete coronary system) remained stable. At baseline, it was 164, and 14 months later, it was 171.

with this density factor, yielding the individual lesion score.[25] If the maximum density measures 302 Hounsfield Units (HU), the density factor is 3. If the maximum density measures 298 HU, the density factor is 2, by definition generating a score reduced by one-third compared with a density factor of 3. To overcome the limitations of the Agatston score, a volumetric score was devised using isotropic interpolation.[26] To generate this score, the input data set is sampled at several intermediate cross sections between the original 3 mm thick sections ('EBCT single slice mode'). Voxels are interpolated on the basis of these intermediate cross sections and assigned a numeric value which depends on their distance from the reference section. This reconstruction can be performed automatically by dedicated software programs. The volumetric scoring system has been used in the majority of randomized trials of pharmacologic modification of CAC progression and in many studies on the natural history of CAC progression. However, despite offering theoretical advantages over the Agatston score, a clear superiority of the volumetric score has not been demonstrated.

Determination of the calcium mass appears to gain more and more clinical acceptance, as it can be exactly determined by using a calibration system and is independent of the type of CT scanner used. It should enable internationally comparable – and reproducible – CAC measurements. According to comparative studies, even with different image acquisition protocols, varying slice thickness and image acquisition time, repeated measurements of calcium mass remain stable, whereas the Agatston score shows in part substantial variability.[27] Coronary calcium mass (reported in mg) and the dimensionless Agatston score share a relationship of approximately 1:4.5, depending on the image acquisition protocol.

Due to the rapid development of the technology, modern multi-slice computed tomography has only infrequently been used for longitudinal studies. The actual scanner generations in conjunction with calcium mass determination probably allow for improved reproducibility of CAC measures.[28]

4 NATURAL HISTORY OF CORONARY ARTERY CALCIUM PROGRESSION

Most studies have reported the annual progression of the CAC score (Agatston, volumetric, or calcium area)[26,29–32] Absolute changes in CAC scores are calculated as

$$\left(\frac{X_2 - X_1}{t_{months}}\right) * 12,$$

where X is the value of the CAC score and t is the time interval between the 2 scans, measured in months. Relative (percent) changes are calculated as

$$\frac{\left(X_2 - X_1\right) * 12 * 100}{X_1 * t_{months}}.$$

In patients from the general population examined in the community setting with a mean age of 46 ± 7 years, Maher et al. reported a mean annual CAC progression of 24%.[30] In asymptomatic patients with several risk factors, Budoff et al. observed a mean annual CAC progression of 33% which was lower in patients on lipid-lowering therapy than in the total group.[31] In both reports, patients with negative EBCTs (that is, a CAC score of 0) were included.[30,31]

Callister et al. included asymptomatic high-risk individuals with a baseline CAC score ≥ 30.[26] In this group, they observed a mean and median annual CAC progression of 52% and 44%, respectively.

We analyzed CAC progression in symptomatic patients who mostly underwent pharmacological treatment and who had a CAC score > 0.[32] The mean annual CAC progression was 51% for total calcium scores (Agatston score) and 42% for total calcium areas. The median values were 32% and 27%, respectively. We also noted that the baseline CAC burden appeared to influence the rate of progression (Figure 11.3).[32] This was later confirmed in other reports.[33] Patients with extensive CAC had the greatest absolute rate of progression, whereas in patients with lower CAC scores, absolute progression was much less. In the latter group (with lower CAC scores), relative progression was significantly higher. This reflects in part a mathematical phenomenon in that an increase in the CAC score from 30 to 60 is an increase by 100%, whereas from 1,030 to 1,060, it is only an increase by 3%. Nevertheless, it appears clinically relevant that opposite trends in absolute and relative (percent) measures of progression can be seen. Achenbach et al. extended this observation by analyzing long time intervals up to 6 years.[34] Over time, relative CAC progression was less than would be anticipated on the basis of shorter time intervals, again demonstrating lower relative CAC progression for higher CAC scores. Accordingly, the initial extent of CAC needs to be accounted for when interpreting CAC progression rates. Finally, absolute CAC score increases appear to be relatively stable over time and are usually higher in the presence of extensive CAC.

In an early study, Janowitz et al. compared CAC progression over 14 months in 10 patients with angiographically proven coronary artery disease (CAD) and 10 asymptomatic

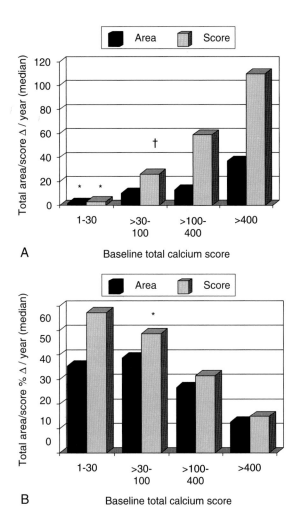

Figure 11.3 Annual coronary artery calcium progression (median) in the complete coronary system in 102 patients with a positive coronary artery calcium score. Classification according to baseline total calcium scores demonstrates opposite trends in absolute and relative (percent) measures of progression with lower relative calcium progression for higher calcium scores.
Adapted from Schmermund et al. Arterioscler Thromb Vasc Biol 2001; 21:421–6, with permission.
(a) Absolute changes. *p<0.05 vs. ">30–100," ">100–400," and ">400"; ‡p<0.05 vs. ">400"
(b) Percent changes. *p<0.05 vs. ">400"

patients and found a significant difference of 48% vs. 22%.[35] It is unlikely that luminal obstruction per se predicts accelerated progression of coronary artery disease. Rather, it would indicate an angiographically appreciable advanced stage of coronary atherosclerotic plaque disease and increased susceptibility to further progression of disease in the absence of adequate treatment. In our above noted series, 85 patients underwent coronary angiography, and CAC progression was not increased in patients with coronary stenoses.[32] Again, as noted above, the baseline amount of CAC needs to be considered in this kind of analysis.

To summarize, the annual rate of CAC progression in asymptomatic patients or symptomatic patients with medical therapy is in the order of 20–30% and tends to slow down with higher CAC scores. Absolute CAC score increases appear to be relatively stable over time. Patients who have no CAC at baseline mostly also have no CAC upon a follow-up scan within the next 5 years or, if CAC appears, the score is low.[31,36] Obviously, first appearance of CAC and progression will depend on patient selection and age, and no general statement can currently be made. More definitive data on the natural history of CAC progression in asymptomatic subjects are to be expected beginning in the year 2008 from the Multi-Ethnic Study of Atherosclerosis (MESA) and Heinz Nixdorf Recall Study in Germany.[37,38]

Regarding the topographic distribution, changes in CAC appear to be similar in the major coronary arteries, left anterior descending, left circumflex, and right coronary artery.[32] The most consistent and greatest progression of CAC can be observed in the segments with the most prominent initial involvement (Figure 11.4). Consistent with previous pathologic and angiographic studies on the natural history of atherosclerosis,[39] the rate of CAC progression is greatest in the proximal left coronary system and shows a more even distribution from proximal to distal in the RCA. The progression or stabilization of CAC occurs in a uniform pattern at different predilection sites in the coronary tree, suggesting that the development of CAC is a coronary systemic process.

5 ACCELERATED CORONARY ARTERY CALCIUM PROGRESSION IN END-STAGE RENAL DISEASE

In the setting of end-stage renal disease, severe soft tissue calcification frequently occurs. Vascular calcification is not only associated with atherosclerotic changes of the vessel intimal layer. Rather, extraskeletal calcification as a result of disturbed calcium homeostasis can lead to extensive medial calcification which is not found in patients with normal renal function.[40] This is thought to be a major determinant of the adverse cardiovascular outcome associated with renal failure and chronic kidney disease.

CAC measurements in dialysis patients have confirmed that the amount of CAC is greatly elevated in these patients and even surpasses the amount seen in patients with established coronary artery disease by a factor of 2.5–5.[41] Also, the progression of CAC is greatly increased and has

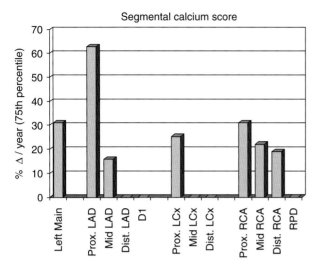

Figure 11.4 Relative annual progression (75th percentile) of coronary artery calcium in 12 coronary artery segments. Progression concentrates on the typical predilection sites of coronary atherosclerosis in the proximal left coronary artery system and, distributed more evenly, the right coronary artery. Left main = left main stem, LAD = left anterior descending coronary artery, LCx = left circumflex coronary artery, RCA = right coronary artery, RPD = right posterior descending coronary artery, Prox. = proximal, Dist. = distal.
Adapted from Schmermund et al. Arterioscler Thromb Vasc Biol 2001; 21: 421–6, with permission.

whereas it was 17% in the patients with no AMI (p <0.0001). Patients with an annual CAC progression ≥15% had a 17.2-fold increased AMI-risk (Figure 11.5). This risk appeared to be modified depending on the baseline CAC score. In particular, patients with a high baseline score *and* an increased progression had an increased AMI-risk, underlining the importance of the relationship between the baseline amount of CAC and the rate of progression.[45]

In the St. Francis Heart Study reported by Arad et al., 4,613 subjects without known CAD underwent EBCT scanning at baseline and sequentially after 2 and 4 years.[12] Subjects were prospectively followed over a mean of 4.3 years after the baseline EBCT scan. After the second EBCT scan (after 2 years), 49 subjects suffered a cardiovascular event. Mean CAC progression between the baseline and the 2-year scan in these subjects was 247, whereas it was 4 in the subjects with no event. In multivariate logistic regression analysis, CAC progression – together with CAC baseline scores – was the strongest predictor of cardiovascular events.[12]

In summary, the limited data available to date indicate that CAC progression has a similar prognostic impact as described for angiographic CAD progression.

been estimated to reach 100% in 2 years.[41–43] Although a link between CAC progression and increased cardiovascular mortality in patients with renal failure appears plausible, no data are available to directly validate this.

6 PROGNOSTIC SIGNIFICANCE OF CORONARY ARTERY CALCIUM PROGRESSION

It has been proposed that patients with increased CAC progression (and normal renal function) have a higher rate of acute myocardial infarction (AMI), independent of statin treatment.[44,45] Raggi et al. conducted a retrospective analysis of 495 patients who had no clinical coronary artery disease but were all treated with statins because of CAC and who underwent sequential EBCT scans with a mean interval of 1.9 ± 1 years (range 1–6 years).[45] The mean time between the baseline EBCT scan and the follow-up contact with the patients was 3.2 years. 41 patients suffered a fatal or nonfatal AMI during this interval. Although the baseline amount of CAC was comparable, patients who later suffered an AMI had a mean CAC progression of 42%,

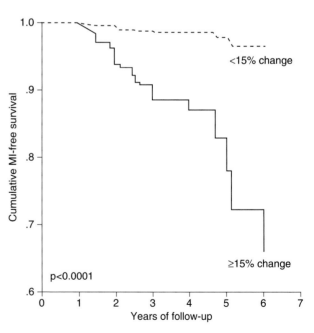

Figure 11.5 Cox proportional hazards survival curves of time to acute myocardial infarction for patients with a yearly calcium volume score change =15% or <15%. All patients received statin therapy. Increased coronary artery calcium progression was associated with a largely increased event rate.
Adapted from Raggi et al. Thromb Vasc Biol 2004; 24: 1272–77, with permission.

7 FACTORS INFLUENCING CORONARY ARTERY CALCIUM PROGRESSION

A number of observational trials have analyzed factors which might potentially influence CAC progression.[29,31,46–48] Early data found an interrelationship between low-density lipoprotein cholesterol (LDL), statin therapy, and CAC progression.[29,31] Callister et al. reported that successful pharmacological LDL cholesterol reduction led to a significant mitigation of CAC progression in asymptomatic high-risk individuals.[29] In untreated patients with a mean LDL cholesterol level of 147 mg/dl, the mean annual CAC progression was 52%. In patients treated pharmacologically with statins but whose LDL cholesterol level remained >120 mg/dl (at a mean value of 139 mg/dl), mean annual progression was 25%. In patients with LDL cholesterol values <120 mg/dl, stabilization of CAC scores was observed (on average, −7%) (Figure 11.6). There was an approximately linear relationship between on-treatment LDL cholesterol levels and CAC progression. Similar findings were made in another observational study involving 299 patients of whom 62 were on statin therapy.[31] Whereas their mean annual CAC progression was 15%, it was 39% in patients receiving no treatment.

Confirmation of these results came from the first published study with a prospective design.[49] Asymptomatic patients from 2 institutions who had undergone EBCT scanning at least 12 months before the study were asked to undergo sequential follow-up EBCT scanning if they had an Agatston CAC score >20 in the baseline scan, an LDL cholesterol value >130 mg/dl and were not receiving lipid-lowering medications. The second EBCT was performed a mean of 14 months after the first scan. All patients then received 0.3 mg cerivastatin for 12 months before undergoing a final EBCT scan. Because of the withdrawal of cerivastatin from the market, the study had to be terminated prematurely after completion of 66 patients. LDL cholesterol was lowered from a mean of 162 ± 36 mg/dl to a mean at follow-up of 108 ± 27 mg/dl. Compared with the first interval, during which no lipid lowering therapy was delivered, annual CAC progression during cerivastatin therapy was significantly reduced from 24.3 ± 21% to 10.5 ± 20% (CAC volume score). LDL cholesterol levels <100 mg/dl were achieved in a total of 32 patients, whose LDL cholesterol was lowered from 152 ± 88 mg/dl to 88 ± 17 mg/dl. Of note, CAC progression was halted in these patients. Measuring initially 27.3 ± 23%, it was reduced to −3.4 ± 12% during cerivastatin therapy.[49]

Hecht and Harman later reported on their experience in asymptomatic high-risk patients who received lipid-lowering therapy with atorvastatin (n = 103, mean dose 14 mg) or with simvastatin (n = 46, mean dose 24 mg).[50] Approximately 50% of all patients also received niacin. LDL-cholesterol values at baseline were higher in the patients treated with atorvastatin, and their CAC scores also were slightly higher when analyzing the percentile values. The mean interval between baseline and follow-up EBCT scan was 1.2 years. During this interval, both groups had dramatic improvements in their lipid levels and reached similar mean non high-density lipoprotein (HDL) cholesterol values of approximately 99 mg/dl. CAC progression was similar in both patient groups and measured 8–11% depending on which scoring system was used.

These observational studies, one of which had a prospective design, were all consistent with the notion of a significant influence of LDL cholesterol levels on the progression of CAC. Importantly, a relationship between on-treatment LDL cholesterol levels and CAC progression was seen. Independent of LDL cholesterol lowering, possible effects of statin treatment by itself or differential effects of various statins did not appear to be of significance. On the basis of these data, LDL cholesterol was believed to be an important modifier of CAC progression.

However, it is notable that some observational reports failed to detect an association between LDL cholesterol

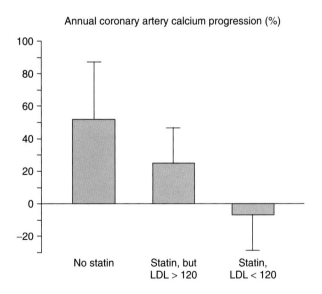

Annual coronary artery calcium progression (%)

Figure 11.6 First observational study on the relationship between low-density lipoprotein (LDL) cholesterol and coronary artery calcium progression. Patients receiving statin treatment had less progression than patients who received no such treatment, and patients who reached LDL cholesterol levels <120 mg/dl had, as a group, no coronary artery calcium progression. On the basis of data from Callister TQ et al. New Engl J Med 1998; 339: 1972–78.

levels and CAC progression.[51,52] Hecht and Harman analyzed CAC progression over 1.2 years in a total of 182 asymptomatic patients regarding the intensity of statin treatment and on-treatment LDL cholesterol levels.[51] Both in patients with intensive statin treatment (80 mg/d) and in the others, annual CAC progression was approximately 9%. In contradistinction to the above noted studies, no relationship was seen between LDL cholesterol levels and CAC progression. Similarly, Wong et al. did not observe differences in CAC progression over 7 years in a total of 761 patients, regardless of whether they had optimal, intermediate, or higher risk LDL cholesterol levels according to the National Cholesterol Education Program.[52] Only decreased high-density lipoprotein (HDL) cholesterol appeared to relate to an increased rate of CAC progression.

8 NON-LIPID INFLUENCES ON CORONARY ARTERY CALCIUM PROGRESSION

Apart from LDL cholesterol, only a few factors which may also influence CAC progression have been proposed. In 2001, Motro and Shemesh reported on a substudy of INSIGHT comprising 201 patients with systemic hypertension (International Nifedipine Study: Intervention as Goal for Hypertension Therapy).[46] CAC was measured using 2-slice spiral computed tomography without electrocardiographic gating, a technique with severe limitations compared with today's standard. Annual CAC progression with blood pressure lowering by diuretic therapy was 26% and significantly higher than the 14% observed with prolonged-release nifedipine. In other studies, systemic hypertension or its pharmacologic treatment has not been reported to influence CAC progression.

Cassidy et al. reported EBCT serial scanning in a community-sample of unselected subjects who underwent the second scan a mean of almost 9 years after the first.[47] Of a total of 443 subjects, the majority (n = 329) had relatively low 10-year Framingham risk <10% of suffering a cardiovascular event. In this group, but not in the subjects with an intermediate or high 10-year Framingham risk, obesity was associated with an increased CAC progression. Finally, a recent report utilizing serial EBCT scanning also found an association between homocysteine levels and CAC progression, whereas C-reactive protein levels did not appear to be related to CAC progression.[48]

To put this in perspective, plausible risk factor correlations of CAC have been confirmed in numerous cross-sectional studies, whereas this has been more difficult in longitudinal studies. Some studies, but not all, proposed a linear relationship between LDL cholesterol and CAC progression. Otherwise, only obesity in a subset of patients and, with many questions, systemic hypertension and homocysteine levels have been discussed. Large epidemiological studies, such as the MESA and Heinz Nixdorf Recall studies, are awaited to resolve the discrepancy between clear risk factor associations of CAC when measured at one point in time and the apparent lack of such clear associations in serial CAC measurements.[37,38]

9 FACTORS INFLUENCING CORONARY ARTERY CALCIUM PROGRESSION IN PATIENTS WITH END-STAGE RENAL DISEASE

In patients with *end-stage renal disease*, a number of factors were identified which correlated with an increased CAC progression. These were, in particular, age, diabetes, higher serum concentrations of calcium and phosphorus, and, perhaps most importantly, duration of dialysis treatment.[42] The longer dialysis therapy had been necessary, the greater the progression of calcification.

10 PHARMACOLOGIC MODULATION OF CORONARY ARTERY CALCIUM PROGRESSION – RANDOMIZED STUDIES

Lowering of LDL cholesterol levels has been established as an effective therapy for patients with ischemic heart disease or equivalent high-risk status. In particular, recent evidence from large clinical trials demonstrated a reduction of cardiovascular events with intensive lipid lowering in a target range <80 mg/dl.[53–58] The *Pravastatin or Atorvastatin Evaluation and Infection Therapy* (PROVE-IT) trial compared clinical cardiovascular events in patients who had just suffered an acute coronary syndrome and who were treated with 80 mg atorvastatin or 40 mg pravastatin.[55] A significant event reduction by 16% was observed in the 80 mg atorvastatin group over the course of approximately 2 years. The *Treating to New Targets* (TNT) trial compared the effect on cardiovascular events of 80 mg versus 10 mg atorvastatin in mostly stable patients with coronary artery disease and observed a significant event reduction by 22% in the 80 mg atorvastatin group over a period of almost 5 years.[57] In addition, a surrogate endpoint study which used intravascular ultrasound observed a stop of coronary plaque progression over 18 months in patients treated with 80 mg atorvastatin compared with a progression of plaque volume in patients treated with 40 mg pravastatin.[56]

The progression of coronary atherosclerosis has frequently been used as a surrogate endpoint in clinical studies. The underlying rationale was provided by the above mentioned studies, demonstrating that the angiographic progression of coronary artery disease was one of the most important predictors of future coronary events.[15,16,21] Along these lines, CAC progression in several studies was predictive of cardiovascular event risk.[12,43,44] Observational studies suggested that LDL cholesterol influenced CAC progression with an increased rate of CAC progression in patients with increased LDL cholesterol levels.[29,31] After prospective initiation of LDL cholesterol lowering, CAC progression was mitigated.[34] As noted above, there have been suggestions that the mechanisms which underlie the acute coronary syndromes, in particular coronary plaque rupture, also have an important role in the progression of coronary atherosclerosis (Figure 11.1).[20] Accordingly, the hypothesis that lipid-lowering therapy would reduce CAC progression was addressed in several randomized trials.

In a subgroup of participants in the *St. Francis Heart Study* who were all asymptomatic and whose CAC score (Agatston method) was in the highest quintile of the distribution, CAC progression was examined over a mean duration of 4.3 years.[59] The treatment group received atorvastatin 20 mg/d, vitamin C 1 g/d, and vitamin E 1,000 U/d, and aspirin 81 mg/d. The placebo group received aspirin 81 mg/d. In the group treated with atorvastatin, the mean baseline LDL cholesterol value of 146 mg/dl was lowered by 47% over the course of the study. Despite the comparatively long treatment period and a trend for a lower event rate in the atorvastatin group, no difference in the progression of CAC (Agatston method) was observed. Overall, the Agatston CAC score increased by 331 in the atorvastatin group (+81%) and by 323 (+73%) in the control group treated with aspirin alone.[59]

In the *Beyond Endorsed Lipid Lowering with EBT Scanning* (BELLES) trial, EBCT scanning to track CAC progression was performed in hyperlipidemic post-menopausal women.[60] In a multicenter study, they were randomized to therapy with 80 mg/d atorvastatin or 40 mg/d pravastatin. Intensive statin therapy with 80 mg

atorvastatin over 1 year lowered LDL cholesterol from 175 mg/dl to 92 mg/dl (−47%), whereas 40 mg pravastatin lowered LDL cholesterol from 174 mg/dl to 129 mg/dl (−25%). However, median CAC progression did not differ and was approximately 20% in both treatment groups.

We analyzed CAC progression in patients who had no coronary artery disease but ≥2 cardiovascular risk factors and at least moderate CAC.[61] In a randomized, double-blind multicenter trial, patients were assigned to receive 80 mg or 10 mg atorvastatin per day over 12 months. CAC progression was determined by EBCT and could be analyzed in 366 patients. After pretreatment with 10 mg atorvastatin for 4 weeks, 12-months study medication reduced mean LDL cholesterol from 106 to 87 mg/dl in the group randomized to receive 80 mg atorvastatin (p <0.001), whereas the levels remained stable in the group randomized to receive 10 mg atorvastatin (108 mg/dl at baseline, 109 mg/dl at the end of the study). Mean CAC progression was similar in both treatment groups. Corrected for the baseline CAC volume score, it was 27% in the 80 mg atorvastatin group and 25% in the 10 mg atorvastatin group (p = 0.65). There was no relationship of CAC progression with on-treatment LDL cholesterol levels (Figure 11.7).

Houslay et al. assessed the effect of high-dose atorvastatin (80 mg) compared with placebo on CAC progression in a double blind randomized trial.[62] Patients with calcific aortic stenosis and CAC were followed over approximately 24 months. Atorvastatin reduced LDL cholesterol by 53% and C-reactive protein by 49%, whereas there was no change with placebo. With 39 patients completing the trial in the atorvastatin group and 49 in the control group, there was no difference in annual CAC progression (26% vs. 18%). Again, as opposed to the earlier observational trials, no relationship between LDL cholesterol concentrations with the rate of CAC progression was seen.

Taken together, these studies suggest that the relationship between lipid lowering therapy, LDL cholesterol levels, CAC progression, and total atherosclerotic plaque is indeed more complex than previously thought. Currently, lipid-lowering therapy cannot be expected to significantly influence CAC progression. No randomized trial observed a relationship between LDL cholesterol levels and CAC progression. The discrepancy with most of the observational trials can perhaps be explained by confounding factors influencing the relationship between LDL cholesterol and CAC progression which were not accounted for. It is possible, for example, that patients who received statins and reached target cholesterol levels in general received a better treatment than their counterparts who had no statin treatment or

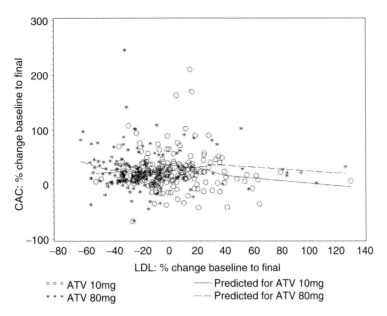

Figure 11.7   Relationship between changes in low-density lipoprotein cholesterol levels and coronary artery calcium progression in patients treated with atorvastatin. Despite more intensive low-density lipoprotein cholesterol reduction with 80 mg compared with 10 mg atorvastatin, coronary artery calcium progression was similar, and there was no association between online low-density lipoprotein cholesterol values and coronary artery calcium progression. Adapted from Schmermund et al. Circulation 2006; 113: 427–37, with permission.

did not reach sufficiently low LDL cholesterol levels. In the prospective study by Achenbach et al., the patients served as their own controls, and it is possible that overall treatment during the second year (during which cerivastatin therapy was commenced) was improved compared with the first year which was purely observational.[49] An additional explanation lies in the increase in CAC scores found between the baseline EBCT scan and the end of the first year of observation in that study.[34] Because relative CAC progression is reduced with higher baseline CAC scores, one would expect less progression during the second than during the first year.

11 PHARMACOLOGIC MODULATION OF CORONARY ARTERY CALCIUM PROGRESSION IN CHRONIC KIDNEY DISEASE

In patients with chronic kidney disease, 2 randomized trials have been performed which analyzed CAC progression as a function of treatment with sevelamer versus calcium salts for phosphorus binding. In both these studies, Treat to Goal (TTG) and Renagel in New Dialysis (RIND), a significant

attenuation of CAC progression was observed in patients receiving sevelamer.[63,64] Interestingly, sevelamer is currently the only substance which appears to attenuate CAC progression. However, this holds true only for patients with end-stage renal disease, and a number of caveats are related to the alternative mechanisms of soft tissue calcification which apply to this group of patients, compared with patients with normal renal function.

12 PROGRESSION OF CORONARY ARTERY CALCIUM – CURRENT STATE

CAC progression can be reliably determined in small groups of patients. Using up-to-date scanner technology, inter-scan variability is smaller than annual CAC progression in such groups, which is usually in the order of 20–30%.[26,30–34] In individual patients, only substantial CAC changes are beyond measurement variability.[24,36] In analogy with angiographic measures of coronary atherosclerosis, increased CAC progression conveys an increased risk of suffering acute myocardial infarction and other cardiovascular events.[12,44,45] Although this might have clinical consequences for selected patients, no factors have been reliably identified which modify CAC progression. In particular, several randomized studies failed to detect an effect of lipid-lowering therapy on CAC progression, even though medications proven to reduce cardiovascular event rates were used.[59–62] Thus, despite the prognostic implications of accelerated CAC progression, possible therapeutic implications remain unclear. Currently, no clinical applications have been established for serial CAC measurements. Large epidemiologic studies (Multi-Ethnic Study of Atherosclerosis, Heinz Nixdorf Recall Study) will help to resolve some of the remaining issues regarding natural history and risk factor correlates of CAC progression.[37,38]

REFERENCES

1. Rumberger JA, Simons DB, Fitzpatrick LA, Sheedy PF, Schwartz RS. Coronary artery calcium area by electron-beam computed tomography and coronary atherosclerotic plaque area. A histopathologic correlative study. Circulation 1995; 92: 2157–62.
2. Sangiorgi G, Rumberger J, Severson A et al. Arterial calcification and not lumen stenosis is correlated with atherosclerotic plaque burden in humans: A histologic study of 723 coronary artery segments using nondecalcifying methodology. J Am Coll Cardiol 1998; 31: 126–33.
3. Rumberger JA, Sheedy PF, Breen JF, Schwartz RS. Electron beam computed tomographic calcium score cutpoints and severity of associated angiographic lumen stenosis. J Am Coll Cardiol 1997; 29: 1542–48.
4. Guerci AD, Spadaro LA, Goodman KJ et al. Comparison of electron beam computed tomography scanning and conventional risk factor assessment for the prediction of angiographic coronary artery disease. J Am Coll Cardiol 1998; 32: 673–9.
5. Schmermund A, Denktas AE, Rumberger JA et al. Independent and incremental value of coronary artery calcium for predicting the extent of angiographic coronary artery disease: Comparison with cardiac risk factors and radionuclide perfusion imaging. J Am Coll Cardiol 1999; 34: 777–86.
6. Haberl R, Becker A, Leber A et al. Correlation of coronary calcification and angiographically documented stenoses in patients with suspected coronary artery disease: results of 1,764 patients. J Am Coll Cardiol 2001; 37: 451–7.
7. Baumgart D, Schmermund A, Görge G et al. Comparison of electron beam computed tomography with intracoronary ultrasound and coronary angiography for the detection of coronary atherosclerosis. J Am Coll Cardiol 1997; 30: 57–64.
8. Schmermund A, Baumgart D, Adamzik M et al. Comparison of electron-beam computed tomography and intracoronary ultrasound in detecting calcified and non-calcified plaques in patients with acute coronary syndromes and no or minimal to moderate angiographic coronary artery disease. Am J Cardiol 1998; 81: 141–6.
9. He ZX, Hedrick TD, Pratt CM et al. Severity of coronary artery calcification by electron beam computed tomography predicts silent myocardial ischemia. Circulation 2000; 101: 244–51.
10. Berman DS, Wong ND, Gransar H et al. Relationship between stress-induced myocardial ischemia and atherosclerosis measured by coronary calcium tomography. J Am Coll Cardiol 2004; 44: 923–30.
11. Pletcher MJ, Tice JA, Pignone M, Browner WS. Using the coronary artery calcium score to predict coronary heart disease events: a systematic review and meta-analysis. Arch Intern Med 2004; 164: 1285–92.
12. Arad Y, Goodman KJ, Roth M, Newstein D, Guerci AD. Coronary calcification, coronary disease risk factors, C-reactive protein, and atherosclerotic cardiovascular disease events: the St. Francis Heart Study. J Am Coll Cardiol 2005; 46: 158–65.
13. Vliegenthart R, Oudkerk M, Hofman A et al. Coronary calcification improves cardiovascular risk prediction in the elderly. Circulation 2005; 112: 572–7.
14. Schmermund A, Möhlenkamp S, Erbel R. Coronary calcium and its relationship with coronary artery disease. Cardiol Clin 2003; 21: 521–34.
15. Waters D, Craven TE, Lespérance J. Prognostic significance of progression of coronary atherosclerosis. Circulation 1993; 87: 1067–75.
16. Kaski JC, Chester MR, Chen L et al. Rapid angiographic progression of coronary artery disease in patients with angina pectoris. The role of complex stenosis morphology. Circulation 1995; 92: 2058–65.
17. Little WC, Constantinescu M, Applegate RJ et al. Can coronary angiography predict the site of a subsequent myocardial infarction in patients with mild-to-moderate coronary artery disease? Circulation 1988; 78: 1157–66.
18. Ambrose JA, Tannenbaum MA, Alexopoulos D et al. Angiographic progression of coronary artery disease and the development of myocardial infarction. JACC 1988; 12: 56–62.
19. Virmani R, Kolodgie FD, Burke AP, Farb A, Schwartz SM. Lessons from sudden coronary death. A comprehensive morphological classification scheme for atherosclerotic lesions. Art Thromb Vasc Biol 2000; 20: 1262–75.
20. Burke AP, Kolodgie FD, Farb A et al. Healed plaque ruptures and sudden coronary death: evidence that subclinical rupture has a role in plaque progression. Circulation 2001; 103: 934–40.
21. Buchwald H, Matts JP, Fitch LL et al. Changes in sequential coronary arteriograms and subsequent coronary events. Surgical Control of the Hyperlipidemias (POSCH) Group. JAMA 1992; 268: 1429–33.
22. Achenbach S, Ropers D, Möhlenkamp S et al. Variability of repeated coronary artery calcification measurements by electron beam tomography. Am J Cardiol 2001; 87: 210–13.
23. Möhlenkamp S, Behrenbeck TR, Pump H et al. Reproducibility of two coronary calcium quantification algorithms in patients with different degrees of calcification. Int J Cardiovasc Imaging 2001; 17: 133–42.
24. Bielak LF, Sheedy PF II, Peyser PA. Coronary artery calcification measured at electron-beam CT: agreement in dual scan runs and change over time. Radiology 2001; 218: 224–9.
25. Agatston AS, Janowitz WR, Hildner FJ et al. Quantification of coronary artery calcium using ultrafast computed tomography. J Am Coll Cardiol 1990; 15: 827–32.
26. Callister TQ, Cooil B, Raya SP et al. Coronary artery disease: Improved reproducibility of calcium screening with an electron-beam CT volumetric method. Radiology 1998; 208: 807–14.
27. Hong C, Becker CR, Schoepf UJ et al. Coronary artery calcium: Absolute quantification in nonenhanced and contrast-enhanced multi-detector row CT studies. Radiology 2002; 223: 474–80.

28. Hoffmann U, Siebert U, Bull-Stewart A et al. Evidence for lower variability of coronary artery calcium mineral mass measurements by multi-detector computed tomography in a community-based cohort – consequences for progression studies. Eur J Radiol 2006; 57: 396–402.

29. Callister TQ, Raggi P, Cooil B, Lippolis NJ, Russo DJ. Effect of HMG-CoA reductase inhibitors on coronary artery disease as assessed by electron-beam computed tomography. New Engl J Med 1998; 339: 1972–8.

30. Maher JE, Bielak LF, Raz JA et al. Progression of coronary artery calcification: A pilot study. Mayo Clin Proc 1999; 74: 347–55.

31. Budoff MJ, Lane KL, Bakhsheshi H et al. Rates of progression of coronary calcium by electron beam tomography. Am J Cardiol 2000; 86: 8–11.

32. Schmermund A, Baumgart D, Möhlenkamp S et al. Natural history and topographic pattern of progression of coronary calcification in symptomatic patients: an electron-beam CT study. Arterioscler Thromb Vasc Biol 2001; 21: 421–6.

33. Yoon H-C, Emerick AM, Hill JA, Gjertson DW, Goldin JG. Calcium begets calcium: Progression of coronary artery calcification in asymptomatic subjects. Radiology 2002; 224: 236–41.

34. Achenbach S, Schmid M, Frimmel S et al. Attenuation of the progression of coronary calcification over the course of time: a long-term observation. Circulation 2005; 112: II–419.

35. Janowitz WR, Agatston AS, Viamonte M Jr. Comparison of serial quantitative evaluation of calcified coronary plaque by ultrafast computed tomography in persons with and without obstructive coronary artery disease. Am J Cardiol 1991; 68: 1–6.

36. Gopal A, Nasir K, Liu ST et al. Coronary calcium progression rates with a zero initial score by electron beam tomography. Int J Cardiol. 2006 Jul 25; [Epub ahead of print].

37. Bild DE, Bluemke DA, Burke GL et al. Multi-ethnic study of atherosclerosis: objectives and design. Am J Epidemiol. 2002; 156: 871–81.

38. Schmermund A, Möhlenkamp S, Stang A et al, for the Heinz Nixdorf Recall Study Investigative Group. Assessment of clinically silent atherosclerotic disease and established and novel risk factors for predicting myocardial infarction and cardiac death in healthy middle-aged subjects: Rationale and design of the Heinz Nixdorf Recall study. Am Heart J 2002; 144: 212–18.

39. Halon DA, Sapoznikov D, Lewis BS et al. Localization of lesions in the coronary circulation. Am J Cardiol 1983; 52: 921–6.

40. Moe SM, Chen NX. Pathophysiology of vascular calcification in chronic kidney disease. Circ Res 2004; 95: 560–7.

41. Braun J, Oldendorf M, Moshage W et al. Electron beam computed tomography in the evaluation of cardiac calcification in chronic dialysis patients. Am J Kidney Dis 1996; 27: 394–401.

42. Goodman WG, Goldin J, Kuizon BD et al. Coronary-artery calcification in young adults with end-stage renal disease who are undergoing dialysis. N Engl J Med 2000; 342: 1478–83.

43. Raggi P, Boulay A, Chasan-Taber S et al. Cardiac calcification in adult hemodialysis patients. A link between end-stage renal disease and cardiovascular disease? J Am Coll Cardiol 2002; 39: 695–701.

44. Raggi P, Cooil B, Shaw LJ et al. Progression of coronary calcium on serial electron beam tomographic scanning is greater in patients with future myocardial infarction. Am J Cardiol 2003; 92: 827–9.

45. Raggi P, Callister TQ, Shaw LJ. Progression of coronary artery calcium and risk of first myocardial infarction in patients receiving cholesterol-lowering therapy. Arterioscler Thromb Vasc Biol 2004; 24: 1272–7.

46. Motro M, Shemesh J. Calcium channel blocker nifedipine slows down progression of coronary calcification in hypertensive patients compared with diuretics. Hypertension 2001; 37: 1410–13.

47. Cassidy AE, Bielak LF, Zhou Y et al. Progression of subclinical coronary atherosclerosis: does obesity make a difference? Circulation 2005; 111: 1877–82.

48. Rasouli ML, Nasir K, Blumenthal RS, Park R, Aziz DC et al. Plasma homocysteine predicts progression of atherosclerosis. Atherosclerosis 2005; 181: 159–65.

49. Achenbach S, Ropers D, Pohle K et al. Influence of lipid-lowering therapy on the progression of coronary artery calcification: a prospective evaluation. Circulation 2002; 106: 1077–82.

50. Hecht HS, Harman SM. Comparison of the effects of atorvastatin versus simvastatin on subclinical atherosclerosis in primary prevention as determined by electron beam tomography. Am J Cardiol 2003; 91: 42–5.

51. Hecht HS, Harman SM. Relation of aggressiveness of lipid-lowering treatment to changes in calcified plaque burden by electron beam tomography. Am J Cardiol 2003; 92: 334–6.

52. Wong ND, Kawakubo M, LaBree L et al. Relation of coronary calcium progression and control of lipids according to National Cholesterol Education Program guidelines. Am J Cardiol 2004; 94: 431–6.

53. Smilde TJ, van Wissen S, Wollersheim H et al. Effect of aggressive versus conventional lipid lowering on atherosclerosis progression in familial hypercholesterolaemia (ASAP): a prospective, randomised, double-blind trial. Lancet 2001; 357(9256): 577–81.

54. Taylor AJ, Kent SM, Flaherty PJ et al. ARBITER: Arterial Biology for the Investigation of the Treatment Effects of Reducing Cholesterol: a randomized trial comparing the effects of atorvastatin and pravastatin on carotid intima medial thickness. Circulation 2002; 106: 2055–60.

55. Cannon CP, Braunwald E, McCabe CH et al. Pravastatin or Atorvastatin Evaluation and Infection Therapy-Thrombolysis in Myocardial Infarction 22 Investigators. Intensive versus moderate lipid lowering with statins after acute coronary syndromes. N Engl J Med 2004; 350: 1495–504.

56. Nissen SE, Tuzcu EM, Schoenhagen P et al. REVERSAL Investigators. Effect of intensive compared with moderate lipid-lowering therapy on progression of coronary atherosclerosis: a randomized controlled trial. JAMA 2004; 291: 1071–80.

57. Larosa JC, Grundy SM, Waters DD et al. Intensive lipid lowering with atorvastatin in patients with stable coronary disease. N Engl J Med 2005; 352: 1425–35.

58. Cannon CP, Steinberg BA, Murphy SA et al. Meta-analysis of cardiovascular outcomes trials comparing intensive versus moderate statin therapy. J Am Coll Cardiol 2006; 48: 438–45.

59. Arad Y, Spadaro LA, Roth M, Newstein D, Guerci AD. Treatment of asymptomatic adults with elevated coronary calcium scores with atorvastatin, vitamin C, and vitamin E. The St. Francis Heart Study randomized clinical trial. J Am Coll Cardiol 2005; 46: 166–72.

60. Raggi P, Davidson M, Callister TQ et al. Aggressive versus moderate lipid-lowering therapy in hypercholesterolemic post-menopausal women: Beyond Endorsed Lipid Lowering with EBT Scanning (BELLES). Circulation 2005; 112: 563–71.

61. Schmermund A, Achenbach S, Budde T et al. Effect of intensive versus standard lipid-lowering treatment with atorvastatin on the progression of calcified coronary atherosclerosis over 12 months: a multicenter, randomized, double-blind trial. Circulation 2006; 113: 427–37.

62. Houslay ES, Cowell SJ, Prescott RJ et al. Progressive coronary calcification despite intensive lipid-lowering treatment: a randomised controlled trial. Heart 2006; 92: 1207–12.

63. Chertow GM, Burke SK, Raggi P. Treat to Goal Working Group. Sevelamer attenuates the progression of coronary and aortic calcification in hemodialysis patients. Kidney Int 2002; 62: 245–52.

64. Block GA, Spiegel DM, Ehrlich J et al. Effects of sevelamer and calcium on coronary artery calcification in patients new to hemodialysis. Kidney Int 2005; 68: 1815–24.

12

How to Perform and Interpret Computed Tomography Coronary Angiography

Nico R. Mollet, Niels Van Pelt, Willem B. Meijboom, Annick Weustink, Francesca Pugliese, Filippo Cademartiri, Koen Nieman, Gabriel P. Krestin, and Pim J. de Feyter

1 INTRODUCTION

Computed tomographic coronary angiography is an emerging technique able to noninvasively detect significant coronary stenoses as well as nonsignificant coronary plaques. Rapid developments in Multislice CT technology has resulted in a markedly improved image quality when imaging the small and rapidly moving coronary arteries. However, CT coronary angiography remains challenging, even using the latest generation Multislice CT scanners. In this chapter we will describe limitations and pitfalls in cardiac CT as well as tips and tricks on data acquisition and image reconstruction when performing CT coronary angiography.

2 DATA ACQUISITION

2.1 Patient selection and preparation

Which patients are most appropriate for CT coronary angiography on a clinical basis is a debatable and contentious issue, and will be discussed in other chapters. Patient selection criteria from a technical perspective though are well defined. First, the patient should be carefully screened for any contraindications to contrast-enhanced CT which include pregnancy, known allergy to

iodinated contrast material and impaired renal function. Patients should be fully briefed about the CT scan to reduce any apprehension. The examination is well tolerated and even patients who are unable to complete a magnetic resonance imaging scan due to claustrophobia are generally able to complete the much shorter CT scan.

Breathing artefacts remain an important issue, and patients must be able to perform a breath hold maneuver at least as long as the scan time. The total scan time is dependent on several CT scanner features (e.g. number of detectors, pitch and rotation time) and will vary between approximately 10 (64-slice) to 20 seconds (16-slice). Patients should not perform a Valsalva maneuver as this reduces the contrast attenuation within the coronary arteries during the CT scan. Patients must be thoroughly instructed how to perform a breath hold maneuver and a mid-inspiration breath hold usually gives the best results. Test breath holds are not only practical for the patient but also useful to evaluate the effect of the apnoea on heart rate (see below).

Patients must have a regular heart rate whereas data of different beats need to be combined to obtain a volume dataset. Mismatch of heart beats will result in combination of data obtained during different phases of the cardiac cycle resulting in step and/or or motion artefacts. CT coronary angiography is not suitable for patients with severe arrhythmia for these reasons. However, image quality in patients with mild arrhythmia (e.g. occasional premature beats or atrial fibrillation with a low ventricular response) is preserved by manual repositioning of the reconstruction windows, so called 'ECG-editing' (see Image Reconstruction section). However, it is necessary to strictly exclude all patients with arrhythmia if this feature is not supported by the vendor to avoid unnecessary radiation exposure and contrast load in patients with a high likelihood of a nondiagnostic scan.

We are careful to warn the patients about the warm feeling resulting from the injection of iodinated contrast material, and to reiterate the importance of following the breath hold instructions which follows shortly after the contrast injection. We use automated breath-hold instructions and these are available in different languages.

An intravenous cannula of 18 or 20 gauge is placed in the anticubital fossa. Smaller veins are avoided to reduce the risk of contrast extravasation. The calibre of the vein is carefully evaluated with a saline test bolus of minimum 10 ml prior to contrast administration.

The optimization of a patient's heart rate is an important issue. CT coronary angiography suffers from motion artefacts related to movement of the coronary arteries during a heart beat. Therefore, the data used for image reconstruction is preferentially obtained from a relative motion-free period of the cardiac cycle, which occurs mostly during the mid-to-end diastolic phase of the cardiac cycle. Optimal, nearly motion-free images are especially obtained in low (<70 beats/minute) heart rates, whereas the diastolic phase is longer in these patients. Therefore β-blockers are usually given prior to the CT scan to reduce the heart rate preferably below 70 beats/minute in patients with higher heart rates. Generally an oral β-blocker such as metoprolol 50–100 mg may be given 45 minutes to 1 hour before the scan. The majority of patients usually have the desired effect of reducing the heart rate to <70 beats/minute. Some institutions give intravenous β-blockers, either as an infusion or as a bolus injection. However the response to injectable β-blockers is variable and it may take some time before the heart rate is optimized while the patient remains on the table. It also requires monitoring of blood pressure and a short stay in the hospital until the effect of the intravenous β-blocker is resolved. Radiologists in particular may also have little experience in injecting β-blockers. Contraindications to β-blockers are atrioventricular heart block, hypotension, decompensated heart failure and asthma. Mild sedation may be used in addition to the use of β-blockers, e.g. a single oral dose of 1 mg lorazepam. Administration of a short acting benzodiazepine lowers anxiety due to the warm feeling after injection of contrast material, thereby preventing an increase in heart rate. Such approach is of

particular use in very anxious patients and patients with an acute coronary syndrome, especially when the use of β-blockers is contraindicated. Some investigators advocate the use of nitroglycerin just before scanning in the absence of contraindications (e.g. hypotension and severe aortic stenosis). Nitroglycerin induces a small increase in coronary lumen diameter and may theoretically lead to more comparable results with conventional coronary angiography in which intracoronary injection of nitroglycerin routinely is performed when evaluating coronary stenoses. We do not routinely use sublingual nitroglycerin using 16- or 64-slice CT scanners, as it may induce a blood pressure drop and a reflex tachycardia. However, we routinely use nitroglycerin when performing CT coronary angiography on the recently introduced dual-source scanner since higher heart rates are more reliably visualized using this scanner. A disadvantage of the use of nitroglycerin is the severe headache it may induce in some patients.

We also check for significant heart rate variability during apnoea prior to the scan. In some patients a decrease of >10 seconds is observed with inspiration and we adjust our scan protocol accordingly. We manually select lower pitch values in case of a significant heart rate drop in scanners which require a variable pitch adapted to the heart rate. This is an important issue, whereas higher pitch values in patients with low heart rates will result in impaired image quality due to interpolation artefacts.

Table 12.1 summarizes common pitfalls during CT coronary angiography data acquisition.

2.2 Contrast administration protocols

Two techniques are currently used to optimize synchronization between the arterial passage of contrast material and CT data acquisition. A test bolus of 20 mL contrast material can be administered to monitor the arrival of the contrast bolus in the ascending aorta. The delay which provides the highest attenuation (the peak of the contrast bolus) within the aorta will be chosen as a fixed delay after which the scan will be started. The bolus tracking technique can also be used to synchronize contrast arrival and the start of the scan. Bolus tracking techniques are widely available nowadays and standard installed on all currently available 16-, 64-, and dual-source CT scanners. In this technique a region of interest (ROI) is positioned in the ascending aorta (Figure 12.1). After injection of the contrast bolus, monitoring scans at the level of the ascending aorta are obtained and attenuation values within

Table 12.1 Potential pitfalls during CT coronary angiography data acquisition

	Limitation	Artefact	Possible solution
Breath hold	Severe dyspnoea (e.g. COPD)	Step artefacts (thoracic motion due to breathing)	Oxygen therapy, Hyperventilation maneuver prior to scan
	Valsalva maneuver	Low contrast-to-noise ratio (low contrast)	Thorough patient instruction and practice breath hold maneuver
	Incorrect timing (breath hold maneuver not finished when scan starts)	Thoracic motion (breathing)	Add delay between end of breath hold instruction and start scan
Heart rate	Severe arrhythmia (e.g. atrial fibrillation with fast ventricular response)	Coronary motion	Abort scanning
	Mild arrhythmia (e.g. occasional premature beat)	Coronary motion Step artefacts (mismatch of reconstruction windows)	Manual reposition of reconstruction windows (ECG-editing)
	Fast (=70 beats/min) heart rate[1]	Coronary motion	β-blockers and/or sedation
Anxiety	Claustrophobia (rare) Due to flush when injecting Iodinated contrast (common)	Thoracic motion (voluntary motion and/or coronary motion)	Sedation
Patient movement	Parkinson's disease etc.	Thoracic motion (involuntary motion)	Specific treatment
Body mass index	Obesity	Low contrast-to-noise ratio (high noise)	Higher tube current

[1]Not applicable to Dual-Source CT systems.

the ROI are measured. Once a certain predefined threshold within the ROI is reached (generally +100 HU), the patient is automatically instructed to perform a breath hold maneuver after which the scan will start. Both contrast administration algorithms are widely used and each site will have its own preference. Using a test bolus is a very robust approach, but requires administration of an additional small amount of contrast material and is more sensitive to the Valsalva maneuver, resulting in low intra-coronary enhancement when compared to bolus tracking techniques. Bolus tracking requires less contrast material; however, it is more sensitive to premature triggering of the scan if the ROI is positioned incorrectly. First, the ROI should be positioned just below the aortic arch where the ascending aorta moves relatively little during the respiratory cycle. This approach minimizes the risk of premature triggering of the scan if the ROI is displaced into e.g. the contrast-enhanced pulmonary trunk as a result of breathing-related shift of the contents of the chest, although the contrast bolus has not yet arrived in the ascending aorta. Streak artefacts arising from the mixture of blood and contrast in the superior vena cava can be a cause of premature triggering if the attenuation values

within the ROI in the adjacent ascending aorta are artificially raised above the predefined threshold. The ROI should consequently be positioned as far away from the vena cava as possible and the ROI should not be too small, because streak artefacts will be averaged out in larger ROIs. We believe that bolus tracking is a very robust technique if the ROI is carefully selected. Moreover, we found a higher intracoronary attenuation using the bolus tracking technique as compared to test bolus technique with identical injection parameters.[1] This is an important feature because we observed a higher diagnostic accuracy of CT coronary angiography to detect significant stenoses and assessment with more confidence in patients with high intracoronary attenuation. We therefore recommend the use of contrast material with a high iodine content, injected with a high flow rate to obtain maximum intracoronary enhancement. However, higher flow rates require administration of a larger amount of contrast material to maintain sufficient enhancement throughout the entire scan. The use of a 40 mL saline bolus chaser injected immediately after the contrast bolus results in a more compact contrast bolus resulting in a more effective utilization of contrast material. The use of a bolus chaser allowed reduction with 35% of the total amount of contrast material administered in a 16-slice CT coronary angiography study.[2] Whether such contrast protocol should be used for the purpose of plaque detection and classification remains controversial, as small calcifications located at the vessel wall may be masked by the adjacent contrast-enhanced coronary lumen.

2.3 Scan parameters

Multislice CT scanning is carried out either in the spiral mode or in the sequential mode. Spiral CT is performed with the patient on the couch continuously moving at a pre-defined speed through the scanner while the X-ray tube and detectors rotate continuously around the patient. Thus a volumetric dataset is acquired from which cross-sectional images can be reconstructed. In the sequential mode the table, and thus the patient, is moved incrementally between successive rotations of the X-ray tube ('step and shoot' approach). Spiral scanning is standard use for CT coronary angiography scans, while sequential scanning can be used for coronary calcium scoring. Scan parameters of a 16-slice, 64-slice, and dual-source CT system are summarized in Table 12.2. The maximum tube current which can be delivered is dependent on the scan time; the longer the scan time, the lower the maximum tube current will be. This is an important issue in the evaluation of arterial coronary bypasses, especially using 16-slice technology; the operator needs to choose whether he wants to visualize the entire mammary artery and an overall lower tube current or to leave out the proximal mammary artery (generally not diseased) and a higher tube current with favorable contrast-to-noise ratio.

The radiation exposure of CT coronary angiography is of concern and approximately 3–5 times as high when compared to conventional coronary angiography. The radiation exposure can be limited by using prospectively ECG-triggered X-ray tube modulation. This feature reduces the tube current by 80% in systole while a full dose is given during diastole, which lowers the radiation exposure by up to 40% in patients with low heart rates.[3,4] This technique, however, limits the possibility of reconstructing images in the end-systolic phase (see Image Reconstruction section). We use end-systolic datasets in up to 35% of patients, which is especially useful in patients with a heart rate <70 beats/min.[5,6] Furthermore, the use of prospective tube modulation requires a regular heart rhythm throughout the scan since the tube modulation is based on the R-R interval

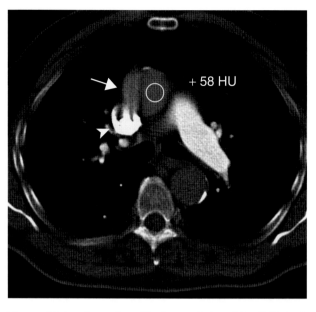

Figure 12.1 Correct positioning and size of the ROI positioned at the ascending aorta. Note the streak artefacts (arrow) originating from the mixture of blood and contrast material within the vena cava superior (arrowpoint) which are avoided.

of the previous heart beats. A sudden change in R-R interval resulting from a single extra-systole though may result in miss-triggering of the tube modulation and a low tube current, thus unfavorable signal-to-noise ratio in diastole, while this is the best phase for image reconstruction in the majority of patients. The tube modulation software is recently updated and is now able to recognize a sudden change in R-R interval, after which the tube modulation is switched off and maximum tube current is given throughout the entire cardiac cycle until the R-R interval is stabilized. We therefore routinely use tube modulation, with full dose radiation between 30–60% of the cardiac cycle, encompassing both end-systole and mid-to-end diastole. This allows good quality image reconstructions in the majority of cases and significantly lowers the radiation exposure.

3 IMAGE RECONSTRUCTION

Imaging of the heart requires data acquisition that is synchronized to the motion of the heart, to be able to reduce cardiac motion artefacts. This is achieved by simultaneously recording the ECG during the scan, which is used to synchronize prospective data acquisition or retrospective data reconstruction. In the sequential CT mode the reconstruction window is determined by prospective triggering of the patient's ECG and data is obtained only during a certain predefined phase of the cardiac cycle. In the spiral mode the ECG signal is used to retrospectively select datasets with optimal image quality thus least motion artefacts. In spiral CT, datasets can be flexibly reconstructed at different phases of the cardiac cycle, because data is obtained during the entire cardiac cycle. Two ECG gating algorithms can be applied to obtain optimal motion-free image quality with spiral CT. A single-segment algorithm can be used in which only data obtained during a single heart beat is used for image reconstruction. The temporal resolution using such algorithm is equal to half of the rotation time (e.g. 165 ms in case of a rotation time of 330 ms). However, the temporal resolution can be further reduced by use of bisegmental or multisegmental reconstruction algorithms that combine data from 2 or more consecutive heart beats, which theoretically should prevent the occurrence of motion artefacts. However, these algorithms require a constant heart rate, a reliable ECG signal, and no arrhythmias, whereas they rely on an identical cardiac contraction pattern with time-consistent positioning of the cardiac structures during each consecutive heart cycle. Moreover, multisegment reconstruction algorithms require a lower pitch, thus longer scan times, more contrast material, and a higher radiation exposure.

Three different techniques can be used to position the reconstruction windows within the cardiac cycle (Figure 12.2). A percentage approach is most commonly used, in which the reconstruction windows are positioned at a certain percentage of the R-R cycle, e.g. 60%. Reconstruction windows can also be positioned using an absolute reverse approach (e.g. 350 ms before the next R-wave; mid-to-end diastole) or an absolute forward approach (e.g. 300 ms after the last R-wave; end-systole). No published data is currently available supporting the preferential use of 1 of those 3 algorithms.

Moreover, these algorithms can be flexibly used and the operator can select the best dataset on a per patient basis. However, a percentage approach is more sensitive to arrhythmia when compared to the other 2 algorithms. The absolute forward approach is useful to determine end-systolic datasets, which is particularly useful in patients with high heart rates and arrhythmia because the position of the end-systolic phase varies less while the diastolic phase may vary significantly.[5,7] The absolute backward approach is commonly used to define optimal image quality during the mid-to-end diastole, which is the best phase for image reconstruction in the majority of patients, especially in patients with low heart rates. The position of the reconstruction windows should be carefully checked to prevent step artefacts which occur when reconstruction windows are not equally positioned within different heart beats. If the ECG leads are not well positioned, resulting in a low voltage R-wave or if the R-wave has an abnormal morphology (e.g. bundle branch block), the CT software designed to detect the R-wave may fail and the position of the reconstruction windows needs to be manually repositioned. However, not all vendors allow manual repositioning of the reconstruction windows, while this is also an important feature which can be applied to preserve image quality in the presence of occasional arrhythmic beats. An example of ECG editing is shown in Figure 12.3. It is of note that ECG editing can only be used with absolute forward or backward algorithms. Reconstruction of consecutive datasets during the entire heart beat, e.g. every 10% of the cardiac cycle, allows evaluation of functional parameters such as left ventricular function (see chapter on Assessment of Left Ventricular Function).

The reconstructed slice thickness can be chosen by the operator and generally is slightly thicker then the individual detector width with an increment of approximately 50%, to obtain a favorable contrast-to-noise ratio (Table 12.2). Dedicated datasets with a reconstructed slice thickness equal to the individual detector width are sometimes used to evaluate coronary stents. Spatial resolution is dependent on the field of view (FOV). We therefore select a FOV which is as small as possible and include only the heart and surrounding structures to obtain optimal spatial resolution for the evaluation of the small sized coronary arteries. Dedicated datasets with a broad FOV can be reconstructed to evaluate part of the lungs and mediastinum. Different image reconstruction filters or kernels are available and vary among different vendors. Medium smooth kernels (e.g. B26f or B30f) are generally used to evaluate native coronary arteries, while sharp kernels (e.g. B46f) are used to evaluate high-density structures such as severely calcified coronary vessels and stents.

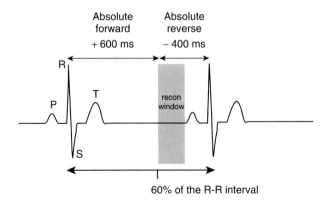

Figure 12.2 Three different algorithms can be applied to position the reconstruction windows within the cardiac cycle in a patient with a heart rate of 60 beats/minute: a percentage of the R-R interval, an absolute forward, or an absolute backward approach.

ECG-STD   ECG-EDIT

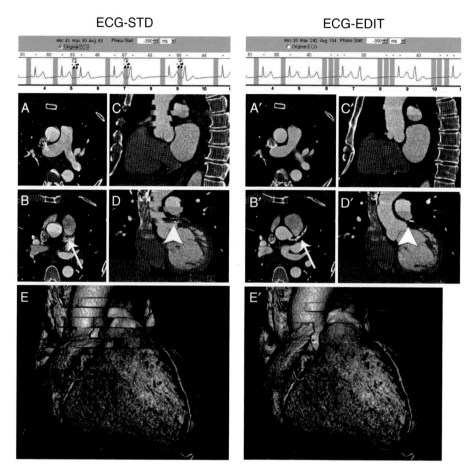

Figure 12.3   Example of manual repositioning of the reconstruction windows (ECG-editing) in a patient with a premature beat during the CT scan. From: Cademartiri, Invest Radiology 2006; 186(3): 634–8.

Table 12.2   Scan protocol and image reconstruction parameters with 16-slice, 64-slice, and Dual-Source CT systems

	16-slice CT	64-slice CT	Dual-source CT
Number of slices	16	64	2 × 64
Individual detector width	0.75 mm	0.5–0.6 mm	0.6 mm
Scan time	18–25 s	6–12 s	6–12 s
Temporal resolution	250–185 ms	210–165 ms	83 ms
Pitch	0.251	0.21	0.2–0.451
Tube voltage	120 kV	120 kV	120 kV
Tube current	Max 750 mAs	Max 950 mAs	Max 1050 mAs
Tube modulation	Possible	Possible	Possible
Contrast load	100–140 mL	80–100 mL	60–100 mL
Flow	4–5 mL/s	4–5 mL/s	4–5 mL/s
Reconstructed slice thickness	1.0 mm	0.6–0.75 mm	0.6–0.75 mm
Increment	0.5 mm	0.3–0.4 mm	0.3–0.4 mm
Kernel	Medium smooth	Medium smooth	Medium smooth

[1]Pitch values may vary among different vendors, especially when the pitch is adapted to the heart rate (standard used in Dual-Source CT).

4 IMAGE EVALUATION AND POST-PROCESSING TECHNIQUES

The entire coronary tree can be visualized in the majority of patients with low heart rates using a single dataset. However, some patients require the use of multiple datasets to visualize the entire coronary tree, e.g. an end-systolic dataset to evaluate the right coronary artery and a mid-to-end diastolic dataset to evaluate the left coronary artery. Several post-processing techniques can be used to evaluate the presence of significant coronary stenoses (Figure 12.4). Volume rendered images are useful to evaluate complex coronary anatomy or bypasses, but should not be used to evaluate the presence

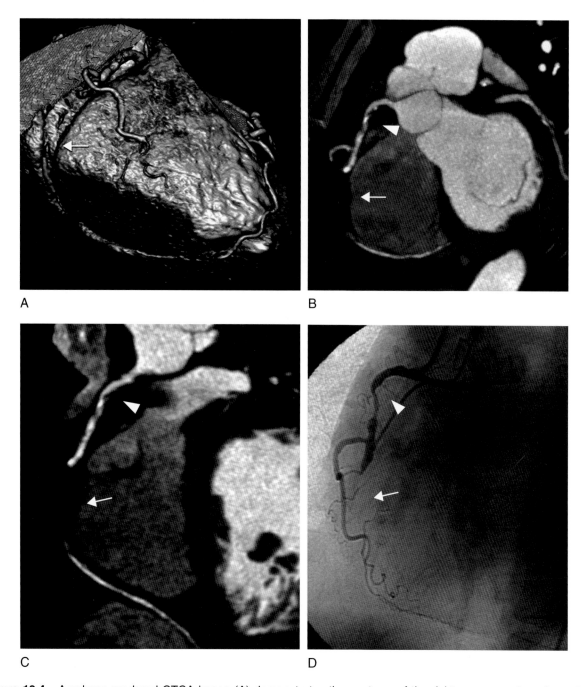

A

B

C

D

Figure 12.4 A volume-rendered CTCA image (A) demonstrates the anatomy of the right coronary artery. A maximum intensity projected image (B) and a curved multiplanar reconstructed image (C) disclose proximally a significant coronary stenosis (arrowhead) followed by a chronic total occlusion (arrow) of the mid right coronary artery which was confirmed by invasive coronary angiography (D).

of significant coronary stenoses, as the diameter of the coronary lumen can easily be manipulated using this technique.[8] However, it is an excellent technique for communicating findings of the investigation to patients and referring physicians. Maximum intensity projections (MIP) also provide a good anatomical overview, however these can only be used for stenosis detection in the absence of any calcifications, as the blooming effect of coronary calcifications is significantly enhanced using this post-processing technique. Multiplanar reconstructions (MPR) or curved multiplanar reconstructions (cMPR) are the most reliable postprocessing tools to evaluate the presence of significant coronary stenoses. Axial scrolling using multiplanar reconstructions is the first step in the evaluation of the coronary arteries, providing a quick anatomical overview, and is particularly useful to detect any image degrading artefacts, which may induce false positive or false negative results in the assessment of coronary stenoses. Thereafter, dedicated (curved) MPRs can be used to evaluate the entire coronary tree on a per segment basis. Unfortunately, evaluation of all coronary segments can be a time-consuming process, especially in the presence of advanced coronary artery disease. We advocate the flexible use of all available postprocessing tools, which requires a dedicated workstation, whereas evaluation of standard projections on a simple picture archiving and communication (PACS) workstation will result in a lower sensitivity to detect significant coronary stenoses.[9]

5 DISCUSSION

CT coronary angiography has developed rapidly and is now poised to become a clinically reliable and useful diagnostic tool. However CT coronary imaging is fraught with limitations and pitfalls. The CT examination gives just one opportunity to obtain the volume of data from which the cardiac reconstructions are made. It is therefore vital that scan protocols are optimized and the patient is well prepared to optimize the data obtained. Because of its rapid development, experience may be limited in any particular institution. Cardiologists often have little experience with CT technology whereas radiologists may have limited experience in the clinical implications of cardiac findings. Training of future cardiac CT (and magnetic resonance) imaging experts should ideally incorporate the acquisition of both radiology and cardiology knowledge and expertise. Consequently a collaborative approach to cardiac CT by both cardiologists and radiologists may provide the best opportunity to improve the quality of the examination and interpretation of findings, and eventually improvement in patient care.

REFERENCES

1. Cademartiri F, Nieman K, van der Lugt A et al. Intravenous contrast material administration at 16-detector row helical CT coronary angiography: test bolus versus bolus-tracking technique. Radiology 2004; 233(3): 817–23.
2. Cademartiri F, Mollet N, van der Lugt A et al. Non-invasive 16-row multislice CT coronary angiography: usefulness of saline chaser. Eur Radiol 2004; 14(2): 178–83.
3. Jakobs TF, Becker CR, Ohnesorge B et al. Multislice helical CT of the heart with retrospective ECG gating: reduction of radiation exposure by ECG-controlled tube current modulation. Eur Radiol 2002; 12(5): 1081–6.
4. Trabold T, Buchgeister M, Kuttner A et al. Estimation of radiation exposure in 16-detector row computed tomography of the heart with retrospective ECG-gating. Rofo 2003; 175(8): 1051–5.
5. Herzog C, Arning-Erb M, Zangos S et al. Multi-detector row CT coronary angiography: influence of reconstruction technique and heart rate on image quality. Radiology 2006; 238(1): 75–86.
6. Mollet NR, Cademartiri F, van Mieghem CA et al. High-resolution spiral computed tomography coronary angiography in patients referred for diagnostic conventional coronary angiography. Circulation 2005; 112(15): 2318–23.
7. Leschka S, Wildermuth S, Boehm T et al. Noninvasive coronary angiography with 64-section CT: effect of average heart rate and heart rate variability on image quality. Radiology 2006; 241(2): 378–85.
8. Vogl TJ, Abolmaali ND, Diebold T et al. Techniques for the detection of coronary atherosclerosis: multi-detector row CT coronary angiography. Radiology 2002; 223(1): 212–20.
9. Cademartiri F, Mollet N, Lemos PA et al. Standard versus user-interactive assessment of significant coronary stenoses with multislice computed tomography coronary angiography. Am J Cardiol 2004; 94(12): 1590–3.

13

Computed Tomographic Angiography for the Detection of Coronary Artery Stenoses

Fabian Bamberg, Shawn DeWayne Teague, and Udo Hoffmann

1 BACKGROUND

Invasive coronary angiography is currently the standard for the diagnosis of obstructive coronary artery disease (CAD) in symptomatic patients. However, about 30–40% of all invasive coronary angiograms (ICA) in the United States are performed for diagnostic purposes only.[1] This is of concern, especially as diagnostic ICA poses small but serious risks (i.e., major vascular complications in approximately 0.40%)[2] yielding an overall mortality of 0.13%.[3–7] Moreover, the economic burden with an average charge for patients hospitalized for diagnostic catheterization of $16,838 in 2000 is considerable.[8]

Despite its invasive nature with complications and inconvenience for the patient and considerable costs, the number of performed ICA remains high. An estimated number of >2 million procedures were performed in 2000[8] and the numbers increased consistently.[9]

A reliable noninvasive imaging method that accurately detects or excludes the presence of obstructive CAD would have enormous implications for patient management. However, as the expectations are high, diagnostic tests are often inadequately appraised and widespread use of tests with uncertain diagnostic efficacy pose significant risks to individuals that include delays in appropriate diagnosis and increase the costs of care.

Over the last 5 years much of the research focus on noninvasive detection of CAD has shifted from magnetic resonance imaging (MRI) to coronary multidetector computed tomography (MDCT). With the recent introduction of 64-slice MDCT we now have a technology available that permits accurate and reproducible detection of coronary atherosclerotic plaque and stenosis, as well as it offers en passant information on global and regional ventricular function and potentially myocardial perfusion. In fact, cardiac MDCT provides an unprecedented opportunity to assess the natural history of CAD. However, the potential benefits of cardiac MDCT remain unclear till its promise is scientifically studied and proven by well-designed investigations.

The rapid advances in cardiac MDCT present a challenge to the medical community; like for virtually every aspect of cardiovascular medicine it is conceivable that MDCT provides information beyond current diagnostics, but its clinical utility by means of patient safety and cost effectiveness needs to be proven. In the event that 64-slice MDCT is not accurate for CAD diagnosis, considerable harm could result by its untested use as a substitute for coronary angiography.

Standards for demonstrating the value of diagnostic tests have the same role as randomized controlled trials for evaluating therapy. The following steps for developing a new diagnostic test have been proposed: (1) elaboration and standardization of technical aspects of a new test, (2) comparison of the new test characteristics with an accepted diagnostic reference standard to define sensitivity and specificity in studies adhering to rigorous methodological criteria, and

(3) validation of the new test in real-life setting outcome studies in which the tests are used for clinical decision making and the outcomes are compared with those of patients managed according to the reference diagnostic test.

There is now a narrow window of opportunity to determine the clinical indications where MDCT may not only provide additional information but also improve patient management and standard health outcomes while being cost-effective.

This chapter will review the currently available data on the utilization of coronary computer tomography angiography (coronary MDCT) for the assessment of significant stenosis of the coronary arteries and evaluate the diagnostic impact on different patient populations.

1.1 Technical development

In 1973, the first CT scanner was introduced by Hounsfield,[10] representing the start point of a rapid integration of CT imaging into medical practice. Due to relatively long ganty rotation times in the range of 1 to 5 seconds, cardiac imaging was only feasible to roughly visualize cardiac morphology. In the early 1980s, Electron Beam Computed Tomography (EBCT) was firstly introduced as an imaging modality. EBCT was characterized by a very high temporal resolution of 100 ms,

permitting motion-free imaging of the cardiac anatomy in the diastolic phase, even at high heart rates. EBCT provided appropriate features for visualization of coronary calcification of the coronary arteries and thus the diagnosis of CAD.[11–14] Since 1999, 4-slice MDCT systems have been studied for the detection of CAD.[15–18] Due to improved scanning speed with four sections, scanning of the heart within one breath-hold became feasible. Despite cardiac motion and calcified plaque rendering a substantial number of scans unassessable, nevertheless, in selected exams a good accuracy for the noninvasive detection of significant coronary stenosis was shown.[19–21] Impact of motion artifacts on image evaluation decreased with the introduction of 16-slice MDCT scanners in 2001. As a result, feasibility studies in high-risk populations reported better diagnostic accuracy.[22–24] Latest MDCT technology nowadays permits simultaneous acquisition of 64-slices enabling scanning of the entire coronary artery tree in between 10 to 13 seconds, less segments with limited interpretability due to motion artifacts, and an isovolumetric spatial resolution of 0.4 mm^3 (Figure 13.1).[25–27] Using 2 x-ray sources and 2 detector arrays offset at 90 degrees, dual-source CT (DSCT) is a novel approach to further decrease temporal resolution in order to achieve good image quality at higher heart rates. Initial results, in a small population with a mean heart rate of 71 bpm, suggest further decrease of motion artifacts as compared to earlier scanner generations.[28]

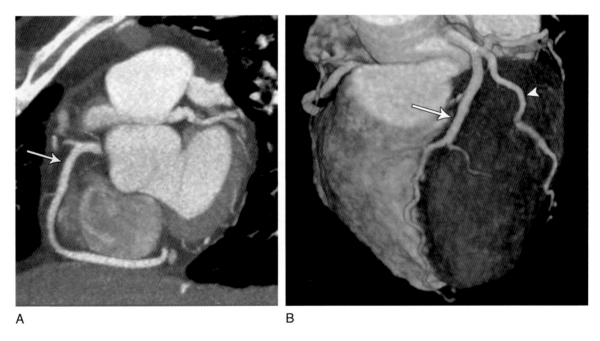

A   B

Figure 13.1   Normal finding of a 48-year-old female patient who presented with chest pain to the emergency room. (A) Maximum-intense projection (MIP) of the right coronary artery (arrow) showing a patent lumen without any luminal narrowing and the absence of any non-stenotic coronary atherosclerotic plaque. (B) 3-dimensional volume rendered coronary MDCT showing the left coronary artery. The LAD (arrow) and LCX (arrowhead) is clearly wide and patent, no evidence of any coronary atherosclerotic plaque.

2 DIAGNOSTIC ACCURACY OF CORONARY CTA FOR THE DETECTION OF SIGNIFICANT CORONARY ARTERY STENOSIS

2.1 Data overview

The fast improvement in scanner technology provides a fast moving target for clinical researchers. So far, feasibility and validation studies were performed comparing the new test (coronary MDCT) with an accepted diagnostic reference gold standard (ICA). A meta-analysis by Stein et al. restricted analysis to 33 studies in which coronary MDCT was compared to ICA and that applied specific patient selection criteria.[29] Based on these initial analysis, recently Hoffmann et al. extended the analysis to 41 studies, including EBCT, 4/8 slice, 16 slice, and 64 slice MDCT scanner technology published in peer-reviewed literature from January 1, 1990, through March 15, 2006.[30] Inclusion criteria were that studies used coronary MDCT or EBCT, evaluated native coronary arteries, used ICA as the reference standard independently of CT findings, and that raw data (i.e., numbers that allowed recalculation of the 2×2 contingency table) were reported.

2.2 Study population

Most of the available literature on coronary MDCT stems from single center investigations (sample size: 20–133 patients). Studies were usually performed at centers with high technical and interpretative expertise in MDCT technology where clinical studies are performed on a daily basis.

The patient population consisted largely of elderly male patients (mean age: 59 years, range 53–65; percent male: mean 75%, range 50–96%) with a high prevalence of CAD (mean 57%) resulting in a considerable selection bias. As is often the case in feasibility studies, the number of outcomes was maximized and all patients were selected to undergo invasive angiography due to the high likelihood of disease (validation bias).

2.3 Study methodology

2.3.1 Definition of stenosis

Most studies defined a significant stenosis as luminal narrowing of ≥50% in diameter, most likely to increase the sensitivity

of the test. In contrast, current clinical practice applies a threshold of <70% diameter loss to define hemodynamically significant lesions (threshold in the left main coronary artery: ≥50%).

2.3.2 Segment versus patient-based analysis

Matching between findings in coronary MDCT and ICA has been performed on a per-segment and/or per-patient basis. Austen et al. developed a classification of 16 coronary segments that have been in widespread use to describe localization of distinct lesions or structures within the coronary artery tree.[31] Most of the research on the diagnostic accuracy of coronary CTA has been done using these 16 segments (or 17 segments including the Ramus Intermedius, if present, as segment 17). Analysis on a per-patient basis includes findings on all coronary segments and puts the subject as the standard of reference.

In fact, it is important to emphasize the differences between a segment-based and a patient-based approach based on all 17 coronary segments. Although segment-based analysis may be useful to demonstrate the feasibility of MDCT to detect significant CAD by revealing the portion of nonevaluable segments due to impaired image quality, it is rather obvious that a per-segment analysis does not reflect clinical applicability of the technique. For clinicians, the patient-based analysis, including all segments and vessels, is more suitable to demonstrate diagnostic accuracy and thus indicate incremental value for clinical practice. While the patient-based assessment (patient has significant or no-disease) correlates with the prevalence of significant CAD in the distinct population, the segment-based analysis differentiates between all segments and may thus represent a different prevalence population.

Limiting the analysis to the proximal segments of the coronary artery tree represents a new approach which is related to the fact that acute coronary events tend to cluster within the proximal third of the coronary arteries.[32] Within these sections, the cross-sectional diameter of the vessels is greater and motion artifacts occur less frequently which will lead to improved diagnostic accuracy.

2.3.3 Assessable and unassessable segments

The majority of studies reported test characteristics of coronary MDCT for the detection of significant stenosis restricted to coronary segments with high image quality.

This practice is known from evaluations of other imaging modalities such as nuclear stress perfusion imaging. However, this approach is inappropriate to assess the clinical value of the technology, as the clinician is required to make a recommendation or diagnosis for the patient even if the image quality is not optimal in all segments. In addition, the decision whether a segment is 'assessable' for stenosis or not has usually been determined by the same observer who interpreted the study for the presence of a significant stenosis introducing additional bias. Therefore, in order to provide clinically relevant results, research studies need to present the analysis in a systematic fashion, including the best-case scenario – test characteristics in segments with optimal image quality – as well as the worst-case scenario – test characteristics including all segments.

2.3.4 Imaging artifacts rendering segments unassessable

There are several artifacts that may, depending on the experience level of the CT reader, render coronary segments, vessels, or entire exams unassessable. In such cases the presence of a significant coronary stenosis or plaque cannot be determined affecting the PPV of the technology.

While earlier scanner generations with limited spatial and temporal resolution and longer scan times were prone to artifacts, it has been observed that the number of segments determined unassassable for image interpretation decreased significantly with advancements of the MDCT technology. The studies reported in the meta-analysis with the least amount of evaluable segments resulted in up to 43% unassessable segments in 4-slice,[33] 18% in 16-slice,[34] and 12% in 64-slice[25] coronary MDCT.

It is clear that an adequate knowledge of the different artifacts is of critical importance, both for reviewing available literature in the field and the clinical setting.

Misregistration or slab artifacts can occur due to inadequate lowering of the heart rate, variability of the RR-interval, and in the presence of extrasystolic beats (Figure 13.2). Sometimes, dedicated reconstruction at several points within the RR-cycle, especially during end-systole, may improve image quality. In the presence of extrasystolic beats, it is sometimes possible to exclude any data acquired during this interval if the resulting data gap can be covered from the adjacent beats (usually <2 seconds can be covered, depending on the pitch). Reconstructing data using a multisegment reconstruction (multiple heart beats at the same anatomic location) results in better temporal resolution and thus may improve image quality in patients scanned at high heart rates, given the absence of significant beat to beat variation.[35,36]

Beam hardening occurs as a result of the absorption of low energy x-rays by very dense objects such as stents and calcified plaque (Figure 13.3). It is visible as an area of low attenuation adjacent to a very dense object. This artifact can be difficult to differentiate from noncalcified plaque. Therefore, the evaluation of the in-stent lumen and areas adjacent to calcified plaque is limited.

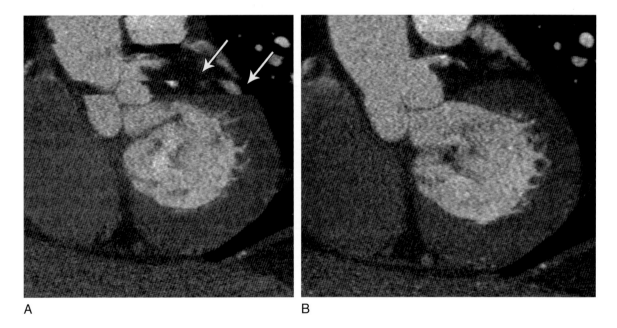

A   B

Figure 13.2   (A) Example of a slab artifact (arrows) which is corrected after ECG editing (B).

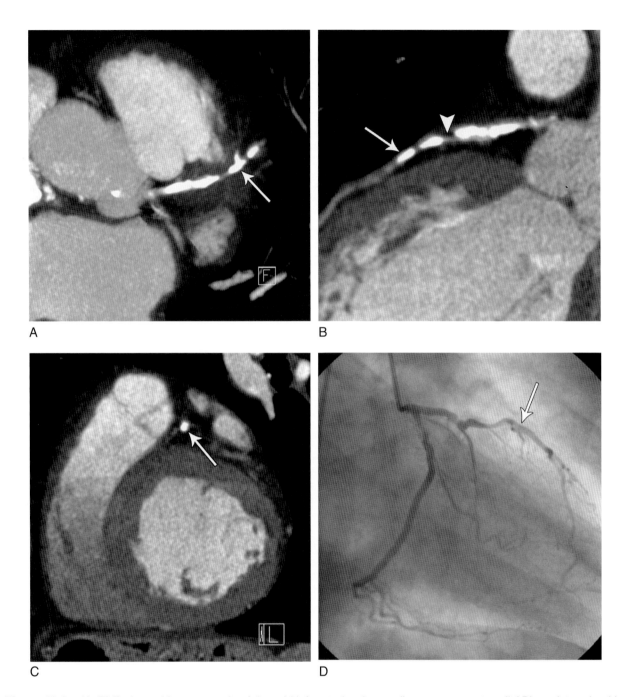

Figure 13.3   (A–D) Patient without stenosis of the mid left anterior descending coronary artery (LAD) as determined by selective coronary angiography. (A) Axial thin slice MIP (5mm) MDCT image demonstrates significant calcified plaque in the mid LAD (arrow). (B) Curved multiplanar reconstructuion image of the LAD demonstrating extensive coronary calcification in the proximal and intermediate portion of the vessel. Arrow indicates section in which the stenosis was suspected. Arrowhead demonstrates beam hardening artifact adjacent to the calcified plaque. (C) Cross sectional reconstruction perpendicular to the centerline of the LAD demonstrates massive calcification apparently without residual contrast filled coronary lumen. (D) Invasive selective coronary angiography demonstrates a normal angiogram without luminal obstruction of the mid LAD.

Respiratory artifacts rarely impair image quality as the scan times have decreased rapidly (Figure 13.4). They are most commonly observed at the end of the image acquisition sometimes leading to diaphragmatic artifacts. An inward motion of the posterior margin of the sternum can objectively determine the presence of an inadequate breath hold. Emphasis on patient preparation and accurate breathing instructions are of critical importance to avoid these artifacts.

Coronary calcification is frequently present in the coronary arteries, especially in proximal segments of elderly

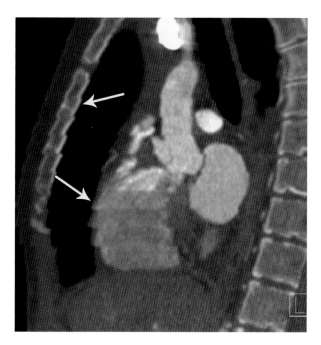

Figure 13.4 Example of a respiratory artifact (arrows) shown in a saggital multiplanar reconstruction (MPR). Characteristic are the steps in the sternum.

patients and patients at increased risk for cardiovascular events (Figure 13.3). Because of the limited spatial resolution of MDCT these objects 'bloom' and thus appear larger than they actually are. This so-called *blooming artifact* is the major reason for the moderate specificity and PPV of current coronary MDCT imaging. For the observer, a calcified plaque may appear to lead to significant narrowing of the coronary lumen even if it is, in reality, confined to the wall of the artery while the lumen is well preserved. Thinner slices and reconstruction using sharper kernels may help to reduce the blooming artifact. Blooming from calcified plaques is the most limiting factor in coronary MDCT today and may result in false positive referrals to invasive selective coronary angiography. Some investigators and clinicians have suggested to perform a noncontrast enhanced CT scan to screen for the presence of severe coronary calcification prior to a contrast enhanced coronary MDCT.[33] In fact, studies have demonstrated that the diagnostic performance of coronary MDCT for the detection of significant stenosis improves if subjects with an Agatston Score >400 are excluded from the analysis.[37] While these data indicate that screening for coronary calcification may improve the overall efficacy of contrast enhanced CT scanning, sometimes the decision whether a noncontrast CT scan should be performed prior to coronary MDCT needs to be made on an individual basis. For example, in a female patient with a differential diagnosis of suspected anterior wall perfusion defect vs. breast attenuation,

a coronary MDCT may still be diagnostic despite an Agatston score >1000, indicating a very high amount of coronary calcification, if the coronary calcification is located outside the mid/distal the LAD segment. Because coronary calcium screening can be performed without contrast and adds only 1–2 mSv of radiation exposure, it may be useful to be performed in patients with a high likelihood of a high burden of coronary calcification such as high age.[38]

3 RESULTS FROM THE CURRENT LITERATURE

3.1 Overall population

For all 41 studies included in the meta-analysis from Hoffmann et al., independent of whether the segment was assessable in CT or not, 1,771 of 2,323 stenotic lesions were correctly detected by coronary MDCT (sensitivity of 76%). A stenosis was correctly ruled out in 12,205 of 13,917 segments (specificity of 88%). For segments that were assessable in MDCT, 2,078 of 2,471 stenotic lesions (84%) were correctly detected. A significant coronary stenosis was correctly ruled out in 14,053 of 14,738 segments (95%). MDCT correctly identified 738 of 813 patients (91%) as having significant CAD. Significant CAD was correctly ruled out in 457 of 621 patients (74%).

3.2 Scanner specific analysis

3.2.1 EBCT

For all segments included, 443 of 623 stenotic lesions were correctly detected by MDCT (sensitivity: 71%) and the presence of a significant stenosis was correctly ruled out in 2,751 of 3,590 segments (specificity: 77%). In assessable segments 414 of 497 stenotic lesions were correctly detected (sensitivity: 83%) while a significant stenosis was correctly ruled out in 2,064 of 2,283 segments (specificity: 90%). On a per patient basis, 142 of 174 patients were correctly identified by EBCT as having significant CAD (sensitivity: 82%) and significant CAD was correctly ruled out in 128 of 218 patients (specificity: 59%).

3.2.2 4/8-slice MDCT

For all segments included, 386 of 620 stenotic lesions were correctly detected by MDCT (sensitivity: 62%) while stenosis and the presence of a significant stenosis was correctly ruled out in 3,082 of 3,671 segments (specificity: 84%). In segments assessable by 4 and 8-slice MDCT, 510 of 623 stenotic lesions were correctly detected (sensitivity: 82%) while stenosis was correctly ruled out in 3,040 of 3,174 segments (specificity: 96%). On a per patient basis, 138 of 160 patients were correctly identified by 4/8-slice MDCT as having significant CAD (sensitivity: 86%) and significant CAD was correctly ruled out in 64 of 80 patients (specificity: 81%).

3.2.3 16-slice MDCT

For all segments, 524 of 625 stenotic lesions were correctly detected by MDCT (sensitivity: 84%) and a significant stenosis was correctly ruled out in 3,353 of 3,518 segments (specificity: 95%). In segments assessable by 16-slice MDCT 683 of 761 stenotic lesions were correctly detected (sensitivity: 90%) while stenosis was correctly ruled out in 4,685 of 4,881 segments (specificity: 96%). On a per patient basis 388 of 404 patients were correctly identified by 16-slice MDCT as having significant CAD (sensitivity: 96%) and significant CAD was correctly ruled out in 172 of 208 patients (specificity: 83%).

3.2.4 64-slice MDCT

Included studies are presented in Table 13.1. For all segments, 63 of 64 stenotic lesions were correctly detected by MDCT (sensitivity: 98%) and the presence of a significant stenosis was correctly ruled out in 21 of 23 segments (specificity: 91%). In assessable segments, 442 of 471 stenotic lesions were correctly detected (sensitivity: 94%) while a stenosis was correctly ruled out in 3,626 of 3,771 segments (specificity: 96%). On a per patient basis, 173 of 178 patients were correctly identified by 16-slice MDCT as having significant CAD (sensitivity: 97%) and significant CAD was correctly ruled out in 118 of 129 patients (specificity: 92%).

4 IMPLICATIONS OF CURRENT DATA FOR THE CLINICAL USE OF CORONARY MDCT

According to recent recommendations, CT angiography of the pulmonary arteries is performed to detect or exclude the presence of pulmonary emboli (PE).[39,40] In fact, only a couple of years ago invasive pulmonary artery angiography

was the established gold standard for the detection of PE. Due to the diagnostic setting in patients with suspected PE, CT angiography, as a noninvasive diagnostic alternative, was investigated in order to replace the gold standard and improve patient care. In contrast, in the field of cardiac imaging, ICA as the established gold standard for the detection of significant CAD allows, if indicated, therapeutic intervention (percutaneous coronary intervention, i.e., stent placement) during the same session. Therefore, clinical application of coronary MDCT as a purely diagnostic alternative to ICA needs to be investigated to complement current medical practice and avoid the portion of ICA that remains diagnostic. In fact, as a purely diagnostic tool, positive findings (true positive and false positive) in coronary MDCT result in additional procedures for interventional/therapeutic purposes.

4.1 Impact of coronary MDCT on different patient populations

There have been widespread efforts to develop predictors of probability for significant CAD according to previously known patient characteristics.[41–45] By combing data from a series of angiography studies performed in the 1960s and the 1970s, Diamond and Forrester showed that simple clinical observations of pain type, age, and gender were powerful predictors of the likelihood of CAD.[41] Data from this work have been combined with those published in the Coronary Artery Surgery Study (CASS)[45] in a pretest probability table (Table 13.2). Clinically, based on a comprehensive assessment, an estimate of the probability of significant CAD for the patient is made (pretest probability of having significant CAD). Diagnostic tests should be chosen according to their ability to revise the pretest probability significantly upwards (positive test result) or downwards (negative test result).

Using Bayesian probability revision the impact of coronary MDCT on different patient populations can be studied.[46] Bayes' formula combines test characteristics (sensitivity, specificity) and the pretest likelihood of disease in the specific population in order to yield a new probability of disease (Table 13.3).

Applying test characteristics of coronary MDCT (sensitivity of 97% and a specificity of 92%) to a high-risk population with a pretest probability of 73%, a positive test result increases the probability by 24% to 99%. A negative test result in the same patient would decrease the probability by 65% to 8%. By applying MDCT test characteristics to the pretest probability of a 49-year-old male who presents with

Table 13.1 Characteristics of study methodology and results of available studies using 64-slice coronary MDCT. Empty cells correspond to data not reported or not available.

First author	Journal	Year	No. of patients	Proportion of segments deemed assessable	Prevalence of significant CAD*	% male subjects	Mean age	Beta-blocker administration	Mean heart rate	Positivity criterion on ICA
Leschka	Eur Heart J	2005	67	100%	70%	75%	60	yes	66	50%
Raff	JACC	2005	70	88%	57%	76%	59	yes	65	50%
Mollet	Circulation	2005	52	100%	75%	65%	60	yes	58	50%
Pugliese	Eur Radiol	2006	35	100%	71%	60%	61	yes	58	50%
Ropers	Am J Cardiol	2006	84	96%	31%	62%	58	yes	59	50%

First author	Journal	Year	Assessable segments only		All segments		Per patient	
			Sensitivity	Specificity	Sensitivity	Specificity	Sensitivity	Specificity
Leschka	Eur Heart J	2005	94%	97%			99%	98%
Raff	JACC	2005	86%	95%			95%	90%
Mollet	Circulation	2005	99%	95%	99%	95%	99%	92%
Pugliese	Eur Radiol	2006	99%	96%	99%	96%	98%	90%
Ropers	Am J Cardiol	2006	93%	97%			96%	91%

*Prevalence of CAD: as assessed by ICA.

Table 13.2 Pretest likelihood of CAD in symptomatic patients according to age and sex. Each value represents the percent with significant CAD on catheterization (Combined Diamond/Forrester and CASS data[41,45]). From Gibbons et al.[92]

Age (years)	Nonanginal chest pain		Atypical angina		Typical angina	
	Men	Women	Men	Women	Men	Women
30–39	4	2	34	12	76	26
40–49	13	3	51	22	87	55
50–59	20	7	65	31	93	73
60–69	27	14	72	51	94	86

atypical chest pain, the diagnostic value in a mid-risk population at intermediate risk can be assessed. A pretest probability of significant CAD of 51% can be assumed according to the Diamond/Forrester and CASS table. In this mid-risk population, a positive MDCT result increases the probability of a significant CAD by 42% to 93%, a negative MDCT result decreases the probability of a significant CAD by 48% to 3%.

Clearly, the diagnostic impact of MDCT imaging for the detection of significant CAD is strongly dependent on the prevalence of disease within a population. Thus, MDCT would probably be most useful in an intermediate/low-risk population. In those patients, not only the prevalence of coronary calcification, a major contributor to false positive findings, is lower, but in addition a high positive rather than a high negative predictive value of MDCT would result in significant changes in patient management, i.e. referral for coronary angiography.

According to this risk stratification scheme, men and women with atypical chest pain and women age 30–49 with typical chest pain who have intermediate pretest probabilities for significant CAD (26 to 72%) may be an attractive target population for coronary MDCT, especially since the prevalence of coronary calcification, a major contributor to

false positive findings, is relatively low in these patients, potentially improving the specificity of CT. However, the value of CT may be limited in these patients, also the risk of radiation-exposure cannot be ignored in younger populations and the test characteristics of coronary CT are unknown in this population.

4.2 Cost-effectiveness of cardiac MDCT

As with all economic goods and services, the provision of health care consumes resources and resources available for health care are limited in supply. Furthermore, health resources are consumed in order to produce health benefits. Therefore, any medical decision or policy decision that entails the use of resources implicitly excludes those resources from alternative possible uses. Cost-effectiveness analysis provides a well-validated decision analytic technique that can be applied to assess the utility of available resources and technologies in order to gain the most health benefit.

From a decision analytic perspective, one has to consider whether coronary MDCT for the detection of a significant

Table 13.3 Summary of probability revision for different prevalence populations (risk populations). Pretest probability according to Diamond/Forrester/ACC.[41,45] Diagnostic test accuracy (sensitivity: 97%, specificity: 92%) is based on pooled diagnostic accuracy from 64- slice MDCT studies as provided in Table 13.1.

Population	Pretest probability P(CAD+)	Positive post-test probability P(CAD+/CTA+)	Negative post-test probability P(CAD+/CTA-)
High-risk	0.93	0.99	0.28
High-risk	0.73	0.97	0.08
Intermediate risk	0.51	0.93	0.03
Low-risk	0.20	0.75	0.01
Low-risk	0.07	0.47	0.0

coronary stenosis is cost effective as compared to ICE. A recent study showed that if a new test was meant to replace a previously established test certain costs as well as sensitivity and specificity criteria would need to be met.[47] In this study, if the cost accepted by society for a new test was $50,000 per QALY and the test cost <$500 (which is currently less than the cost of a coronary MDCT including both technical and professional charges) the test would have to have a sensitivity and specificity of 99% to replace invasive selective coronary angiography. The multitude of data that is available in a patient population which is best suited for coronary invasive selective coronary angiography demonstrates that the test does not reach the sensitivity and specificity required even if the cost was lowered to <$500. Therefore, it seems unreasonable from both a clinical and a cost effective point of view that coronary MDCT will replace ICA using current technology.

In a patient population with low probability of disease, some sensitivity can be lost while maintaining a high specificity and still allow the test to be cost effective.[47] However, another consideration is the test in this patient population is not in direct competition with another test and, therefore, has the potential to provide new patient management information with much less strict criteria on cost, sensitivity, and specificity.

4.3 Potential clinical applications of cardiac MDCT

4.3.1 Assessment of bypasses

There is growing evidence that coronary MDCT permits assessment of coronary bypass graft occlusion and patency with high diagnostic accuracy (approaching 100% to detect bypass occlusion).[48–52] From a clinical perspective, it is also reasonable not only to assess the patency of the graft but also the presence of coronary stenoses in the course of the bypass graft or at the anastomotic site. In fact, due to smaller caliber of these vessels, the presence of artifacts caused by metal clips, and the often heavy coronary calcification, render limited image quality. Recent data from Ropers et al. in 50 patients with a total of 138 grafts indicate that all CABG were evaluable and were correctly classified as occluded or patent and the sensitivity for stenosis detection in patent grafts was 100% with a specificity of 94%.[52] In this study, a per-patient basis, classifying patients with at least one detected stenosis in a graft, a distal runoff vessel, or a nongrafted artery or with at least one unevaluable segment as 'positive,' MDCT yielded a sensitivity of 97% and specificity of 86%.

4.3.2 Anomalous coronary arteries

Anomalous coronary arteries are important differential diagnoses in patients with suspected coronary disease, chest pain, or syncope. So far, assessment has been related to ICA, however, more detailed evaluation of anomalous coronary arteries concerning their origin and course is limited. Due to the 3-dimensional nature of the technique, studies indicate that coronary MDCT permits accurate and straightforward analysis of the coronary course.[53,54] However, as opposed to MRI, another imaging alternative for the assessment of coronary anomalies, coronary MDCT requires radiation and a contrast administration but provides high-resolution datasets with fast image acquisition times.

4.3.3 Acute chest pain

Early and accurate triage of patients presenting with acute chest pain to the emergency department (ED) remains difficult because neither the chest pain history,[55,56] a single set of established biochemical markers for myocardial necrosis (Troponin I, Troponin T, CK- MB),[57,58] or initial 12-lead electrocardiogram (ECG) alone or in combination identifies a group of patients that can be safely discharged without further diagnostic testing.[59–61] Moreover, current strategies fail to identify patients with a high probability of acute coronary syndromes (ACS) who have myocardial ischemia but no objective evidence for myocardial necrosis at ED presentation. As a consequence, the threshold to admit chest pain patients to the hospital remains low and >85% of these patients are discharged after additional observation and testing without a diagnosis of ACS.[62,63] The admission and evaluation of these patients has enormous economic implications for the US health care system, estimated at an annual cost of $8 billion.[64] Despite this conservative practice, 2–8% of patients who are discharged from the ED ultimately develop an ACS within the next 30 days.[55,67–69] Thus, there is a clear need to improve the early triage of patients with acute chest pain.

For the first time, there are now initial data showing that noninvasive assessment of CAD by coronary MDCT has excellent performance characteristics for excluding ACS in subjects presenting with possible myocardial ischemia to the ED (NPV: 100%), and may be useful to improve early triage.[70,71] In those two studies, coronary MDCT was performed subsequent to the inconclusive work up in the ED (nondiagnostic ECG changes and negative biomarkers) and the MDCT images were evaluated for the presence of a

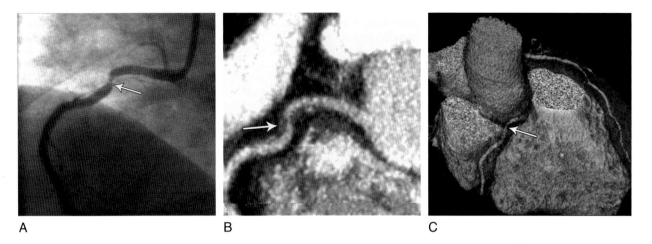

Figure 13.5 (A–C) A 48-year old male patient with recent onset of chest pain. (A) Selective invasive coronary angiography demonstrates a proximal moderate to significant stenosis of the right coronary artery (RCA) (arrow). (B and C) Contrast-enhanced MDCT reveals a concentric noncalcified plaque of the proximal RCA (arrows) in multiplanar reconstruction (B) and in 3-dimensional volume rendered image (C).

significant coronary stenosis and/or plaque. None of the subjects who achieved diagnostic image quality, and in whom no significant coronary artery stenosis was detected, developed ACS during index hospitalization and six month follow-up. However, coronary MDCT was limited in a significant portion of subjects because the exams remain inconclusive, as the presence of a significant stenosis cannot be completely ruled out due to coronary calcification and/or motion artifacts or the inability to assess the hemodynamic significance of a detected stenosis. Both scenarios may potentially lead to additional testing. Figure 13.5 demonstrates the finding of a 48-year-old male patient with recent onset of chest pain with a moderate to significant stenosis of the right coronary artery.

4.3.4 Preoperative assessment

Preoperative assessment prior to noncardiac surgery is another potential application in which coronary MDCT may enhance current standard of care. These patients typically are deemed at low to intermediate risk, do not warrant an invasive procedure, and receive a stress test either with or without imaging. However, standard treadmill has a relative low diagnostic accuracy for the detection of significant CAD (sensitivity and specificity of 65–70% and 70–75%, respectively) which improves to 80–90% sensitivity and specificity if pharmacological myocardial perfusion SPECT imaging is performed.[72] As shown, available data suggest that coronary MDCT may provide similar sensitivities with potentially higher specificities and therefore may be an appealing alternative for the evaluation of patients prior to noncardiac surgery.

Further research is necessary to determine the incremental diagnostic value in this population, also considering side effects of contrast-administration and radiation exposure.

4.3.5 Equivocal stress test

Inconclusive or equivocal stress tests represent a limitation in the management of patients with suspected CAD in current clinical practice. While a normal stress test eliminates the need for further imaging because the patient is at low risk for subsequent cardiac events,[73,74] there is the scenario of an inconclusive or equivocal test in which a coronary CTA could be potentially helpful. Diaphragm attenuation, breast attenuation,[75–77] and left bundle branch block[78–80] can all lead to false positive perfusion defects on nuclear medicine studies. A diagnostic test, characterized by a high negative predictive value in order to eliminate the possibility of a significant coronary lesion, would represent an ideal follow-up.

4.4 Detection and characterization of coronary atherosclerotic plaque

The clinical impact of quantification of nonsignificant and assessment of noncalcified plaque burden remains questionable. Although some groups investigated the feasibility of 16- and 64-slice MDCT to detect and quantify nonsignificant CAD, analysis was limited to high-quality exams in small cohorts.[81–83] However, the potential value for risk stratification is striking. There is evidence that the probability of experiencing an acute coronary event is directly proportional to the total burden of coronary artery calcification (CAC) as quantified by EBCT/MDCT[84,85] and that CAC scores correlate well with the total amount of atherosclerotic burden.[86,87] A very high calcium score has a high positive predictive value for future hard cardiac events; a very low CAC score nearly excludes the occurrence of events. However, about 80% of the overall plaque burden has been shown to be noncalcified[88] and most investigators agree that that portion of noncalcified plaque is related to plaque instability.[89,90] In addition to CAC, MDCT provides the opportunity to quantify noncalcified CAD, which may potentially be a stronger predictor for cardiac events. Consequently, plaque burden of calcified and non-calcified CAD as quantified by MDCT may be established as a novel local biomarker for cardiac risk. Quantification of the overall amount of non-calcified CAD – comparable to CAC scores – may conceivably, in the future, enable percentile-based risk stratification and subsequent better identification of patients at risk.[91]

Despite these encouraging concepts, feasibility data available show little evidence that calcified and noncalcified plaque quantification can be transferred into clinical practice soon. A recent study from Leber et al. in 19 subjects showed that MDCT correctly detected 83% of noncalcified plaque, 94% of mixed plaque, and 95% of calcified plaque as compared to intravascular ultrasound (IVUS).[82] However, plaque volume measurement revealed an underestimation of noncalcified and mixed plaque whereas calcified plaque was systematically overestimated and, more importantly, interobserver variability was 37%. Although these results suggest that noninvasive plaque detection by MDCT is feasible, a moderate concordance to IVUS and insufficient reproducibility may encumber clinical use of plaque quantification using current technology. Perhaps, a semi-quantitative approach related to coronary segments in which non-calcified and/or calcified plaque can be detected may facilitate reliability and enable assessment of coronary plaque burden not restricted to CAC. Further large-scale studies, similar to initial CAC trails, are necessary to determine the longitudinal association between the amounts of nonsignificant CAD – quantitatively or semiquantitatively – and hard cardiac outcomes.

5 FUTURE DIRECTIONS

In order to determine a technology's clinical utility enormous efforts need to be undertaken. The first step on a long road is to assess feasibility demonstrating the accuracy and reproducibility of a new technology. If general feasibility of a technology is met, observational studies can conclude whether the selected patient population and the clinical end points are appropriate. In the majority of these observational studies, a preliminary assessment of safety, cost, and cost effectiveness can be performed, information that is critical to rationalize costly randomized diagnostic trials as the final step of the process. Only technology assessment at this level permits recommendations by national and international societies and would potentially justify reimbursement by third party payers in the context of evidenced-based medicine.

Applying these principles to the technology and clinical application of coronary MDCT there are numerous studies that have demonstrated the high sensitivity and specificity of both 16- and 64-slice MDCT for the detection and quantification of coronary stenosis and initial experience for the detection and quantification of nonsignificant CAD. Beyond feasibility assessment in single-center studies, there has not been much effort to advance to observational studies and define the population that will potentially benefit of coronary MDCT. This may be related to a continuous rapid technical improvement with the promotion of a new scanner generation almost every year. In this context, obviously it has been the outmost difficulty to perform large-scaled prospective trials which implement state of the art technology as the diagnostic intervention. Those studies require a longer period of time to complete and acquired results may not apply to technology on the market by then.

Nevertheless, diagnostic accuracy of coronary MDCT is excellent independent of scanner type if analysis is restricted to assessable segments. Diagnostic accuracy of MDCT based on all segments, the clinically relevant measure, increases from EBCT to 4/8-, 16- to 64-slice MDCT, reflecting the improvement in scanner technology. However, probability revision on a patient-based analysis reveals that the clinical utility may be limited in a population of high risk for significant CAD.

There is now a window of opportunity to provide these data and to potentially demonstrate that coronary MDCT improves patient management in terms of diagnostic accuracy, clinical decision-making, and cost effectiveness. Because this window might be narrow, these ambitious goals may only be achieved in a major collaborative effort between cardiologists, radiologists, and public health researchers.

REFERENCES

1. Johnson LW et al. Coronary arteriography 1984–1987: a report of the Registry of the Society for Cardiac Angiography and Interventions. I. Results and complications. Cathet Cardiovasc Diagn 1989; 17(1): 5–10.

2. Laskey W, Boyle J, and Johnson LW. Multivariable model for prediction of risk of significant complication during diagnostic cardiac catheterization. The Registry Committee of the Society for Cardiac Angiography & Interventions. Cathet Cardiovasc Diagn 1993; 30(3): 185–90.

3. Chandrasekar B et al. Complications of cardiac catheterization in the current era: a single-center experience. Catheter Cardiovasc Interv 2001; 52(3): 289–95.

4. Duncan R, Coles MAS, Ian S, Negus et al. Comparison of Radiation Doses From Multislice Computed Tomography Coronary Angiography and Conventional Diagnostic Angiography. J Am Coll Cardiol 2006. April 17 epub.

5. Smith LD, Spyer G, and Dean JW. Audit of cardiac catheterisation in a district general hospital: implications for training. Heart 1999; 81(5): 461–4.

6. Wyman RM et al. Current complications of diagnostic and therapeutic cardiac catheterization. J Am Coll Cardiol 1988; 12(6): 1400–6.

7. Zanzanico P, Rothenberg LN, and Strauss HW. Radiation Exposure of Computed Tomography and Direct Intracoronary Angiography: Risk Has its Reward. J Am Coll Cardiol 2006. April 17 epub.

8. Association AH. Heart Disease and Stroke facts: 2003 Statistical supplement. 2003, American Heart Association: Dallas TX. 1–46.

9. Kozak LJ, DeFrances CJ, and Hall MJ. National hospital discharge survey: 2004 annual summary with detailed diagnosis and procedure data. Vital Health Stat 13 2006; (162): 1–209.

10. Hounsfield GN. Computerized transverse axial scanning (tomography). 1. Description of system. Br J Radiol 1973; 46(552): 1016–22.

11. Achenbach S et al. Value of electron-beam computed tomography for the noninvasive detection of high-grade coronary-artery stenoses and occlusions. N Engl J Med 1998; 339(27): 1964–71.

12. Becker CR et al. Detection and quantification of coronary artery calcification with electron-beam and conventional CT. Eur Radiol 1999; 9(4): 620–4.

13. Schmermund A et al. Intravenous electron-beam computed tomographic coronary angiography for segmental analysis of coronary artery stenoses. J Am Coll Cardiol 1998; 31(7): 1547–54.

14. Chernoff DM, Ritchie CJ, and Higgins CB. Evaluation of electron beam CT coronary angiography in healthy subjects. AJR Am J Roentgenol 1997; 169(1): 93–9.

15. Ohnesorge B et al. Cardiac imaging by means of electrocardiographically gated multisection spiral CT: initial experience. Radiology 2000; 217(2): 564–71.

16. Achenbach S et al. Noninvasive coronary angiography by retrospectively ECG-gated multislice spiral CT. Circulation 2000; 102(23): 2823–8.

17. Becker CR et al. Imaging of noncalcified coronary plaques using helical CT with retrospective ECG gating. AJR Am J Roentgenol 2000; 175(2): 423–4.

18. Nieman K et al. Coronary angiography with multi-slice computed tomography. Lancet 2001; 357(9256): 599–603.

19. Achenbach S et al. Detection of coronary artery stenoses by contrast-enhanced, retrospectively electrocardiographically-gated, multislice spiral computed tomography. Circulation 2001; 103(21): 2535–8.

20. Knez A et al. Usefulness of multislice spiral computed tomography angiography for determination of coronary artery stenoses. Am J Cardiol 2001; 88(10): 1191–4.

21. Nieman K et al. Usefulness of multislice computed tomography for detecting obstructive coronary artery disease. Am J Cardiol 2002; 89(8): 913–18.

22. Nieman K et al. Reliable noninvasive coronary angiography with fast submillimeter multislice spiral computed tomography. Circulation 2002; 106(16): 2051–4.

23. Heuschmid M et al. [Visualization of coronary arteries in CT as assessed by a new 16 slice technology and reduced gantry rotation time: first experiences]. Rofo Fortschr Geb Rontgenstr Neuen Bildgeb Verfahr 2002; 174(6): 721–4.

24. Flohr T et al. New technical developments in multislice CT – Part 1: Approaching isotropic resolution with sub-millimeter 16-slice scanning. Rofo Fortschr Geb Rontgenstr Neuen Bildgeb Verfahr 2002; 174(7): 839–45.

25. Raff GL et al. Diagnostic accuracy of noninvasive coronary angiography using 64-slice spiral computed tomography. J Am Coll Cardiol 2005; 46(3): 552–7.

26. Cademartiri F et al. Non-invasive coronary angiography with 64-slice computed tomography. Minerva Cardioangiol 2005; 53(5): 465–72.

27. Mollet NR et al. High-resolution spiral computed tomography coronary angiography in patients referred for diagnostic conventional coronary angiography. Circulation 2005; 112(15): 2318–23.

28. Achenbach S et al. Contrast-enhanced coronary artery visualization by dual-source computed tomography – initial experience. Eur J Radiol 2006; 57(3): 331–5.

29. Stein PD et al. Multidetector computed tomography for the diagnosis of coronary artery disease: a systematic review. Am J Med 2006; 119(3): 203–16.

30. Hoffmann U JH, Dunn E, d'Janne Othee B. Is CT angiography ready for prime time? A meta-analysis. JACC 2004; 43 (Supplement A) (5): 312A.

31. Austen WG et al. A reporting system on patients evaluated for coronary artery disease. Report of the Ad Hoc Committee for Grading of Coronary Artery Disease, Council on Cardiovascular Surgery, American Heart Association. Circulation 1975; 51(4 Suppl): 5–40.

32. Wang JC et al. Coronary artery spatial distribution of acute myocardial infarction occlusions. Circulation 2004; 110(3): 278–84.

33. Kuettner A et al. Diagnostic accuracy of multidetector computed tomography coronary angiography in patients with angiographically proven coronary artery disease. J Am Coll Cardiol 2004; 43(5): 831–9.

34. Hoffmann U et al. Predictive value of 16-slice multidetector spiral computed tomography to detect significant obstructive coronary artery disease in patients at high risk for coronary artery disease: patient-versus segment-based analysis. Circulation 2004; 110(17): 2638–43.

35. Dewey M et al. Multisegment and halfscan reconstruction of 16-slice computed tomography for detection of coronary artery stenoses. Invest Radiol 2004; 39(4): 223–9.

36. Hoffmann MH et al. Noninvasive coronary angiography with multislice computed tomography. Jama 2005; 293(20): 2471–8.

37. Kuettner A et al. Image quality and diagnostic accuracy of non-invasive coronary imaging with 16 detector slice spiral computed tomography with 188 ms temporal resolution. Heart 2005; 91(7): 938–41.

38. Budoff MJ et al. Assessment of coronary artery disease by cardiac computed tomography: a scientific statement from the American Heart Association Committee on Cardiovascular Imaging and Intervention, Council on Cardiovascular Radiology and Intervention, and Committee on Cardiac Imaging, Council on Clinical Cardiology. Circulation 2006; 114(16): 1761–91.

39. Quiroz R et al. Clinical validity of a negative computed tomography scan in patients with suspected pulmonary embolism: a systematic review. Jama 2005; 293(16): 2012–17.

40. Winer-Muram HT et al. Suspected acute pulmonary embolism: evaluation with multi-detector row CT versus digital subtraction pulmonary arteriography. Radiology 2004; 233(3): 806–15.

41. Diamond GA, Forrester JS. Analysis of probability as an aid in the clinical diagnosis of coronary-artery disease. N Engl J Med 1979; 300(24): 1350–8.

42. Pryor DB et al. Estimating the likelihood of significant coronary artery disease. Am J Med 1983; 75(5): 771–80.

43. Sox HC Jr et al. Using the patient's history to estimate the probability of coronary artery disease: a comparison of primary care and referral practices. Am J Med 1990; 89(1): 7–14.

44. Pryor DB et al. Value of the history and physical in identifying patients at increased risk for coronary artery disease. Ann Intern Med 1993; 118(2): 81–90.

45. Chaitman BR et al. Angiographic prevalence of high-risk coronary artery disease in patient subsets (CASS). Circulation 1981; 64(2): 360–7.

46. Rembold CM, and Watson D. Posttest probability calculation by weights. A simple form of Bayes' theorem. Ann Intern Med 1988; 108(1): 115–20.

47. Hunink MG et al. Noninvasive imaging for the diagnosis of coronary artery disease: focusing the development of new diagnostic technology. Ann Intern Med 1999; 131(9): 673–80.

48. Malagutti P et al. Use of 64-slice CT in symptomatic patients after coronary bypass surgery: evaluation of grafts and coronary arteries. Eur Heart J 2006.

49. Nieman K et al. Evaluation of patients after coronary artery bypass surgery: CT angiographic assessment of grafts and coronary arteries. Radiology 2003; 229(3): 749–56.

50. Chiurlia E et al. Follow-up of coronary artery bypass graft patency by multislice computed tomography. Am J Cardiol 2005; 95(9): 1094–7.

51. Achenbach S et al. Noninvasive, three-dimensional visualization of coronary artery bypass grafts by electron beam tomography. Am J Cardiol 1997; 79(7): 856–61.

52. Ropers D et al. Diagnostic accuracy of noninvasive coronary angiography in patients after bypass surgery using 64-slice spiral computed tomography with 330-ms gantry rotation. Circulation 2006; 114(22): 2334–41; quiz 2334.

53. Schmid M et al. Visualization of coronary artery anomalies by contrast-enhanced multi-detector row spiral computed tomography. Int J Cardiol 2006; 111(3): 430–5.

54. Ropers D et al. Visualization of coronary artery anomalies and their anatomic course by contrast-enhanced electron beam tomography and three-dimensional reconstruction. Am J Cardiol 2001; 87(2): 193–7.

55. Lee TH et al. Clinical characteristics and natural history of patients with acute myocardial infarction sent home from the emergency room. Am J Cardiol 1987; 60(4): 219–24.

56. Swap CJ, Nagurney JT. Value and limitations of chest pain history in the evaluation of patients with suspected acute coronary syndromes. Jama 2005; 294(20): 2623–9.

57. Limkakeng A Jr et al. Combination of Goldman risk and initial cardiac troponin I for emergency department chest pain patient risk stratification. Acad Emerg Med 2001; 8(7): 696–702.

58. Zimmerman J et al. Diagnostic marker cooperative study for the diagnosis of myocardial infarction. Circulation 1999; 99(13): 1671–7.

59. Fesmire FM et al. The Erlanger chest pain evaluation protocol: a one-year experience with serial 12-lead ECG monitoring, two-hour delta serum marker measurements, and selective nuclear stress testing to identify and exclude acute coronary syndromes. Ann Emerg Med 2002; 40(6): 584–94.

60. Hedges JR et al. Serial ECGs are less accurate than serial CK-MB results for emergency department diagnosis of myocardial infarction. Ann Emerg Med 1992; 21(12): 1445–50.

61. Selker HP et al. Use of the acute cardiac ischemia time-insensitive predictive instrument (ACI-TIPI) to assist with triage of patients with chest pain or other symptoms suggestive of acute cardiac ischemia. A multicenter, controlled clinical trial. Ann Intern Med 1998; 129(11): 845–55.

62. Hollander JE et al. Effects of neural network feedback to physicians on admit/discharge decision for emergency department patients with chest pain. Ann Emerg Med 2004; 44(3): 199–205.

63. McCaig LF, and Burt CW. National Hospital Ambulatory Medical Care Survey: 2002 emergency department summary. Adv Data 2004; (340): 1–34.

64. Tosteson AN et al. Cost-effectiveness of a coronary care unit versus an intermediate care unit for emergency department patients with chest pain. Circulation 1996; 94(2): 143–50.

65. Reference removed.

66. Reference removed.

67. Pope JH et al. Missed diagnoses of acute cardiac ischemia in the emergency department. N Engl J Med 2000; 342(16): 1163–70.

68. Lee TH, Goldman L. Evaluation of the patient with acute chest pain. N Engl J Med 2000; 342(16): 1187–95.

69. Goldman L et al. Prediction of the need for intensive care in patients who come to the emergency departments with acute chest pain. N Engl J Med 1996; 334(23): 1498–504.

70. Hoffmann U et al. Coronary multidetector computed tomography in the assessment of patients with acute chest pain. Circulation 2006; 114(21): 2251–60.

71. Goldstein JA et al. A randomized controlled trial of multislice coronary computed tomography for evaluation of acute chest pain. J Am Coll Cardiol 2007; 49(8): 863–71.

72. Abrams J. Clinical practice. Chronic stable angina. N Engl J Med 2005; 352(24): 2524–33.

73. Fuster V, Alexander RW, O'Rourke RA. Hurst's the heart. 11th ed. 2004, New York: McGraw-Hill, Medical Pub. Division. 2 v. (xxvii 2472, 65).

74. Hachamovitch R, Shaw L, Berman DS. Methodological considerations in the assessment of noninvasive testing using outcomes research: pitfalls and limitations. Prog Cardiovasc Dis 2000; 43(3): 215–30.

75. Detrano R et al. Factors affecting sensitivity and specificity of a diagnostic test: the exercise thallium scintigram. Am J Med 1988; 84(4): 699–710.

76. Iskandrian AE, Heo J, Nallamothu N. Detection of coronary artery disease in women with use of stress single-photon emission computed tomography myocardial perfusion imaging. J Nucl Cardiol 1997; 4(4): 329–35.

77. Taillefer R et al. Comparative diagnostic accuracy of Tl-201 and Tc-99m sestamibi SPECT imaging (perfusion and ECG-gated SPECT) in detecting coronary artery disease in women. J Am Coll Cardiol 1997; 29(1): 69–77.

78. Braat SH et al. Thallium-201 exercise scintigraphy and left bundle branch block. Am J Cardiol 1985; 55(1): 224–6.

79. DePuey EG, Guertler-Krawczynska E, Robbins WL. Thallium-201 SPECT in coronary artery disease patients with left bundle branch block. J Nucl Med 1988; 29(9): 1479–85.

80. Hirzel HO et al. Thallium-201 scintigraphy in complete left bundle branch block. Am J Cardiol 1984; 53(6): 764–9.

81. Achenbach S et al. Detection of Calcified and Noncalcified Coronary Atherosclerotic Plaque by Contrast-Enhanced, Submillimeter Multidetector Spiral Computed Tomography: A Segment-Based Comparison With Intravascular Ultrasound. Circulation 2004; 109(1): 14–17.

82. Leber AW et al. Accuracy of 64-slice computed tomography to classify and quantify plaque volumes in the proximal coronary system: a comparative study using intravascular ultrasound. J Am Coll Cardiol 2006; 47(3): 672–7.

83. Moselewski F et al. Measurement of cross-sectional coronary atherosclerotic plaque and vessel areas by 16-slice multi-detector CT: comparison to IVUS. Am J Cardiol 2004; 94: 1294–1297.

84. Arad Y et al. Prediction of coronary events with electron beam computed tomography. J Am Coll Cardiol 2000; 36(4): 1253–60.

85. Raggi P et al. Identification of patients at increased risk of first unheralded acute myocardial infarction by electron-beam computed tomography. Circulation 2000; 101(8): 850–5.

86. Agatston AS, Janowitz WR. Ultrafast computed tomography in coronary screening. Circulation 1994; 89(4): 1908–9.

87. Breen JF et al. Coronary artery calcification detected with ultrafast CT as an indication of coronary artery disease. Radiology 1992; 185(2): 435–9.

88. Rumberger JA et al. Coronary artery calcium area by electron-beam computed tomography and coronary atherosclerotic plaque area. A histopathologic correlative study. Circulation 1995; 92(8): 2157–62.

89. Rosenfeld ME et al. Advanced atherosclerotic lesions in the innominate artery of the ApoE knockout mouse. Arterioscler Thromb Vasc Biol 2000; 20(12): 2587–92.

90. Schmermund A, Erbel R. Unstable coronary plaque and its relation to coronary calcium. Circulation 2001; 104(14): 1682–7.

91. Greenland P et al. Prevention Conference V: Beyond secondary prevention: identifying the high-risk patient for primary prevention: noninvasive tests of atherosclerotic burden: Writing Group III. Circulation 2000; 101(1): E16–22.

92. Gibbons RJ et al. ACC/AHA 2002 guideline update for the management of patients with chronic stable angina–summary article: a report of the American College of Cardiology/American Heart Association Task Force on Practice Guidelines (Committee on the Management of Patients With Chronic Stable Angina). Circulation 2003; 107(1): 149–58.

14

Computed Tomographic Angiography of Coronary Artery Anomalies

Phillip M. Young, Ronald S. Kuzo, and Thomas C. Gerber

Anomalies of the coronary vasculature have gained increasing attention in recent years. The medical significance of anomalous coronary arteries lies in the risk of sudden cardiac death in young, previously asymptomatic individuals, which is associated with certain variants of such anomalies. Typically, coronary anomalies are either recognized as incidental findings in patients undergoing invasive, selective coronary angiography, or are diagnosed at autopsy. Given the limited number of suitable diagnostic modalities, these uncommon but potentially lethal conditions are rarely detected and probably frequently under-recognized or incorrectly characterized in live patients.

However, modern multidetector row CT scanning (MDCT), with ECG gating, allowing exquisite delineation of cardiac and vascular anatomy, offers a widely available method for accurately delineating incidentally discovered coronary artery anomalies; it also has the ability to noninvasively investigate individuals with signs or symptoms, suggesting the presence of coronary artery anomalies with the potential to cause adverse cardiac events.

1 PREVALENCE OF ANOMALOUS CORONARY ARTERIES

Coronary artery anomalies have been described with a frequency of approximately 0.3% to 1.3% in angiographic studies[1,2] and approximately 0.3% to 0.5% in large autopsy series.[3,4] There is some overlap between variants of normal coronary anatomy and true anomalies, and many "anomalies" are of little clinical significance and have little potential for causing adverse events.[5,6] However, anomalous coronary arteries have been implicated as the cause of sudden death in 5% to 35% of young athletes.[7] Retrospective analysis of 27 cases of sudden death associated with anomalous coronary arteries demonstrated that 55% had no premonitory symptoms.[8] Of those who had symptoms, the prior investigations, including 12-lead ECG, stress ECG with maximal exercise, and left ventricular wall motion and cardiac dimensions by two-dimensional echocardiography were all normal.

2 CLASSIFICATION AND CLINICAL SIGNIFICANCE OF CORONARY ARTERY ANOMALIES

Angelini[5] has suggested classifying coronary anomalies into three categories: abnormalities of the coronary ostia, abnormalities of the coronary stems, and abnormalities in the terminus of the artery.

2.1 Abnormalities of coronary ostia

Typically, there are 2 coronary ostia (right and left) located centrally in the right and left coronary sinus of

Valsalva, respectively. However, as many as 3 or 4 coronary ostia, including separate origins of the circumflex and left anterior descending arteries, or a separate origin of the conus branch, are considered normal variants without clinical significance.

Although anomalies of caliber or morphology of the coronary ostia can be hemodynamically significant, premorbid anatomic delineation of these anomalies is quite difficult. Yet, ostial abnormalities, particularly the concept of the "slit-like orifice", may play an important role in the pathophysiology of sudden death in patients with abnormal coronary stems, as will be discussed later. The coronary ostium is usually at least equal in size to the caliber of the proximal portion of the coronary artery. Normally, the ostium is located within 1 cm cranial to the aortic valve plane. Origin of a coronary artery above this level is usually not clinically important, but knowledge that such a variation is present may help anticipate the degree of difficulty of catheter-based invasive procedures or avoid problems or errors during cardiac and thoracic surgery. Rarely, a coronary artery may arise from the pulmonary artery. Although pulmonary arterial origin of the right coronary artery (RCA), left anterior descending artery (LAD), and left circumflex coronary artery (LCX) have been described, they are extremely rare and usually not clinically significant. The condition of *a*nomalous *l*eft *c*oronary *a*rtery from the *p*ulmonary *a*rtery (ALCAPA), also known as Bland-White-Garland syndrome, is slightly more common and will be discussed in the section on coronary anomalies with shunt physiology.

2.2 Abnormalities of the coronary stem

Although rare in absolute terms, anomalous path of the coronary artery stem presents a much more common clinical dilemma. The most frequently encountered anomaly of clinical significance involves abnormal origin from the contralateral coronary sinus (e.g., LCA originating from the right coronary sinus of Valsalva or RCA originating from the left coronary sinus). In traveling to its perfusion territory, the artery must course either posteriorly to the aorta (retroaortic), anteriorly to the pulmonary outflow tract (prepulmonic), between the main pulmonary artery and the aorta (interarterial), or through the interventricular septum.

The risk of adverse events is highest in anomalous arteries that take an interarterial course. The proposed mechanism of pathology is compression of the artery between the

adjacent great vessels, which is most likely to occur during vigorous exercise. Although based on skewed patient populations from multiple sources, the mortality rate for patients with these anomalies has been estimated at 30%.[9] This risk of adverse outcomes has resulted in the designations of "malignant coronary artery anomaly" for those with an interarterial course, versus "benign coronary artery anomaly" for those with prepulmonic and retroaortic courses.

Some authors propose that tortuosity or angulation of the vessel with respect to the aorta can have adverse hemodynamic consequences.[10–12] It has been suggested at necropsy that angulation of the vessel with respect to the aorta can cause a valve-like "ridge" in the ostium which is accentuated with dilatation of the aortic root while the coronary stem is fixed in place (Figure 14.1). Virmani et al.[12] suggested that even arteries with normally located ostia may be at risk of sudden cardiac death if the angle of the artery with respect to the aorta is less than 45 degrees. Kragel and Roberts, in a series of 32 necropsy cases, could not establish statistical

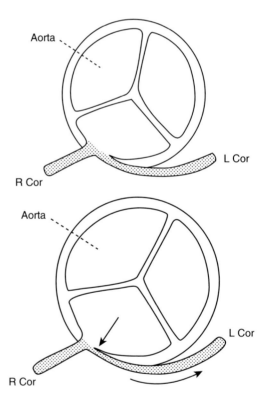

Figure 14.1 Mechanisms of compression of anomalous coronary arteries. Example of a coronary artery originating at an acute angle from the aorta show in diastole (top). The narrow, slit-like orifice may be compressed (arrow) as the aorta expands in systole (bottom). With permission from: Cheitlin MD, DeCastro CM, McAllister HA. Sudden death as a complication of anomalous left coronary origin from the anterior sinus of Valsalva: a not-so-minor congenital anomaly. Circulation 1974; 50: 780–7.

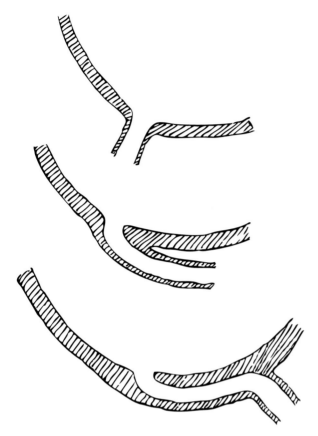

Figure 14.2 Various forms of coronary artery origin from the aorta. *Top*, Normal origin at nearly right angle. *Middle*, origin at acute angle. *Bottom*, intramural course of the very proximal portion of a coronary artery. With permission from: Angelini P. Normal and anomalous coronary arteries: definitions and classification. American Heart Journal 1989; 117: 418–34.

significance of a slit-like shape of the ostium, but did note an association between clinical outcome and dominance or non-dominance of the anomalous artery. It has been noted on pathologic investigation as well as intravascular ultrasound that some arteries take a path that actually travels through the wall of the aorta, causing variable degrees of compression (Figure 14.2).[9]

The clinical significance of a septal course is not entirely clear, but at least 1 case of near-complete occlusion of the abnormal coronary artery was documented during systole by angiography.[14] This has also been noted in at least one reported case on CT.[15]

2.3 Myocardial bridging

In myocardial bridging, an epicardial segment of a coronary artery tunnels through a portion of myocardium. Typically this abnormality involves the middle segment of the LAD,

and generally has an excellent prognosis.[16–20] Although conventional angiography may confirm as much as 50% luminal narrowing of the affected artery during systole, most coronary blood flow normally occurs in diastole and the anomaly rarely has hemodynamic significance. Interestingly, the tunneled arterial segment frequently demonstrates sparing of atherosclerotic plaque.[16]

Juilliere et al.[17] followed 61 patients with myocardial bridges detected on coronary angiography for a mean of 11 years. None of the patients developed a myocardial infarction, and adverse outcomes were not seen to correlate with the degree of systolic compression. Although myocardial bridging is typically a benign anomaly, the diminished caliber could affect myocardial reserve if there is infarction in another vascular distribution, and this may play a role in selected cases of multivessel disease.[21]

Rare clinical sequelae have been reported, usually secondary to compression and ischemia.[19–21] The risk of hemodynamic compromise in these cases is probably related to the length, depth, and location of the intramyocardial segment, as well as the amount of coronary reserve.

2.4 Abnormalities of termination

Abnormalities of termination include coronary artery fistulae and coronary arteriovenous malformations (AVMs), both of which pose quite rare but potentially important problems which are increasingly well-visualized with CT. The distinction between fistulae and AVMs in the literature is blurry, and the terms are sometimes used interchangeably. Coronary artery fistulae have been described in up to 0.5% of coronary angiograms, but are the most common indication for repair of a coronary anomaly.[22]

Most fistulae are small, and the shunt volume is not sufficient to cause symptoms. In one review of 51 Dutch adult patients with isolated coronary artery fistulae, 13 had symptoms of angina pectoris without angiographic evidence of significant atherosclerotic disease, and 7 had evidence for ischemia on stress testing. The 5-year cardiac mortality was 4%, in a population in which the mean age at catheterization was 60.3 years.[23]

Coronary arterial steal phenomenon has been described, which may lead to myocardial ischemia but only rarely to infarction.[24] Increasing left-to-right shunt may occur and may eventually cause elevation of pulmonary artery and right ventricular pressures. Generally, symptoms from such coronary shunts do not arise until adulthood, and early surgical repair and catheter-based coil embolization in the pediatric population remain controversial. Some authors favor early intervention to prevent potential complications.[25–27] However, others note a large preponderance of small, hemodynamically insignificant fistulae in the adult population, for which surgery or catheter-based therapy is not warranted.[28] Currently, the consensus statement from the American Heart Association considers coronary fistulae a Class II indication (coil occlusion may be appropriate) for intervention in the pediatric population.[29]

2.5 Acquired coronary anomalies: coronary aneurysms

Coronary artery aneurysms are defined as dilation of the artery to 1.5 times the diameter of the largest "normal" portion of the artery in the adjacent segment or the diameter of the patient's largest coronary artery.

Coronary artery aneurysms are uncommon, with an incidence of 1.4% in an autopsy study of 694 patients[30] and an incidence of 4.9% on angiography in the Coronary Artery Surgery Study (CASS) registry.[31] It should be noted that CASS was a retrospective study that relied on angiography performed at multiple centers, and review of images by the authors led them to believe that aneurysms were overdiagnosed in the study population.

The main etiology of coronary artery aneurysms is atherosclerosis. This probably accounts for the slight male preponderance of coronary aneurysms.[32] Inflammatory disorders such as Kawasaki disease, endocarditis, connective tissue disorders such as Marfan's Syndrome, and iatrogenic causes (complications of angioplasty and prior cardiac surgery) are also important causes. Congenital aneurysms have also been described. In a review of the literature from 1963, 52% of coronary artery aneurysms were caused by atherosclerosis, 17% were congenital, and 11% mycotic.[30] Coronary fistulae may cause significant aneurysmal dilation of the involved coronaries, with one transesophageal echocardiographic study measuring an average coronary diameter of 7.1 mm.[33] However, the etiology varies with geographic location, with Kawasaki's disease being more common in East Asian populations.[34]

Because of the low prevalence of coronary artery aneurysms, the prognostic implications of their presence are not well understood. In CASS, the authors found no significant difference in 5-year mortality between patients with and without aneurysmal disease who were matched for the degree of atherosclerotic luminal narrowing. The degree of ectasia likely affects the prognosis, and

some authors consider "giant coronary artery aneurysms," implying severe ectasia (on the order of 20 mm diameter or greater), to be a distinct entity.[34] However, there are no established criteria for what constitutes a giant coronary artery aneurysm. Giant aneurysms are probably at higher risk of serious complication, including rupture, thrombosis, and distal embolization, but their natural history is not well understood.

3 CT ANGIOGRAPHY OF CORONARY ARTERY ANOMALIES

Along with cardiac magnetic resonance (CMR), coronary computed tomographic angiography (CCTA) is indicated for the investigation of coronary artery anomalies because of its potential to noninvasively delineate anomalous anatomy and help in planning potential management.[35] Currently, the most frequent reason to use CCTA in this setting is to delineate the proximal course of coronary arteries with anomalous origins. The indirect, two-dimensional projectional nature of invasive, catheter-based angiography can make this a difficult task. A number of studies have shown that, in contrast to CCTA, invasive angiography could only in 31–55% of cases delineate the course of anomalous arteries, and CCTA in each study was felt to be more accurate.[36–42]

In addition to characterizing the origin of the anomalous vessel and its path relative to the aorta and pulmonary artery, it is also important to note the relationship of the vessel to the aortic wall and the overall coronary dominance pattern. Careful analysis of the proximal anomalous coronary artery with respect to the aortic wall, including tortuosity, angulation, and mural tunneling, as well as the overall coronary dominance pattern, can provide useful prognostic information and may help in presurgical planning.

3.1 Right coronary artery arising from the left coronary cusp, left main coronary artery, or left anterior descending artery

RCAs originating from the left coronary sinus most frequently course interarterially. To date, 70 such cases have been described on MDCT or electron beam computed tomography (EBCT)[15,36–55] (Figure 14.3). All but 2 of these cases demonstrated an interarterial course of the anomalous artery. In one

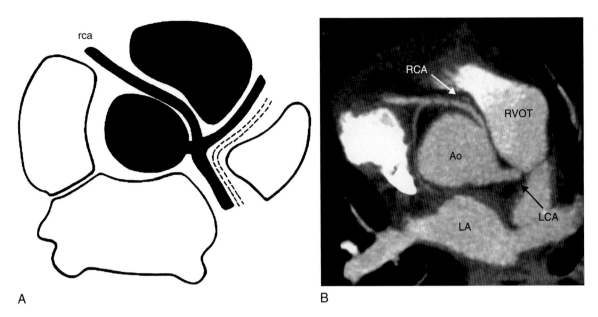

Figure 14.3   Interarterial course of an anomalous right coronary artery (RCA). Schematic (*left*) and maximum intensity projection image (*right*) oriented approximately in the horizontal plane demonstrate the RCA arising from the left sinus of Valsalva and traveling between the aorta (Ao) and the right ventricular outflow tract (RVOT) and pulmonary artery to its perfusion territory. LA, left atrium; LCA, left coronary artery. Left panel with permission from: Bunce NH et al. Coronary artery anomalies: Assessment with free-breathing three-dimensional coronary MR angiography. Radiology 2003; 227: 201–8.

case, cine loop reconstruction demonstrated 35% diameter reduction in the RCA during systole, correlating with evidence of inferior wall ischemia on dobutamine stress echocardiography.[55]

In three of these cases, conventional angiography had previously misinterpreted the course of the arteries as "benign."[39–41] One case has been described in which the RCA arose from the left coronary cusp, and the course was implied to be benign but not specificied.[49] Another case has been described of the RCA arising from the noncoronary sinus, with a tortuous but benign course posterior to the aorta.[38] In 1 case, the RCA was not detected during emergent invasive angiography, and CT was successfully used to evaluate for the presence of an anomalous artery.[51] A single case has been described of origin of the RCA from the LAD in the setting of tetralogy of Fallot.[52]

3.2 Left main coronary artery arising from the right coronary cusp, right coronary artery, or sharing a common origin with the right coronary artery

The course of an anomalous left main coronary artery arising from the right coronary sinus, from the RCA, or sharing

a common origin with the RCA, is variable. Fifty-one cases of this anomaly have been described on MDCT or EBCT, with 29 taking an interarterial course or having a branch with an interarterial component (Figure 14.4). Of the remainder, 6 followed a septal course, 9 followed a retroaortic course, and 7 followed a purely prepulmonic course.[14,36–38,40–42,46,49–50,53–61] An example of a left coronary artery arising from the RCA with a retroaortic proximal course is shown in Figure 14.5.

In one series of 10 cases, 3 were misinterpreted on invasive angiography blinded to CT results. Two cases which had been thought to have an interarterial course were shown to have a benign retroaortic course on CT, while another case that had been thought to have a benign course was upgraded when CT demonstrated interarterial course of the LCA.[42] Two cases have been described in which the left anterior descending and circumflex arteries arose from separate ostia in the right coronary sinus. In one case, both arteries took a benign course.[40] In the other, the LAD took a prepulmonic course but gave off a septal branch which traveled an interarterial course. The circumflex coronary artery took a retroaortic course.[60] Similarly, another early case report demonstrated a single coronary artery arising from the right sinus of Valsalva. MDCT clearly demonstrated that the LAD took a prepulmonic course and the LCX took a retroaortic course (Figure 14.6).[61]

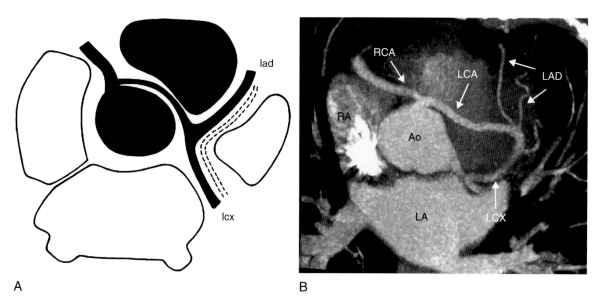

Figure 14.4 Interarterial course of an anomalous left coronary artery (LCA). Schematic (*left*) and maximum intensity projection image (*right*) demonstrate origin of the left main coronary artery from the right sinus of Valsalva and traveling an interarterial path, partly through the septum, to its perfusion territory. Small branches course anteriorly to supply the left anterior descending (LAD) territory, while the circumflex (LCX) is quite robust and tortuous. RA, right atrium; RCA, right coronary artery; Ao, aorta; LA, left atrium. Left panel with permission from: Bunce NH et al. Coronary artery anomalies: Assessment with free-breathing three-dimensional coronary MR angiography. Radiology 2003; 227: 201–8.

3.4 Left circumflex coronary artery arising separately from the right coronary cusp or right coronary artery

The left circumflex may arise separately from the LAD, or may originate from the right coronary cusp or RCA (Figure 14.7). This anomaly is invariably benign and no cases of this anomaly presenting with an interarterial course have ever been described in the CT or angiographic literature. Fifty-one cases of this anomaly have so far been described on MDCT or EBCT.[36,38–42,53–54,62–63] All cases of the anomalous right-sided origin of the circumflex artery, whether arising from the coronary sinus or the right

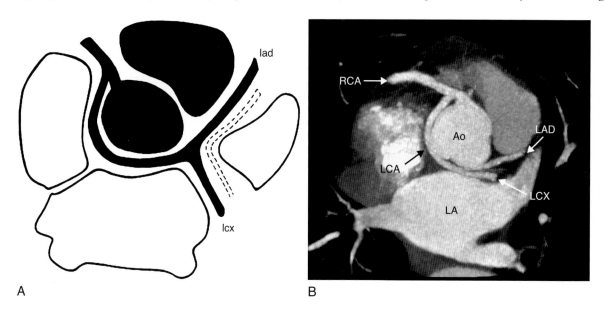

Figure 14.5 Retroaortic course of an anomalous left coronary artery (LCA). Schematic (*left*) and maximum intensity projection image (*right*) oriented approximately in the horizontal plane demonstrate a single coronary artery arising from the right sinus of Valsalva, with the LCA coursing posterior to the aorta (Ao) to its perfusion territories. LA, left atrium; LAD, left anterior descending artery; LCX, circumflex coronary artery; RCA, right coronary artery. Left panel with permission from: Bunce NH et al. Coronary artery anomalies: Assessment with free-breathing three-dimensional coronary MR angiography. Radiology 2003; 227: 201–8.

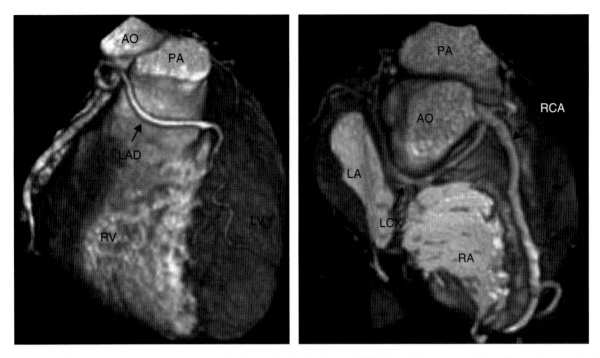

Figure 14.6   Single coronary artery originating from the right sinus of Valsalva. Volume rendering demonstrates the left anterior descending artery (LAD) coursing in front of the pulmonary artery (PA). The left circumflex coronary artery (LCX) courses behind the aorta. RV, right ventricle; LV, left ventricle; AO, aorta; LA, left atrium; RA, right atrium; RCA, right coronary artery. With permission from: Deibler AR et al. Imaging of congenital coronary anomalies with multislice computed tomography. Mayo Clinic Proceedings 2004; 79(80): 1017–23.

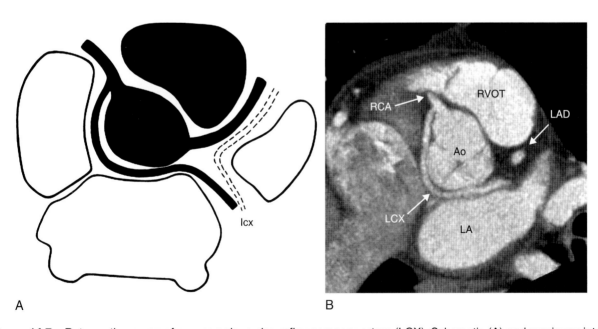

A   B

Figure 14.7   Retroaortic course of an anomalous circumflex coronary artery (LCX). Schematic (A) and maximum intensity projection image (B) oriented approximately in the horizontal plane demonstrate the circumflex coronary artery arising from the proximal portion of the right coronary artery (RCA), and coursing posterior to the aorta (Ao) to its perfusion territory. The left anterior descending artery (LAD) has a separate, normal origin in the left sinus of Valsalva. LA, left atrium; RVOT, right ventricular outflow tract. Left panel with permission from: Bunce NH et al. Coronary artery anomalies: Anomalies with free-breathing three-dimensional coronary MR angiography. Radiology 2003; 227: 201–8.

coronary artery, traveled a retroaortic path to their perfusion territory.

3.5 Left anterior descending artery arising from the right coronary sinus or right coronary artery

Eleven cases of the left anterior descending artery arising from the right coronary sinus have been reported on CT.[40–42,54,60,62] In a series of 3 patients, 1 patient demonstrated an interarterial course and 2 demonstrated a septal course.[60] In the other 8 cases, the artery took a prepulmonic course to the anterior wall of the left ventricle. One case has been reported in which the LAD was duplicated (the anomalous prepulmonic LAD coexisted with a diminutive native LAD arising from the LCA along with a robust ramus intermedius).[54]

3.6 Myocardial bridging

Intramyocardial course of the LAD is frequently seen on CT (Figure 14.8). In analysis of 118 consecutive patients, 30.5% had some degree of myocardial bridging.[64] In this study, 55% of the patients with muscular bridges had no evidence of coronary atherosclerosis, and only 22% had evidence of stenosis greater than 50%. Half of the patients referred were asymptomatic and scanned because of coronary risk factors; of the remainder, 27% had known coronary disease and 22% had chest pain and equivocal results on prior tests.

The first case report on CT described a patient with atypical chest pain who had this anomaly incidentally detected, and the patient was managed conservatively.[65] Another interesting case series described 3 patients who were imaged for atypical chest pain who demonstrated concomitant bridging in both the LAD and RCA territories.[66] It is likely that increasing use of CT and CMR for cardiac imaging will increase the number of patients found to have this typically benign condition.

3.7 Coronary artery anomalies with shunt physiology

A few case reports have described CT findings of anomalous termination of coronary arteries with shunt physiology.

In one series, 4 cases of fistulae connecting a coronary artery (2 LAD, 1 LCA, and 1 RCA) to a pulmonary artery and 1 fistula from the circumflex to the right atrium were all clearly defined.[42] Another report illustrated a patient with a suspected coronary artery fistula who declined conventional angiography. CT demonstrated a single coronary artery arising from the left coronary sinus. After giving off the LAD and circumflex arteries, the artery coursed caudad in the right atrioventricular groove and terminated in the basal surface of the right ventricle.[67] Although CT does not yet offer the opportunity to quantify flow and shunt physiology, as does angiography or CMR, CT may be a helpful investigative tool if, as in this case, angiography is contraindicated or declined by a patient.

There may also be a complementary role in characterizing the anatomy of certain cases Datta et al.[49] described a case of fistula between the circumflex artery and great cardiac vein in which the anatomy of the fistula was difficult to ascertain during angiography due to the high flow state. CT clearly identified the origin and termination of the fistula, as well as the tortuous vessels. CT can clearly demonstrate the relationship of the fistula to adjacent structures and may be used to demonstrate associated abnormalities not otherwise evident. Yoshimura et al.[68] described 2 cases of RCA-LV fistula, 1 case of RCA-RV fistula, and 1 case of LCA-RV fistula. In all cases the drainage pattern was clearly delineated, and in 1 case cine reconstructions demonstrated focal decrease in wall motion at the fistula drainage site in the RV.

Anomalous origin of the LCA from the pulmonary artery (Bland-White-Garland syndrome) is a rare coronary artery anomaly that usually presents with left-to-right shunt physiology. Eight cases of this anomaly have been described on CT.[68–72] Many of these patients become symptomatic during childhood, but incidental discovery in adults has been described. CT imaging of these anomalies can be quite striking, and demonstrates coronaries which are dilated and tortuous due to increased flow (Figure 14.9).

In all cases of cardiac anomalies with a potential for shunt physiology, careful attention should be paid to secondary signs of pulmonary hypertension and right heart strain, including morphologic enlargement of the right ventricle and right atrium, enlargement of the central pulmonary arteries, paradoxical bowing of the interventricular septum, and reflux of contrast into the inferior vena cava and hepatic veins. Such information can provide valuable clues to the physiologic significance of the anatomical findings.

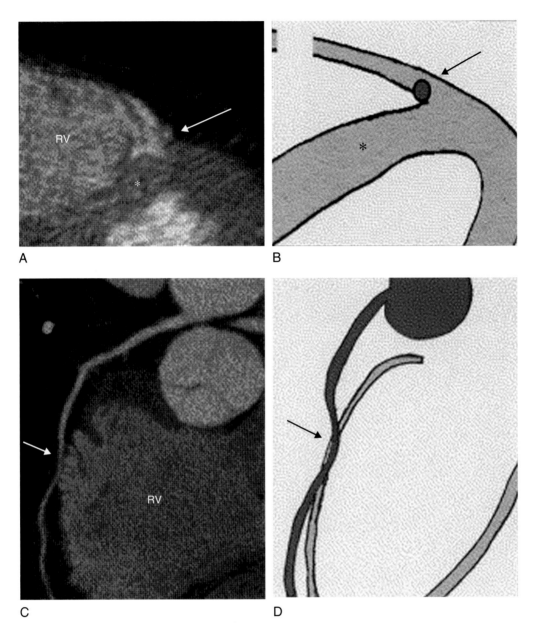

Figure 14.8 Myocardial bridge. Multiplanar reformations (A) and schematics (B). *Top panel,* an approximate short axis view shows an intramyocardial position of the left anterior descending artery (*arrow,* LAD) traveling deep into the anterior interventricular sulcus and disappearing into the right ventricular trabeculae. *Asterisk,* interventricular septum. A reformation which follows the course of the LAD (*bottom panel*) shows the short intramyocardial segment (arrow). RV, right ventricle. With permission from: Konen E et al. The prevalence and anatomical patterns of intramuscular coronary arteries: a coronary computed tomography angiographic study. Journal of the American College of Cardiology 2007; 49(5): 587–93.

3.8 CTA of acquired coronary anomalies

Coronary artery aneurysms are often characterized on CT as markedly dilated and tortuous vessels, which may have areas of luminal thrombus and/or calcification, as well as mural thickening. Aneurysms may be short, elongated, or even fusiform. Some authors have attributed high attenuation plaque (70–90 Hounsfield units) to mural fibrosis.[73]

Calcification may cause significant blooming artifact and limit evaluation of the vessel lumen. However, CT often can be useful in evaluating areas of stenosis, thrombosis, positive remodeling, and presence of developed collateral vessels. An example of a symptomatic coronary aneurysm of obscure etiology in a young woman is shown in Figure 14.10.

CT imaging of aneurysms associated with Kawasaki disease presents some unique challenges to CT, including small size of the coronary arteries, relatively high heart

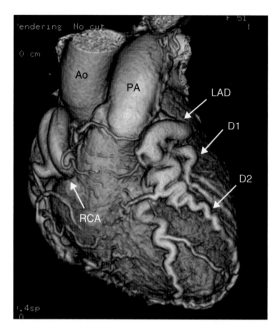

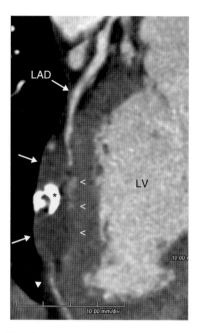

Figure 14.9   Anomalous left coronary artery arising from the pulmonary artery (PA), also known as Bland-White-Garland syndrome. The volume-rendered image demonstrates dilatation and tortuosity of the left anterior descending artery (LAD), first and second diagonal branches (D1, D2), and right coronary artery (RCA), along with extensive collateral vessel formation, indicative of shunt pathology. The anomalous origin of the left coronary artery is not well seen. Ao, aorta. Image courtesy of Dr. Eric E Williamson, Mayo Clinic, Rochester.

Figure 14.10   Coronary artery aneurysm (arrows) of the mid portion of the left anterior descending artery (LAD). Multiplanar reformation following the course of the LAD. The aneurysm is filled with thrombus. Partial calcification of the thrombus (asterisk) suggests chronicity. The LAD is occluded at the level of the aneurysm (open arrows) but the distal portion (arrowhead) is filled via ipsicollaterals. LV, left ventricle.

rates, reduced compliance with breath-holding in young children, and risks of radiation to a generally young patient population. However, in certain cases CT may provide a useful noninvasive adjunct to echocardiography, and diagnostic quality images have been obtained in patients as young as 7 years old.[74]

3.9 Associations of anomalous coronary arteries with other pathology

Attention to the origin of the coronary arteries during investigations performed for other indications may also provide useful information.[75] Anomalous origins of the right and circumflex coronary arteries have been noted in association with anomalies of the aortic root, and particularly bicuspid aortic valves; preoperative detection of such anatomy may help the surgeon to avoid injury to these vessels during cardiac surgery.[13,76–78] Case reports have described postoperative compression of anomalous arteries by bioprosthetic valve rings,[79–81] and preoperative awareness of coronary anomalies may help in surgical planning or postoperative evaluation.

4 POTENTIAL PITFALLS IN CT IMAGING OF CORONARY ANOMALIES

Caution must be used when interpreting scans not optimized for evaluation of the heart and coronary arteries (e.g., CT pulmonary angiography performed to evaluate for pulmonary emboli). Motion artifact on scans performed without ECG-gating can mimic anomalous coronary arteries with an interarterial course (Figure 14.11) in as many as 6–20% of patients, with some of this variation related to the number of detectors and the temporal resolution of the CT images.[82,83]

5 HOW AND WHEN TO MAKE THE DIAGNOSIS OF A CONGENITAL CORONARY ANOMALY

In addition to conventional angiography, other techniques, including echocardiography, intravascular ultrasound, and CMR, have been used to evaluate coronary artery

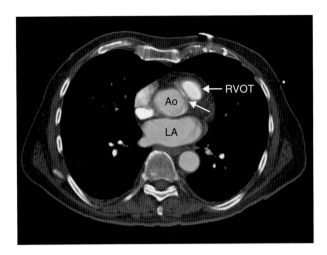

Figure 14.11 Motion artifact simulating an interarterial course of the right coronary artery (*arrow*). The transaxial source image from a nongated computed tomographic pulmonary angiogram study performed for chest pain in the emergency department shows a tubular opacity between the right ventricular outflow tract (RVOT) and the ascending aorta (Ao). The patient underwent further investigation with transesophageal echocardiography, which demonstrated normal origin of the coronary arteries. LA, left atrium.

anomalies.[84–87] CT has distinct advantages when compared with these techniques, including wide availability and the brief duration of the scan. Disadvantages include the need for iodinated contrast agents (with potential nephrotoxicity and allergic reactions) and the radiation dose. This last disadvantage, in particular, might lead the physician to consider CMR as the first-line noninvasive diagnostic tool in young patients in whom coronary or cardiac anomalies are suspected. Although CT often delineates the mid and distal segments of the coronary arteries more clearly than CMR, the important clinical consequences of most coronary artery anomalies result from abnormalities in the proximal course of the arterial stem and can be well characterized on CMR.

Given the exquisite anatomic detail that CT can quickly and noninvasively provide, the question arises when to initiate a CT workup for coronary artery anomalies. Although few clinical indications are defined, a multidisciplinary task force spearheaded by the American College of Cardiology Foundation considers CCTA appropriate for the investigation of known or suspected coronary anomalies.[35] CCTA is particularly useful if the proximal course is unclear, as in anomalies in which there is variability in course (e.g., origin of the LCA or LAD from the right coronary sinus), or in which the course is typically (but not always) malignant (e.g., RCA arising from the left coronary sinus).

The role of CT coronary angiography in noninvasively screening individuals is less clear. A trial of screening 3,650 young athletes (mean age 30) with transthoracic echocardiography revealed only 3 (0.09%) in whom anomalous coronary arteries were suspected and confirmed on selective angiography.[88] Such a low-yield rate suggests a need for criteria to identify asymptomatic individuals who should undergo further investigation, particularly when using a relatively costly technique with a high radiation dose. The American Heart Association has published a set of recommendations for pre-participation screening of high school and college athletes.[89] This list includes items from personal history, family history, and physical examination; it does not make recommendations regarding specific methods of investigation. It is important to remember that there can be substantial legal implications both for failing to identify individuals who may be at risk of sudden cardiac death on the one hand, and to groundlessly barring athletes from a fulfilling and potentially lucrative career on the other.[90]

Screening techniques are typically employed for diseases

1. which have significant morbidity and/or mortality
2. can be detected in the premorbid state, and
3. for which therapeutic intervention may prevent adverse events.

In addition, the benefits of the screening procedure should outweigh the risks, and the procedure should be sufficiently cost effective to justify screening of a defined population. Given the rarity of clinically significant anomalies, potential cost, and radiation dose, screening for coronary anomalies by CT appears unreasonable, especially in a population as poorly defined as "young athletes."

CT imaging, however, may be useful for confirming a diagnosis in selected symptomatic individuals with a high pre-test probability of a congenital coronary anomaly. Such individuals might include young athletes who experience otherwise unexplained anginal chest pain, syncope, or cardiac arrest during exercise, or individuals with a family history of sudden cardiac death.

Although the indications for the evaluation for congenital coronary anomalies will no doubt evolve, the availability of MDCT and its established utility for noninvasively detecting and characterizing such anomalies should make this an accepted first- or second-line method for the investigation of this rare but potentially lethal condition.

REFERENCES

1   Click RL, Holmes DR Jr, Vlietstra RE, Kosinski AS, Kronmal RA. Anomalous coronary arteries: location, degree of atherosclerosis and effect on survival – a report from the Coronary Artery Surgery Study. Journal of the American College of Cardiology 1989; 13: 531–7.

2. Yamanaka O, Hobbs RE. Coronary artery anomalies in 126,595 patients undergoing coronary arteriography. Catheterization and Cardiovascular Diagnosis 1990; 21: 28–40.

3. Alexander RW, Griffith GC. Anomalies of the coronary arteries and their clinical significance. Circulation 1956; 14: 800–5.

4. Lipsett J, Cohle SD, Berry PJ, Russell G, Byard RW. Anomalous coronary arteries: a multicenter pediatric autopsy study. Pediatric Pathology 1994; 14: 287–300.

5. Angelini P. Normal and anomalous coronary arteries: definitions and classification. American Heart Journal 1989; 117: 418–34.

6. Angelini P, Velasco JA, Flamm S. Coronary anomalies: incidence, pathophysiology, and clinical relevance. Circulation 2002; 105: 2449–54.

7. Corrado D, Thiene G, Cocco P et al. Nonatherosclerotic coronary artery disease and sudden death in the young. British Heart Journal 1992; 68: 601–7.

8. Basso C, Maron BJ, Corrado D, Thiene G. Clinical profile of congenital coronary artery anomalies with origin from the wrong aortic sinus leading to sudden death in young competitive athletes. Journal of the American College of Cardiology 2000; 35(6): 1493–501.

9. Angelini P. Coronary artery anomalies – current clinical issues. Texas Heart Institute Journal 2002; 29(4): 271–8.

10. Cheitlin MD, DeCastro CM, McAllister HA. Sudden death as a complication of anomalous left coronary origin from the anterior sinus of Valsalva: a not-so-minor congenital anomaly. Circulation 1974; 50: 780–7.

11. Roberts WC, Siegel RJ, Zipes DP. Origin of the right coronary artery from the left sinus of Valsalva and its functional consequences: analysis of 10 necropsy patients. American Journal of Cardiology 1982; 49: 863–8.

12. Virmani R, Chun PKC, Goldstein RE, Robinowitz M, McAllister HA. Acute takeoffs of the coronary arteries along the aortic wall and congenital coronary ostial valve-like ridges: association with sudden death. Journal of the American College of Cardiology 1984; 3(3): 766–71.

13. Kragel AH, Roberts WC. Anomalous origin of either the right or left main coronary artery from the aorta with subsequent coursing between aorta and pulmonary trunk: analysis of 32 necropsy cases. American Journal of Cardiology 1988; 62: 771–7.

14. Schiele TM, Weber C, Rieber J et al. Septal course of the left main coronary artery originating from the right sinus of Valsalva. Circulation 2002; 105(12): 1511–12.

15. Sato Y, Ichikawa M, Masubuchi M et al. MDCT of the anomalous origin of the right coronary artery from the left sinus of Valsalva as a single coronary artery. International Journal of Cardiology 2006; 109: 125–6.

16. Angelini P, Tivellato M, Donis J, Leachman RD. Myocardial bridges: a review. Progress in Cardiovascular Diseases 1983; 26: 75–88.

17. Juilliere Y, Berder V, Suty-Selton C et al. Isolated myocardial bridges with angiographic milking of the left anterior descending coronary artery: a long-term follow-up study. American Heart Journal 1995; 129: 663–5.

18. Kramer JR, Kitazume H, Proudfit WL, Sones, FM Jr. Clinical significance of isolated coronary bridges: benign and frequent condition involving the left anterior descending artery. American Heart Journal 1982; 103: 283–8.

19. Alegria JR, Herrmann J, Holmes DR, Lerman A, Rihal CS. Myocardial bridging. European Heart Journal 2005; 26: 1159–68.

20. Moehlenkamp S, Hort W, Ge J, Erbel R. Update on myocardial bridging. Circulation 2002; 106: 2616–22.

21. Yano K, Yoshino H, Taniuchi M et al. Myocardial bridging of the left anterior descending coronary artery in acute inferior wall myocardial infarction. Clinical Cardiology 2001; 24: 202–8.

22. Reul RM, Cooley DA, Hallman GL, Reul GJ. Surgical treatment of coronary artery anomalies: report of 37.5 year experience at the Texas Heart Institute. Texas Heart Institute Journal 29: 299–307.

23. Said SA, van der Werf T. Dutch survey of coronary artery fistulas in adults: congenital solitary fistulas. International Journal of Cardiology 2006; 106: 323–32.

24. Brueck M, Bandorski D, Vogt PR, Kramer W, Heidt MC. Myocardial ischemia due to an isolated coronary fistula. Clinical Research in Cardiology 2006; 95: 550–3.

25. Karagoz HY, Zorlutuna YI, Babacan KM et al. Congenital coronary artery fistulas: Diagnostic and surgical considerations. Japanese Heart Journal 1989; 30(5): 685–94.

26. Kamiya H, Yasuda T, Nagamine H et al. Surgical treatment of congenital coronary artery fistulas: 27 years experience and a review of the literature. Journal of Cardiac Surgery 2002; 17: 173–7.

27. Liberthson RR, Sagar K, Berkoben JP, Weintraub RM, Levine FH. Congenital Coronary Arteriovenous Fistula: Report of 13 patients, review of the literature, and delineation of management. Circulation 1979; 59(5): 849–54.

28. Gillebert C, Van Hoof R, Van De Werf F, Piessens J, De Geest H. Coronary artery fistulas in an adult population. European Heart Journal 1986; 7: 437–43.

29. Allen HD, Beekman RH, Garson A et al. Pediatric therapeutic cardiac catheterization: A statement for healthcare professionals from the council on cardiovascular disease in the young, American Heart Association. Circulation 1998; 97: 609–25.

30. Daoud A, Pankin D, Tulgan H, Florentin R. Aneurysms of the coronary artery. Report of ten cases and review of the literature. American Journal of Cardiology 1963; 11: 228–37.

31. Swaye PS, Fisher LD, Litwin P et al. Aneurysmal coronary artery disease. Circulation 1983; 67(1): 134–8.

32. Syed M, Lesch M. Coronary artery aneurysm: a review. Progress in Cardiovascular Diseases 1997; 40(1): 77–84.

33. Vitarelli A, De Curtis G, Conde Y et al. Assessment of congenital coronary artery fistulas by transesophageal color Doppler echocardiography. The American Journal of Medicine 2002; 113(2): 127–33.

34. Li D, Wu Q, Sun L et al. Surgical treatment of giant coronary artery aneurysm. Journal of Thoracic and Cardiovascular Surgery 2004; 130(3): 817–21.

35. Hendel RC, Patel MR, Kramer CM et al., American College of Cardiology Foundation Quality Strategic Directions Committee Appropriateness Criteria Working Group, American College of Radiology, Society of Cardiovascular Computed Tomography, Society for Cardiovascular Magnetic Resonance, American Society of Nuclear Cardiology, North American Society for Cardiac Imaging, Society for Cardiovascular Angiography and Interventions, Society of Interventional Radiology. ACCF/ACR/SCCT/SCMR/ASNC/NASCI/SCAI/SIR 2006 appropriateness criteria for cardiac computed tomography and cardiac magnetic resonance imaging: a report of the American College of Cardiology Foundation Quality Strategic Directions Committee Appropriateness Criteria Working Group, American College of Radiology, Society of Cardiovascular Computed Tomography, Society for Cardiovascular Magnetic Resonance, American Society of Nuclear Cardiology, North American Society for Cardiac Imaging, Society for Cardiovascular Angiography and Interventions, and Society of Interventional Radiology. Journal of the American College of Cardiology 2006; 48(7): 1475–97.

36. Schmitt R, Froehner S, Brunn J et al. Congenital anomalies of the coronary arteries: imaging with contrast-enhanced, multidetector computed tomography. European Radiology 2005; 15: 1110–21.

37. von Ooijen PMA, Dorgelo J, Zijlstra F, Oudkerk M. Detection, visualization and evaluation of anomalous coronary anatomy on 16-slice multidetector-row CT. European Radiology 2004; 14: 2163–71.

38. Shi H, Aschoff AJ, Brambs HJ, Hoffmann MHK. Multislice CT imaging of anomalous coronary arteries. European Radiology 2004; 14: 2172–81.

39. Deibler AR, Kuzo RS, Vöhringer M et al. Imaging of Congenital Coronary Anomalies With Multislice Computed Tomography. Mayo Clinic Proceedings 2004; 79(80): 1017–23.

40. Memisoglu E, Hobikoglu G, Tepe MS, Norgaz T, Bilsel T. Congenital coronary anomalies in adults: comparison of anatomic course visualization by catheter angiography and electron beam CT. Catheterization and Cardiovascular Interventions 2005; 66: 34–42.

41. Ropers D, Moshage W, Daniel WG et al. Visualization of coronary artery anomalies and their anatomic course by contrast-enhanced electron beam tomography and three-dimensional reconstruction. American Journal of Cardiology 2001; 87: 193–7.

42. Schmid M, Achenbach S, Ludwig J et al. Visualization of coronary artery anomalies by contrast-enhanced multi-detector row spiral computed tomography. International Journal of Cardiology 2006; 111: 430–5.

43. Coles DR, Wilde P, Baumbach A. An anomalous right coronary artery shown by multislice CT coronary angiography. BMJ Heart 2004; 90(10): 1188.

44. Ghersin E, Litmanovich D, Ofer A et al. Anomalous origin of right coronary artery: diagnosis and dynamic evaluation with multidetector computed tomography. Journal of Computer Assisted Tomography 2004; 23(2): 293–4.

45. Dirksen M, Bax J, Blom N et al. Detection of malignant right coronary artery anomaly by multi-slice CT coronary angiography. European Radiology 2002; 12(3): S177–80.

46. Mousseaux E, Hernigou A, Sapoval M et al. Coronary arteries arising from the contralateral aortic sinus: Electron beam computed tomographic demonstration of the initial course of the artery with respect to the aorta and the right ventricular outflow tract. Journal of Thoracic and Cardiovascular Surgery 1996; 112(3): 836–40.

47. Kim CK, Park CB, Jin U, Lee BY, Son KS. Evaluation of unroofing procedure of anomalous origin of right coronary artery from left coronary sinus between aorta and pulmonary trunk by multidetector computed tomography. Journal of Computer Assisted Tomography 2005; 29(6): 752–5.

48. Gilkeson RC, Markowitz A, Sachs P. Evaluation of the cardiac surgery patient with MSCT. Journal of Thoracic Imaging 2005; 20(4): 265–72.

49. Datta J, White CS, Gilkeson RC et al. Anomalous coronary arteries in adults: depiction at multi-detector row CT angiography. Radiology 2005; 235(3): 812–18.

50. Khouzam R, Marshall T, Lowell D, Siler JR. Left coronary artery originating from right coronary sinus with diagnosis confirmed by CT. Angiology 2003; 54: 499–502.

51. Ichikawa M, Komatsu S, Asanuma H et al. Acute myocardial infarction caused by "malignant" anomalous right coronary artery detected by multidetector row computed tomography. Circulation Journal 2005; 69: 1564–7.

52. Gulati GS, Singh C, Kothari SS, Sharma S. An unusual coronary artery anomaly in tetralogy of Fallot shown on MDCT. American Journal of Roentgenology 2006; 186(4): 1192–3.

53. Berbarie RF, Dockery WD, Johnson KB et al. Use of multi-slice computed tomographic coronary angiography for the diagnosis of anomalous coronary arteries. American Journal of Cardiology 2006; 98(3): 402–6.

54. Duran C, Kantarci M, Subasi ID et al. Remarkable anatomic anomalies of coronary arteries and their clinical importance: A multidetector computed tomography angiographic study. Journal of Computer Assisted Tomography 2006; 30(6): 939–48.

55. Ghersin E, Litmanovich D, Ofer A et al. Anomalous origin of right coronary artery: Diagnosis and dynamic evaluation with multidetector computed tomography. Journal of Computer Assisted Tomography 2004; 28(2): 293–4.

56. Hong C, Woodard PK, Bae KT. Congenital coronary artery anomaly demonstrated by three dimensional 16 slice spiral CT angiography. BMJ Heart 2004; 90(5): 478.

57. Ropers D, Gehling G, Pohle K et al. Anomalous course of the left main or left anterior descending coronary artery originating from the right sinus of valsalva. Circulation 2002; 105: e42–e43.

58. Sapoval MR, Mosseaux E, Desnos M. Anomalous origin of the left coronary artery from the right coronary sinus diagnosed by electron beam computerized tomography. Circulation 1995; 91(7): 2093.

59. Sevrukov A, Aker N, Sullivan C, Jelnin V, Candipan RC. Identifying the course of an anomalous left coronary artery using contrast-enhanced electron beam tomography and three-dimensional reconstruction. Catheterization and Cardiovascular Interventions 2002; 57: 532–6.

60. Karadag B, Spieker LE, Wildermuth S, Boehm T, Corti R. Cardiac arrest in a soccer player: a unique case of anomalous coronary origin detected by 16-row multislice computed tomography coronary angiography. Heart and Vessels 2005; 20: 116–19.

61. Gerber TC, Kuzo RS, Safford RE. Computed tomographic imaging of anomalous coronary arteries. Circulation 2002; 106(15): e67.

62. Gaudio C, Nguyen BL, Tanzilli G, Mirabelli F, Catalano C. Anomalous "benign" coronary arteries detected by multidetector computed tomography. International Journal of Cardiology 2006; 109: 417–19.

63. Weininger M, Beer M, Hahn D, Beissert M. Images in cardiology: Multislice cardiac computed tomographic images of anomalous origin of the left circumflex artery from the right coronary sinus. Heart 2006; 92(11): 1634.

64. Konen E, Goitein O, Sternik L et al. The prevalence and anatomical patterns of intramuscular coronary arteries: A coronary computed tomography angiographic study. Journal of the American College of Cardiology 2007; 49(5): 587–93.

65. Goitein O, Lacomis JM. Myocardial bridging: noninvasive diagnosis with multidetector CT. Journal of Computer Assisted Tomography 2005; 29(2): 238–40.

66. Rychter K, Salanitri J, Edelman RR. Multifocal coronary artery myocardial bridging involving the right coronary and left anterior descending arteries detected by ECG-gated 64 slice multidetector CT coronary angiography. The International Journal of Cardiovascular Imaging 2006; 22(5): 713–7.

67. Soon KH, Selvanayagam J, Bell KW et al. Giant single coronary system with coronary cameral fistula diagnosed on MSCT. International Journal of Cardiology 2006; 106: 276–8.

68. Yoshimura N, Hamada S, Takamiya M, Kuribayashi S, Kimura K. Coronary artery anomalies with a shunt: evaluation with electron-beam CT. Journal of Computer Assisted Tomography 1998; 22(5): 682–6.

69. Mesurolle B, Qanadli SD, Merad M et al. Anomalous origin of the left coronary artery arising from the pulmonary trunk: report of an adult case with long-term follow-up after surgery. European Radiology 1999; 9: 1570–3.

70. Khanna A, Torigian DA, Ferrari VA, Bross RJ, Rosen MA. Anomalous origin of the left coronary artery from the pulmonary artery in adulthood on CT and MRI. American Journal of Roentgenology 2005; 185: 326–9.

71. Girish R. Images in cardiology. Multislice cardiac computed tomographic images of anomalous origin of the left coronary artery from the pulmonary artery (ALCAPA). Heart 2006; 92(1): 2.

72. Coche E, Muller P, Gerber B. Images in cardiology: Anomalous origin of the left main coronary artery from the main pulmonary artery illustrated before and after surgical correction on ECG-gated 40-slice computed tomography. Heart 2006; 92(9): 1193.

73. Renzulli, M, Piovaccari, G, Fattori, R. Potential of multislice CT in the follow-up of Kawasaki coronary disease. European Heart Journal 2006; 27(20): 2384.

74. Chu WCW, Mok GCF, Lam WWM, Yam M, Sung RYT. Assessment of coronary artery aneurysms in paediatric patients with Kawasaki disease by multidetector row CT angiography: feasibility and comparison with 2D echocardiography. Pediatric Radiology 2006; 36(11): 1148–53.

75. Uppot RN, Dam A, Wills JS, Blackwell RA, Boyle K. Evaluation of anomalous coronary artery anatomy using multi-detector CT. Delaware Medical Journal 2004; 76(4): 165–8.

76. Doty DB. Anomalous origin of the left circumflex coronary artery associated with a bicuspid aortic valve. Journal of Thoracic and Cardiovascular Surgery 2001; 122: 842–3.

77. Palamo AR, Schrager BR, Chahine RA. Anomalous origin of the right coronary artery from the ascending aorta high above the left posterior coronary sinus of a bicuspid aortic valve. American Heart Journal 1995; 109: 902–4.

78. Gaudino M, Glieca F, Bruno P et al. Unusual right coronary artery anomaly with major implication during cardiac operations. Annals of Thoracic Surgery 1997; 64(3): 838–9.

79. Roberts WC, Marrow AG. Compression of anomalous left circumflex coronary arteries by prosthetic valve fixation rings. Journal of Thoracic and Cardiovascular Surgery 1969; 57: 834–8.

80. Roberts WC, Sullivan MF. Clinical and necropsy observations early after simultaneous replacement of the mitral and aortic valves. American Journal of Cardiology 1986; 58: 1067–84.

81. de Marchena EJ, Russo CD, Wozniak PM, Kessler KM. Compression of an anomalous left circumflex coronary artery by a bioprosthetic valve ring. Journal of Cardiovascular Surgery 1990; 31: 52–4.

82. Katoh M, Wildberger JE, Guenther RW, Buecker A. Malignant right coronary artery anomaly simulated by motion artifacts on MDCT. AJR American Journal of Roentgenology 2005; 185: 1007–10.

83. Barriales-Villa R, Moris C. Usefulness of helical computed tomography in the identification of the initial course of coronary anomalies. American Journal of Cardiology 2001; 88: 719.

84. Fernandes F, Alam M, Smith S, Khaja F. The role of transesophageal echocardiography in identifying anomalous coronary arteries. Circulation 1993; 88: 2532–40.

85. Nanda NC, Bhambore MM, Jindal A et al. Transesophageal three-dimensional echocardiographic assessment of anomalous coronary arteries. Echocardiography 2000; 17: 53–60.

86. Post JC, van Rossum AC, Bronzwaer JC et al. Magnetic resonance angiography of anomalous coronary arteries: a new gold standard for delineating the proximal course? Circulation 1995; 92: 3163–71.

87. Bunce NH, Lorenz CH, Keegan J et al. Coronary artery anomalies: assessment with free-breathing three-dimensional coronary MR angiography. Radiology 2003; 227: 201–8.

88. Zeppili P, dello Russo A, Santini C et al. In vivo detection of coronary artery anomalies in asymptomatic athletes by echocardiographic screening. Chest 1998; 114: 89–93.

89. Maron BJ, Thompson PD, Puffer JC et al. Cardiovascular preparticipation screening of competitive athletes: a statement for health professionals from the Sudden Death Committee (clinical cardiology) and Congenital Cardiac Defects Committee (cardiovascular disease in the young), American Heart Association. AHA medical/scientific statement. Circulation 1996; 94: 850–6.

90. Paterick TE, Paterick TJ, Fletcher GF, Maron BJ. Medical and legal issues in the cardiovascular evaluation of competitive athletes. JAMA 2005; 294(23): 3011–18.

15

Noninvasive Evaluation of Coronary Artery Bypass Grafts with Multislice Computed Tomography

Christof Burgstahler, Anja Reimann, Harald Brodoefel, Martin Heuschmid, Andreas F. Kopp, and Stephen Schroeder

1 INTRODUCTION

Coronary artery bypass graft (CABG) surgery is usually performed in patients with advanced coronary artery disease (CAD). Recurrence of angina pectoris in these patients is a common problem, and early graft occlusion is described in up to 23% of all patients,[1] with a large number of patients developing angina pectoris within the initial three months. Surgical revascularization is done usually with either arterial or venous grafts or the combination of both. Arterial grafts (left or right internal mammarian artery or free arterial grafts) are preferable as they have a higher graft patency rate than venous grafts in short- and mid-time follow-up.[2] Five years after coronary artery bypass surgery approximately 90% of arterial grafts are patent, in contrast to 80% of venous grafts. The gold standard for direct visualization of coronary artery vessels is invasive X-ray coronary angiography. However, due to its invasive character and possible complications, there is a need for non-invasive tools to assess coronary artery bypass vessels.

Former CT scanners were not able to provide sufficient spatial and temporal resolution to visualize coronary arteries and coronary bypass grafts. Since 1999, multislice computed tomography (MSCT) scanners are available, allowing the visualization and assessment of coronary arteries with good overall image quality.

2 TECHNICAL REQUIREMENTS

Noninvasive imaging of coronary vessels is complicated by several factors. First, coronary vessels are characterized by a rapid and complex motion during the heart cycle. Depending on the coronary artery, velocity ranges between 20 mm/sec and 110 mm/sec, with the highest velocity for the right coronary artery.[3] Thus, high temporal resolution is essential for coronary imaging. Second, the coronary arteries are small structures with an average diameter of approximately 4–5 mm of the proximal parts,[4] thus demanding a high spatial resolution.

The first CT scanners to provide high spatial resolution were electron beam computed tomography scanners, enabling the physician to image the heart and the coronary arteries noninvasively. In 1999, with the introduction of MSCT scanners with 4 slices and a gantry rotation time of 500 ms, a second type of CT scanner was available for noninvasive cardiac imaging. Over the last several years, EBCT has become less important due to the rapid technical improvement of MSCT and the relatively low spatial resolution of EBCT. Today, noninvasive coronary imaging is the domain of multislice computed tomography.

3 BYPASS IMAGING WITH EBCT

Electron beam computed tomography is a cross-sectional imaging method originally designed to detect and quantify coronary calcifications. In contrast to multislice computed tomography, which is characterized by the rotation of the X-ray tube, EBCT is a stationary gun running at a constant tube current of 625 mAs and a tube voltage of 130 kV. The generated electron beam is deflected and focused on one of several target rings, then reflected towards one of two detector rings located on the opposite site. Due to the constant tube current an individual dose adaptation (e.g., in obese patients) is not possible. This might hamper the diagnostic accuracy of EBCT due to a reduction of image quality. While coronary calcium scoring is performed on native scans, the application of contrast media is necessary to visualize coronary arteries and coronary bypass grafts in both modalities, EBCT and MSCT.

3.1 Detection of coronary bypass graft occlusion and stenosis with EBCT

In 1997, Achenbach[5] published a study evaluating 56 bypass grafts by EBCT. The results were compared to invasive angiography. Two bypass grafts were not assessable by EBCT. Of the remaining 54 bypass graft vessels 13 grafts were occluded and all of them were correctly classified by EBCT (sensitivity and specificity 100%). In 36 of 43 patent grafts the evaluation of hemodynamically relevant stenosis was possible (sensitivity, 100%; specificity, 97%).[5] Besides breathing artifacts, the misplacement of the imaging volume was the main reason for non-diagnostic images.

4 CORONARY ARTERY BYPASS GRAFTS VISUALIZATION WITH MSCT

The assessment of coronary artery bypass graft patency using computed tomography was already described in 1981 with a single row scanner.[6] Even with this timeworn

scanner type graft patency was assessable correctly in 79 of 100 grafts.

Today multi-slice computer tomography scanners with at least 16 to 64 rows are used in clinical routine. Dedicated algorithms for postprocessing the acquired raw data (multi-planar reformation, maximum intensity projection, 3-dimensonal volume rendering) have been developed to ease the evaluation coronary arteries and coronary bypass grafts (Figures 15.1 and 15.2).

Non invasive imaging of coronary artery bypass grafts by modern MSCT scanners enables graft patency and stenosis to be detected with high sensitivity and specificity. Four-row scanners already detect or rule out the obstruction of grafts with high overall accuracy. In a pilot study, we evaluated 14 venous and 7 arterial grafts with MSCT in comparison to invasive angiography. The sensitivity and specificity for the detection of graft stenosis was 86% and 100%, respectively. However, 2 of 21 grafts could not be evaluated by MSCT.[7] Ropers et al.[8] reported on a series of 65 patients, in which MSCT showed a sensitivity of 97% and a specificity of 98% for detection of graft obstruction. These promising results were demonstrated by the success of visualization in larger vessels, and by the low number of calcifications in coronary artery bypass grafts. The initial data were

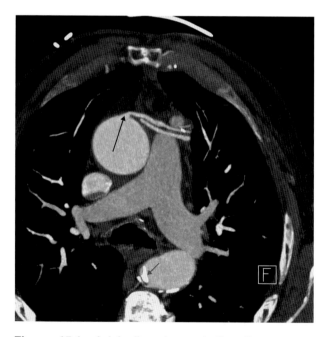

Figure 15.1 Axial slice demonstrating the contrast-enhanced ascending aorta and two venous bypass grafts (origin of one bypass marked with the arrow). This image might be used for diagnostic purposes and represent the basis for further views generated by special post processing software tools. The calcification of the descending aorta (gray arrow) is an additional finding.

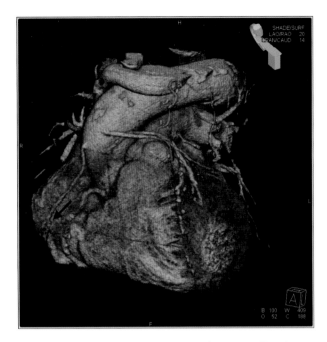

Figure 15.2 Three-dimensional volume rending image generated from the axial slice stack (same patient as in Figure 15.1). The two venous grafts to the first diagonal branch and the right circumflex artery have their origin distally from the venous bypass graft to the right coronary artery. Stepladder artifact leads to a mismatch of the vertical part of the right coronary artery and the bypass graft (arrow) to the right coronary artery.

confirmed in future studies with 16-slice scanners in larger patient cohorts. Besides graft patency, improvement of the spatial and temporal resolution allowed evaluation of large lesions in arterial or venous bypass grafts. Martuscelli et al.[9] enrolled 93 patients with previous coronary artery bypass graft surgery in their study. In contrast to the above mentioned studies, lesions of more than 50% diameter stenosis were

included in the analysis. A total of 285 grafts were evaluated and in 84 of 93 patients all grafts were of diagnostic image quality. Among these 84 patients, MSCT correctly diagnosed 54 occluded grafts and 4 significant stenoses within the bypass body and 15 of 17 significant lesions of the anastomotic region were correctly diagnosed. For the 84 patients, diagnostic accuracy of MSCT was 99%, sensitivity was 97%, and specificity was 100%. When all 93 patients originally enrolled in the study were considered, the sensitivity of MSCT in diagnosing significant stenoses was 96%. Comparable results were published by Schlosser et al.[10] with a sensitivity of 96%, a specificity of 95%, a positive predictive value of 81%, and a negative predictive value of 99% for bypass stenosis/occlusion.

The latest data for the noninvasive assessment of coronary bypass grafts with 64-slice scanners were published in 2006.[11] Malagutti et al.[11] performed 64-slice MSCT in 52 symptomatic patients 10 ± 5 years after bypass surgery and compared the results to invasive angiography. One hundred and nine grafts were analyzed. The per-segment detection of graft disease yielded a sensitivity of 99% (71/72) and a specificity of 96% (106/110). These results confirmed a outperformed data from Pache et al.[12] using the same scanner generation (sensitivity of 97.8%, a specificity of 89.3%, a positive predictive value of 90%, and a negative predictive value of 97.7% in 96 bypass grafts / 31 patients).

In summary, there is good evidence that the noninvasive detection of coronary bypass graft occlusion is possible, even with former CT generations with an overall high accuracy. Sixteen or 64-slice scanners are able to evaluate bypass grafts and bypass stenosis in a larger cohort of patients.

Table 15.1 summarizes some of the recent literature concerning bypass graft visualization with MDCT.

Table 15.1 Diagnostic accuracy of MDCT to detect bypass occlusion or bypass stenosis

Author/rows	Patients/grafts	Assessibility	Sensitivity%	Specificity%	PPV%	NPV%
Burgstahler[7] 4-slice	10/21	86% grafts	86	100	75	86
Ropers[8] 4-slice	65/182	77% grafts	97	98	97	98
Burgstahler[13] 16-slice	13/43	95% grafts	100	93	89	100
Martuscelli[9] 16-slice	96/285	84/96 patients	97	100		
Schlosser[10] 16-slice	51/131	48/51 patients	96 100*	95 100*	83	99
Pache[12] 64-slice	31/96	94% (distal anastomosis)	98	89	90	98
Malagutti[11] 64-slice	52/109	100%	100	98	98	100

*Bypass occlusion. NPV, negative predictive value; PPV, positive predictive value.

4.1 Evaluation of native coronary arteries in patients with history of coronary artery bypass grafts

Despite the fact that coronary artery bypass grafts are quite easily assessed by MSCT, the evaluation of native coronary arteries remains a problem in patients who have previously undergone bypass surgery because of severe calcifications in diffusely diseased coronary arteries. The impact of severe calcifications on image quality and diagnostic accuracy has been reported in several studies.[14,15] Highly calcified lesions hamper to differentiate between a high-grade stenosis and the sole presence of nonobstructive calcified plaque.

Data about the diagnostic accuracy of MDCT for native vessels in patients with coronary artery bypass are rare. Own data, generated with a 16-slice scanner, revealed a sensitivity of 83% and a specificity of 59% for the presence of a relevant stenosis (diameter reduction of at least 50%, positive predictive value of 78%, negative predictive value of 67%)[13] which is much lower than in patients without coronary bypass graft in their history. Malagutti et al.[11] evaluated native vessels as well as the distal run-off in their bypass study. With 64-slice computed tomography the sensitivity and specificity in non-grafted vessels was high (97% and 86%, respectively) but the results for the evaluation of the distal run-off was lower (sensitivity and specificity to detect run-off disease 89% and 93%, positive predictive value 50%).

This remains one of the main limitations of non-invasive imaging with MDCT in patients with coronary artery bypass grafts, as the treatment and the proceeding depends on clinical presentation of the patient, graft status and status of the native vessels, and the verification of a myocardial ischemia.

4.2 Multislice computed tomography in comparison to invasive angiography

Although invasive angiography is still the gold standard for the assessment of coronary artery bypass grafts, multislice computed tomography is superior in some regards. First, the origin of coronary bypass grafts can easily be visualized by MSCT. In clinical routine, some bypass grafts are difficult to intubate or localize with standard catheters. Even with special catheters, some grafts cannot be visualized selectively. This is associated with an increase of procedural

costs, radiation exposure, and contrast media application. In that case, pre-invasive MSCT angiography might help to localize the bypass graft vessels. Second, radiation and contrast media exposure is almost similar in patients with or without coronary artery bypass grafts applying MSCT. Finally, MSCT reveals information on vessel wall morphology, and the morphology of a lesion (extent of calcification, diameter of the vessel). This might be helpful to plan an intervention in bypass grafts.

4.3 Radiation exposure

Noninvasive coronary imaging with multislice computed tomography is associated with considerable exposure to radiation. For noninvasive imaging of coronary arteries, radiation values of 6.4 ± 1.9 and 11.0 ± 4.1 mSv for 16- and 64-slice scanners are reported. The radiation exposure can be markedly reduced, if ECG-gated tube current modulation – i.e. prospective reduction of the tube current during systole – and a tube voltage of 100 kV, instead of 120 kV, is applied. These steps may reduce radiation exposure at 57 to 64%.[16]

Although larger data about radiation exposure and its impact on image quality in bypass grafts are missing, at least ECG-gated tube current modulation should be applied in all patients.

In contrast to patients without coronary bypass grafts the field of view has to be increased in some cases for bypass imaging, especially to visualize the proximal part of the left or right internal mammarian artery. The majority of patients with LIMA graft dysfunction have stenosis at the site of insertion of the native coronary.[17] Lesions of the proximal part of the vessel might appear soon after surgery caused by kinking of the left internal mammarian artery during surgical mobilization[18] or by a surgical clip.[19] However, as stenosis or occlusion of the proximal part is quite rare, it has to be decided in each individual case whether the scan range has to be extended to the subclavian artery.

4.4 Contrast media

Assessment of coronary arteries and coronary artery bypass grafts with multislice computed tomography is only possible by applying contrast media. Thus, contraindications to coronary CTA might be known allergic reaction to contrast media, renal failure and hyperthyroidism.

4.5 Impact of heart rate and heart rhythm

Elevated heart rates have shown to reduce image quality due to motion artifacts.[20,21] Thus, elevated heart rates prior to the scan are lowered by administration of beta-blockers, which might be given orally (e.g., 50 to 100 mg metoprolol po. 30 minutes prior to the CT scan) or intravenously. For 16- and 64-slice scanners heart rates of approximately 60 beats per minutes are preferable.[22]

With dual source computed tomography, which has been available since 2006, diagnostic image quality can be achieved even with elevated heart rates.[23] At present it remains unclear whether beta-blockers are mandatory if the patient is examined by dual-source CT.

For bypass imaging, heart rate is not that important than for visualization of the native arteries, as bypass grafts do not move much during the heart cycle. Therefore, efforts for special imaging protocols are in progress. Theoretically, untriggered images of the proximal part of the coronary bypass graft arteries might be sufficient to diagnose by pass occlusion or stenosis. This would lead to a significant reduction of radiation exposure. However, by origin of the native coronaries, ECG-triggered image acquisition is absolutely mandatory. Currently there is no commercial scan protocol combining both acquisition modes in one examination.

Most studies comparing invasive angiography with cardiac multi-slice computed tomography excluded patients with irregular heart rates from analysis. For excellent image quality a stable sinus rhythm is one precondition. Although there are reports that a dedicated postprocessing algorithm improves image quality in patients with nonsinus rhythm or atrial fibrillation,[24,25] the diagnostic accuracy in patients with irregular heart rhythms is unforeseeable and moderate in most cases.

4.6 Idiosyncrasy of bypass imaging

In contrast to native coronary arteries, bypass grafts are characterized by a larger vessel diameter and less motion during the heart cycle, facilitating visualization by multi-slice computed tomography. On the other hand, bypass imaging is complicated by several aspects.

Surgical clips may influence image quality in the adjacent bypass graft segment. This has no impact in the diagnosis of a bypass graft occlusion which can normally still be easily diagnosed. However, artifacts caused by clips may

pretend or mask the presence of a stenosis (e.g., by beam hardening).

The trickiest part of the bypass graft to evaluate is the insertion into the native vessel. On the one hand, there is a discrepancy of the gauge between the bypass graft vessel and native vessel in most cases. On the other hand, the ankle between the graft and the coronary artery causes some kind of banding, complicating the assessment of the insertion. Adjacent metal clips sometimes inhibit the evaluation of the insertion.[12] Figure 15.3 demonstrates an insertion of a graft without stenosis.

4.6.1 Difference between venous and arterial bypass grafts

Although arterial grafts have a smaller diameter than venous grafts, the sensitivity and specificity for the detection of significant stenosis in both types of bypass grafts do not differ significantly, at least if the images are acquired by 64-slice computed tomography. Malagutti et al.[11] reported a 100% sensitivity and specificity for arterial grafts (100% and 96% for venous grafts), whereas Pache et al.[12] described the sensitivity and specificity for venous bypass grafts (98% and 97%) to be better than for arterial grafts (83% and 75% with three false positive results due to metal clip artifacts).

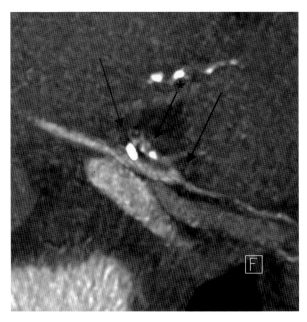

Figure 15.3 Insertion of venous bypass graft. Small diameter of the native vessel with coronary calcifications (*) proximal to the bypass graft insertion. The dark arrow marks the insertion, the gray arrow indicates a clip.

5. PRACTICAL MANAGEMENT: HOW TO PERFORM NONINVASIVE BYPASS IMAGING WITH MULTISLICE CT

The CT scanning of patients with coronary bypass grafts is comparable to the imaging technique for patients without prior heart surgery. A careful preparation and instruction of the patient is demandable for accurate image quality and diagnostic performance. Blood testing to exclude hyperthyroidism and renal failure is necessary to avoid severe complications of the contrast media administration. Moreover, the patient should be asked whether they had any prior allergic reaction to contrast media.

To reduce motion artefacts caused by elevated heart rate[20,21] β-blockade (e.g., with 50–100 mg metoprolol po) should be performed within 30 minutes prior to the CT scan. Sometimes additional intravenous administration of a beta-blocker is necessary to achieve a heart rate of less than 65 bpm. Although dual-source CT has shown to be able to visualize coronary arteries with good image quality even in patients with higher heart rates, the administration of beta-blockers should be taken into account for bypass imaging. Patients with a history of bypass grafts have advanced coronary artery disease with prior myocardial infarctions and a high probability of heart beat irregularities that might be at least partially suppressed by beta-blockers.

5.1 CT scanning

The patient has to be placed comfortably on the examination table. An 18-gauge catheter should be placed into an antecubital vein to inject the contrast medium. During the scan, the arms of the patient have to be placed overhead. Moreover, the patient has to be carefully instructed on how to perform the breath hold. ECG electrodes are placed on the thorax and the ECG signal has to be checked carefully (no artifacts). Cables of the ECG should not intersect.

For planning of the contrast enhanced scan, a low dose of radiation topogram is acquired. The field of view for the contrast enhanced scan is adjusted for each patient (depending whether the proximal part of the left internal mammarian artery should be scanned). A test bolus of 20 mL of contrast medium and a chaser bolus of 20 mL of physiological saline solution is injected through an 18-gauge catheter into an antecubital vein to determine the circulation time.

For the coronary angiography a total of 60 to 80 mL of contrast media is injected through the catheter, and the scan starts with the delay of the circulation time. Immediately before the start of the scan, the patient is asked to breath in and hold their breath until the scan is finished (depending on the type of scanner, approximately 10–15 seconds). A total of 150 to 250 axial slices are acquired (raw data). Image reconstruction is normally performed in the diastolic phase, with a relative retrospective gating of 60% for all coronary arteries in a first step.[15] In case of impaired image quality additional image reconstruction has to be performed at different RR intervals after a test series. For further postprocessing, the data are transferred to a work station. The analyses are done interpreting axial slices (origin of the bypass grafts from the ascending aorta, probably button like shaped in case of a proximal occlusion), 3-dimensional volume rendering images (helps to locate the vessels that are connected to the bypass grafts) and maximal intensity protection (MIP) with different slice thickness and multiplanar reformation images (MPR). In case of impaired image quality, additional reconstructions at different RR-intervals and/or different kernels may help to reassess the anatomy of the lesion. In the case of a total occlusion of a bypass graft, remaining metal clips indicate the previous course of the vessel. Indirect signs indicating the patency of a graft are likely clear contrast enhancement of the distal run off and/or better contrast enhancement of the native vessel distal to the insertion than

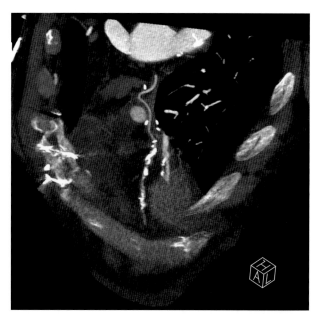

Figure 15.4 Curved multiplanar reformation (curved MPR) of a left internal mammarian artery bypass graft to the left anterior descending artery (LAD). The native vessel is severely calcified.

proximal of the insertion. However, the distinction between retrograde or antegrade filling via collaterals is not possible.

5.2 Patient preparation and CT scanning

1. Patient history
   - prior infarctions? number of bypass grafts? surgery records available? angina pectoris?
   - contraindications for contrast media (allergy? hyperthyroidism? renal failure?)
   - instruction of the patient (breath hold)
2. Physical examination (blood pressure, heart rate)
   - lowering of the heart rate with beta-blockers (contraindications?) if necessary
   - application of nitroglycerin possible?
   - irregular heart beat (impaired image quality)
3. Positioning of the patient on the table
   - application of the ECG (correct contact of the electrodes, no intersection of the cables)
   - iv catheter (antecubital) and connection to the contrast medium
   - placement of the arms overhead
   - nitroglycerin (optional)
4. CT scanning
   - topogram and adjustment of the field of view
   - determination of the circulation time (test bolus)
   - application of the contrast medium
   - breath hold-start of the scan
5. Postprocessing
   - diastolic reconstruction (60% of the RR interval, additional reconstructions if necessary)
   - transfer of the raw data to the work station
   - image interpretation using axial slices, 3-dimensional images, MIP and MPR
   - storage of the raw data and/or the reconstructed images
   - report of the findings

6 CONCLUSION

Although there are some limitations, noninvasive bypass imaging by MSCT is safe and provides additional information, especially about graft wall morphology. Invasive angiography is associated with the risk of possible graft dissection from direct cannulation and contrast injection. Thus, MSCT might be useful, particularly in patients in whom early graft occlusion is suspected or in patients for whom the history of bypass grafts is unavailable.

REFERENCES

1. Rifon J, Paramo JA, Panizo C et al. The increase of plasminogen activator inhibitor activity is associated with graft occlusion in patients undergoing aorto-coronary bypass surgery. Br J Haematol 1997; 99: 262–7.
2. Cho KR, Kim JS, Choi JS et al. Serial angiographic follow-up of grafts one year and five years after coronary artery bypass surgery. Eur J Cardiothorac Surg 2006; 29: 511–16.
3. Mao S, Lu B, Oudiz RJ et al. Coronary artery motion in electron beam tomography. J Comput Assist Tomogr 2000; 24: 253–8.
4. Dodge JT Jr., Brown BG, Bolson EL et al. Lumen diameter of normal human coronary arteries. Influence of age, sex, anatomic variation, and left ventricular hypertrophy or dilation. Circulation 1992; 86: 232–46.
5. Achenbach S, Moshage W, Ropers D et al. Noninvasive, three-dimensional visualization of coronary artery bypass grafts by electron beam tomography. Am J Cardiol 1997; 79: 856–61.
6. Kahl FR, Wolfman NT, Watts LE. Evaluation of aortocoronary bypass graft status by computed tomography. Am J Cardiol 1981; 48: 304–10.
7. Burgstahler C, Kuettner A, Kopp AF et al. Non-invasive evaluation of coronary artery bypass grafts using multi-slice computed tomography: initial clinical experience. Int J Cardiol 2003; 90: 275–80.
8. Ropers D, Ulzheimer S, Wenkel E et al. Investigation of aortocoronary artery bypass grafts by multislice spiral computed tomography with electrocardiographic-gated image reconstruction. Am J Cardiol 2001; 88: 792–5.
9. Martuscelli E, Romagnoli A, D'Eliseo A et al. Evaluation of venous and arterial conduit patency by 16-slice spiral computed tomography. Circulation 2004; 110: 3234–8.
10. Schlosser T, Konorza T, Hunold P et al. Noninvasive visualization of coronary artery bypass grafts using 16-detector row computed tomography. J Am Coll Cardiol 2004; 44: 1224–9.
11. Malagutti P, Nieman K, Meijboom WB et al. Use of 64-slice CT in symptomatic patients after coronary bypass surgery: evaluation of grafts and coronary arteries. Eur Heart J 2006.
12. Pache G, Saueressig U, Frydrychowicz A et al. Initial experience with 64-slice cardiac CT: non-invasive visualization of coronary artery bypass grafts. Eur Heart J 2006; 27: 976–80.
13. Burgstahler C, Beck T, Kuettner A et al. Non-invasive evaluation of coronary artery bypass grafts using 16-row multislice computed tomography with 188 ms temporal resolution. Int J Cardiol 2006; 106: 244–9.
14. Kuettner A, Kopp AF, Schroeder S et al. Diagnostic accuracy of multidetector computed tomography coronary angiography in patients with angiographically proven coronary artery disease. J Am Coll Cardiol 2004; 43: 831–9.
15. Kuettner A, Trabold T, Schroeder S et al. Noninvasive detection of coronary lesions using 16-detector multislice spiral computed tomography technology: initial clinical results. J Am Coll Cardiol 2004; 44: 1230–7.
16. Hausleiter J, Meyer T, Hadamitzky M et al. Radiation dose estimates from cardiac multislice computed tomography in

daily practice: impact of different scanning protocols on effective dose estimates. Circulation 2006; 113: 1305–10.

17. Dimas AP, Arora RR, Whitlow PL et al. Percutaneous transluminal angioplasty involving internal mammary artery grafts. Am Heart J 1991; 122: 423–9.

18. Rerkpattanapipat P, Ghassemi R, Ledley GS et al. Use of stents to treat kinks causing obstruction in a left internal mammary artery graft. Catheter Cardiovasc Interv 1999; 46: 223–6.

19. Klein AL, Marquis JF, Higginson LA. Percutaneous transluminal angioplasty of a surgically obstructed left internal mammary artery graft. Cathet Cardiovasc Diagn 1988; 14: 46–8.

20. Schroeder S, Kopp AF, Kuettner A et al. Influence of heart rate on vessel visibility in noninvasive coronary angiography using new multislice computed tomography: experience in 94 patients. Clin Imaging 2002; 26: 106–11.

21. Giesler T, Baum U, Ropers D et al. Noninvasive visualization of coronary arteries using contrast-enhanced multidetector CT: influence of heart rate on image quality and stenosis detection. AJR Am J Roentgenol 2002; 179: 911–16.

22. Ferencik M, Moselewski F, Ropers D et al. Quantitative parameters of image quality in multidetector spiral computed tomographic coronary imaging with submillimeter collimation. Am J Cardiol 2003; 92: 1257–62.

23. Achenbach S, Ropers D, Kuettner A et al. Contrast-enhanced coronary artery visualization by dual-source computed tomography—initial experience. Eur J Radiol 2006; 57: 331–5.

24. Cademartiri F, Mollet NR, Runza G et al. Improving diagnostic accuracy of MDCT coronary angiography in patients with mild heart rhythm irregularities using ECG editing. AJR Am J Roentgenol 2006; 186: 634–8.

25. Kovacs A, Probst C, Sommer T et al. [CT coronary angiography in patients with atrial fibrillation]. Rofo 2005; 177: 1655–62.

16

Assessment of Coronary Artery Stents by Coronary Computed Tomograpic Angiography

David Maintz and Harald Seifarth

1 INTRODUCTION

Stents are wire mesh tubes used to prop open a coronary artery during angioplasty. Stents reduce the acute risk of a coronary intervention and reduce the risk of restenosis afterwards. Stents have become by far more widely accepted compared to other interventional techniques such as atherectomy or rotablation.

Coronary CT angiography in the presence of stents is a controversial topic. CT represents a possible noninvasive method for the detection of in-stent restenosis, but in the presence of stents imaging is impeded by artifacts. Knowledge of the clinical background of the patient, stent type, location of the stent, scanner technology, scan protocols and image reconstruction methods is crucial to define an indication for the exam and to correctly interpret scan results.

1.1 History

The first coronary stents were implanted in 1986 by J. Puel and U. Sigwart in Europe and G. Roubin and R. Schatz in the USA. Since then, several generations of bare metal stents were developed being more flexible and easier to deliver to the narrowed artery. Early results highlighted problems associated with the use of stents, in particular a high incidence of subacute occlusions and bleeding complications.[1] In 1993, two important clinical trials,

BENESTENT[2] and STRESS,[3] demonstrated that intracoronary stents significantly reduced the incidence of angiographic restenosis, establishing the elective placement of stents as a standard treatment.

Since then, an exponential increase of stent procedures can be observed. The rate of coronary stent insertion increased 147% between 1996 and 2000. In 2004, 615,000 stent procedures were performed in the United States.[4]

1.2 Stent patency – clinical results

At the time of the STRESS and BENESTENT trials, subacute stent occlusion occurred in 3.7% of patients, a value higher than that seen with balloon angioplasty alone. The use of dual antiplatelet therapy with aspirin and clopidogrel resulted in a lower incidence of subacute thrombosis. While the reduction of restenosis and repeated intervention achieved with stenting in comparison to balloon angioplasty alone has been proven in multiple studies,[5] neointimal hyperplasia with recurrent stenosis remains an issue for bare metal stents (BMS). In-stent restenosis rates ranging from 11% to 46% after 6 months have been reported for BMS.[6] The need to treat restenosis with repeated percutaneous or surgical revascularization procedures was 14% for BMS.[7]

To reduce restenosis rates, drug-eluting stents (DES) have been introduced. DES are coated with antiproliferative substances such as sirolimus (Cyper, Cordis, Johnson & Johnson)

or paclitaxel (Taxus, Boston Scientific). The use of drug-eluting stents has reduced the occurrence of restenosis and the need of repeated revascularization procedures by 50–70%.[8,9]

This success has led to a rapid increase of the use of DES vs. BMS. However, implantation rates for DES vary regionally. In 2006, approximate implantation rates were 80% in the USA and 45% in Europe.

However, there is an ongoing debate as to whether DES lead to higher rates of late stent thrombosis due to impaired healing of coronary arteries. Scientific data are conflicting: One meta-anlaysis has suggested that rates of death and myocardial infarction may be increased in patients who have received DES in comparison to BMS,[10] while others report no significant differences between the two treatments.[11,12]

1.3 Stent types

Stents can be classified according to their geometry (slotted tube, monofilament, multicellular, modular, helical-sinusoidal), underlying material (stainless steel, tantalum, cobalt-alloys, platinum, nitinol, titanium), modus of application (self expandable, balloon expandable), covering (phosphorylcholine, carbon), drug elution (rapamycin, paclitaxel, actinomycin). Other features include flexibility, strut thickness, profile, radial stability, shortening. The most important characteristics influencing the radioopacity of stents are the material (atomic number, e.g. titanium = 22, chromium = 24,

steel = 26, cobalt = 27, nickel = 28, tantalum = 73) and the relative amount of metal per stent area.

1.4 Imaging

While invasive coronary angiography (ICA) remains the gold standard for coronary stent evaluation, noninvasive assessment of coronary stents would be highly desirable. Such an alternative to ICA would ideally have to address the three following clinical problems: (1) stent occlusion (Figure 16.1), (2) stent restenosis (Figure 16.2), (3) disease progression in other coronary arteries.

A combination of beam-hardening and partial-volume artifacts causes artificial thickening of the stent struts during CT, so-called 'blooming' of stents. This 'blooming' is responsible for the artificial lumen narrowing of stents. The magnitude of artifacts and consequently the degree of lumen narrowing depends on the type of stent, the stent diameter and various scan and reconstruction parameters.

2 RESULTS OF CORONARY STENT IMAGING OBTAINED WITH DIFFERENT CT SCANNER TYPES

Before the era of Multidetector Computed Tomography (MDCT) attempts were made to use Electron Beam CT

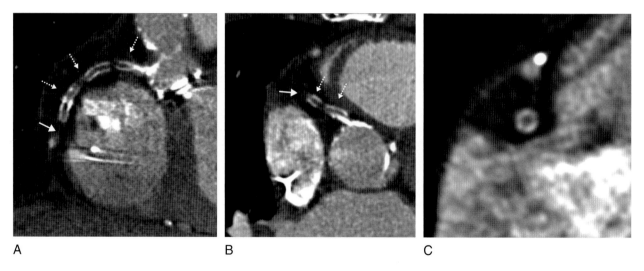

A   B   C

Figure 16.1   Stent occlusion, 4-slice MDCT. 69-year-old patient with three implanted stents in the right coronary artery. (A) shows a longitudinal reformation along the RCA with all three stents visible (dotted arrows). (B) A transverse reformation depicting the proximal two stents (dotted arrows). (C) A reformatted image perpendicular to the most distal stent. Missing contrast distal to the stents (continuous arrows) indicates stent occlusion. The thrombotic material inside the stents appears hypodense.

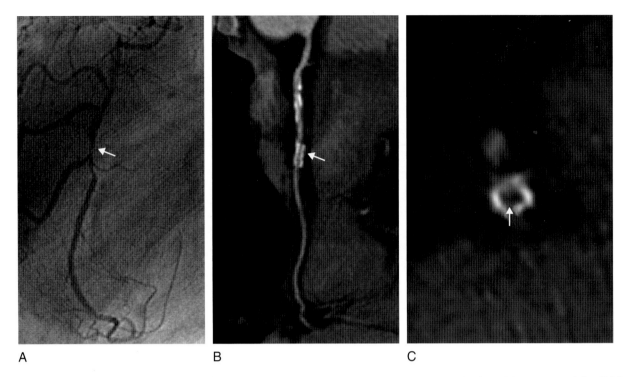

A   B   C

Figure 16.2   Stent restenosis, dual-source MDCT. 58-year-old patient with 8-mm stent in the mid segment of the RCA. Catheter angiography reveals a significant luminal stenosis at the stent location (A). (B) A curved MIP along the RCA demonstrating the stent location. (C) MPR perpendicular to the stent revealing the instent stenosis with hypodense plaque (arrow) and contrasted remaining lumen.

(EBCT) for the imaging of stents. EBCT enabled exact localization of coronary stents and indirect evaluation of stent patency by cine loop evaluation and time-attenuation curve analysis.[13–16]

Since the turn of the century, EBCT has been increasingly replaced by Multidetector CT, offering higher spatial resolution. First results of coronary stent imaging using *4-slice MDCT* revealed that reliable lumen assessment was not possible due to severe blooming artifacts. In an in-vitro study evaluating 19 different stents, the percentage of artificial stenosis from blooming ranged from 62% to 100%.[17] Three patient studies are published that report 100% correct assessment of stent patency (stent occluded or not occluded, decision based on the indirect sign of contrast in the vessel distal to the stent), but insufficient stent lumen visibility and stenosis assessment.[18–20] Figure 16.1 demonstrates a case with stent occlusion diagnosed by a lack of in-stent contrast and lack of contrast distal to the stent.

The introduction of *16-slice MDCT* systems with increased spatial and temporal resolution effected improvement of general image quality and stent assessability. Furthermore, stent-optimized reconstruction kernels were provided (see paragraph on reconstruction methods). A number of in-vitro studies have been performed that

compared different stent products with regard to lumen visibility and stenosis assessment with different scan and reconstruction parameters. Depending on stent type, scanner hardware, and convolution kernel, artificial lumen narrowing ranged from 20% to 100%.[21,22]

In a clinical study by Schuijf et al. 50/65 stents (77%) were evaluable. In these 7/9 stenoses were detected and absence of stenosis was correctly identified in all 41 patent stents, resulting in a sensitivity and specificity of 78% and 100%.

In the largest series of coronary stents investigated by CT so far, Gilard et al. report a lumen visibility depended on stent diameter: on average 64% (126/190 stents) were visible, of stents with diameter >3 mm 81% were visible, but only 51% of stents with a diameter ≤3 mm.[23] Likewise, restenosis detection sensitivity and specificity were 54% and 100% for small stents ≤3 mm and 86% and 100% for larger stents >3 mm. In another study, the detection rates of instent stenoses were assessed in comparison to the detection rates of stenoses in unstented coronaries and, somewhat surprisingly, similar sensitivities and specificities (67% vs. 67% and 98% vs. 99%) were found.[24]

64-slice MDCT offers a further increase of spatial and temporal resolution and larger volume coverage when compared to previous scanner generations. Detection rates of coronary artery stenoses in the native coronary arteries were reported to be as high as 99%.[25–27] However, evaluation of stents still constitutes a problem because of the blooming artifacts. The difference of the magnitude of stent artifacts using 16-slice CT and 64-slice CT in comparison has been quantified by two in-vitro studies. Mahnken et al. found an improvement of 5.9% lumen diameter visibility and Seifarth et al. found an improvement of lumen diameter visibility in the range of 2.5% to 8%, depending on the orientation of the stent axis relative to the z-axis of the scanner.[28,29] After these promising results a number of in-vivo studies were performed with varying results. Rist et al. report a sensitivity and specificity of 75% and 92% for the detection of significant in-stent disease in 45 patients with 6 instent stenoses and 2 occlusions.[30] The largest series using 64-slice CT so far investigated 102 coronary stents.[31] Only 58% of these were evaluable regarding lumen visibility. In the evaluable stents, six of seven instent stenoses were correctly detected, and the absence of instent stenosis was correctly identified in 51 of 52 cases (sensitivity 86%, specificity 98%). The most recently published study reports a sensitivity and specificity of 64-slice CT for the detection of instent stenoses and occlusions of 89% and 95% in a collective of 30 patients with 39 stents, of which 9 were occluded, 20 patent and 10 stenosed.[32]

Of all referenced studies using 64-slice CT for the assessment of coronary stents, the one by Rixe et al.[31] gives the most realistic picture of clinical practice and confirms the own experiences of the author's: A high number of coronary stents are not evaluable even with advanced CT technology. However, in the evaluable ones, detection of significant in-stent disease is possible (Figure 16.2).

Dual source MDCT (DSCT) offers the same qualities with regard to spatial resolution as 64-slice MDCT and even higher temporal resolution (=83 ms). The use of a dual-energy mode is not yet implemented for cardiac applications. However, increased soft tissue contrast with a low tube current (e.g. 80 kV) and reduced artifacts and noise with a higher current of 140 kV, for example, give perspective for further improvements of stent imaging using DSCT.[33]

3 INFLUENCE OF IMAGE RECONSTRUCTION METHODS ON STENT VISUALIZATION

The influence of image reconstruction algorithms on stent visualization is at least as important as the influence of the scanner type. In general, the sharper the kernel the higher percentage of the stent lumen becomes visible (Figure 16.3).

However, using very sharp kernels the lumen attenuation might be artificially decreased. Therefore, stent-dedicated convolution kernels (e.g. B46f for Siemens scanners) have been developed that have less overshoot in the low-frequency region of the modulation-transfer function and consequently offer more reliable lumen attenuation assessment. In-vitro and in-vivo studies have reported the superiority of a stent-optimized kernel (B46f) in comparison to the conventional medium-soft (B30f) convolution kernel.[21,22,34] The increase of image noise using a stent-optimized kernel can be retrospectively compensated for by smoothening filters.[35] To account for optimal image quality in both the stented and unstented parts of coronary arteries, it is recommended to routinely obtain conventional medium-soft kernel and stent-optimized sharp kernel reconstructions.

4 VISUALIZATION OF DIFFERENT STENT TYPES

More than 100 different coronary stent types are known. Many of them are still available, others have been suspended but can still be found in patients that were treated in the past. Stents can be composed of different material. Most products are made from stainless steel. Cobalt-chromium is another frequently used material. Tantalum and nitinol (nickel titanium alloy) are also being used but less frequently. Stents from biodegradable materials such as magnesium are being evaluated in phase 3 studies. The degree of artifacts produced by stents from different materials largely depends on the atomic number of the material. Consequently, tantalum causes the strongest artifacts, followed by steel, cobalt-chromium and nitinol. Magnesium stents exhibit only minor artifacts. Some stents bear radioopaque markers at the stent ends. These markers can cause additional artifacts superimposing the stent lumen at the ends. Besides the underlying material, the appearance of steel stents varies depending on the individual design (see Figure 16.4).

5 INFLUENCE OF STENT DIAMETER AND LOCATION OF STENTS

The diameter of the stent is another important factor influencing the lumen visibility. The larger the stent diameter the higher the visible percentage of the lumen. Stents with a diameter of ≥3.0 mm can often be evaluated.[36] In the study by Schuif et al., 28% of stents with a diameter ≤3.0 mm, but

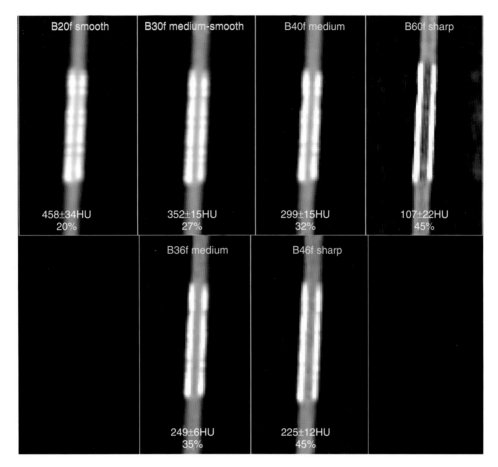

Figure 16.3 Differences of lumen visibility depending on the convolution kernel used for reconstruction. In-vitro experiment with a stent implanted in a 3 mm coronary phantom, vessel contrast 230 HU. The upper image row shows images reconstructed with conventional smooth, medium-smooth, medium and sharp convolution kernels. Note increased lumen diameter visibility with sharp kernel (45%). The drawback with this sharp kernel is an artificially low instent attenuation of 107 HU. The two images in the lower row were reconstructed using stent-optimized convolution kernels. The advantage of these kernels is an increase of lumen diameter visibility when compared to the corresponding conventional kernels while preserving a 'relialistic' attenuation.

only 10% of stents with a diameter >3 mm, were unevaluable.[37] Stent implantation in the left main (LM) and proximal left anterior descending/proximal left circumflex coronary artery provides the 'best case scenario' for the use of MSCT in the detection of in-stent restenosis. This is because of the relatively large stent diameters (usually approximately 3.9 mm in the LM), the fact that scan orientation is parallel to the stent axis and the relatively low motion in this area. Excellent results in patient studies confirm these considerations: in a series of 114 patients with 131 proximal stents (3.25 mm) Chabbert et al. found lumen evaluability in 121 stents (92.4%) and correct identification of in-stent restenosis in 91.7% (prevalence of restenosis 22.5%) using 16-slice CT.[38] Gilard et al. were able to evaluate the stent lumen of LM coronary stents (average diameter 3.9 mm) in 27/29 cases and to identify 4/4 instent restenoses.[36] Identification of neointimal hyperplasia with

lumen reduction of less than 35% was not possible in this 16-slice MDCT study.

Van Mieghem evaluated a large collective of patients with left main coronary stents using 16-slice CT (n = 27) or 64-slice CT (n = 43).[39] All 10 of 70 in-stent restenoses were correctly identified. However, there were also 5 false-positive results (sensitivity 100%, specificity 91%).

6 INDICATIONS FOR A CT EXAMINATION AFTER STENT TREATMENT

Stent assessment shall not be regarded as an accepted indication for a CT examination in general. It is important to define whether the purpose of a CT scan is the assessment of stent patency (= to exclude stent occlusion), assessment of

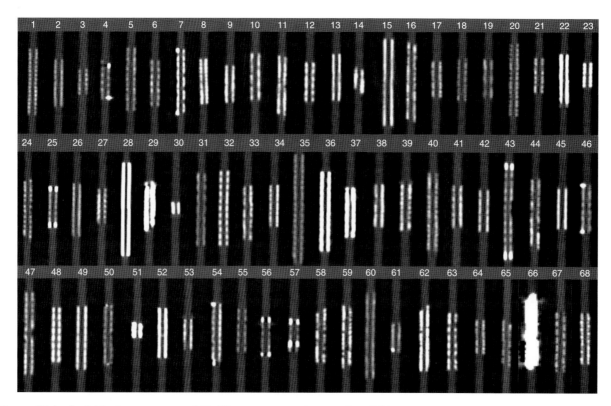

Figure 16.4   Individual appearance of 68 different stents using 64-slice CT (in-vitro experiment, lumen contrast 250 HU). The numbers of the stents correspond to Table 16.1. Name of the stent, manufacturer and underlying material can be derived from there as well as a rough classification according to the magnitude of artifacts into low, medium and high. Note that some stents (number 4, 7, 25, 43, 46, 54, 56, 57, 61) have hyperdense markers at the stent ends that cause additional artifacts.

stent restenosis or evaluation of disease progression in non-stented coronary vessels.

1. Stent patency: Exclusion of a stent occlusion may be possible by indirect evaluation of the contrast distal of the stent. If high contrast in the coronary segment distal to the stent is present, stent occlusion can be regarded unlikely. However, one must bear in mind that in some cases with occluded stents collateral flow might cause contrast distal to the stent.

2. Stent restenosis: To exclude stent stenosis, the stent lumen must be visible. This is only possible in certain stent types (Figure 16.4 might be helpful to identify these) and in stents in proximal coronary vessels (≥3 mm diameter). Intimal hyperplasia within a stent with lumen reduction of >30% may not even be detected these cases.

3. Disease progression in nonstented coronary arteries: To exclude a significant stenosis in coronary segments other than the stented one is another condition. In these cases all general considerations for coronary CTA apply (see different chapter).

7 OTHER IMPORTANT CONSIDERATIONS BEFORE EXAMINING A STENT PATIENT

As a consequence of the up to date available data from studies evaluating CT of coronary stents, the following recommendations can be given:

1. Stent type: The stent type must be suitable for CT imaging. A catalogue of the appearance of different stent-types in CT as provided in Figure 16.4 might be helpful for this decision. Information that reliably excludes a stent restenosis larger than 50% diameter reduction can only be expected in stents with low or medium artifacts.

2. The stent diameter should be ≥3 mm.

3. 64-slice MDCT (or Dual source MDCT) is the recommended scanner technology that should be available if stent restenosis is the question of interest.

4. A stent-optimized convolution kernel must be available for image reconstruction. In all patients that are treated

Table 16.1 Name, manufacturer, material and magnitude of artifacts of different coronary stent. The stent numbers correspond to Figure 6.4

No.	Name	Manufacturer	Material	CT artifacts
1	Arthos-Inert	AMG International	Stainless steel 316L	medium
2	Arthos-Pico	AMG International	Cobalt-Cromium Alloy	low
3	Axxion	Krauth CardioVascular	Stainless steel 316L + Paclitaxel on synthetic glycocalix coating	low
4	be-Stent 2	Medtronic	Stainless steel 316L	medium
5	BiodivYsio	Abbott Vascular Devices	Stainless steel 316L + Phosphorylcholine-coating	medium
6	CCSV	Micro Science Medical	Stainless steel 316L, Tantalcoating	medium
7	Chrono	Sorin Biomedica	Cobalt-Cromium Alloy + Carbofilm coating	medium
8	Coroflex Blue	B. Braun	Cobalt-Cromium Alloy (L605)	medium
9	Coroflex Delta	B. Braun	Stainless steel 316L	medium
10	Coroflex Theca	B. Braun	Stainless steel 316L + PTFEP-Polyzene-F coating	low
11	Crossflex	Cordis	Stainless steel 316L	medium
12	Cypher	Cordis	Stainless steel 316L	medium
13	Driver	Medtronic	Cobalt-Cromium Alloy	low
14	Duett	Guidant	Stainless steel 316L	high
15	Endeavor	Medtronic	Cobalt-Cromium Alloy + phosphorylcholine + ABT 578 coating	low
16	Express 2	Boston Scientific	Stainless steel 316L	medium
17	F1 Medium (009FF12)	Abbott Vascular Devices	Stainless steel 316L	medium
18	F1 Small (006FF16)	Abbott Vascular Devices	Stainless steel 316L	medium
19	Flex AS	Phytis	Stainless steel 316L + DLC-coating	medium
20	Flex Small (006F26)	Abbott Vascular Devices	Stainless steel 316L	low
21	Flex Standard (010F12)	Abbott Vascular Devices	Stainless steel 316L	low
22	Herculink	Guidant	Stainless steel 316L	high
23	Jograft	Abbott Vascular Devices	Stainless steel 316L + PTFE-graft	medium
24	Jostent	Abbott Vascular Devices	Stainless steel 316L	medium
25	Lekton	Biotronik	Stainless steel 316L, silicon-carbide coating	medium
26	Liberté	Boston Scientific	Stainless steel 316L+PTFE	medium
27	MAC	AMG International	Stainless steel 316L	medium
28	Magic Wallstent	Boston Scientific	Cobalt alloy with titanium core (33%)	high
29	Mansfield Coronary Stent	Mansfield	Tantalum	high
30	MicroStent	Medtronic-AVE	Stainless steel 316L	high
31	Mini	Cordis	Stainless steel 316L	medium
32	MSM Coronary Stent	Micro Science Medical	Stainless steel 316L, Tantalcoating	medium
33	Nexus	Occam International	Stainless steel 316L	medium
34	Nexus 2	Occam International	Stainless steel 316L	low
35	NIR Primo	Boston Scientific	Stainless steel 316L	medium
36	NIR Royal	Boston Scientific	Stainless steel 316LS + Gold-coating	high
37	NIR Royal Adv	Boston Scientific	Stainless steel 316LS + Gold-coating	high
38	Palmaz	Cordis	Stainless steel 316L	medium
39	Penta	Guidant	Stainless steel 316L	medium
40	Pixel	Guidant	Stainless steel 316L	medium
41	Pro-Kinetik	Biotronik	Cobalt-Cromium Alloy + PROBIO, SiC coating	medium
42	Radius	Boston Scientific	Nitinol	low
43	Rithron-XR	Biotronik	Stainless steel 316L	medium
44	R-Stent	Orbus Medical Technologies	Stainless steel 316L	medium
45	S 7	Medtronic	Stainless steel 316L	low
46	Sirius Carbostent	Sorin Biomedica	Stainless steel 316L + Carbon-coating + 2 Platinum markers	medium
47	Sito Stent S	Sitomed	Stainless steel 316L	medium
48	Sonic Bx	Cordis	Stainless steel 316L	high

Continued

Table 16.1 Name, manufacturer, material and magnitude of artifacts of different coronary stent. The stent numbers correspond to Figure 6.4.—cont'd

No.	Name	Manufacturer	Material	CT artifacts
49	Symbiot	Boston Scientific	Nitinol	low
50	Syncro	Sorin Biomedica	Stainless steel 316L + Carbon-coating + 2 Platinum markers	medium
51	Tantal	Abbott Vascular Devices	Tantalum based alloy	high
52	Tantal Sandwich	Abbott Vascular Devices	316L (inside), Ta (intermediate), 316L (outside)	high
53	Taxus	Boston Scientific	Stainless steel 316L	medium
54	Tecnic	Sorin Biomedica	Stainless steel 316L + Carbon-coating + 2 Platinum markers	medium
55	Tenax-complete	Biotronik	Stainless steel 316L	low
56	Tenax-XR	Biotronik	Stainless steel 316L, Gold-markers	medium
57	Teneo	Biotronik	Stainless steel 316L	low
58	Tetra	Guidant	Stainless steel 316L	medium
59	Tristar	Guidant	Stainless steel 316L	medium
60	Tsunami	Terumo	Stainless steel 316L	medium
61	Tsunami Gold	Terumo	Stainless steel 316L	medium
62	Ultra	Guidant	Stainless steel 316L	medium
63	VelocityBx	Cordis	Stainless steel 316L	medium
64	Vision	Guidant	Cobalt-Cromium Alloy	low
65	V-Flex	Cook	Stainless steel 316L	medium
66	Wiktor	Medtronic	Tantalum	high
67	Yukon Choice	Translumina	Stainless steel 316L	low
68	Zeta	Guidant	Stainless steel 316L	medium

with coronary stents, scan reconstruction with both a stent optimized kernel and a conventional kernel shall be routinely obtained for optimal assessment of stented and nonstented coronary segments.

5. General requirements that apply for standard CTA (contraindications, heart rate, etc.) must be considered.

REFERENCES

1. Serruys PW, Strauss BH, Beatt KJ et al. Angiographic follow-up after placement of a self-expanding coronary-artery stent. N Engl J Med 1991; 324(1): 13–17.
2. Serruys PW, de Jaegere P, Kiemeneij F et al. A comparison of balloon-expandable-stent implantation with balloon angioplasty in patients with coronary artery disease. Benestent Study Group. N Engl J Med 1994; 331(8): 489–95.
3. Fischman DL, Leon MB, Baim DS et al. A randomized comparison of coronary-stent placement and balloon angioplasty in the treatment of coronary artery disease. Stent Restenosis Study Investigators. N Engl J Med 1994; 331(8): 496–501.
4. Heart and stroke statistical update, 2007. Dallas: American Heart Association, 2007.
5. Bertrand ME, Rupprecht HJ, Urban P, Gershlick AH. Double-blind study of the safety of clopidogrel with and without a loading dose in combination with aspirin compared with ticlopidine in combination with aspirin after coronary stenting:
the clopidogrel aspirin stent international cooperative study (CLASSICS). Circulation 2000; 102(6): 624–9.
6. Antoniucci D, Valenti R, Santoro GM et al. Restenosis after coronary stenting in current clinical practice. Am Heart J 1998; 135(3): 510–18.
7. Williams DO, Holubkov R, Yeh W et al. Percutaneous coronary intervention in the current era compared with 1985–1986: the National Heart, Lung, and Blood Institute Registries. Circulation 2000; 102(24): 2945–51.
8. Moses JW, Leon MB, Popma JJ et al. Sirolimus-eluting stents versus standard stents in patients with stenosis in a native coronary artery. N Engl J Med 2003; 349(14): 1315–23.
9. Stone GW, Ellis SG, Cox DA et al. A polymer-based, paclitaxel-eluting stent in patients with coronary artery disease. N Engl J Med 2004; 350(3): 221–31.
10. Nordmann AJ, Briel M, Bucher HC. Mortality in randomized controlled trials comparing drug-eluting vs. bare metal stents in coronary artery disease: a meta-analysis. Eur Heart J 2006; 27(23): 2784–814.
11. Kastrati A, Mehilli J, Pache J et al. Analysis of 14 Trials Comparing Sirolimus-Eluting Stents with Bare-Metal Stents. N Engl J Med 2007.
12. Spaulding C, Daemen J, Boersma E, Cutlip DE, Serruys PW. A Pooled Analysis of Data Comparing Sirolimus-Eluting Stents with Bare-Metal Stents. N Engl J Med 2007.
13. Mohlenkamp S, Pump H, Baumgart D et al. Minimally invasive evaluation of coronary stents with electron beam computed tomography: In vivo and in vitro experience. Catheter Cardiovasc Interv 1999; 48(1): 39–47.

14. Pump H, Moehlenkamp S, Sehnert C et al. Electron-beam CT in the noninvasive assessment of coronary stent patency. Acad Radiol 1998; 5(12): 858–62.

15. Pump H, Mohlenkamp S, Sehnert CA et al. Coronary arterial stent patency: assessment with electron-beam CT. Radiology 2000; 214(2): 447–52.

16. Schmermund A, Rensing BJ, Sheedy PF, Bell MR, Rumberger JA. Intravenous electron-beam computed tomographic coronary angiography for segmental analysis of coronary artery stenoses. J Am Coll Cardiol 1998; 31(7): 1547–54.

17. Maintz D, Juergens KU, Wichter T et al. Imaging of coronary artery stents using multislice computed tomography: in vitro evaluation. Eur Radiol 2003; 13(4): 830–5.

18. Kruger S, Mahnken AH, Sinha AM et al. Multislice spiral computed tomography for the detection of coronary stent restenosis and patency. Int J Cardiol 2003; 89(2–3): 167–72.

19. Ligabue G, Rossi R, Ratti C et al. Noninvasive evaluation of coronary artery stents patency after PTCA: role of Multislice Computed Tomography. Radiol Med (Torino) 2004; 108(1–2): 128–37.

20. Maintz D, Grude M, Fallenberg EM, Heindel W, Fischbach R. Assessment of coronary arterial stents by multislice-CT angiography. Acta Radiol 2003; 44(6): 597–603.

21. Mahnken AH, Buecker A, Wildberger JE et al. Coronary artery stents in multislice computed tomography: in vitro artifact evaluation. Invest Radiol 2004; 39(1): 27–33.

22. Maintz D, Seifarth H, Flohr T et al. Improved coronary artery stent visualization and in-stent stenosis detection using 16-slice computed-tomography and dedicated image reconstruction technique. Invest Radiol 2003; 38(12): 790–5.

23. Gilard M, Cornily JC, Pennec PY et al. Assessment of coronary artery stents by 16 slice computed tomography. Heart 2006; 92(1): 58–61.

24. Kefer JM, Coche E, Vanoverschelde JL, Gerber BL. Diagnostic accuracy of 16-slice multidetector-row CT for detection of in-stent restenosis vs detection of stenosis in non-stented coronary arteries. Eur Radiol 2006.

25. Leschka S, Alkadhi H, Plass A et al. Accuracy of MSCT coronary angiography with 64-slice technology: first experience. Eur Heart J 2005; 26(15): 1482–7.

26. Mollet NR, Cademartiri F, van Mieghem CA et al. High-resolution spiral computed tomography coronary angiography in patients referred for diagnostic conventional coronary angiography. Circulation 2005; 112(15): 2318–23.

27. Ropers D, Rixe J, Anders K et al. Usefulness of multidetector row spiral computed tomography with 64- × 0.6-mm collimation and 330-ms rotation for the noninvasive detection of

28. significant coronary artery stenoses. Am J Cardiol 2006; 97(3): 343–8.

29. Mahnken AH, Muhlenbruch G, Seyfarth T et al. 64-slice computed tomography assessment of coronary artery stents: a phantom study. Acta Radiol 2006; 47(1): 36–42.

30. Seifarth H, Ozgun M, Raupach R et al. 64- Versus 16-slice CT angiography for coronary artery stent assessment: in vitro experience. Invest Radiol 2006; 41(1): 22–7.

31. Rist C, von Ziegler F, Nikolaou K et al. Assessment of coronary artery stent patency and restenosis using 64-slice computed tomography. Acad Radiol 2006; 13(12): 1465–73.

32. Rixe J, Achenbach S, Ropers D et al. Assessment of coronary artery stent restenosis by 64-slice multi-detector computed tomography. Eur Heart J 2006; 27(21): 2567–72.

33. Oncel D, Oncel G, Karaca M. Coronary stent patency and in-stent restenosis: determination with 64-section multidetector CT coronary angiography – initial experience. Radiology 2007; 242(2): 403–9.

34. Maintz D, Seifarth H, Leidecker C et al. Implications for Visualization of Coronary Artery Stents and Instent Stenoses using Dual Energy CT in phantom experiments. European Radiology 2007, 17(suppl 1): 143.

35. Hong C, Chrysant GS, Woodard PK, Bae KT. Coronary artery stent patency assessed with in-stent contrast enhancement measured at multi-detector row CT angiography: initial experience. Radiology 2004; 233(1): 286–91.

36. Seifarth H, Raupach R, Schaller S et al. Assessment of coronary artery stents using 16-slice MDCT angiography: evaluation of a dedicated reconstruction kernel and a noise reduction filter. Eur Radiol 2005; 15(4): 721–6.

37. Gilard M, Cornily JC, Rioufol G et al. Noninvasive assessment of left main coronary stent patency with 16-slice computed tomography. Am J Cardiol 2005; 95(1): 110–12.

38. Schuijf JD, Bax JJ, Jukema JW et al. Feasibility of assessment of coronary stent patency using 16-slice computed tomography. Am J Cardiol 2004; 94(4): 427–30.

39. Chabbert V, Carrie D, Bennaceur M et al. Evaluation of in-stent restenosis in proximal coronary arteries with multidetector computed tomography (MDCT). Eur Radiol 2006.

40. Van Mieghem CA, Cademartiri F, Mollet NR et al. Multislice spiral computed tomography for the evaluation of stent patency after left main coronary artery stenting: a comparison with conventional coronary angiography and intravascular ultrasound. Circulation 2006; 114(7): 645–53.

17

Computed Tomography of the Myocardium, Pericardium, and Cardiac Chambers

James F. Glockner

1 INTRODUCTION

Recent developments in cardiac CT technology have been employed primarily to investigate coronary artery disease, whether to detect and quantify coronary artery calcification or to directly image coronary artery luminal narrowing with CT angiography. Considering that coronary artery disease is the major cause of death in the western world, this is an eminently reasonable approach. It is worth noting, however, that not all cardiac pathology involves the coronary arteries, and that many of the CT techniques used to image the coronary arteries are equally applicable to detecting and characterizing non-coronary pathology. This chapter offers a brief overview of the use of CT to image the myocardium, pericardium, and cardiac chambers.

2 TECHNICAL CONSIDERATIONS

While in theory it is best to determine an imaging protocol based on the cardiac abnormality to be examined, in practice myocardial or pericardial abnormalities are often noted as incidental findings on routine chest CT or CTA of the pulmonary arteries or aorta. Image quality in these typically non-gated acquisitions can be quite variable, but it is often surprisingly good, and more than adequate to detect and characterize many cardiac pathologies.

Ideally, however, images are acquired using state-of-the-art equipment after careful consideration of the appropriate protocol. Cardiac CT has traditionally been performed either using electron beam CT (EBCT) or multidetector row CT (MDCT) in conjunction with prospective or retrospective ECG gating. Electron beam CT has some important advantages relative to multidetector CT: faster temporal resolution and lower radiation doses. However, the latest generation of MDCT systems approaches the temporal resolution of EBCT, has much higher spatial resolution, and much shorter acquisition times. EBCT also suffers in terms of its ability to perform general cross sectional imaging, and therefore MDCT has become the dominant platform for cardiac CT.

Any dedicated CT examination of the heart should employ either prospective or retrospective ECG gating. Prospective gating offers the advantage of reduced radiation dose; however acquisition times are generally longer, spatial resolution is reduced, and images are somewhat more susceptible to cardiac arrhythmias. Prospectively gated images may be all that is necessary to detect and characterize a calcified or fatty mass, for example. Retrospectively gated images, acquired in spiral mode with a low pitch, require a higher radiation dose, but can be reconstructed at any phase of the cardiac cycle (allowing creation of cine loops) and can be acquired with submillimeter isotropic spatial resolution, so that any imaging plane can be viewed without loss of spatial resolution.

Cardiac examinations, particularly those performed with low pitch spiral MDCT and retrospective gating, generate large amounts of data, and should always be interpreted at a workstation where reconstructions can be performed in a variety of planes. Long and short axis cardiac planes are often helpful in appreciating the relationship of masses to the cardiac chambers as well as in detecting myocardial and pericardial abnormalities, but traditional axial, coronal, and sagittal planes occasionally provide the most helpful images. Three-dimensional reconstructions using volume rendering or maximum intensity projection techniques are probably less useful in evaluation of the myocardium and pericardium in comparison to the coronary arteries, but are occasionally informative.

3 PERICARDIUM

3.1 Anatomy and physiology

The pericardium is a double-walled sac containing the heart and roots of the great vessels. An external fibrous layer surrounds the inner serous pericardium, which consists of an outer parietal layer and an inner visceral layer. The parietal and visceral pericardium are separated by a potential space, the pericardial cavity. The inner surface of the serous pericardium is lined by a layer of mesothelial cells which produce the small amount of fluid normally present in the pericardial cavity.[1]

The physiologic role of the pericardium is somewhat mysterious: it may serve as a barrier to the spread of inflammation and infection from adjacent mediastinal structures. Other potential functions include reducing friction of cardiac motion, and limiting acute distention of the heart in the setting of rapid venous return of large amounts of blood. Nevertheless, normal cardiac function is not impeded in post-pericardectomy patients.

The pericardial cavity normally contains 15–50 ml of fluid. While the amount and location of this fluid is variable, it tends to collect in dependent regions and at sites of pericardial reflection. Visualization of the pericardium as it overlies the posterior right atrium, left atrium, and lateral wall of the left ventricle is limited because of its close proximity to the atrial walls and myocardium. The pericardium is most clearly visualized over the free wall of the right ventricle and the inferior apical left ventricle, where it is outlined by mediastinal and subpericardial fat. The normal thickness of the pericardium on CT ranges from 1–3 mm; the true thickness is probably slightly less than this, due to motion induced blurring and volume averaging (Figure 17.1).[2–3] The pericardium can appear erroneously thickened in the presence of a small effusion, or if measurement is performed in a non-orthogonal projection, for example on axial images near the superior or inferior margin as it changes orientation from vertical to horizontal.

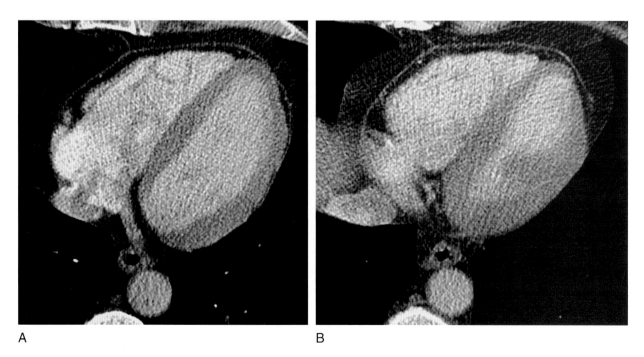

A   B

Figure 17.1 Normal pericardium. Axial prospectively gated contrast-enhanced CT images reveal normal thin pericardium best seen anterior to the right ventricular free wall.

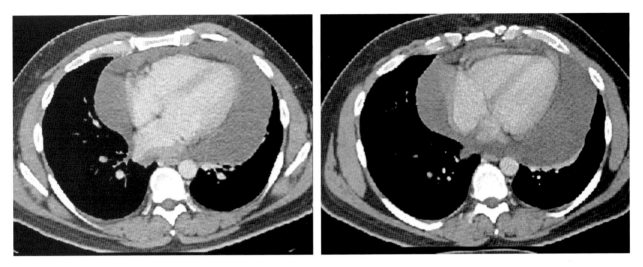

Figure 17.2 Pericardial effusion. Axial contrast-enhanced CT reveals a large fluid attenuation pericardial effusion surrounding the heart.

3.2 Pericardial effusion

Significant pericardial effusions are easily detected with CT, generally as low attenuation, non-enhancing fluid separating the parietal and visceral pericardial surfaces (Figure 17.2). Small amounts of fluid may be difficult to distinguish from pericardial thickening, particularly without administration of contrast. Care must also be taken to avoid mistaking normal amounts of pericardial fluid as pathological: fluid often accumulates in the pericardial recesses (sites of pericardial reflection) or along the inferior border of the pericardium. Small amounts of fluid commonly accumulate in the superior pericardial recess between the ascending aorta and pulmonary artery on axial images: this normal variant should not be mistaken for mediastinal mass or adenopathy, or a focal aortic dissection[4–5] (Figure 17.3).

Pericardial effusions may occur as a response to a large number of systemic or cardiac diseases. Some of the more common underlying conditions include viral or idiopathic pericarditis, postinfarction syndrome, neoplasia, uremia, trauma, prior radiation therapy, collagen vascular disease, and AIDS. Pericardial fluid in excess of 50 ml is considered abnormal, and this will generally correspond to a pericardial width in excess of 4 mm.

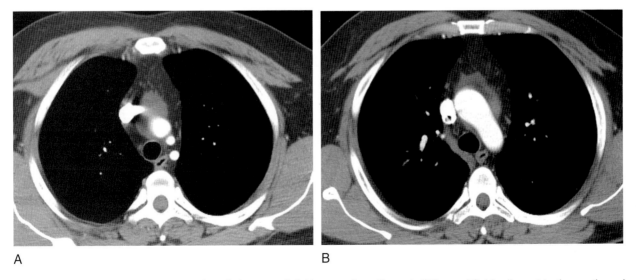

A   B

Figure 17.3 Fluid in the superior pericardial recess. Axial images from thoracic CT reveal fluid adjacent to the aortic arch and great vessels in the superior pericardial recess. This is a normal variant which should not be mistaken for a mass or focal dissection.

3.3 Pericarditis

Pericarditis, or inflammation of the pericardium, is also associated with a large number of diseases, and there is considerable overlap with causes of pericardial effusion. One large pathologic series revealed that in most cases (68%) the cause of pericarditis was unknown. Previous pericardiotomy and irradiation each accounted for 9% of cases.[6] CT findings of pericarditis include thickening and enhancement of the pericardium, often associated with a simple or complex pericardial effusion.

Constrictive pericarditis occurs when cardiac function is impaired by a thickened or fibrotic pericardium. The clinical presentation of constrictive pericarditis is often nonspecific, and can be confused with restrictive cardiomyopathy, heart failure, and hepatic cirrhosis. Patients often present with signs and symptoms of right sided heart failure disproportionate to the extent of left ventricular dysfunction or valvular disease. The most important diagnostic challenge in this setting is to distinguish between constrictive pericarditis, a surgical disease, and restrictive cardiomyopathy, which generally requires medical therapy. A wide range of etiologies have been implicated in constrictive pericarditis.[7,8] A series from the Mayo Clinic examined 143 surgical specimens with constrictive pericarditis and found that pericardial constriction was idiopathic in 49% of cases.[9] The two most prevalent known causes were both iatrogenic: previous pericardiotomy (30%) and irradiation (11%). Additional etiologies included viral pericarditis, connective tissue disease, neoplasm, and uremia. The presence of gross calcification was relatively uncommon in constrictive pericarditis, occurring in only 28% of specimens.

The diagnostic hallmark of constrictive pericarditis is pericardial thickening with or without calcifications in the setting of clinical signs and symptoms suggestive of the diagnosis (Figures 17.4 and 17.5).[10,11] Secondary signs of constrictive pericarditis include focal distortion of the contour of the ventricles or atria by the thickened pericardium, atrial enlargement, tubular ventricles, dilatation of the IVC and hepatic veins, ascites, and pleural effusions. The presence of pericardial calcification is suggestive but not diagnostic of constrictive pericarditis. The use of intravenous contrast is not always necessary for the diagnosis of constrictive pericarditis; however, in conjunction with thin section, retrospectively gated CT, cine images can be reconstructed in long or short axis projections which may then be assessed for evidence of diastolic dysfunction. Most characteristic is the presence of paradoxical septal motion in early diastole

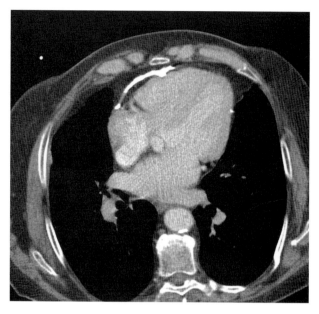

Figure 17.4 Constrictive pericarditis. Contrast-enhanced prospectively gated image reveals a sheet of confluent pericardial calcification overlying the right ventricle in a patient with symptoms of pericardial constriction.

(septal bounce) related to elevated diastolic filling pressures in the right ventricle.[12]

Constrictive pericarditis can be seen in the setting of normal pericardial thickness. One investigation, for example, found that only 58% of patients with surgically confirmed constrictive pericarditis had pericardial thickening or calcification.[13] Fairly often in these cases, however, there

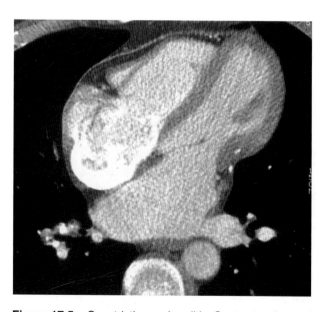

Figure 17.5 Constrictive pericarditis. Contrast-enhanced retrospectively gated image shows focal contour deformity of the lateral basal left ventricle with two small foci of pericardial calcification. Note also enlarged left and right atria.

are subtle secondary signs of constrictive pericarditis – in our experience it is rare to see a completely normal CT in the setting of pericardial constriction.

3.4 Pericardial cysts

Pericardial cysts are benign lesions which occur when a portion of embryonic pericardium is pinched off during development. Most contain simple fluid, and are most commonly located in the anterior right cardiophrenic angle. Most patients are asymptomatic, and the lesions are detected incidentally as a cardiophrenic mass on chest x-ray. Pericardial cysts are easily demonstrated on CT as well circumscribed cystic lesions containing simple fluid (Figure 17.6). Pericardial cysts may occasionally contain proteinaceous or hemorrhagic fluid, in which case differentiation from a solid mass may be more difficult. In these cases, administration of contrast and verification of a lack of enhancement can confirm the diagnosis.

3.5 Congenital absence of the pericardium

Complete or partial absence of the pericardium is a rare developmental abnormality. Complete absence is relatively uncommon, occurring in approximately 10% of cases, and partial absence is more frequently left-sided. Pericardial agenesis may be associated with additional congenital heart defects in up to one third of cases, including atrial septal defect, patent ductus arteriosus, and tetralogy of Fallot.[14] Partial or complete pericardial agenesis is usually asymptomatic, and is detected incidentally on chest x-ray by noting a shift of the heart to the left with an unusually prominent left atrial appendage or pulmonary artery segment.

CT may reveal complete or partial absence of the pericardium; however, portions of the pericardium overlying the left atrium and lateral left ventricle may not normally be visualized. In cases of partial absence, the bulging left atrial appendage and leftward protuberance of the pulmonary artery are appreciated. Herniation of the left atrial appendage or left ventricle through a partial defect has been described,[15,16] and this can result in sudden death from cardiac strangulation.

3.6 Pericardial malignancies

Metastatic pericardial disease is much more common than primary malignancy, and is generally associated with a poor prognosis.[17] While metastatic involvement of the pericardium is not unusual in autopsy series,[18,19] it is a relatively uncommon finding on CT. Lung and breast carcinoma,

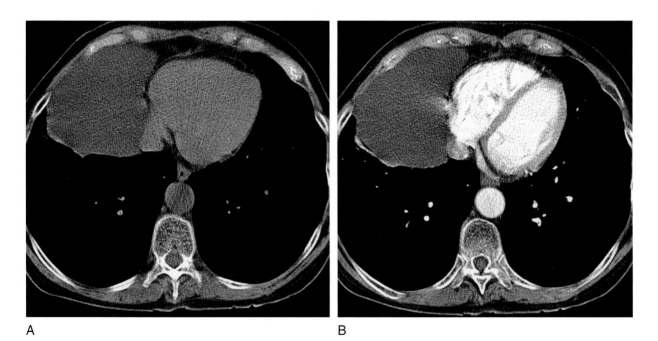

A   B

Figure 17.6 Pericardial cyst. Pre (a) and post (b) contrast images demonstrate a cystic lesion adjacent to the right heart border without enhancement.

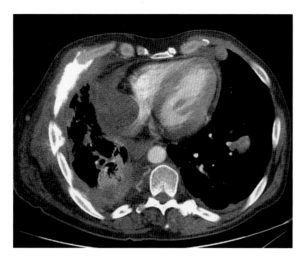

Figure 17.7 Pericardial metastasis. Contrast-enhanced CT image reveals a focal pericardial mass extending into the right atrium in this patient with rectal carcinoma. Note also pleural, pulmonary, and bone metastases.

renal cell carcinoma, lymphoma, and melanoma are some of the most frequent primary sources. Spread to the pericardium can occur via hematogenous, lymphatic, or transvenous extension, or by direct extension from lung or mediastinal tumors.

Pericardial metastatic disease may manifest as a focal pericardial mass, diffuse thickening, or a simple or complex effusion (Figure 17.7). In patients with a known malignancy and pericardial effusion, the differential diagnosis includes malignant effusion as well as benign idiopathic, radiation-induced or drug-induced pericarditis.

Primary tumors of the pericardium are rare. Benign tumors of the pericardium include lipoma, teratoma, fibroma, and hemangioma. Malignant neoplasms include mesothelioma, lymphoma, and sarcoma.[17,20]

4 MYOCARDIUM

CT can be a valuable technique in assessing patients with myocardial disease, including cardiomyopathies, myocadial ischemia, congenital anomalies, and masses. Examination protocols are not always straightforward, and should be tailored to the particular patient and clinical question. Much useful information, for example, can be obtained from retrospectively gated coronary CTA data: cine images can be reconstructed to assess myocardial function, complications of previous myocardial infarction demonstrated, and incidental anomalies noted. However, a contrast-enhanced coronary CTA protocol may not be suitable for all patients: if the clinical question is a possible mass, for example, pre- and post-contrast images might be required. Additionally, consideration

should always be given to limit the radiation dose as much as possible while still obtaining a diagnostic exam.

4.1 Cardiomyopathies

Cardiomyopathies are defined as diseases of the heart muscle associated with cardiac dysfunction, and are classified as dilated cardiomyopathy (DCM), hypertrophic cardiomyopathy (HCM), restrictive cardiomyopathy, and arrhythmogenic right ventricular cardiomyopathy or dysplasia (ARVD).[21] Specific entities such as amyloidosis, sarcoidosis, myocarditis, muscular dystrophies, etc., generally fall into one or more of these classifications. MRI is more often performed than CT to evaluate patients with cardiomyopathies, a result of its superior myocardial tissue characterization, lack of ionizing radiation, and its ability to detect myocardial scarring and infarction with delayed enhancement pulse sequences. There are a number of situations, however, where CT might be preferred. Patients with pacemakers or AICD devices, for example, are unable to undergo MRI. MRI can be quite limited in patients with significant arrythmias; CT image quality also deteriorates in these cases, but often to a lesser degree. Finally, claustrophobic, unstable, or hypoxic patients unable to tolerate the longer examination times and multiple breath holds typically required in MRI may benefit from CT.

Dilated cardiomyopathy is characterized by dilatation of the cardiac chambers with increased myocardial mass, reduced wall thickness, and reduced contractility. Causes of dilated cardiomyopathy include familial/genetic, viral, immune, toxic, or metabolic; however idiopathic dilated cardiomyopathy is probably the most common cause, with an estimated prevalence of 36/100,000 in the United States.[22]

Findings on cardiac CT include dilated cardiac chambers with increased LV and RV volumes and reduced ejection fractions on cine images. Coronary CTA may be helpful to distinguish patients with ventricular dysfunction resulting from coronary atherosclerosis and myocardial ischemia from those with dilated cardiomyopathy.

Hypertrophic cardiomyopathy (HCM) is characterized by left ventricular hypertrophy (occasionally with involvement of the right ventricle), impaired diastolic function, a relatively small ventricular cavity, and increased risk of sudden cardiac death. HCM is a fairly common disorder, with an estimated incidence of 1/500, and is inherited in an autosomal dominant pattern with variable penetrance, although sporadic cases are frequent.[23] Hypertrophic myocardium histologically demonstrates myofibril disarray, various sizes of myofibrils, and myocardial fibrosis. The basal septum is most often involved, resulting in systolic anterior motion (SAM) of the anterior mitral valve leaflet and concomitant mitral regurgitation directed posteriorly and laterally. This in turn causes subvalvular obstruction of the LV outflow tract as the mitral leaflet contacts the hypertrophic basal septum in mid systole. The appearance of HCM is quite variable, however, and may involve any portion of the left ventricle, including the apex, and can result in mid cavitary rather than LV outflow tract obstruction. Patients with large gradients (>30 mm Hg) have a significantly higher risk of cardiovascular morbidity and mortality.[23] Other risk factors include the extent of hypertrophy and myocardial scarring. CT can provide accurate measurements of myocardial mass and myocardial thickness, assess myocardial function, and evaluate the extent of LVOT obstruction by planimetry. The recent emergence of delayed enhancement imaging in CT may also allow accurate assessment of the volume of myocardial fibrosis to aid in risk stratification.

Restrictive cardiomyopathies are characterized by left ventricular diastolic dysfunction (and variable right ventricular involvement) with relatively preserved systolic function. Causes include infiltrative diseases such as amyloidosis, hemochromatosis, and endomyocardial fibrosis. While MRI has shown promise in distinguishing specific etiologies of restrictive cardiomyopathies, CT probably has less to offer in this regard, since soft tissue characterization is limited. However, abnormal myocardial delayed enhancement has

been noted on cardiac MRI in amyloid patients; this may have a correlate in CT delayed enhancement. Likewise, a thickened interatrial septum or posterior atrial wall of greater than 6 mm is a fairly specific finding for amyloid and can aid in distinguishing between amyloid and hypertrophic cardiomyopathy.[24,25] This observation is easily applicable to CT studies. Patients with eosinophilic endomyocarditis may develop confluent left or right ventricular thrombus in a subendocardial location, a classic finding demonstrable either on MRI or CT (Figure 17.8).

Since the clinical signs and symptoms of restrictive cardiomyopathy often mimic those of constrictive pericarditis, the distinction between these two entities is important. As noted above, cardiac CT is an excellent test for constrictive pericarditis, and can usually make the distinction between constrictive and restrictive disease.

Arrhythmogenic Right Ventricular Dysplasia (ARVD) is a genetic cardiomyopathy characterized by fibro-fatty replacement of the right ventricular myocardium, resulting in arrhythmias and right ventricular failure. ARVD is thought to account for up to 5% of sudden deaths in individuals younger than 35 years in the United States, with an estimated prevalence of 1/5000.[26,27] Symptoms usually first appear in the second and third decades of life, consisting of ventricular arrhythmias, syncope, or sudden cardiac death. Inheritance is autosomal dominant in 30–50% of cases, and a diagnosis often prompts evaluation of first degree relatives.[28]

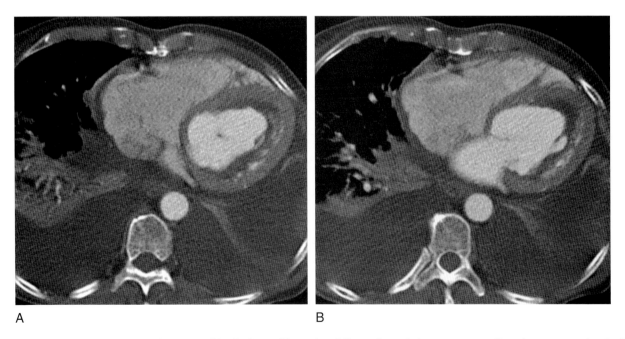

A   B

Figure 17.8   Eosinophilic endomyocarditis. Patient with eosinophilia and restrictive symptoms. Gated contrast-enhanced CT reveals low attenuation confluent subendocardial thrombus in the left ventricle as well as large pleural effusions and basilar atelectasis.

Clinical diagnosis of ARVD is quite challenging, and is based on a set of major and minor criteria proposed by the Task Force of Cardiomyopathies in 1994[29] encompassing electrical, anatomic, and functional abnormalities. Non-invasive imaging often plays an important role in fulfilling these diagnostic criteria. Classic imaging features of ARVD include focal fatty replacement of the right ventricular free wall, focal thinning of the RV wall, RV dilatation and hypokinesis, aneurysmal outpouchings along the RV myocardium, hypertrabeculation and trabecular disarray of the right ventricle, and dilatation of the RV outflow tract. A 'triangle of dysplasia' has been described, consisting of the inferior wall, RV apex, and infundibulum, which are frequent sites of involvement in ARVD.[30]

MRI is performed much more frequently than CT in patients with known or suspected ARVD. Advantages of MRI include its lack of ionizing radiation and iodinated contrast and superior temporal resolution. Nevertheless, CT has been used successfully to detect patients with ARVD.[31–37] Since CT protocols for ARVD generally require cine images (and therefore intravenous contrast) and high spatial resolution, radiation doses can be quite high, and consequently MRI is probably the best choice for evaluating young patients and screening asymptomatic first degree relatives. CT has several advantages, however, including much shorter examination times, limited number and length of breath holds required, and the ability to evaluate patients with pacemakers and AICD devices. Additionally, image quality in CT is generally somewhat less sensitive to degradation by arrhythmias: this can be a frustrating problem with MRI, even using state of the art equipment and pulse sequences. The superior spatial resolution of multidetector CT is also a potential major advantage over MRI: state-of-the-art 64 row MDCT achieves submillimeter isotropic voxels, while most MRI sequences have in-plane resolution approaching 1 mm × 1 mm, and slice thicknesses of 4–8 mm. These differences can be particularly important when searching for subtle anatomic abnormalities in structures as thin as the RV free wall.

CT is able to demonstrate focal fatty infiltration of the RV with an accuracy at least as high as MRI. Care must be taken, however, to distinguish between subpericardial fat and intramyocardial fat. Some authors have noted a clear line of demarcation between subpericardial fat and the RV myocardium in normal patients with disruption of the line in patients with ARVD[30]; in our hands, however, this distinction is quite difficult to make consistently and is of limited practical value. It is also important to remember that fatty infiltration of the right ventricle is not uncommonly seen as a normal variant, more frequently in older patients and in patients with abundant mediastinal and subpericardial fat.[38] The presence of intramyocardial fat should therefore not be interpreted as clear evidence of ARVD without associated functional or morphologic abnormalities (Figure 17.9). Wall thinning is another criteria which in practice is

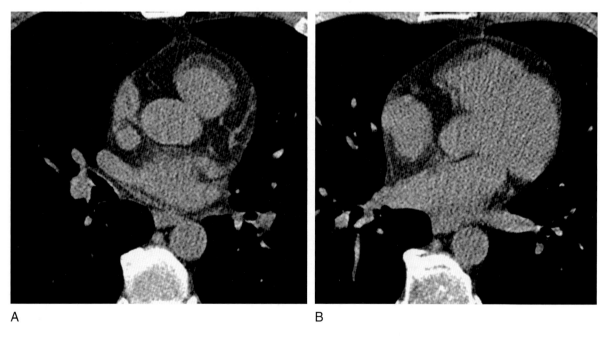

A   B

Figure 17.9 Fatty replacement of the right ventricular free wall as a normal variant. Noncontrast prospectively gated images show a rim of low attenuation fat in the right ventricular outflow tract (a) and the right ventricular free wall (b) in an asymptomatic patient.

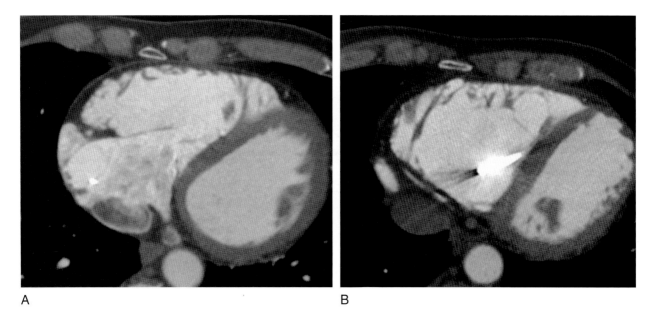

A   B

Figure 17.10   ARVD. Contrast-enhanced prospectively gated images show dilatation of the right ventricle with subtle out-pouchings along the surface of the free wall. Note AICD lead in (B).

difficult to apply, since the normal thickness of the RV free wall ranges from 1–3 mm. Evaluation of reconstructed images in end-systole can be helpful in this regard. The presence of focal aneurysmal outpouchings along the RV free wall with associated hypokinesis or dyskinesis remains the most reliable indication of ARVD in our practice (Figure 17.10).

5 CARDIAC MASSES

Arriving at an exact diagnosis in the setting of a cardiac mass is not always possible with CT, or with any other imaging modality. From a practical standpoint, however, CT is generally very useful.[39] Patients often present with an abnormality detected on echocardiography that might or might not represent a true mass. CT can easily sort out common pseudomasses at echocardiography, such as lipomatous infiltration of the interatrial septum or prominent calcification of the mitral annulus (Figure 17.11). CT is also effective in differentiating mass from thrombus, and can often allow accurate diagnosis of true masses based on location and enhancement characteristics.

Protocols for CT characterization of masses typically include pre and post-contrast gated imaging. Retrospective gating with cine reconstruction may not be required, but is occasionally helpful to assess the functional effect of masses.

Primary cardiac neoplasms are rare, with a cumulative prevalence of 0.002–0.3% in autopsy series. Approximately 75% of primary cardiac tumors are benign, with the most common of these the myxoma, accounting for 30% of all primary tumors. Almost all primary malignant tumors are sarcomas, most often rhabdomyosarcoma and angiosarcoma.[40–42]

Metastatic cardiac disease is 20–40 times more common than primary neoplasms, and may involve the heart by direct extension, hematogenous, or lymphatic spread.[43–47] Bronchogenic carcinoma, breast carcinoma, melanoma, lymphoma, and leukemia are the most frequent primary tumors metastasizing to the heart.

Myxomas are the most common benign primary cardiac tumor, and are typically located in the left atrium (75%), but are occasionally seen in the right atrium (20%). Myxomas typically arise near the fossa ovalis of the interatrial septum from a broad base or a narrow stalk, and are often highly mobile, protruding into the atrioventricular valve during diastole (Figure 17.12). Patients may present with signs and symptoms of embolization or valvular obstruction. Approximately 16% of myxomas have focal calcification, and enhancement is usually heterogeneous. The major differential diagnosis is atrial thrombus.[42,48–51]

Lipomas account for 10% of cardiac tumors. 50% arise from a subendocardial surface, 25% from the epicardium, and 25% have intracavitary extension. Lipomas are easily diagnosed on CT as a lesion with smooth borders showing a density of approximately −100 HU, similar to mediastinal fat (Figure 17.13).[42,52,53] Cardiac lipomas should be differentiated from lipomatous hypertrophy of the interatrial

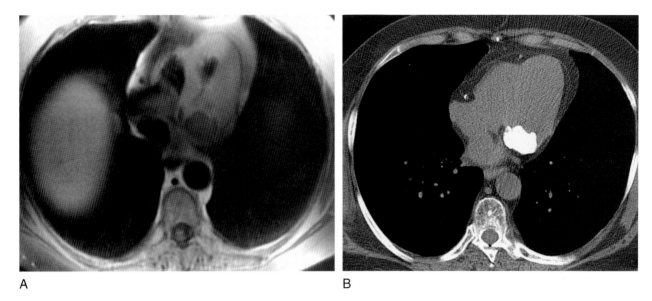

A   B

Figure 17.11   Mitral annular calcification. Patient with mass detected on echocardiography. Axial double inversion recovery MR image (a) reveals a focal mass in the region of the mitral annulus. Noncontrast gated CT image (b) reveals extensive focal calcification of the mitral annulus exactly corresponding to the size of the lesion on MR.

septum (LHIS): this is a normal variant frequently found in older and obese patients. An unusual feature of LHIS is that it may contain brown fat, which can show increased FDG uptake on PET imaging, leading to occasional false positive diagnoses of cardiac metastases.[54,55] LHIS, unlike lipomas, is not encapsulated, and has a characteristic dumbbell shape, with sparing of the foramen ovale (Figure 17.14).

Fibromas are collections of fibroblasts interspersed among large amounts of collagen, and are thought by some pathologists to represent hamartoma rather than true neoplasms. These are most often detected in infants and children, but may be detected in young adults, and are the second most common benign primary cardiac tumor in children after rhabdomyoma.[40] Fibromas are associated with arrhythmias, heart failure, and sudden cardiac death. There is an increased prevalence of cardiac fibromas in Gorlin syndrome, an autosomal dominant disorder associated with basal cell carcinomas, odontogenic keratocysts of the

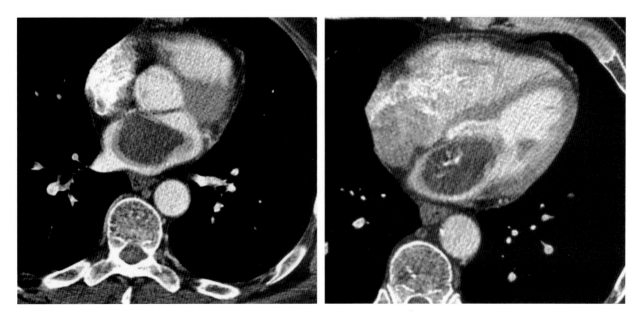

Figure 17.12   Left atrial myxoma. Contrast-enhanced gated CT images reveal a large hypoenhancing mass in the left atrium with some central calcification. Note protrusion of the mass across the mitral valve in (b).

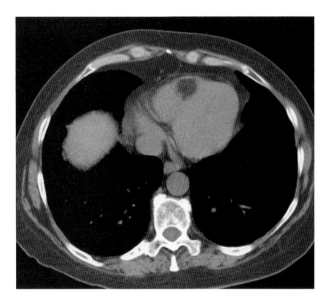

Figure 17.13 Right ventricular lipoma. Non-contrast gated CT image shows a focal mass in the right ventricular apex with signal intensity similar to subcutaneous fat.

mandible, skeletal anomalies, and a tendency toward neoplastic growth in several organ systems. Fibromas typically arise in the myocardium of the interventricular septum and left ventricular free wall. Fibromas may be circumscribed but not truly encapsulated, or infiltrative. On CT, fibromas generally appear as homogeneous masses with soft tissue attenuation, frequently containing calcification.[56,57]

Rhabdomyomas are the most common primary cardiac tumors in children, generally diagnosed in infancy, and are associated with tuberous sclerosis in 50% of cases.[52,58,59] They generally involve the ventricles, and may be large enough to cause obstruction of a valve or cardiac chamber. The majority of rhabdomyomas regress spontaneously, and thus surgery is not required unless the lesions are causing significant symptoms.

Cardiac hemangiomas typically arise from the ventricular myocardium in young to middle aged patients, demonstrate intense enhancement after contrast administration, and may have foci of calcification[59] (Figure 17.15). *Papillary fibroelastomas* are benign endocardial papillomas that predominantly involve cardiac valves. These are probably the second most common benign cardiac neoplasm, but reports of imaging these lesions with CT and MRI are quite rare, due to their small size and rapid motion associated with valve leaflets. Most lesions are detected incidentally on echocardiography as a subcentimeter pedunculated valvular mass.[59–62] *Paragangliomas* are rare vascular tumors arising from intrinsic cardiac paraganglial cells, predominantly located in the atria. Patients may present with hypertension and biochemical evidence of catecholamine overproduction. As many as 20% of patients with cardiac paragangliomas have associated paragangliomas in other locations. Most lesions arise in the left atrium, appear somewhat circumscribed, and show intense contrast enhancement.[42,59,63–65]

Angiosarcoma is the most common primary malignant cardiac tumor, typically occurring in young and middle aged adults who present with right-sided heart failure and

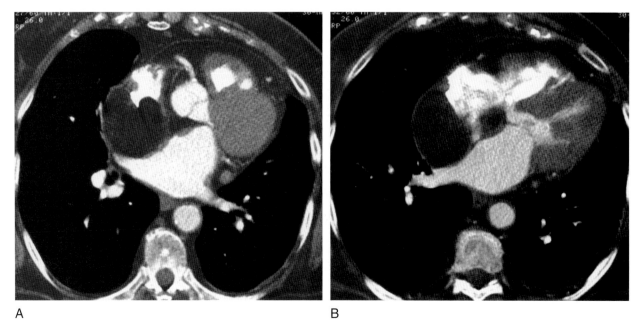

A   B

Figure 17.14 Lipomatous infiltration of the interatrial septum. Contrast-enhanced CT reveals fatty replacement and hypertrophy of the interatrial septum.

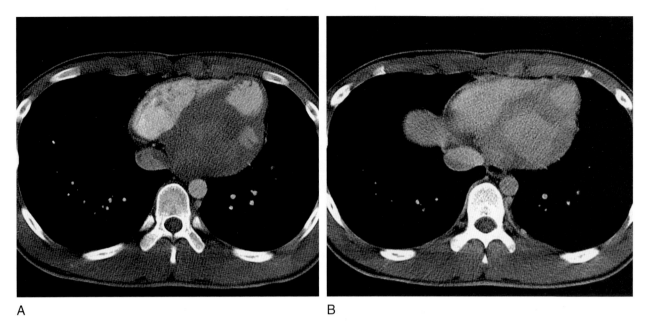

A   B

Figure 17.15   Left ventricular hemangioma. Immediate (a) and 70 second delayed (b) images from contrast-enhanced gated cardiac CT reveal a large lesion in the inferior left ventricle which rapidly enhances and becomes isointense to the ventricular cavity on the delayed image.

tamponade, as the tumor has a striking predilection for the right heart and particularly the right atrium. Angiosarcoma may manifest as a well defined mass projecting into the right atrium or as an infiltrative lesion often invading the RV and pericardium and encasing the right coronary artery. Lesions are typically heterogeneous in appearance, with significant contrast enhancement[66–69] (Figure 17.16).

6 COMPLICATIONS OF MYOCARDIAL ISCHEMIA

Coronary CTA has emerged as an effective technique in many circumstances for direct evaluation of coronary atherosclerosis. Data from coronary CTA may also yield useful information regarding complications of myocardial

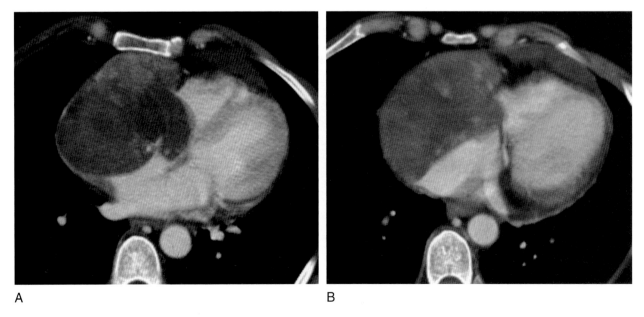

A   B

Figure 17.16   Angiosarcoma. Contrast-enhanced non-gated CT images reveal a large heterogeneously enhancing infiltrative mass invading the right atrium and pericardium.

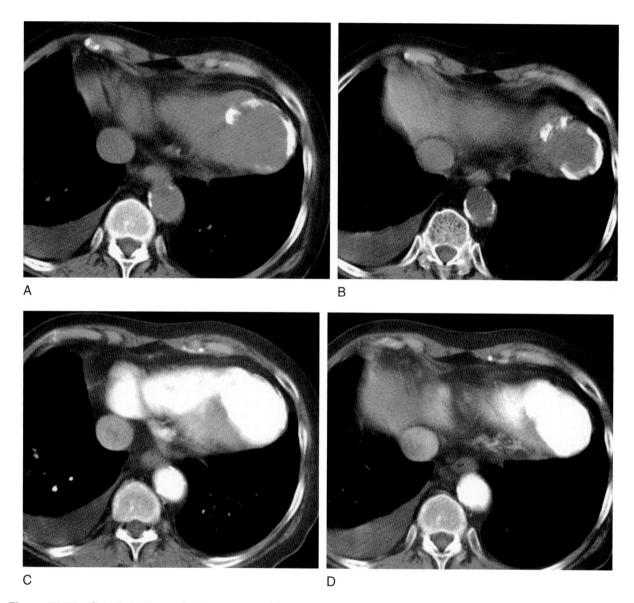

Figure 17.17 Calcified left ventricular aneurysm. Noncontrast (a and b) and post contrast (c and d) gated images reveal focal dilatation of the inferior LV apex with a rim of calcification, representing aneurysm formation following apical infarct.

ischemia. Cine images can be reconstructed in long or short axis views, for example, and examined for evidence of focal wall motion abnormalities or global diminished function. True myocardial aneurysms usually result from prior infarction, are typically anteroapical in location, and have an imaging appearance consisting of a focal bulge in the myocardium, myocardial thinning, and dyskinesis (Figure 17.17). Ventricular pseudoaneurysms represent a contained myocardial rupture, are typically narrow necked and inferolateral in location, and may also occur as a complication of myocardial infarction. Ventricular thrombus occasionally arises in the setting of infarction or ischemia and reduced ventricular function. Thrombus typically arises adjacent to an anterior or apical infarct, and appears as a

filling defect on contrast-enhanced images. In the proper clinical setting, diagnosis of ventricular thombus on CT is usually fairly straightforward (Figure 17.18). Differentiation of thrombus from a focal mass is occasionally problematic; chronic thrombus may partially calcify and can develop granulation tissue which enhances. Mitral insufficiency may result from papillary muscle infarction or rupture, most often occurring in the setting of an inferior infarct disrupting the blood supply of the posteromedial papillary muscle from the posterior descending artery. Mitral insufficiency can be detected and characterized with CT, and the abnormal papillary muscle directly visualized.

Post-infarction pericarditis can occur focally adjacent to the infarct or as a more generalized inflammatory process

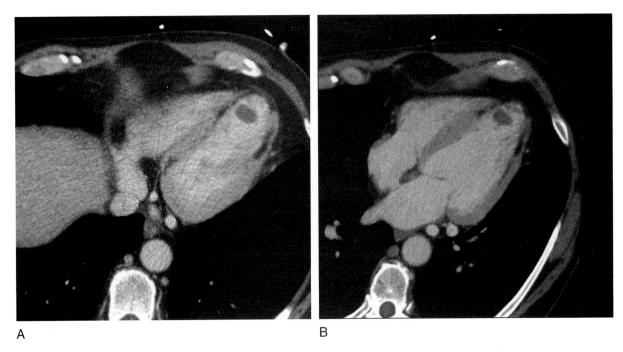

A   B

Figure 17.18   Infarct and left ventricular thrombus. Focal filling defect in the left ventricular apex represents thrombus in a patient with an extensive apical infarct. The old infarct can be seen as a region of subendocardial fatty replacement.

(Dressler's syndrome). CT findings of pericarditis include pericardial thickening, effusion, and enhancement.

7 INCIDENTAL CONGENITAL ANOMALIES

Incidental asymptomatic congenital anomalies are occasionally detected on cardiac CT exams performed for other indications. Small atrial or ventricular septal defects may be seen, for example, or vascular anomalies such as partial anomalous pulmonary venous return, or mild forms of ventricular noncompaction. Careful evaluation of the myocardium, pericardium, and cardiac chambers should always be undertaken whenever cardiac CT is performed, and will occasionally yield interesting and unexpected results (Figure 17.19).

8 CT vs MRI

Whether CT or MRI is the optimal cross-sectional modality to evaluate the myocardium or pericardium depends on a great many factors. Sometimes the decision is easy: equipment for one modality may not be available or may not be state of the art, or technical expertise may be lacking. Patients may not be candidates for a particular technique,

for example, those with pacemakers or AICD devices in the case of MRI or contrast allergies in the case of CT. Radiation doses can be particularly high with gated high resolution CT, particularly if pre and post contrast images are obtained; this should always be a consideration, particularly in radiation-sensitive populations or in those patients who are likely to undergo multiple follow up examinations. On the other hand, some patients are simply unable to tolerate the longer MRI examination with its usual requirement for multiple breath holds, and fare much better with a shorter CT examination. Patients with arrhythmias can be very challenging to image with MRI; while CT image quality is also degraded in the setting of arrhythmias, it is often less affected.

Soft tissue characterization with MRI is superior to CT, and in general this is an advantage for MRI in evaluating cardiac and pericardial masses as well as cardiomyopathies. However, MRI is relatively insensitive to calcium, which is frequently an important finding, and CT is equally sensitive to the presence of fat. CT has superior spatial resolution, a critical consideration when evaluating very small structures. MRI is the gold standard for quantification of cardiac volumes and wall motion; however CT probably has similar accuracy, and cine images from an axial acquisition can be reconstructed in any plane when submillimeter isotropic voxels are acquired. Functional capabilities of MRI include the ability to measure flow and velocity with phase contrast

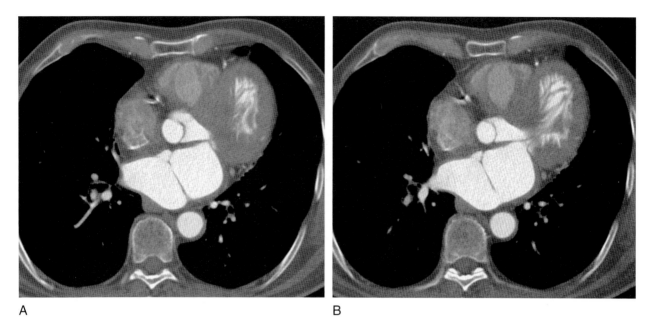

A   B

Figure 17.19   Cor triatriatum. Contrast-enhanced gated CT images demonstrate a septation dividing the anterior and posterior segments of the left atrium.

sequences, which can be useful in assessing valve disease or entities which affect cardiac valves.

9 CONCLUSIONS

Cardiac CT is an important and useful tool in evaluation of the pericardium and myocardium. A wide range of abnormalities can be detected and confidently diagnosed using state of the art cardiac CT. Pericardial effusion, thickening, and calcification are easily demonstrated, as are the morphologic and functional changes of constrictive pericarditis. Pericardial masses can be detected and adequately characterized in most cases, and their anatomic location and invasion of adjacent structures precisely defined. In general MRI is preferred for evaluation of patients with cardiomyopathies due to the superior soft tissue characterization; CT is quite effective in most cases, and is probably equally effective in assessing patients with suspected ARVD. Cardiac masses are also generally well characterized by CT. The presence of fat and/or calcification is frequently the key to distinguishing between benign and malignant etiologies, and CT is an ideal technique in this regard. Since coronary CTA is performed with increasing frequency in the setting of coronary atherosclerosis, myocardial complications of ischemia will be seen with increasing frequency, including aneurysms, infarcts, and functional sequelae of infarctions.

As CT technology continues to improve, additional applications for investigation of myocardial and pericardial pathology will no doubt emerge. Radiation dose and the frequent need for iodinated contrast will remain significant limitations for the foreseeable future; nevertheless, CT is a valuable clinical tool with great flexibility, and the range of clinical applications nicely complements that of MRI.

REFERENCES

1. Moore KL, Dalley AF. Thorax. In: Clinically Oriented Anatomy. New York: Lipincott, Williams and Wilkins, 1999; 60–173.
2. Bull RK, Edwards PD, Dixon AK. CT dimensions of the normal pericardium. Br J Radiol 1998; 71: 923–5.
3. Breen JF. Imaging of the Pericardium. J Thorac Imag 2000; 16: 47–54.
4. Oyama N, Oyama N, Komuro K et al. Computed tomography and magnetic resonance imaging of the pericardium: anatomy and pathology. Magn Reson Med Sci 2004; 3: 145–52.
5. Choi YW, McAdams HP, Jeon SC, Seo HS, Hahm CK. The "high riding" superior pericardial recess: CT findings. AJR 2000; 175: 1025–8.
6. Mulvagh SL, Rokey R, Vick GW, Johnston DL. Usefulness of nuclear magnetic resonance imaging for evaluation of pericardial effusions, and comparison with two-dimensional echocardiography. Am J Cardiol 1989; 64(16): 1002–9.
7. Nishimura RA. Constrictive pericarditis in the modern era: a diagnostic dilemma. Heart 2001; 86: 619–23.

8. Cameron J, Oesterle SN, Baldwin JC, Hancock EW. The etiologic spectrum of constrictive pericarditis. Am Heart J 1987; 113(2 Pt 1): 354–60.

9. Oh KY, Shimizu M, Edwards WD et al. Surgical pathology of the pericardium: a study of 344 cases (1993–1999). Cardiovasc Path 2001; 10: 157–68.

10. Ling LH, Oh JK, Breen JF et al. Calcific constrictive pericarditis: is it still with us? Ann Intern Med 2000; 132: 444–50.

11. Masui T, Finck S, Higgins CB. Constrictive pericarditis and restrictive cardiomyopathy: evaluation with MR imaging. Radiology 1992; 182(2): 369–73.

12. Ghersin E, Lessick J, Litmanovich D et al. Septal bounce in constrictive pericarditis: diagnosis and dynamic evaluation with multidetector CT. J Comput Assist Tomogr 2004; 28: 676–8.

13. Hurrell DG, Nishimura RA, Higano ST et al. Value of dynamic respiratory changes in left and right ventricular pressures for the diagnosis of constrictive pericarditis. Circulation 1996; 93: 2007–13.

14. Spodick DH. Pericardial disease. In: Braunwald E, ed. Heart disease: a textbook of cardiovascular medicine, 6th ed. Philadelphia, PA: Saunders, 2001; 1823–76.

15. Rusk RA, Kenny A. Congenital pericardial defect presenting as chest pain. Heart 1999; 81: 327–8.

16. Gassner I, Judmaier W, Fink C et al. Diagnosis of congenital pericardial defects, including a pathognomic sign for dangerous apical ventricular herniation, on magnetic resonance imaging. Br Heart J 1995; 74: 60–6.

17. Hancock EW. Neoplastic pericardial disease. Cardiol Clin 1990; 8(4): 673–82.

18. Abraham KP, Reddy V, Gattuso P. Neoplasms metastatic to the heart: review of 3314 consecutive autopsies. Am J Cardiovasc Pathol 1990; 3: 195–8.

19. Klatt EC, Heitz DR. Cardiac metastases. Cancer 1990; 65: 1456–9.

20. Wang ZJ, Reddy GP, Gotway MB et al. CT and MR imaging of pericardial disease. Radiographics 2003; 23: S167–S180.

21. Richardson P et al. Report of the 1995 World Health Organization/International Society and Federation of Cardiology Task Force on the definition and classification of cardiomyopathies. Circulation 1996; 93: 841–2.

22. Hughes SE, McKenna WJ. New insights into the pathology of inherited cardiomyopathy. Heart 2005; 91: 257–64.

23. Maron BJ et al. American College of Cardiology/European Society of Cardiology clinical expert consensus document on hypertrophic cardiomyopathy. A report of the American College of Cardiology Foundation Task Force on clinical expert consensus documents and the European Society of Cardiology Committee for practice guidelines. J Am Coll Cardiol 2003; 42: 1687–1713.

24. Fattori R et al. Contribution of magnetic resonance imaging in the differential diagnosis of cardiac amyloidosis and symmetric hypertrophic cardiomyopathy. Am Heart J 1998; 136: 824–30.

25. Maceira AM, Joshi J, Prasad SK et al. Cardiovascular magnetic resonance in cardiac amyloidosis. Circulation 2005; 111: 186–93.

26. Marcus FI, Fontaine GH, Guiraudon G, et al. Right ventricular dysplasia: a report of 24 adult cases. Circulation 1982; 65: 384–98.

27. Laurent M, Descaves C, Biron Y et al. Familial form of arrhythmogenic right ventricular dysplasia. Am Heart J 1987; 113: 827–29.

28. Hamid MS, Gimeno JR, Valdes M, Elliott PM. Prospective evaluation of relatives for familial arrhythmogenic right ventricular cardiomyopathy/dysplasia reveals a need to broaden diagnostic criteria. J Am Coll Cardiol 2002; 40: 1445–50.

29. McKenna WJ, Thiene G, Nava A et al. Diagnosis of arrhythmogenic right ventricular dysplasia/cardiomyopathy. Task force of the working group myocardial and pericardial disease of the European Society of Cardiology and of the Scientific Council on cardiomyopathies of the International Society and Federation of Cardiology. Br Heart J 1994; 71: 215–18.

30. Tandri H, Bomma C, Calkins H, Bluemke DA. Magnetic resonance and computed tomography imaging of arrhythmogenic right ventricular dysplasia. J Magn Reson Imaging 2004; 19: 848–58.

31. Dery R, Lipton MJ, Garrett JS et al. Cine-computed tomography of arrhythmogenic right ventricular dysplasia. J Comput Assist Tomogr 1986; 10: 120–3.

32. Villa A, Di Guglielmo L, Salerno J et al. Arrhythmogenic dysplasia of the right ventricle. Evaluation of 7 cases using computerized tomography. Radiol Med 1998; 75: 28–35.

33. Sotozono K, Imahara S, Masuda H et al. Detection of fatty tissue in the myocardium by using computerized tomography in a patient with arrhythmogenic right ventricular dysplasia. Heart Vessels Suppl 1990; 5: 59–61.

34. Hamada S, Takamiya M, Ohe T, Ueda H. Arrhythmogenic right ventricular dysplasia: evaluation with electron-beam CT. Radiology 1993; 187: 723–7.

35. Tada H, Shimizu W, Ohe T et al. Usefulness of electron-beam computed tomography in arrhythmogenic right ventricular dysplasia. Circulation 1996; 94: 437–44.

36. Kimura F, Sakai F, Sakomura Y et al. Helical CT features of arrhythmogenic right ventricular cardiomyopathy. Radiographics 2002; 22: 1111–24.

37. Bomma C, Tandri H, Nasir K et al. Role of helical CT in qualitative and quantitative evaluation of arrhythmogenic right ventricular dysplasia. Pacing Clin Electrophysiol 2003; 26(Suppl 1): 965.

38. Burke AP, Farb A, Tashko G, Virmani R. Arrhythmogenic right ventricular cardiomyopathy and fatty replacement of the right ventricular myocardium: are they different disease? Circulation 1998; 97: 1571–80.

39. Mousseaux E, Hernigou A, Azencot M et al. Evaluation by electron beam computed tomography of intracardiac masses suspected by transesophageal echocardiography. Heart 1996; 76: 256–63.

40. Burke A, Virmani R. Tumors of the heart and great vessels. In: Atlas of tumor pathology: fasc 16, ser 3. Washington DC: Armed Forces Institute of Pathology, 1996; 1–98.

41. Perchinsky MJ, Lichtenstein SV, Tyers GF. Primary cardiac tumors: forty years' experience with 71 patients. Cancer 1997; 79: 1809–15.

42. Araoz, PA, Mulvagh SL, Tazelaar HD, Julsrud PR, Breen JF. CT and MR imaging of benign primary cardiac neoplasms with echocardiographic correlation. Radiographics 2000; 20: 1303–19.

43. Abraham KP, Reddy V, Gattuso P. Neoplasms metastatic to the heart: review of 3314 consecutive autopsies. Am J Cardiovasc Pathol 1990; 3: 195–8.

44. Klatt EC, Heitz DR. Cardiac metastases. Cancer 1990; 65: 1456–59.

45. Lam KY, Dickens P, Chan AC. Tumors of the heart: a 20 year experience with a review of 12,458 consecutive autopsies. Arch Pathol Lab Med 1993; 117: 1027–31.

46. Nakayama R, Yoneyama T, Takatani O, Kimura K. A study of metastatic tumors to the heart, pericardium, and great vessels. Jpn Heart J 1966; 7: 227–34.

47. Chiles C, Woodard PK, Gutierrez FR, Link KM. Metastatic involvement of the heart and pericardium: CT and MR imaging. Radiographics 2001; 21: 439–49.

48. Reynen K. Cardiac myxomas. N Engl J Med 1995; 333: 1610–17.

49. Tazelaar HD, Locke TJ, McGregor CG. Pathology of surgically excised primary cardiac tumors. Mayo Clin Proc 1992; 67: 957–65.

50. Grebenc ML, Rosado-de-Christenson ML, Green CE, Burke AP, Galvin JR. Cardiac myxoma: imaging features in 83 patients. Radiographics 2002; 22: 673–89.

51. Obeid AI, Marvasti M, Parker F, Rosenberg J. Comparison of transthoracic and transesophageal echocardiography in diagnosis of left atrial myxomas. Am J Cardiol 1989; 63: 1006–8.

52. Schvartzman PR, White RD. Imaging of cardiac and paracardiac masses. J Thoracic Imaging 2000; 15: 265–73.

53. Kamiya H, Ohno M, Iwata H et al. Cardiac lipoma in the interventricular septum: evaluation by computed tomography and magnetic resonance imaging. Am Heart J 1990; 119: 1215–17.

54. Heyer CM et al. Lipomatous hypertrophy of the interatrial septum: a prospective study of incidence, imaging findings, and clinical symptoms. Chest 2003; 124: 2068–73.

55. Chaithiraphan V, Abbara S. MRI of cardiomyopathies and cardiac masses. In: Ho VB, Kransdorf MJ, Reinhold C, eds. Body MRI Categorical Course Syllabus. American Roentgen Ray Society 2006; 125–42.

56. Burke AP, Rosado-de-Christenson M, Templeton PA, Virmani R. Cardiac fibroma: clinico-pathologic correlates and surgical treatment. J Thorac Cardiovasc Surg 1994; 108: 862–70.

57. Beghetti M, Gow RM, Haney I, Mawson J et al. Pediatric primary benign cardiac tumors: a 15 year review. Am Heart J 197; 134: 1107–14.

58. Fenoglio JJ, Callister HA, Ferrans VJ. Cardiac rhabdomyoma: a clinicopathologic and electron microscopic study. Am J Cardiol 1976; 38: 241–51.

59. Grebenc ML, Rodado de Christenson ML, Burke AP, Green CE, Galvin JR. Primary cardiac and pericardial neoplasms: radiologic-pathologic correlation. Radiographics 2000; 20: 1073–11103.

60. Al-Mohammad A, Pambakian H, Young C. Fibroelastoma: case report and review of the literature. Heart 1998; 79: 301–4.

61. Shiraishi J, Tagawa M, Yamada T et al. Papillary fibroelastoma of the aortic valve. Jpn Heart J 2003; 44: 799–803.

62. Wintersperger BJ, Becker CR, Gulbins H et al. Tumors of the cardiac valves: imaging findings in magnetic resonance imaging, electron beam computed tomography, and echocardiography. Eur Radiol 2000; 10: 443–9.

63. Hamilton BH, Francis IR, Gross BH et al. Intrapericardial paragangliomas (pheochromocytomas): imaging features. AJR 1997; 168: 109–13.

64. Nonaka K, Makuuchi H, Naruse Y, Kobayashi T, Goto M. Surgical excision of malignant pheochromocytoma in the left atrium. Jpn J Throrac Cardiovasc Surg 2000; 48: 126–8.

65. Sahdev A, Sohaib A, Monson JP et al. CT and MR imaging of unusual locations of extra-adrenal paragangliomas (pheochromocytomas). Eur Radiol 2005; 15: 85–92.

66. Matheis G, Beyersdorf F. Primary cardiac angiosarcoma: a case report. Cardiology 1995; 86: 83–5.

67. Shin MS, Kirklin JK, Cain JB, Ho KJ. Primary angiosarcoma of the heart: CT characteristics. AJR 1987; 148: 267–8.

68. Bruna J, Lockwood M. Primary heart angiosarcoma detected by computed tomography and magnetic resonance imaging. Eur Radiol 1998; 8: 66–8.

69. Araoz PA, Eklund HE, Welch TJ, Breen JF. CT and MR imaging of primary cardiac malignancies. Radiographics 1999; 1: 1421–34.

18

Assessment of Global and Regional Left Ventricular Function by Computed Tomography

Kai Uwe Juergens, Walter Heindel, and Roman Fischbach

1 INTRODUCTION

Ischemic heart disease is the leading cause of morbidity and mortality in industrialized countries.[1] For clinical diagnosis and risk stratification in patients with suspected or documented heart disease, the accurate and reproducible determination of left ventricular (LV) myocardial function is of utmost importance, as LV volumes and myocardial mass are independent predictors of morbidity and mortality in patients with coronary heart disease.[2,3] Global LV function is considered the strongest determinant of heart failure and death due to myocardial infarction.[4] Furthermore, the evaluation of LV function provides valuable information for treatment planning, monitoring of the efficacy of treatment as well as prognostic parameters in patients with ischemic and nonischemic cardiomyopathy.[3–5]

Currently, global and regional LV function can be assessed using different invasive modalities, i.e. mono- and biplane cineventriculography, and noninvasive imaging modalities, i.e. echocardiography,[6–8] cine magnetic resonance imaging (CMR),[9–18] electron-beam computed tomography (EBCT)[19–23] as well as ECG-gated single photon emission computed tomography (SPECT) and positron emission tomography (PET).[22–25] In clinical practice, the assessment of LV volumes and function is most commonly accomplished with echocardiography as a quick and widely available bedside test as well as with CMR that is currently considered the modality of reference for assessment of cardiac function.[8–10,14]

In 1998, ECG-gated multi-detector row computed tomography (MDCT) was introduced as a noninvasive cardiac imaging technique primarily aiming at the detection of coronary artery stenoses and cardiac morphology. Retrospective ECG gating of a cardiac MDCT study allows for MDCT image reconstruction in any phase of the cardiac cycle, thus end-diastolic and end-systolic images can be produced. Using 4- and 16-slice MDCT LV volumes and global function parameters is assessed in good agreement with cine ventriculography, echocardiography, and CMR. The fast technical development of scanner hardware has lead to a rapid improvement of spatial and temporal resolution, which has made coronary MDCT angiography a robust and widely available technique. Post-processing tools have emerged that allow fast and semiautomatic determination of LV function parameters from MDCT data.[26–44]

229

2 ASSESSMENT OF LV FUNCTION: PHYSIOLOGY AND METHODOLOGY

2.1 Global LV function

During the cardiac cycle, electrical excitation causes a mechanical contraction of the myocardium, resulting in changes of the LV volume: the mechanical cycle starts with an isovolumetric contraction of LV myocardium at the end of the ventricular filling. The increase in ventricular pressure results in the ejection of blood into the systemic and pulmonary circulation that is followed by isovolumetric ventricular relaxation, resulting in the ventricular filling period. Volume changes of the left and the right ventricle within one cardiac cycle are quantitatively comparable (Figure 18.1). LV volumes (LV_{Vol}) are determined using different methodological approaches, the *area-length method*, the *Simpson's method*, and *threshold-based direct volume measurements* (Figure 18.2):

- the *area-length method* is based on a vertical or horizontal long-axis view is primarily used in mono- and biplane cineventriculography as well as in echocardiography according to the formula

$$LV_{Vol} = \frac{8}{3} \times \frac{A^2}{\pi \cdot L}$$ (*A*: ventricular area; *L*: length from apex to mitral valve plane)

- *Simpson's method* primarily used in CMR, EBCT, and MDCT and employs contiguous short-axis images of the left ventricle:
$LV_{Vol} = \Sigma \ A_N \times S$ (*A*: cross-sectional areas; *S*: section thickness)

- the *threshold-based three-dimensional direct volume measurements* from MDCT data sets are achieved by a segmentation technique depicting attenuation or signal intensity differences between myocardium and cardiac chambers; the sum of all contiguous voxels exceeding a predefined attenuation threshold represents the total chamber volume.[45]

Other than the area-length method, threshold-based direct volumetry and Simpson's method do not rely on geometric assumptions and provide more accurate and reproducible results for determination of LV diastolic (EDV) and systolic (ESV) volumes, which are defined as the volumes of the LV cavity determined at end-diastolic and end-systolic phase of the cardiac cycle. From the acquired LV volumes, secondary function parameters are calculated. LV ejection fraction (LVEF) describes the relative change of EDV to ESV during the cardiac cycle: the normal ventricle ejects about two-thirds of its end-diastolic volume during systolic contraction (see reference values in Table 18.1).

$$LVEF = \frac{(EDV - ESV)}{EDV} \times 100 \ [\%].$$

The stroke volume is defined as the absolute change in the LV volume during the cardiac cycle according to the equation SV = EDV − ESV [mL]. The cardiac output (CO) represents the pumped blood volume per minute equaling the stroke volume times heart rate, i.e. CO = SV × heart rate [mL / min].

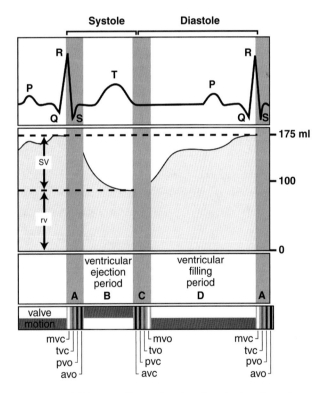

Figure 18.1 Diagram illustrating the electrical and mechanical events during the cardiac cycle; left ventricular volume curve, electrocardiogram and valvular events are depicted:
A: *isovolumetric contraction* phase,
B: *ventricular ejection* period,
C: *isovolumetric relaxation* phase,
D: *ventricular filling* period
(mvc/mvo: mitral valve closing/opening; tvc/tvo: tricuspid valve closing/opening; pvo/pvc: pulmonary valve opening/closing; avo/avc: aortic valve opening/closing; sv: stroke volume, rv: residual volume).

2.2 Regional LV function

The determination of regional LV function parameters refers to the subtle analysis of LV wall segments. In accordance with

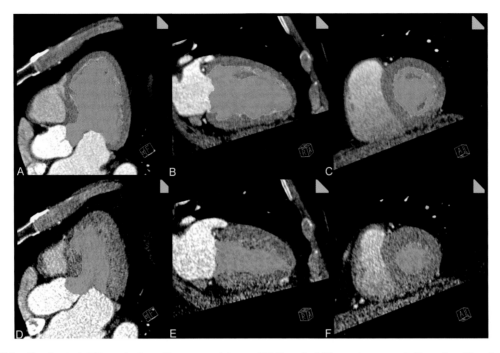

Figure 18.2   Dedicated CT analysis software applying a 3D threshold-based segmentation algorithm for determination of left-ventricular volumes and ejection fraction from diastolic (A-C) and systolic (D-F) Dual Source CT angiography image reformations in a 66-year-old man with suspected coronary artery disease; consecutive blurring of the systolic images due to the application of online dose modulation.

Table 18.1 *Global* (A) and *regional* left ventricular (B) volumetric and functional parameters as determined using Cine Magnetic Resonance Imaging as imaging modality of reference in healthy volunteers (adapted from references 8–10*, and 51)

A

	Male		Female	
Left ventricle	*Range of normal values*	*Mean **	*Range of normal values*	*Mean **
LV-EDV [ml]	102–235	169 ± 33	96–174	135 ± 19
LV-ESV [ml]	29–93	61 ± 16	27–71	49 ± 11
LV-SV	66–148	108 ± 21	62–110	86 ± 12
LV-EF [%]	55–73	64 ± 5	54–74	64 ± 5
LV mass [g]	85–181	133 ± 24	37–67	90 ± 12

B

	Male	Female
Left ventricle		
EDWT [mm]	7.6 ± 1.4	6.3 ± 1.0
ESWT [mm]	13.2 ± 1.8	12.2 ± 1.6
SWT [mm]	5.5 ± 0.8	5.8 ± 1.2
% WT [%]	75 ± 16	96 ± 24

LV: left ventricle/ventricular; EDV: end-diastolic volume, ESV: end-systolic volume; SV: stroke volume; EF: ejection fraction; EDWT: end-diastolic wall thickness; ESWT: end-systolic wall thickness; SWT: systolic wall thickening; % WT: percentual wall thickening.

other cross-sectional imaging modalities, the use of the 17-segment model of the American Heart Association (AHA) is advisable when reporting regional LV wall motion studies.[46] The model is based on short-axis image reformations with six LV segments in the basal and mid-ventricular and four LV segments in the apical section; an additional 17th segment is assigned to the LV apex (Figure 18.3).

The thickness of the normal LV myocardium measures between 6 and 8 mm in diastole and 10 to 14 mm in systole. Systolic contraction within the cardiac cycle results in a thickening of the ventricular myocardium and, thus, a significant reduction of ventricular volume. The normal systolic wall thickening of the LV myocardium measures approximately 5 to 8 mm (Table 18.1).

The continuous change in wall thickness due to LV contraction and relaxation during the cardiac cycle can be semi-quantitatively evaluated by visual assessment from cine loop displays of the moving heart, or quantitatively assessed using dedicated analysis software. A myocardial segment with impaired contraction is called *hypokinetic*, whereas absent motion in a myocardial segment is termed *akinesis*; a paradoxical outward motion during systolic contraction is called *dyskinesis* (Figure 18.4).

Regular systolic myocardial contraction requires functional muscle tissue and relies on sufficient regional blood

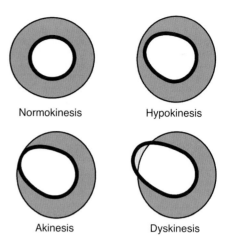

Normokinesis   Hypokinesis

Akinesis   Dyskinesis

Figure 18.4   Four-point scale for qualitative assessment of left ventricular (LV) regional wall motion and graduation of impaired LV function. Regular LV wall motion is classified as normokinesis. LV wall motion disturbance is graded into hypokinesis (reduced regional systolic wall thickening), akinesis (absent regional systolic wall thickening) and dyskinesis (outward movement of the LV wall segment during systolic contraction).

supply. Due to the coronary flow reserve, only high-grade coronary artery obstructions will reduce coronary blood flow below this critical level at rest. Since coronary blood flow increases significantly with exercise, flow obstructing lesions will become symptomatic with regional hypoperfusion and thus a loss of LV contraction. However, scar tissue does not contract and, therefore, does not show systolic wall thickening; wall motion will be affected to various degrees. Stress imaging techniques using exercise or drug induced vasodilatation make use of this fact to diagnose obstructive coronary artery disease based on. Stress imaging requires serial measurements, which are easily achieved with CMR[17,18] and ultrasound, but represent a major limitation for MDCT due to repeated contrast media injections and radiation exposure. Still, MDCT reveals basic information on LV regional wall function at rest and this information comes for free with a coronary CT data set.[41,47,48]

3 MDCT ASSESSMENT OF LV FUNCTION: PRACTICAL APPROACH AND DIAGNOSTIC VALUE

3.1 Global LV function

3.1.1 Global LV function: MDCT protocol

MDCT data acquisition is based on the routine protocols used for coronary artery imaging as LV function assessment

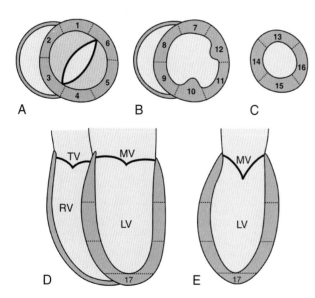

Figure 18.3   Seventeen-segment model used for segment-based MRI and MDCT analysis of regional left ventricular (LV) function (modified from Cerqueira 2002, ref. 46): (A), (B), and (C): short-axis planes (A. basal, B. mid-cavity, C. apical), (D): horizontal long-axis, and (E): vertical long-axis. *LV-Segments (S) 1, 7, and 13*: anterior; *S 2, and 8*: anteroseptal; *S 3, and 9*: inferoseptal; *S 4, 10, and 15*: inferior; *S 5, and 11*: inferolateral; *S 6, and 12*: anterolateral; *S 14*: septal; *S 16*: lateral; *S 17*: apex (RV= right ventricle, TV= tricuspid valve, LV= left ventricle, MV= mitral valve).

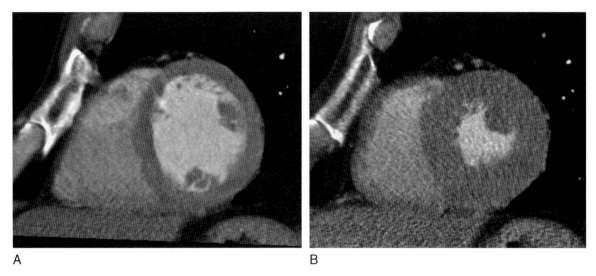

A   B

Figure 18.5   Diastolic (A) and systolic (B) short-axis image reformation in a 59-year-old man undergoing Dual-Source CT angiography for exclusion of coronary artery disease demonstrate the effect of online dose modulation with consecutive blurring of the systolic image: LV-ejection fraction was regular (65.2%).

is usually performed complementary to coronary CT angiography. Depending on the scanner used, scan protocols may differ. With the introduction of advanced MDCT scanners with up to 40-/64- detector rows and Dual-source CT (DSCT) systems, CT scan duration is 6 to 12 seconds.[42,44,59-62] The performance of automatic segmentation algorithms varies with the quality of contrast opacification, which is focused on the coronary arteries and the left ventricle. If functional parameters are to be obtained, delineation of the right atrium and ventricle and the septal myocardium is improved with a modified contrast injection scheme using either a biphasic injection or application of diluted contrast after the initial bolus injection.

Prospective tube current modulation is available with routine coronary artery scan protocols; as tube current is reduced during the systolic phase image noise increases significantly (Figure 18.5). Since LV function studies do not need high resolution images and use thicker section thickness, prospective tube current modulation does not affect accurate endocardial border delineation or LV segmentation in the systolic phase; however, published reports have not included tube current modulation with their imaging protocols.

3.2 Global LV function: MDCT data post-processing and analysis

For accurate and reproducible analysis of LV function, MDCT data postprocessing should enable data reconstruction of the

entire RR interval in 5 to 10% steps. In principle, solely a diastolic and systolic phase reconstruction each is necessary for global LV function assessment. The appropriate reconstruction windows for the systolic and diastolic phases are visually identified as the images showing the minimum ventricular diameter, as well as the maximum ventricular diameter from axial images at a representative mid-ventricular level (Figure 18.6) reconstructed every 5% of the RR-interval.[36] Using dedicated postprocessing software, MDCT data reconstruction is performed either in short-axis orientation to apply the *Simpson's approach* or in axial orientation enabling *threshold-based 3D-volumetry*. The section thickness for short-axis images is set to five to eight millimeters according to recommendations by several studies.[33,34,36,41,52,53]

In principle, diastolic and systolic LV volumes can be calculated using standard MDCT software tools for area and distance measurements when applying the *area-length method*. However, studies performed since 2004 used commercially available dedicated MDCT analysis software packages exclusively, either applying the Simpson's method or enabling threshold-based 3D-volumetry. Performing the Simpson's method on short-axis image MDCT reformations only the delineation of endocardial borders is necessary for global LV function assessment: contours are either automatically detected by the analysis software or/and have to be manually traced/corrected on the diastolic and systolic short-axis image reformations, resulting in a time-consuming procedure. An accurate definition of the basal slice is desired as it contains the largest area of the MDCT image

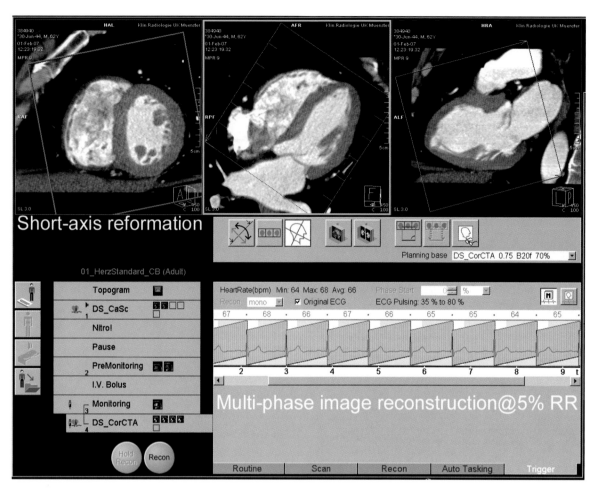

Figure 18.6   Dedicated postprocessing software enable multi-phase MDCT data reconstruction in 5% steps of the entire RR-interval, either in short-axis orientation (as shown) to apply the *Simpson's approach,* or in axial orientation enabling *threshold-based 3D-volumetry*; the section thickness for short-axis images is set to five to eight millimeters.

reformations stack, and a potential error in LV volumetry might be caused from inadequate slice selection. LV papillary muscles are included in the LV lumen and, therefore, do not need additional contouring.[36] Evaluation software for (semi-) automated LV volume and wall thickness measurements helps to standardize and to speed up analysis and reporting.

Recent developments in postprocessing MDCT software enable threshold based 3D-volumetry;[37,53] thus, LV volume assessment accomplished by much faster and with less user interaction compared to a conventional slice-by-slice assessment according to the Simpson's method has become feasible. Artifacts induced by electrodes of pacemakers or implanted cardio-defibrillators (ICD) and contrast-media in the ventricular cavities might cause systematical errors in threshold-based volumetry. To date, however, prospective studies comparing different evaluation software packages for cardiac MDCT are not available.

3.2.1 Global LV function: MDCT accuracy and reproducibility

Multiple single-center studies have been published determining global LV volume and function parameters using 4-, 8- and 16-slice CT;[30–41,53–83] recently, initial experience on LV function assessment with 64-slice CT systems has been reported.[52,84] LV-EDV, LV-ESV and LV-EF determined by MDCT showed a good agreement with measurements from cineventriculography, echocardiography, SPECT and CMR in patients with suspected or manifest CHD; LV-ESV was slightly overestimated by MDCT versus CMR, resulting in a systematic underestimation of LV-EF from 1 to 7%, most likely due to the limited temporal resolution achieved by MDCT systems used, yielding a temporal resolution between 125 and 250 ms with single or bi-segment image reconstruction (Table 18.2). However, a temporal resolution of 30 to 50 ms per image is mandatory to capture the maximum

Table 18.2 Left ventricular end-diastolic and end-systolic volumes and ejection fraction determined from 4- (A) 8-, 16-, and 64-slice (B) spiral Computed Tomography (MDCT) of the heart in comparison to competitive imaging modalities.

A. Comparison of 4-slice MDCT used for determination of LV end-diastolic (LV-EDV) and end-systolic (LV-ESV) volumes as well as ejection fraction (LV-EF) to cineventriculography (CVG), 2D-echocardiography (2D-Echo) and Cine Magnetic Resonance Imaging (CMR) using Turbo gradient-echo (TGrE) and Steady-State free precession (SSFP) Cine sequences. Cc: Correlation coefficient.

Author	N	Modality compared to MDCT	LV-EDV - Cc-	LV-ESV - Cc-	LV-EF - Cc-	Δ LV-EF using MDCT
Hosoi et al. *Radiat Med* 2003	11	CVG	0.95	0.98	0.93	-
Heuschmid et al. *RÖFO* 2003	25	CVG	0.59	0.82	0.88	−17 ± 9%
Hundt et al. *J Comput Assist Tomogr* 2005	30	CVG	0.73	0.88	0.76	−13 ± 22.5 %
Grude et al. *Invest Radiol* 2003	28	TGrE - CMR	0.92	0.90	0.90	−7.9 ± 5.6%
Erhard et al. *RÖFO* 2002	7	SSFP - CMR	0.93	0.95	0.83	−3.8 ± 9.4%
Halliburton et al. *Int J Card Imag* 2003	15	SSFP - CMR	0.26	0.62	0.30	−1.6%
Mahnken et al. *RÖFO* 2003	16	SSFP - CMR	0.99	0.99	0.98	−0.9 ± 3.6%
Juergens et al. *Radiology* 2004	30	SSFP - CMR	0.93	0.94	0.89	−0.2 ± 4.9%

B. Comparison of 8-(Ω), 16-, and 64-slice MDCT used for determination of LV-EDV and LV-ESV, and LV-EF to 2D-echocardiography, ECG-gated SPECT, and Magnetic Resonance Imaging using SSFP Cine sequences (SSFP-CMR). Cc: Correlation coefficient.

Author	N	Modality compared to MDCT	LV-EDV - Cc-	LV-ESV - Cc-	LV-EF - Cc-	Δ LV-EF using MDCT
Koch et al. *RÖFO* 2004	19	SSFP - CMR	0.96	0.98	0.91	−3.0 ± 7.1 %
Heuschmid et al. *RÖFO* 2005	31	SSFP - CMR	0.86	0.91	0.87	1.4 ± 5.2 %
Yamamuro et al. *Radiology* 2005 (Ω)	50	SSFP - CMR	0.97	0.99	0.96	−1.2 ± 4.6 %
Mahnken et al. *Eur Radiol* 2005	21	SSFP - CMR	0.99	0.99	0.99	−0.07 ± 2.0%
Juergens et al. *Am J Roentgenol* 2006	20	SSFP - CMR	0.96	0.95	0.92	−2.1 ± 3.6 %
Schuijf et al. *Int J Cardiol* 2006	70	2D-Echo	0.97	0.98	0.91	1.7 ± 4.9 %
Heuschmid et al. *Eur Radiol* 2006	52	SSFP - CMR	0.83	0.90	0.88	1.8 ± 4.7 %
Belge et al. *Eur Radiol* 2006	40	SSFP - CMR	0.82	0.87	0.96	−0.5 ± 13.0 %
Dewey et al. *Eur Radiol* 2006	33	SSFP - CMR	0.90	0.90	0.86	−2.1 ± 8.2 %
Dewey et al. *J Am Coll Cardiol* 2006	88	SSFP - CMR	0.87	0.92	0.91	−2.1± 5.2 %
Sugeng et al. *Circulation* 2006	31	SSFP - CMR	0.98	0.97	0.93	−1.8 ± 5.4 %
Fischbach et al. *Eur Radiol* 2006	30	SSFP - CMR	0.96	0.94	0.83	−2.5 ± 4.2 %
Henneman et al. *J Nucl Cardiol* 2006	40	2D-Echo	0.97	0.98	0.91	−2.5 ± 9.8 %
Schepis et al. *J Nucl Med* 2006	60	Gated SPECT	0.89	0.95	0.82	1.1 ± 1.7 %

systolic contraction, especially in patients with higher heart rates.[11] Due to improved temporal resolution of 40-, 64- and Dual-Source CT scanners, an even better agreement of MDCT and CMR assessment of LV function is to be expected. To date, no data on DSCT assessment of LV function has been published in the literature.

At present, the clinical experience with MDCT LV function analysis is limited to specialized centers, as well as small numbers of patient and rather homogenous patient populations reported to date with CHD and near normal ranges of LV size, configuration, and function. Since MDCT is a true volumetric modality, the accuracy of the measurements is not supposed to be influenced by

enlarged or grossly deformed hearts; however, the proof of this hypothesis is still pending. Recent studies demonstrated accurate determination of global cardiac function parameters by 16-slice CT in patients with LV dysfunction due to different pathologies, e.g. previous myocardial infarction, or LV dilatation. Reproducibility of global LV function parameters was found within the range of other modalities with the interobserver variability being 0.5 to 11.5 % for LV-EDV and LV-ESV, and 2 to 8.6 % for LV-EF; corresponding values for CMR are 2 to 6 %.[34,38,52,65,77,79,81]

The total evaluation time of MDCT global LV function analysis has been reported as ranging between 30 to 50 minutes on 4-slice MDCT[35] versus 14 to 20 minutes applying software-assisted LV function analysis according to Simpson's method on 16-slice MDCT.[55,79,83] A significant reduction in postprocessing time will be achieved by advanced raw data reconstruction algorithms, allowing interactive planning and direct calculation of multiphase short-axis images, and the use of automatic LV segmentation for volume and ejection fraction determination.

3.3 Regional LV function

3.3.1 Regional LV function: MDCT protocol, data post-processing and analysis

Regional LV function is determined from the identical MDCT data sets as global function parameters. With currently available MDCT reconstruction algorithms developed for coronary artery visualization, a temporal resolution between 100 to 250 ms, as achieved by 4- to 16-slice MDCT, is sufficient to display diastolic and systolic phases in most patients, but fast volume changes during the rapid systolic ventricular filling and ejection phases (Figure 18.1) are not adequately detected. While plain LV volume determination is feasible in good agreement with competitive imaging modalities, regional LV function assessment, especially detection of diastolic dysfunction, is limited. Sixty-four-slice MDCT, as well as currently introduced DSCT systems (Figures 18.7, 18.8) is providing a constant temporal resolution of 83 ms and up to 40 ms using multi-segment data reconstruction algorithms, might help to overcome this limitation.

Therefore, standardized MDCT data postprocessing for regional LV wall motion assessment should include image reconstructions of 20 phases at 5% steps of the RR-interval from CT raw data sets to utilize the full diagnostic potential from the improved temporal resolution. Multiphase MDCT images are reconstructed in short-axis (section thickness 5 to 8 mm), vertical, and horizontal long-axis (section thickness 2 to 3 mm) orientation enabling semi-quantitative analysis of regional LV function parameters: using MDCT analysis software images from corresponding slice positions are visually reviewed in a cine loop to qualitatively assess LV wall motion applying the 17-segment AHA-model and grading segmental LV wall motion according to a 4-point scale.

Quantitative regional LV function assessment requires delineation of endocardial and epicardial LV contours for measuring diastolic and systolic LV wall thickness, systolic wall thickening, and the determination of LV myocardial mass, which is considered to be an important follow-up parameter in patients treated for arterial hypertension. Generation and edition of endo- and epicardial LV contours is supported by dedicated MDCT analysis software applying the Simpson's method on short-axis image reformations or the 3D threshold based region-growing segmentation algorithm based on axial MDCT images. The continuous changes in wall thickness due to LV contraction and relaxation are calculated as myocardial wall thickness over time, i.e. during the cardiac cycle, and expressed as time-volume-curves. Normalization to body-surface-area enables comparison to reference values (Table 18.1 A and B).

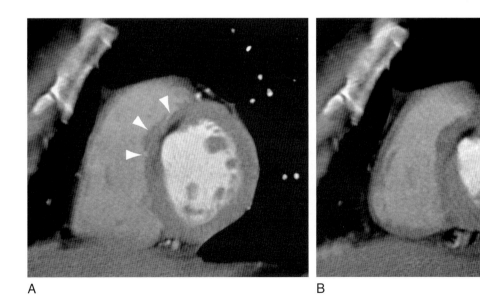

A   B

Figure 18.7 Dual-Source CT study from a 37-year-old man with previous subendocardial anteroseptal infarction (*arrows*), hypokinesis of the antero-septal myocardium and reduced global left ventricular (LV) function (LV-ejection fraction 54.2%).

3.2.2 Regional LV function: MDCT accuracy and reproducibility

To date, semi-quantitative visual analysis and quantification of regional LV function parameters have been reported by a few single-center studies using 4-slice,[31,38,51,56] 16-slice,[54,55,60,61,67,75,82] and 64-slice MDCT.[52,84] MDCT reveals basic information on LV regional wall function at rest, as systolic and diastolic image reconstructions depict changes in wall thickness and multiphase reconstructions[45] allow analysis of the LV wall motion over the cardiac cycle. Normokinetic LV segments are reliably identified with MDCT.[54] Even areas of impaired motion were identified with sufficient reliability in comparison to CMR, echocardiography, and ECG-gated SPECT; however, sensitivity for detection and accurate classification of LV wall motion abnormalities needs to be improved (Table 18.2). Further improvement of the MDCT system's temporal resolution seems to be the most important factor for enhancing MDCT performance.[54] The definitive role and diagnosis value of MDCT in a clinical setting needs to be further defined, once improved postprocessing tools and scanners with improved temporal resolution have become widely available.

Due to significantly improved temporal resolution, an even better agreement of quantitative MDCT and CMR assessment of regional LV function parameters is to be

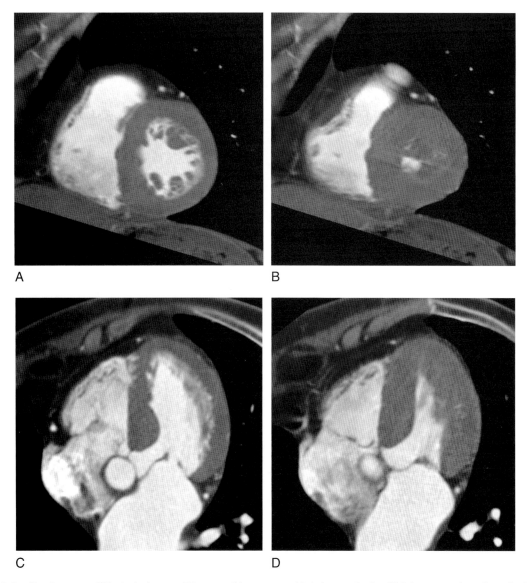

A

B

C

D

Figure 18.8   Dual-source CT study from a 76-year-old woman with left ventricular (LV) hypertrophy: diastolic (A+C) and systolic (B+D) short-axis (A+B) and four-chamber (C+D) image reformations showed myocardial hypertrophy, particularly of the interventricular septum without obstruction of the LV outflow-tract; LV-ejection fraction was normal (72.5%).

expected from DSCT systems. The determination of LV myocardial ischemia and its consecutive regional dysfunction is important with regard to the clinical management of patients with CHD, especially if viable LV myocardium can be detected and myocardial revascularization might lead to improvement in LV function and patient survival. Initial observations made in a study comparing myocardial enhancement patterns seen with MDCT to dual isotope SPECT showed that the extent of an early myocardial enhancement deficit could predict subsequent myocardial wall thickness and wall motion recovery in patients after successful revascularization.[85]

4 CONCLUSIONS

Left ventricular function assessment with MDCT has entered clinical routine as multiple studies on 4- to 64-slice CT systems have demonstrated that MDCT allows for reliable determination of LV volumes and global LV function parameters in good agreement with established imaging modalities. Although MDCT is still not considered a first-line modality for LV function assessment, this technique provides clinically valuable additional information in patients undergoing MDCT coronary angiography, contributing to a combined assessment of cardiac morphology and LV function without the need of additional radiation exposure. As CMR is contraindicated, MDCT enables LV function assessment in patients with implanted pacemakers and ICD, especially in follow-up after cardiac resynchronization therapy. With improvements in dedicated postprocessing and image analysis software, a further increase in clinical applicability of global LV function evaluation has to be expected. Regional LV wall motion analysis at rest is feasible from MDCT data sets in good agreement with competitive imaging modalities; however, sensitivity for detection and accurate classification of LV wall motion abnormalities using 16-slice CT scanners needs to be improved. As provided by 64-slice MDCT and DSCT systems further improvement in temporal resolution seems to be mandatory to match regional LV function analysis obtained from CMR and echocardiography, especially if any stress tests with MDCT are intended.

REFERENCES

1. Murray CJ, Lopez AD. Alternative projections of mortality and disability by cause 1990–2020: global burden of disease study. Lancet 1997; 349: 1498–1504.

2. Hammermeister KE, DeRouen TA, Dodge HT. Variables predictive of survival in patients with coronary disease. Selection by univariate and multivariate analyses from the clinical, electrocardiographic, exercise, arteriographic, and quantitative angiographic evaluations. Circulation 1979; 59: 421–30.

3. White HD, Norris RM, Brown MA et al. Left ventricular end-systolic volume as the major determination of survival after recovery from myocardial infarction. Circulation 1987; 76: 44–51.

4. Shah PK, Maddahi J, Staniloff HM et al. Variable spectrum and prognostic implications of left and right ventricular ejection fraction in patients with and without clinical heart failure after acute myocardial infarction. Am J Cardiol 1986; 58: 387–93.

5. Buck T, Hunold P, Wentz KU et al. Tomographic three-dimensional echocardiographic determination of chamber size and systolic function in patients with left ventricular aneurysm: comparison to magnetic resonance imaging, cineventriculography, and two-dimensional echocardiography. Circulation 1997; 96: 4286–97.

6. Kuhl HP, Spuentrup E, Wall A et al. Assessment of myocardial function with interactive non-breath-hold real-time MR imaging: comparison with echocardiography and breath-hold Cine MR imaging. Radiology 2004; 231: 198–207.

7. Malm S, Frigstad S, Sagberg E, Larsson H, Skjaerpe T. Accurate and reproducible measurement of left ventricular volume and ejection fraction by contrast echocardiography: a comparison with magnetic resonance imaging. J Am Coll Cardiol 2004; 44: 1030–35.

8. Lorenz CH, Walker ES, Morgan VL, Klein SS, Graham Jr TP. Normal human right and left ventricular mass, systolic function, and gender differences by Cine Magnetic Resonance Imaging. J Card Magn Reson 1999; 1: 7–21.

9. Sandstede J, Lipke C, Beer M et al. Age- and gender-specific differences in left and right ventricular cardiac function and mass determined by cine magnetic resonance imaging. Eur Radiol 2000; 10: 438–42.

10 Alfakih K, Plein S, Thiele H et al. Normal human left and right ventricular dimensions for MRI as assessed by turbo gradient echo and steady-state free precession imaging sequences. J Magn Reson Imaging 2003; 17: 323–29.

11 Setser RM, Fischer SE, Lorenz CH. Quantification of left ventricular function with magnetic resonance images acquired in real time. J Magn Reson Imaging 2000; 12: 430–8.

12. Barkhausen J, Ruehm SG, Goyen M et al. MR evaluation of ventricular function: true fast imaging with steady-state precession versus fast low-angle shot cine MR imaging: feasibility study. Radiology 2001; 219: 264–9.

13. Thiele H, Nagel E, Paetsch I et al. Functional cardiac MR imaging with steady-state free precession (SSFP) significantly improves endocardial border delineation without contrast agents. J Magn Reson Imaging 2001; 14: 362–7.

14. Messrroghli DR, Bainbridge GJ, Alfakih K et al. Assessment of regional left ventricular function accuracy and reproducibility of positioning standard short-axis sections in cardiac MR imaging. Radiology 2005; 235: 229–36.

15. Plein S, Smith WHT, Ridgway JP et al. Qualitative and quantitative analysis of regional left ventricular wall dynamics using real-time magnetic resonance imaging: comparison with conventional breath-hold gradient echo acquisition in

volunteers and patients. J Magn Reson Imaging 2001; 14: 23–30.

16 Spuentrup E, Schroeder J, Mahnken AH et al. Quantitative assessment of left ventricular function with interactive real-time spiral and radial MR imaging. Radiology 2003; 227: 870–6.

17. Kuijpers D, Janssen CHC, van Dijkman PRM, Oudkerk M. Dobutamine stress MRI. Part I. Safety and feasibility of dobutamine cardiovascular magnetic resonance in patients suspected of myocardial ischemia. Eur Radiol 2004; 14: 1823–8.

18. Kuijpers D, van Dijkman PRM, Janssen CHC et al. Dobutamine stress MRI. Part II. Risk stratification with dobutamine cardiovascular magnetic resonance in patients suspected of myocardial ischemia. Eur Radiol 2004; 14: 2046–52.

19. Boyd DP, Lipton MJ. Cardiac computed-tomography. Proc IEEE 1983; 71: 298–307.

20. Lipton MJ, Higgins CB, Farmer D et al. Cardiac imaging with a high-speed Cine-CT scanner: preliminary results. Radiology 1984; 152: 579–82.

21. Woo P, Mao S, Wang S, Detrano RC. Left ventricular size determined by electron beam computed tomography predicts significant coronary artery disease and events. Am J Cardiol 1997; 79: 1236–8.

22. Gerber TC, Behrenbeck T, Allison T et al. Comparison of measurement of left ventricular ejection fraction by Tc-99 m sestamibi first-pass angiography with electron beam computed tomography in patients with anterior wall acute myocardial infarction. Am J Cardiol 1999; 83: 1022–6.

23. Manrique A, Faraggi M, Vera P et al. TI-201 and Tc-99m MIBI gated SPECT in patients with large perfusion defects and left ventricular dysfunction: comparison with equilibrium radionuclide angiography. J Nucl Med 1999; 40: 805–9.

24. Bavelaar-Croon CD, Kayser HW, van der Wall EE et al. Left ventricular function: correlation of quantitative gated SPECT and MR imaging over a wide range of values. Radiology 2000; 217: 572–5.

25. Slart RHJA, Bax JJ, de Jong RM et al. Comparison of gated PET with MRI for evaluation of left ventricular function in patients with coronary artery disease. J Nucl Med 2004; 45: 176–82.

26. Nieman K, Cademartiri F, Lemos PA et al. Reliable noninvasive coronary angiography with fast submillimeter multislice spiral computed tomography. Circulation 2002; 106: 2051–4.

27. Ropers D, Baum U, Pohle K et al. Detection of coronary artery stenoses with thin-slice multi-detector row spiral computed tomography and multiplanar reconstruction. Circulation 2003; 107: 664–6.

28. Hoffmann U, Moselewski F, Cury RC et al. Predictive value of 16-slice multidetector spiral computed tomography to detect significant obstructive coronary artery disease in patients at high risk for coronary artery disease: patient-versus-segment-based analysis. Circulation 2004; 110: 2638–43.

29. Dewey M, Laule M, Krug L et al. Multisegment and halfscan reconstruction of 16-slice computed tomography for detection of coronary artery stenoses. Invest Radiol 2004;39: 223–9.

30. Juergens KU, Grude M, Fallenberg EM et al. Using ECG-gated Multidetector CT to evaluate global left ventricular myocardial function in patients with coronary artery disease. Am J Roentgenol 2002; 179: 1545–50.

31. Dirksen MS, Bax JJ, de Roos A et al. Usefulness of dynamic multislice computed tomography of left ventricular function in unstable angina pectoris and comparison with echocardiography. Am J Cardiol 2002; 90: 1157–60.

32. Hosoi S, Mochizuki T, Miyagawa M et al. Assessment of left ventricular volumes using multidetector row computed tomography (MDCT): phantom and human studies. Radiat Med 2003; 21: 62–7.

33. Heuschmid M, Küttner A, Schröder S et al. Left ventricular functional parameters using ECG-gated multidetector spiral CT in comparison with invasive ventriculography. Fortschr Röntgenstr 2003; 175: 1349–54.

34. Grude M, Juergens KU, Wichter T et al. Evaluation of global left ventricular myocardial function with electrocardiogram-gated multidetector computed tomography: comparison with magnetic resonance imaging. Invest Radiol 2003; 38: 653–61.

35. Boehm T, Alkadhi H, Roffi M et al. Time-effectiveness, observer-dependence, and accuracy of measurements of left ventricular ejection fraction using 4-channel MDCT. Fortschr Röntgenstr 2004; 176: 529–37.

36. Juergens KU, Grude M, Maintz D et al. Multi-Detector Row CT of Left Ventricular Function with Dedicated Analysis Software versus MR Imaging: Initial Experience. Radiology 2004: 230: 403–10.

37. Ehrhard K, Oberholzer K, Gast K et al. Multislice CT (MSCT) in cardiac function imaging: threshold-value-supported 3D volume reconstructions to determine the left ventricular ejection fraction in comparison to MRI. Fortschr Röntgenstr 2002; 174: 1566–69.

38. Mahnken AH, Spuentrup E, Niethammer M et al. Quantitative and qualitative assessment of left ventricular volume with ECG-gated multislice Spiral CT: value of different image reconstruction algorithms in comparison to MRI. Acta Radiol 2003; 604–11.

39. Halliburton SS, Petersilka M, Schvartzman PR, Obuchowski N, White RD. Evaluation of left ventricular dysfunction using multiphasic reconstructions of coronary multi-slice computed tomography data in patients with chronic ischemic heart disease: validation against cine magnetic resonance imaging. Int J Card Imaging 2003; 19: 73–83.

40. Mahnken AH, Spüntrup E, Wildberger JE et al. Quantification of cardiac function with multislice spiral CT using retrospective ECG-gating: comparison with MRI. Fortschr Röntgenstr 2003; 175: 83–8.

41. Coche E, Belge B, Vlassenbroeck A et al. Accurate assessment of left ventricular volumes and ejection fraction using retrospectively gated multislice cardiac CT: comparison with cine MRI. Eur Radiol 2004; 14: S2–270.

42. Raff GL, Gallagher MJ, O'Neill WW et al. Diagnostic accuracy of noninvasive coronary angiography using 64-spiral spiral computed tomography. J Am Coll Cardiol 2005; 46: 552–7.

43. Schuijf JD, Bax JJ, Shaw LJ et al. Meta-analysis of comparative diagnostic performance of magnetic resonance imaging and multislice computed tomography for noninvasive coronary angiography. Am Heart J 2006; 151: 404–11.

44. Leschka S, Husmann L, Desbiolles LM et al. Optimal image reconstruction intervals for non-invasive coronary angiography with 64-slice CT. Eur Radiol 2006; 16: 1964–72.

45. Juergens KU, Fischbach R. Left ventricular function studied with MDCT. Eur Radiol 2006; 16: 342–57.

46. Cerqueira MD, Weissman NJ, Dilsizian V et al. Standardized myocardial segmentation and nomenclature for

tomographic imaging of the heart. A statement for healthcare professionals from the Cardiac Imaging Committee of the Council on Clinical Cardiology of the American Heart Association. Circulation 2002; 105: 539–42.

47. Leitlinien der Deutschen Röntgengesellschaft (DRG) für den Einsatz der MR-Tomographie in der Herzdiagnostik. Fortschr Röntgenstr 2004; 176: 1185–93.

48. Juergens KU, Schulze Eilfing B et al. Anatomy and morphology of the heart based on Multidetector-row computed tomography coronary angiography: Morphometric analysis of 60 middle aged asymptomatic male individuals. Eur Radiol 2004; 14: R3.

49. Leber AW, Knez A, von Ziegler F et al. Quantification of obstructive and nonobstructive coronary lesions by 64-slice computed tomography: a comparative study with quantitative coronary angiography and intravascular ultrasound. J Am Coll Cardiol 2005; 46: 147–54.

50. Achenbach S, Ropers D, Kuettner A et al. Contrast-enhanced coronary artery visualization by dual-source computed tomograpyhy – initial experience. Eur J Radiol 2005; 57: 331–5.

51. Johnson TR, Nikolaou K, Wintersperger BJ et al. Dual-source CT cardiac imaging: initial experience. Eur Radiol 2006; 16: 1409–15.

52. Schepis T, Gaemperli O, Koepfli P et al. Comparison of 64-slice CT with gated SPECT for evaluation of left ventricular function. J Nucl Med 2006; 47: 1288–94.

53 Muhlenbruch G, Das M, Hohl C et al. Global left ventricular function in cardiac CT. Evaluation of an automated 3D region-growing segmentation algorithm. Eur Radiol 2006; 16: 1117–23.

54. Fischbach R, Juergens KU, Ozgun M et al. Assessment of regional LV function with Multidetector-row Computed Tomography versus Magnetic Resonance Imaging. Eur Radiol 2007; 17:1009–17.

55. Koch K, Oellig F, Kunz P et al. Assessment of global and regional left ventricular function with a 16-slice Spiral-CT using two different software tools for quantitative analysis and qualitative evaluation of wall motion changes in comparison with Magnetic Resonance Imaging. Fortschr Röntgenstr 2004; 176: 1786–93.

56. Dirksen MS, Jukema JW, Bax JJ et al. Cardiac multidetector-row computed tomography in patients with instable angina. Am J Cardiol 2005; 95: 457–61.

57. Schuijf JD, Bax JJ, Salm LP et al. Noninvasive coronary imaging and assessment of left ventricular function using 16-slice computed tomography. Am J Cardiol 2005; 95: 571–4.

58. Juergens KU, Ozgun M, Maintz D et al. Analyse der globalen und regionalen linksventrikulären Funktion mittels 16-Zeilen-Spiral-Computertomographie des Herzens im Vergleich zur MR-Tomographie. Fortschr Röntgenstr 2005; 177: S273.

59. Schuijf JD, Bax JJ, Jukema JW et al. Noninvasive angiography and assessment of left ventricular function using multi-slice computed tomography in patients with type 2 diabetes. Diabetes Care 2004; 27: 2905–10.

60. Mahnken AH, Koos R, Katoh M et al. Sixteen-slice spiral CT versus MR imaging for the assessment of left ventricular function in acute myocardial infarction. Eur Radiol 2005: 714–20.

61. Schuijf JD, Bax JJ, Jukema JW et al. Noninvasive evaluation of the coronary arteries with multislice computed tomography in hypertensive patients. Hypertension 2005; 45: 1–6.

62. Juergens KU, Maintz D, Grude M et al. Multi-detector row computed tomography of the heart: does a multi-segment

reconstruction algorithm improve left ventricular volume measurements? Eur Radiol 2005; 15: 111–17.

63. Cui W, Kondo T, Anno T et al. The accuracy and optimal slice thickness of multislice helical computed tomography for right and left ventricular volume measurement. Chin Med J 2004; 117: 1283–87.

64. Heuschmid M, Rothfuss J, Schröder S et al. Left ventricular functional parameters: comparison of 16-slice spiral CT with MRI. Fortschr Röntgenstr 2005; 177: 60–6.

65. Yamamuro M, Tadamura E, Kubo S et al. Cardiac functional analysis with multi-detector row CT and segmental reconstruction algorithm: comparison with echocardiography, SPECT, and MR imaging. Radiology 2005; 234: 381–90.

66. Schlosser T, Pagonidis K, Herborn CU et al. Assessment of left ventricular parameters using 16-MDCT and new software for endocardial and epicardial border delineation. Am J Roentgenol 2005; 184: 765–73.

67. Lessick J, Mutlak D, Rispler S et al. Comparison of multidetector computed tomography versus echocardiography for assessing regional left ventricular function. Am J Cardiol 2005; 96: 1011–15.

68. Hundt W, Siebert K, Wintersperger BJ et al. Assessment of global left ventricular function: comparison of cardiac multi-detector-row computed tomography with angiocardiography. J Comput Assist Tomogr 2005; 29: 373–81.

69. Mahnken AH, Katoh M, Bruners P et al. Acute myocardial infarction: assessment of left ventricular function with 16-detector row spiral CT versus MR imaging – study in pigs. Radiology 2005; 236: 112–17.

70. Coche E, Vlassenbroek A, Roelants V et al. Evaluation of biventricular ejection fraction with ECG-gated 16-slice CT: preliminary findings in acute pulmonary embolism in comparison with radionuclide ventriculography. Eur Radiol 2005; 15: 1432–40.

71. Kopp AF, Heuschmid M, Reimann A et al. Evaluation of cardiac function and myocardial viability with 16- and 64-slice multidetector computed tomography. Eur Radiol 2005; 15: D15–20.

72. Utsunomiya D, Awai K, Sakamoto T et al. Cardiac 16-MDCT for anatomic and functional analysis: assessment of a biphasic contrast injection protocol. AJR Am J Roentgenol 2006; 187: 638–44.

73. Heuschmid M, Rothfuss JK, Schroeder S et al. Assessment of left ventricular myocardial function using 16-slice multidetector-row computed tomography: comparison with magnetic resonance imaging and echocardiography. Eur Radiol 2006; 16: 551–9.

74. Mahnken AH, Muhlenbruch G, Koos R et al. Automated vs. manual assessment of left ventricular function in cardiac multidetector row computed tomography: comparison with magnetic resonance imaging. Eur Radiol 2006; 16: 1416–23.

75. Salm LP, Schuijf JD, de Roos A et al. Global and regional left ventricular function assessment with 16-detector row CT: comparison with echocardiography and cardiovascular magnetic resonance. Eur J Echocardiogr 2006; 7: 308–14.

76. Mahnken AH, Hohl C, Suess C et al. Influence of heart rate and temporal resolution on left-ventricular volumes in cardiac multislice spiral computed tomography: a phantom study. Invest Radiol 2006; 41: 429–35.

77. Belge B, Coche E, Pasquet A, Vanoverschelde JL, Gerber BL. Accurate estimation of global and regional cardiac function

by retrospectively gated multidetector row computed tomography: comparison with cine magnetic resonance imaging. Eur Radiol 2006; 16: 1424–33.

78. Henneman MM, Schuijf JD, Jukema JW et al. Comprehensive cardiac assessment with MSCT: evaluation of LV function and perfusion in addition to coronary anatomy in patients with previous myocardial infarction. Heart 2006; 92:1779–85.

79. Juergens KU, Seifarth H, Maintz D et al. Left ventricular function determination with Multidetector-row CT of the heart: Are short-axis image reformations necessary? AJR Am J Roentgenol 2006; 186: S371–8.

80. Dewey M, Muller M, Teige F, Hamm B. Evaluation of a semiautomatic software tool for left ventricular function analysis with 16-slice computed tomography. Eur Radiol 2006; 16: 25–31.

81. Sugeng L, Mor-Avi V, Weinert L. Quantitative assessment of left ventricular size and function. Side-by-side comparison of real-time three-dimensional echocardiography and computed tomography with magnetic resonance reference. Circulation 2006; 114: 654–61.

82. Dewey M, Muller M, Teige F et al. Multisegment and half-scan reconstruction of 16-slice computed tomography for assessment of regional and global left ventricular myocardial function. Invest Radiol 2006; 41: 400–9.

83. Dewey M, Muller M, Eddicks E et al. Evaluation of global and regional left ventricular function with 16-slice computed tomography, biplane cineventriculography, and two-dimensional transthoracic echocardiography. J Am Coll Cardiol 2006; 48: 2034–44.

84. Henneman MM, Schuijf JD, Jukema JW et al. Assessment of global and regional left ventricular function and volumes with 64-slice MSCT: a comparison with 2D echocardiography. J Nucl Cardiol 2006; 13: 480–7.

85. Koyama Y, Matsuoka H, Mochizuki T et al. Assessment of reperfused acute myocardial infarction with two-phase contrast-enhanced helical CT: prediction of left ventricular function and wall thickness. Radiology 2005; 235: 804–11.

19

Assessment of Heart Valve Disease by Computed Tomography

R. van Lingen, N. Manghat, C. Roobottom, and G. Morgan-Hughes

1 INTRODUCTION

The constant technological improvements in CT have seen it merge seamlessly from a research tool in cardiac imaging to mainstream clinical utility in areas such as the assessment of coronary artery disease. Although obviously not currently the accepted gold standard for the assessment of the heart valves over other imaging modalities such as echocardiography, the increase in temporal and spatial resolution with the current generation of 64-slice multidetector CT (MDCT) scanners mean that excellent images can be obtained in most patients of even these thin mobile structures. A huge wealth of information about the heart valves is available from any high specification cardiac MDCT scan regardless of the original indication for the investigation. It is important that this data is analyzed appropriately and commented upon. Electrocardiographic gated MDCT data reconstructed at different phases across the cardiac contraction cycle allows haemodynamic assessment by implication of regurgitant valve lesions and direct measurements of stenotic valve areas. Furthermore MDCT might potentially be the preferred imaging modality in certain clinical situations in which echocardiographic assessment is known to be challenging. In our experience these situations would include the assessment of the aortic root for abscess formation in prosthetic aortic valve infective endocarditis, and the assessment of the pulmonary valve in infective endocarditis and carcinoid syndrome (Figure 19.1). Additionally MDCT is

likely to play an increasingly important role in percutaneous valve procedures such as mitral annuloplasty and aortic stent valve insertion. Accurate preprocedural anatomical assessment is crucial to the success of these two rapidly developing techniques and MDCT would be ideally placed to provide the required imaging.

The following chapter will review the basic causes and pathophysiology of the common heart valve diseases and provide a literature review of up to date published reports on the use of MDCT in the assessment of these diseases. Insights into practical reporting and application of MDCT for the assessment of heart valve disease will be provided. These insights are based around experience gained from a busy clinical cardiac MDCT service, which has been in place since 2003, and an active research programme.

2 CARDIAC CHAMBERS

Ideally, all valve pathology needs to be assessed in the context of the underlying cardiac chambers' size and function. The atria and their associated inflow vessels are all clearly visible on MDCT, including the left atrial (LA) appendage, which needs to be assessed for the presence of thrombus. The utility of CT for the accurate anatomical depiction of the atrial region[1] is best illustrated by its increasing use in atrial fibrillation ablation procedures, including pulmonary vein isolation.

243

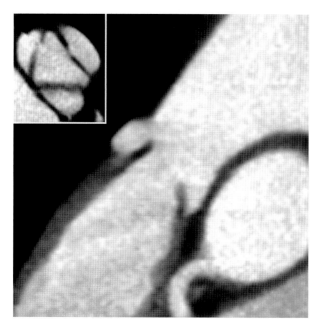

Figure 19.1 Pulmonary valve at end-diastole unable to close due to thickening and restriction of cusp leaflets secondary to carcinoid syndrome, resulting in severe pulmonary regurgitation.

Left ventricular (LV) systolic function is usually the most important associated factor that needs to be considered in valve disease. Not only is LV systolic dysfunction an important clinical parameter, it confers prognostic information, influences treatment decisions and is an aetiological cause of valvular dysfunction (the central mitral regurgitation in a patient with a dilated cardiomyopathy being an example)

(Figure 19.2). LV functional assessment by MDCT has been shown to be accurate compared to a number of alternative imaging modalities, including cardiac magnetic resonance imaging (MRI), echocardiography and Single Photon Emission Computed Tomography (SPECT)[2–10] with good interobserver variability.[3] MDCT appears to correlate most closely with MRI in calculating ejection fraction,[14] although it tends to slightly underestimate measured values of wall thickness and volume.[2,7,8,11] However, there is a predominance of patients with well-preserved LV function in the reported literature, and in those with global or regional wall impairment this underestimation bias might be further exaggerated.[9,12] Right ventricular (RV) function can also be quantified but requires good RV contrast opacification which is not always possible with standard cardiac CT acquisition protocols.[4] As the information required to assess the left ventricle is acquired as part of the standard volume of data in a routine MDCT the semi-automative quantification packages now available should make this an accurate interpretation with little impact on reporting times.[10,12]

3 AORTIC VALVE

3.1 Anatomy and function

The normal aortic valve (AV) is tricuspid with cusps easily visible on MDCT as thin structures (Figure 19.3 – images A,

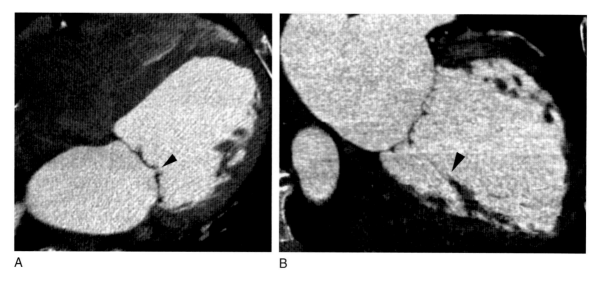

A   B

Figure 19.2 A patient with dilated cardiomyopathy demonstrating end-systolic LV cavity dilatation with consequent mitral annular ring dilation and failure of coaptation of the mitral valve leaflets (A), and the thinned and stretched sub-valvular chordae tendinae and papillary muscles (B) holding the leaflets in place.

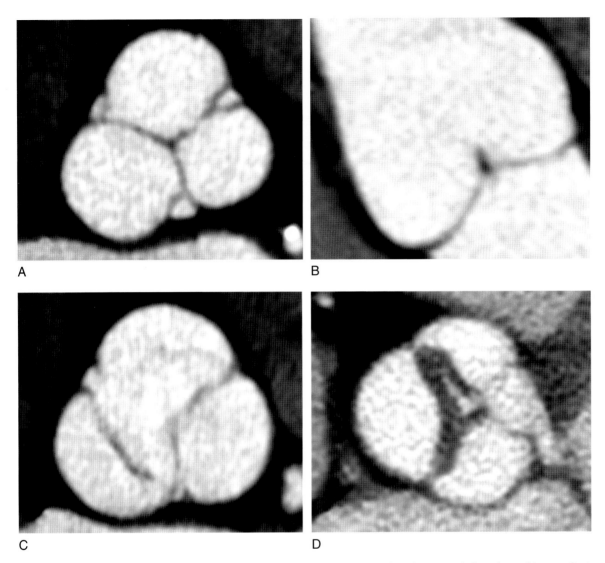

Figure 19.3   Images A and B are orthogonal views of normal tricuspid aortic valve at end-diastole and image C at end-systole. Image D demonstrates thickened and abnormal but non-calcified cusp leaflet tips of stenotic aortic valve at end diastole. Note the failure of full closure which would result in a degree of aortic regurgitation.

B and C). The right and left cusps are below the right and left coronary sinuses, which in turn give rise to the right and left coronary arteries. The third cusp is therefore referred to as the noncoronary cusp. The normal open valve area is 2.5–3.5 cm^2.[13]

4 AORTIC STENOSIS

4.1 Causes

The site of stenosis can be valvular, subvalvular or supravalvular. Valvular aortic stenosis (AS) may be congenital, degenerative or rheumatic (Table 19.1).[13] Numerous

variations on valve cusps number and morphology have been described but congenital bicuspid valves are the most common variant, occurring in 1–2% of people.[14] Bicuspid AV (Figure 19.4 – C) may be identified in patients of any age although stenosis of the valve is usually accelerated and more likely to present in younger persons.[15] Associated congenital abnormalities of either coarctation of the aorta or interrupted aortic arch should always be sought, as well as aortic root dilation[16] (Figure 19.5).

Age-related degenerative calcific AS is the most common cause of AS in adults, can be present in 2–3%[17] and is a leading indication for aortic valve replacement (AVR).[18] Degenerative calcific AS shares common risk factors with aortic and coronary artery atherosclerosis and mitral valve

Table 19.1   Aetiology of aortic valve pathology

Aortic regurgitation	Aortic stenosis
• Rheumatic fever • Degenerative • Infective endocarditis (Figures 19.13, 19.14) • Large ventricular septal defect • Complication of percutaneous aortic balloon valvotomy and radiofrequency catheter ablation[43] • Structural deterioration of a bioprosthetic valve • Trauma Aortic root disease: • Degenerative • Cystic medial necrosis • Aortic dissection • Osteogenesis imperfecta • Systemic hypertension	• Congenital • Degenerative • Rheumatic fever • Rheumatoid arthritis

annular calcification.[19–21] Patients usually present from around the sixth decade with symptoms and/or signs of aortic valve disease. A rheumatic valve is usually both regurgitant and stenotic.

4.2 Pathophysiology and natural history

The classically described natural history of adult aortic stenosis is a gradual decrease in valve area, which is initially well tolerated and asymptomatic. However, once the valve has stenosed to about 50% of it's original area[22] (±1.5 cm^2) a transvalvular pressure gradient between the left ventricle and aorta begins to develop. From that point on even minor diminution of valve area leads to a rapid rise in pressure gradient. This in turn leads to progressive pressure overload on the left ventricle. The compensatory response to pressure loading of the left ventricle is to develop left ventricular hypertrophy (LVH) (Figure 19.6). Initially this allows for increased pressure with normal LV wall stress, but as the disease progresses the hypertrophy increasingly gains pathological features, and this combination of increasing wall thickness and afterload excess leads to progressive diastolic followed by systolic dysfunction. The ultimate reduction in contractile function and cardiac output means that intraventricular pressure falls, resulting in an apparent decrease in the transvalvular gradient despite continuing severe valve stenosis. This can clinically be difficult to distinguish from

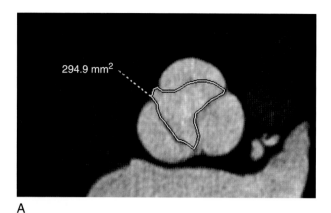

A

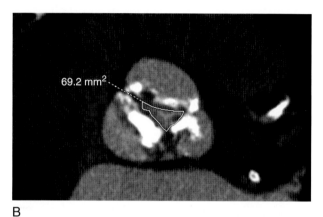

B

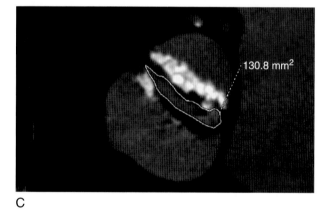

C

Figure 19.4   Image A is a planimetered area of a normal aortic valve fully opened at end-systole, image B the significantly reduced area of a patient with severe calcific aortic stenosis in a tricuspid valve, and image C the reduced area of a patient with a calcified bicuspid aortic valve.

patients with mild aortic valve restriction and an incidental cardiomyopathy.

4.3 MDCT assessment

Degenerative AS has a similar risk factor profile to atherosclerotic coronary artery disease and displays a similar

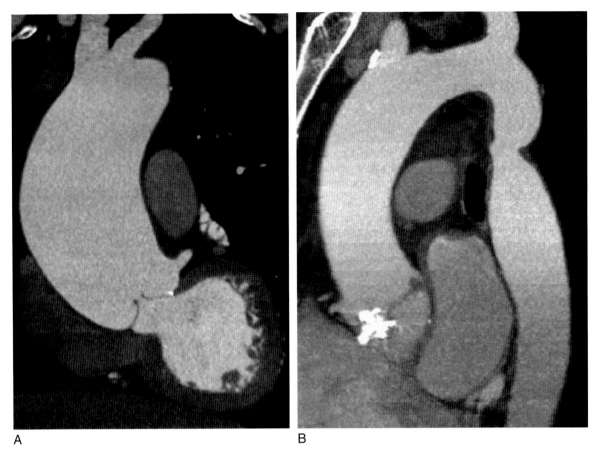

A   B

Figure 19.5   Image A demonstrates a significantly dilated ascending aortic root with resultant failure of diastolic coaptation of the aortic valve and consequent aortic regurgitation. Image B is of a calcified bicuspid aortic valve with associated coarctation of the descending aorta.

tendency to calcify over time. Early MDCT assessment of AS therefore focused on the correlation between increasing levels of AV calcification (AVC) with increasing pressure gradients and decreasing valve area.[23–26] It has been shown that on a 0–4 subjective scoring scale of AVC, grade 3–4 calcification results in 60% of patients having AS, with only 2.4% of patients with scores of 0–2 having AS.[27] However, it appears that the relationship between AVC and gradient is slightly more complex than a simple linear correlation.[24] Although there is a linear relationship of increasing AVC from mild gradients up to the point of severe AS, once a patient has severe AS, calcification volumes can vary widely, although always being high. It has been suggested from echocardioghraphic data that very high levels of AVC might confer an adverse prognosis in even asymptomatic severe AS patients.[28] By extension, therefore, CT scanning is ideally placed to provide similar but more objective data, and this represents an important clinical utility for cardiac MDCT. In particular the two subgroups of patients with AS that can be especially difficult to judge in terms of whether they are

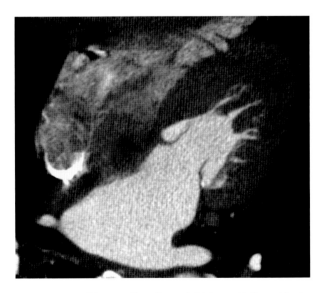

Figure 19.6   The small cavity and thickened left ventricular muscular walls at end-diastole of a patient with left ventricular hypertrophy secondary to hypertrophic cardiomyopathy.

likely to benefit from AVR, are the asymptomatic patients with severe AS and those with AS and poor LV function. Very high levels of AVC suggest an adverse prognosis in the former group. In the second group the actual diagnosis of severe AS can be difficult as a high pressure gradient over the AV will not be generated in the setting of poor LV function. High levels of AVC may assist in making the diagnosis of severe AS in patients such as this. In both situations the information obtained facilitates the decision making process with regards to the timing of, or need for, AVR.

As the resolution of newer generation of MDCT scanners improve, papers are starting to be published on direct comparison between MDCT and echocardiographic valve area assessment.[29,30] Both transthoracic Doppler derived valve areas.[29,30] and transoesophageal echocardiographic (TEE) planimetered valve areas [30] appear to correlate well with MDCT planimetered valve areas (Figure 19.4). Isolated case reports and anecdotal experience demonstrate that aberrations in cusp morphology,[31,32] supravalvular stenosis[33] and associated intrathoracic pathology[32–34] (such as aortic root dilation and coarctation of the aorta) are demonstrated clearly by MDCT (Figure 19.5).

5 AORTIC REGURGITATION

5.1 Causes

Primary disease of the AV leaflets and/or the wall of the aortic root may cause aortic regurgitation (AR). There is separation of the leaflets when the aortic annulus becomes significantly dilated. Dilatation of the aortic root can cause tension and bowing of the individual cusps, which may thicken, retract and become too short to close the aortic orifice. This can cause a downward spiral of worsening AR and increasing ascending aorta dilation. Table 19.1[13] highlights some of the important causes of AR, with AR secondary to dilation of the ascending aorta now being more common than pure primary valve disease in patients undergoing AVR.[35–36]

5.2 Pathophysiology and natural history

Chronic AR results in both pressure and volume overloading of the LV, which can stimulate the development of both concentric and eccentric LVH with a large left ventricular end-diastolic volume. As the LV dilation progresses over time, ejection fraction starts to deteriorate and symptoms usually

intervene. If AVR occurs prior to permanent LV dysfunction then beneficial remodeling can return the LV to normal.

5.3 CT assessment

Although MDCT is excellent for assessing the thoracic aorta and diseases which affect the AV, such as aortic root dilation and dissection, there is very little in the literature regarding calculation of regurgitant valve area. One paper[37] has compared TEE with MDCT in 71 patients, and found a sensitivity and specificity of 95% and 96% respectively for moderate and severe grades of AR. However, heavily calcified valves precluded assessment by MDCT in up to 50% of patients with AR, and mild regurgitation was poorly ruled out with a sensitivity of only 70%.

Despite the lack of literature on the subject AR is straightforward to diagnose with cardiac MDCT. The AV should be closed at end-diastole. Failure of coaptation of the AV is very clear on cardiac MDCT data sets reconstructed at end-diastole (Figure 19.3 – D, and Figure 19.7). The failure of coaptation demonstrated allows the diagnosis of AR by implication. Almost invariably in this situation the aortic root will be dilated or the valve itself abnormal. Further supporting evidence of AR may be evident on the scan. One such example is the differing contrast opacification seen between the LV and the LA in the patient with severe AR but a competent mitral valve (Figure 19.7). These findings should be commented upon when reporting cardiac MDCT and haemodynamic assessment with echocardiography recommended.

5.4 Clinical context of MDCT reporting of the aortic valve

Evidence of AVC on routine thoracic MDCT scanning should prompt a careful evaluation of the aorta and coronary arterial tree for evidence of associated atherosclerosis. A suspected stenotic AV should have a comment made on its degree of calcification. Aortic root and arch calibres should always be measured, and any evidence of congenital abnormalities of the AV must prompt an assessment of the descending thoracic aorta for evidence of associated coarctation. During cardiac MDCT, performed for whatever indication, the number and morphology of the AV leaflets should be assessed, and if abnormal, the end systolic

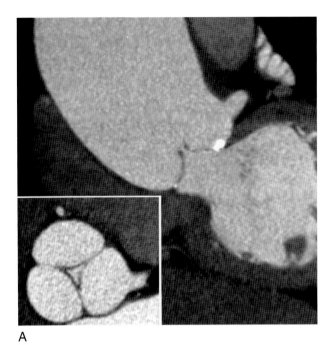

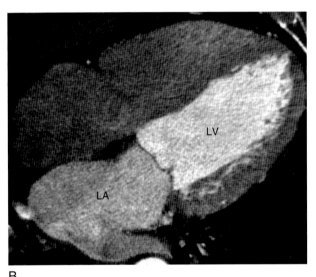

Figure 19.7 Aortic regurgitation in a patient with a dilated aortic root and regurgitant aortic valve visible at end-diastole. Note the interesting differential contrast between the left atrium and left ventricle in the lower image. This is due to contrast accentuation in the LV due to the additive effects of the aortic regurgitant jet, and the competent mitral valve preventing this from occurring in the left atrium.

maximally opened valve leaflet tip area traced around to calculate a planimetered area. The LV wall thicknesses and chamber dimensions in end-diastole and end-systole should be measured for objective evidence of LVH or LV dilatation, and the LV ejection fraction should be calculated.

Similarly, in the regurgitant valve, morphological assessment should be made of the leaflets and an end diastolic

assessment of leaflet coaptation. Careful measurement and assessment of the aortic root and thoracic aorta for associated dilation, dissection or connective tissue abnormalities should be performed. LV chamber size and function is equally important for the assessment of any adverse impact on the LV by the regurgitant AV.

6 MITRAL VALVE

6.1 Anatomy and function

The mitral valve (MV) apparatus involves the mitral valve annulus (MVA), mitral leaflets, chordae tendinae, papillary muscles and the adjacent myocardium. The leaflets and papillary muscles are easily visible on cardiac MDCT, although the thin structures of the chordae tendinae less so depending on scan quality. The normal cross sectional area of the open MV in adults is 4–6 cm^2.[13]

7 MITRAL STENOSIS

7.1 Causes

Rheumatic fever is the predominant cause of mitral stenosis (MS) (Table 19.2).[13,38,39] Rheumatic involvement results in four forms of mitral valve leaflet fusion: commissural, cuspal, chordal and combined.[40] The cusps fuse at their edges and thickening and shortening of the chordae tendinae results in tethering of the valve leaflets with concomitant restriction of cusp excursion. The stenotic MV is typically funnel shaped and the orifice is frequently

Table 19.2 Aetiology of mitral valve pathology

Mitral stenosis	Mitral regurgitation
• Rheumatic heart disease • Congenital • Carcinoid syndrome • Connective tissue disorder • Lutembachers syndrome (when associated with atrial septal defect)	• Rheumatic heart disease • Infective endocarditis • Annular calcification • Cardiomyopathy • Ischemic heart disease • Collagen vascular diseases • Trauma • Hypereosinophilic syndrome • Carcinoid syndrome

shaped like a 'fish mouth.' The thickened leaflets may be so adherent and rigid that they cannot open or shut and lead to combined MS and mitral regurgitation (MR).[13]

7.2 Pathophysiology and natural history

Once the MVA decreases to below 2.0 cm² the pressure begins to rise in the LA and a transvalvular pressure gradient develops. Increasing LA pressure is transmitted back into the pulmonary vasculature resulting in rising pulmonary pressures. This in turn ultimately leads to RV dilation and failure. Thus the majority of the complications of MS such as a dilated LA with thrombus, atrial fibrillation, pulmonary hypertension, pulmonary oedema and haemoptysis are logical consequences of this abnormal haemodynamic state. The LV is protected from this by the stenotic valve and thus is normal in most patients. Posterobasal LV extension of the fibrotic valve process can however result in mild localized hypokinesis. If LV dysfunction is present it is usually related to con-comitant pathology such as ischemic heart disease or additional MR.[41]

7.3 CT assessment

To date there is no publication that we are aware of comparing modern generation MDCT to echocardiography for the assessment of MS. Very early studies in the mid 1990s attempted to use CT in patients undergoing percutaneous mitral balloon commisurotomy to monitor changes in cardiac chamber volumes[42] and to assess MV morphology as a predictor of eventual post procedure valve area.[43] In 2002, MDCT was used to evaluate the different anatomical components of the MV and its apparatus, an important consideration in planning percutaneous or surgical approaches to treatment.[44] Despite using only single slice mid-diastolic images, reasonable visualization was achieved. But a recent feasibility study comparing MDCT with TEE in patients with normal MVs appears promising in terms of dynamic morphological assessment.[45] The long-axis perpendicular plane appears better than short-axis views throughout the cardiac cycle and most valvular and subvalvular structures (with the exception of the thin chordae tendinae) appear well visualized with good interobserver variability (Figure 19.8). This clearly sets the stage for further MDCT studies on abnormal valves, with the higher temporal resolution of

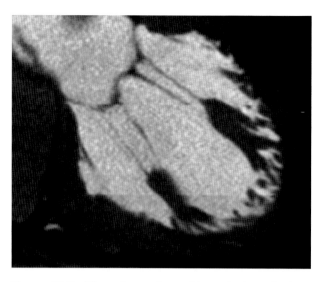

Figure 19.8   The echocardiographic equivalent of a long axis view of the mitral valve demonstrating thin mitral valve leaflets with the normal sub-valvular apparatus of chordae tendinae and papillary muscles clearly visible.

64-slice machines and beyond looking promising in terms of further reducing valve leaflet motion artifact.

8 MITRAL REGURGITATION

8.1 Causes

The important causes of MR are listed in Table 19.2.[13] As previously mentioned, the deformation of valve leaflets in chronic rheumatic heart disease can lead to regurgitation (Figure 19.9), as can infective endocarditis (Figure 19.10). Severe idiopathic (degenerative) calcification of the MVA may also be an important cause of MR.[46,47] With severe annular calcification, a rigid, curved ring of calcium encircles the mitral orifice and calcific spurs may project into the adjacent myocardium.[48] This is perhaps better demonstrated by MDCT than by other imaging modalities, and provides important information for the cardiothoracic surgeon prior to MV repair or replacement, as frequently the annulus has to be extensively decalcified during the procedure. This additional information may have a significant impact on both the nature and timing of any planned cardiothoracic procedure. Excess redundant myxomatous tissue leading to valve enlargement and systolic prolapse is the cardinal feature of the mitral valve prolapse (MVP) syndrome.[41,49] Ischemically mediated MR can either be secondary to acute rupture of a papillary muscle or the altered LV geometry and function secondary to a region of wall motion abnormality. MR resulting from

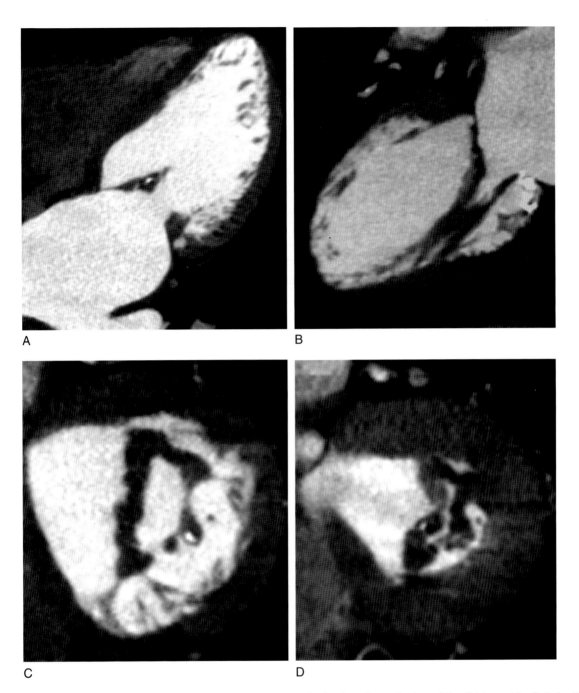

A   B

C   D

Figure 19.9   Cardinal cardiac CT features of a rheumatic mitral valve. A – tethering of the thickened leaflets by the sub-valvular apparatus. B – calcification of the mitral annular ring and subvalvular apparatus. C – restricted opening in the short-axis view of the thickened myxomatous anterior and posterior valve leaflets. D – failure of coaptation and closure at end-systole resulting in mitral regurgitation.

dilatation of the MVA secondary to dilating cardiomy-opathies of any cause is also common[50] (Figure 19.2).

8.2 Pathophysiology and natural history

Chronic MR results in a pure volume overloaded state, as opposed to the combined pressure and volume loading

of aortic regurgitation. Thus both the LA and LV gradually dilate in response to the retrogradely ejected portion of the stroke volume. This can be tolerated for many years, but at the point when ejection fraction starts to decline, diastolic, LA and pulmonary capillary pressures start to rise and symptoms can progress rapidly. Reduced LV function is a serious finding, as the regurgitation back into the low pressure LA confers a 'sparing' effect of afterload reduction, and implies a greater loss of

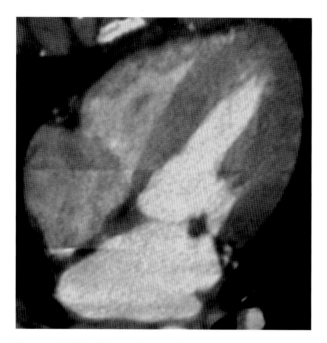

Figure 19.10   Vegetation on the posterior mitral valve leaflet of a patient with infective endocarditis.

myocardial integrity when it occurs than with other valvular conditions.[41]

8.3 CT assessment

There are two potential strategies for attempting to assess the presence and severity of MR using cardiac MDCT. One is to directly planimeter or trace the valve area and the second is to calculate regurgitant volume from forward stroke and LV flow volumes. Before this is considered, however, the structure of the entire MV apparatus needs to be evaluated. The question to be answered is: 'Is there a substrate for MR here?' If the answer is yes, then attempts to confirm the presence of and the severity of the MR should be vigorous.

One set of authors has reported their experience with evaluating MDCT for the first method by measuring planimetered systolic MV regurgitant area in 25 normal and 19 patients with MR and compared the results with TOE and ventriculography.[51] Although only small numbers of patients were involved, results were encouraging in that all patients with no MR were correctly identified by MDCT, and there appeared to be good correlation with the semi-quantitative assessment by the alternative assessment methods of TOE and ventriculography. However, despite this correlation, statistically there was still difficulty in distinguishing

between some grades of MR, such as between mild and moderate regurgitation.

The second method of evaluating MR by MDCT is to calculate a regurgitation volume. This is done by calculating the LV total stroke volume and subtracting from it the forward stroke volume, the difference being the presumed MR volume. An important caveat is that this assumption only holds true in the absence of AR or an intra-cardiac shunt. The LV total volume is the difference between end diastolic and end systolic volumes, and the forward stroke volume is determined by using the indicator dilution method to calculate cardiac output with a region of interest attenuation time curve in the ascending aorta. Lembcke and co-authors have published three papers assessing MR by this method, two using echocardiography and MRI and one using echocardiography and ventriculography as comparators.[52–54] Again, overall, good correlation was found between MDCT grading of the severity of the MR, including normal patients, and echo, MRI and ventriculography. But the method is by no means perfect, and it must be emphasized that in the most robust study,[53] which included 219 patients, there was perfect agreement in 61% of patients between MDCT and echocardiography, but still a mismatch by one grade in 31% and by two grades in 6%.

8.4 Clinical context of MDCT reporting of the mitral valve

As with the AV the finding of MVA calcification on routine MDCT of the thoracic aorta should be commented upon. At cardiac MDCT the MV and its apparatus should be assessed carefully. The MV leaflets should be examined in the short- and long-axis views. Comment should be made on any redundant tissue, thickening, retraction or the unlikely finding of vegetations (Figure 19.10). A planimetered area should be made if any failure of leaflet coaptation and possibly an attempt to infer haemodynamic data by calculating a regurgitant volume. The annular area should be measured, and the extent of any calcification commented on. Similarly, the condition of the two papillary muscles and associated chordae tendinae should be checked, and any ruptured chordae noted. Measurement of atrial dimensions and area (measured by planimetry in the four chamber view), the presence or absence of any LA thrombus, and the LV function and dimensions are further important factors to include in the report.

9 TRICUSPID AND PULMONARY VALVE DISEASE

9.1 Anatomy, causes and pathophysiology

The tricuspid valve (TV) is trileaflet with cusps that occupy a septal anterior, superior and inferior position. It is more difficult to appreciate on CT due to its thinner cusps and contrast protocols usually aimed to maximize left-sided visualization. The pulmonary valve (PV) characteristics are similar to the AV except for the absence of the coronary ostia. The PV cusps, as with the TV, are more difficult to appreciate on CT and the same contrast issues are relevant as with TV imaging. As a general guide, in our experience, if the PV cusps are easily visible then they are likely to be thickened.

Better visualization is obtained if intracardiac contrast opacification timing is chosen that optimizes right heart structures (such as a CT pulmonary angiogram protocol) combined with ECG-gating. During CT coronary angiography a saline bolus chaser is normally employed to help flush contrast from the right side of the heart. This is to reduce contrast dose and prevent beam-hardening artefact from the SVC and right heart, which adversely affects visualization of the right coronary artery. Unfortunately the sequelae of this are that assessment of the TV and PV becomes more difficult. However, using bolus-tracking techniques, the operator may choose to vary the timing of the contrast bolus to optimally opacify both the left and right heart or predominantly the right heart.

The most common cause of tricuspid regurgitation (TR) is not intrinsic involvement of the valve itself but rather dilation of the RV and of the tricuspid annulus causing secondary or functional TR. This is usually as a sequelae of left-sided cardiac or pulmonary disease. Tricuspid stenosis (TS) is almost always rheumatic in origin.[55] Other causes are listed in Table 19.3,[13] but a rheumatic TV is usually both stenotic and regurgitant.

The most common cause of PR is dilation of the valve ring secondary to pulmonary hypertension or right ventricular dilation of any aetiology, or to dilation of the pulmonary artery, either idiopathic or secondary to a connective tissue disorder (Table 19.4).[13] The congenital form is the most common cause of PS and constitutes 10–12% of cases of congenital heart disease in adults.[56] Like AS, it can be supravalvular, valvular and subvalvular,

with valvular being most common and supravalvular being associated with other congenital abnormalities such as Tetralogy of Fallot.[14] Table 19.4[13] lists the important causes of PS.

9.2 Clinical context of MDCT reporting

The classic sign of TR on CT is the early retrograde reflux of intravenous contrast material into the inferior vena cava and/or hepatic veins.[57,58] However, there are a number of factors which can influence the sensitivity and specificity of this, including the rate of contrast injection[58] and in our experience an inadvertent Valsalva maneuver during breath-hold. Previously undiagnosed pericardial constriction (Figure 19.11) or pulmonary hypertension are important diagnoses to entertain in the presence of isolated TR, and

Table 19.3 Aetiology of tricuspid valve pathology

Tricuspid stenosis	Tricuspid regurgitation
• Rheumatic fever • Congenital tricuspid atresia • Right atrial tumors • Carcinoid syndrome • Obstruction to right ventricular inflow: • Endomyocardial fibrosis • TV vegetations • Pacemaker lead • Extracardiac tumors • Ebstein's anomaly	• Causes of RV failure • Rheumatic fever • Infective endocarditis • Congenital • Carcinoid • Rheumatoid arthritis • Trauma • Prolapse (floppy) • Ebstein's anomaly

Table 19.4 Aetiology of pulmonary valve pathology

Pulmonary stenosis	Pulmonary regurgitation
• Congenital – most common • Rheumatic – uncommon • Carcinoid syndrome	• Pulmonary hypertension • Infective endocarditis • Iatrogenic, e.g. TOF repair • Congenital malformations • Trauma • Carcinoid • Rheumatic fever

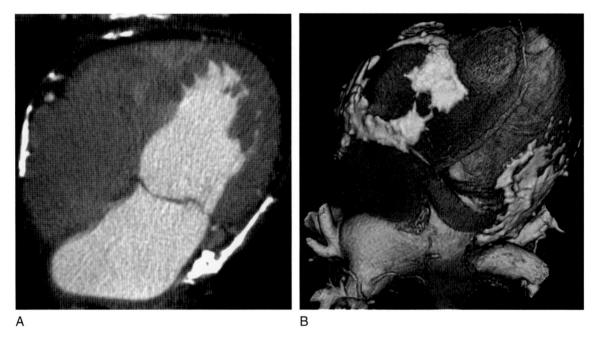

A   B

Figure 19.11   2D and 3D reconstruction of a heart with calcific pericardial constriction.

MDCT has the added advantage of being an excellent modality for assessing the pericardium for thickening and calcification and reviewing the lung windows for disease. If TR is picked up on a thoracic MDCT then specific comment about the pericardium should be made.

There is little in the literature on the MDCT assessment of the PV. It is important to measure the pulmonary artery dimensions, and visually inspect the PV leaflets for thickening and distortion. It is important to remember that the echocardiographic views of the PV, even with TOE, may be significantly suboptimal.

There may be individual cases where it may be appropriate to consider cardiac MDCT imaging specifically for this purpose. It has been used for this reason in our institution to not only successfully rule out abnormalities of the PV, but also to demonstrate them. One such example is in the carcinoid syndrome, the results of which are well documented, with the TV and PV affected.[59] Abnormalities such as this are readily demonstrated with cardiac MDCT and again, as with the AV, PR may be inferred by a lack of coaptation in the end-diastolic images (Figure 19.1).[60]

9.3 Prosthetic valves and infective endocarditis

These two subjects deserve a brief individual review due to their importance. There is little in the literature on cardiac

MDCT imaging of these topics other than case reports and clinical reviews and the majority of advice is based on our own clinical experience.

9.4 Prosthetic valves

There are 2 major groups of artificial valves: mechanical prostheses with almost unlimited lifespan but in whom patients need lifelong anticoagulation, and bioprostheses (tissue valves) which have a lower infective risk profile and no need for anticoagulation, but are traditionally quoted as lasting 10–15 years. Both valve types can be assessed by MDCT (Figure 19.12), with the subvalvular area prone to echocardiographic image drop out in mechanical valves, often being well visualized, and the natural calcification and degeneration of bioprosthetic tissue leaflets readily quantifiable.

9.5 Infective endocarditis

Infective endocarditis (IE) is a microbial infection of the endocardial surface of the heart, most commonly affecting the valves but it can affect septal defects, chordae or mural endocardium. Lesions are characteristically vegetations comprising platelets, fibrin, inflammatory cells and microorganisms[61] and may be detected by MDCT.

Prosthetic heart valve endocarditis (PVE) is associated with high mortality rates, especially if early (within

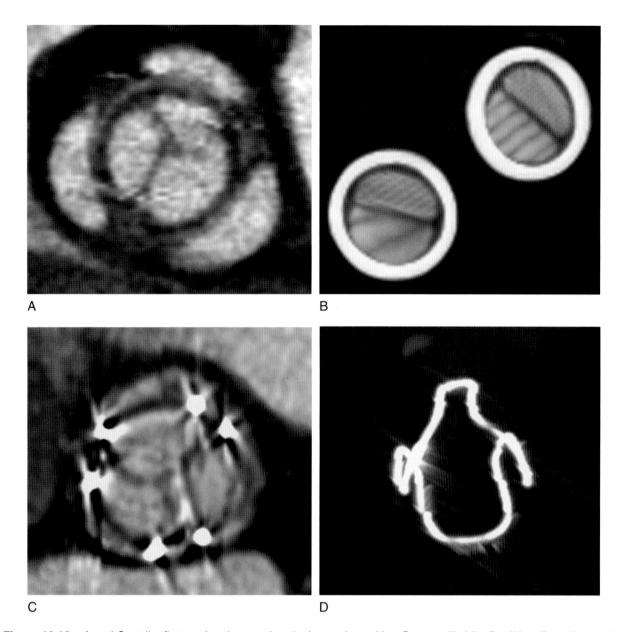

Figure 19.12   A and C – trileaflet porcine tissue valves in the aortic position. B – metallic bileaflet tilting disc valves in the aortic and pulmonary positions. D – underlying metallic scaffolding of a tissue valve.

12 months of surgery), and can lead to valve dehiscence and paravalvular abscesses necessitating valve replacement. Mechanical valves are more at risk from early PVE than bioprostheses, as the infection is more likely to be restricted to valve leaflets in bioprostheses.[62]

9.6 Clinical context of MDCT reporting

There can be considerable artefactual drop out from mechanical valves, even with TOE, and MDCT can therefore be very useful in assessing the subvalvular apparatus of valves as well as any associated vegetations. Similar cardiac MDCT assessment should be undertaken with prosthetic valves as with native valves in the same anatomical position, the size of the sewing ring should be measured and any paraprosthetic dehiscence looked for. Equally important are the complications of IE, such as distant septic emboli, and cardiac MDCT is excellent for the detection of aortic root abscesses in the presence of PVE (Figure 19.13) or native valve IE (Figure 19.14). As has been alluded to previously, the aortic root abscess in the presence of PVE may be difficult to detect with other imaging modalities

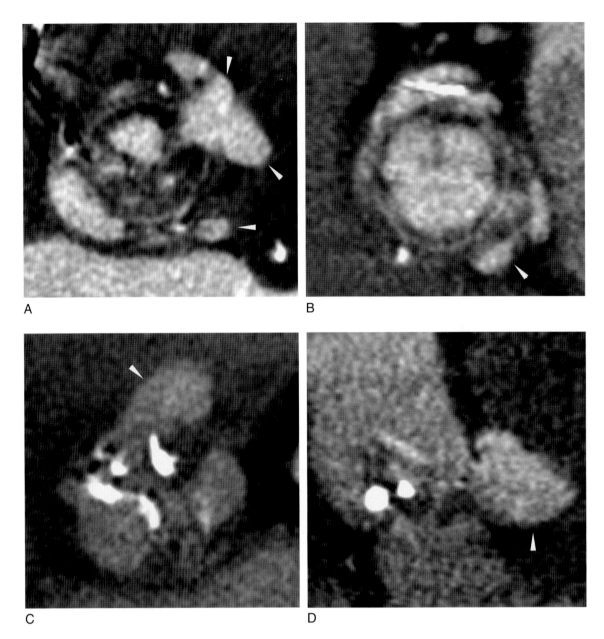

Figure 19.13 Multiple aortic root abscesses (A–D, arrowheads) in different patients with aortic valve replacements.

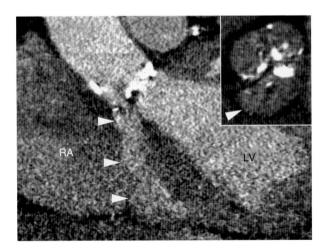

Figure 19.14 Native aortic valve infective endocarditis leading to aortic root abscess. This has eroded into the right atrium and resulted in an aortic to right atrial fistula (jet of contrast from aorta into atrium arrowed).

and may represent a primary indication for cardiac MDCT.

9.7 Future directions

There will be continuing research in the haemodynamic assessment of cardiac function by implication, and newer techniques such as myocardial perfusion scanning will garner more and more ancillary information. Newer percutaneous interventional strategies, such as mitral valve annuloplasty and aortic stent valves, are steadily emerging from the research and palliative care arena into more widespread clinical use, and are likely to increasingly utilize MDCT as part of their perioperative assessment.[63–65] All this in what from a patient's point of view is a single scan with a short breath-hold of 10 seconds or less. The utopian ideal of the 'one stop shop' for complete morphological and functional cardiac assessment by MDCT scanning continues to draw ever nearer.

ACKNOWLEDGEMENTS

We would like to thank Helen Blake in the Department of Medical Photography for all her hard work and patience in assisting us with the preparation of the images for this chapter.

REFERENCES

1. Wongcharoen W, Tsao HM, Wu MH et al. Morphologic characteristics of the left atrial appendage, roof, and septum: implications for the ablation of atrial fibrillation. J Cardiovasc Electrophysiol. 2006 Sep; 17(9): 951–6.
2. Belge B, Coche E, Pasquet A, Vanoverschelde J, Gerber BL. Accurate estimation of global and regional cardiac function by retrospectively gated multidetector row computed tomography: Comparison with cine magnetic resonance imaging. Eur Radiol. 2006 Jul; 16(7): 1424–33.
3. Yamamuro M, Tadamura E, Kubo S et al. Cardiac functional analysis with multi-detector row CT and segmental reconstruction algorithm: comparison with echocardiography, SPECT, and MR imaging. Radiology 2005 Feb; 234(2): 381–90.
4. Raman S, Shah M, McCarthy B, Garcia A, Ferketich A. Multi-detector row cardiac computed tomography accurately quantifies right and left ventricular size and function compared with cardiac magnetic resonance. Am Heart J. 2006 Mar; 151(3): 736–44.
5. Juergens K, Fischbach R. Left ventricular function studied with MDCT. Eur Radiol. 2006 Feb; 16(2): 342–57.
6. Kim IJ, Choo KS, Lee JS et al. Comparison of Gated Blood Pool SPECT and Multi-Detector Row Computed Tomography for Measurements of Left Ventricular Volumes and Ejection Fraction in Patients with Atypical Chest Pain: Validation with Radionuclide Ventriculography. Cardiology. 2006 May 24; 107(1): 8–16.
7. Grude M, Juergens KU, Wichter T et al. Evaluation of global left ventricular myocardial function with electrocardiogram-gated multidetector computed tomography: comparison with magnetic resonance imaging. Invest Radiol. 2003 Oct; 38(10): 653–61.
8. Halliburton SS, Petersilka M, Schvartzman PR, Obuchowski N, White RD. Evaluation of left ventricular dysfunction using multiphasic reconstructions of coronary multi-slice computed tomography data in patients with chronic ischemic heart disease: validation against cine magnetic resonance imaging. Int J Cardiovasc Imaging 2003 Feb; 19(1): 73–83.
9. Lessick J, Mutlak D, Rispler S et al. Comparison of multidetector computed tomography versus echocardiography for assessing regional left ventricular function. Am J Cardiol. 2005 Oct 1; 96(7): 1011–5.

10. Manghat NE, Morgan-Hughes GJ, Roobottom CA. Use of a semi-automated left ventricular "rapid ejection fraction" algorithm with 16-detector row CT and comparison with two-dimensional echocardiography: initial experience in a UK centre. Clin Radiol. 2006 Feb; 61(2): 206–8.
11. Juergens KU, Maintz D, Grude M. Multi-detector row computed tomography of the heart: does a multi-segment reconstruction algorithm improve left ventricular volume measurements? Eur Radiol. 2005 Jan; 15(1): 111–17.
12. Juergens KU, Seifarth H, Maintz D et al. MDCT determination of volume and function of the left ventricle: are short-axis image reformations necessary? Am J Roentgenol. 2006 Jun; 186(6 Suppl 2): S371–8.
13. Bonow RO and Braunwald E. Valvular Heart Disease. 7 ed. Braunwald's Heart Disease: A Textbook of Cardiovascular Medicine, ed. DP Zipes et al. 2005. Philadelphia: Elsevier Saunders, 1553–632.
14. Brickner ME, Hillis LD and Lange RA. Congenital heart disease in adults. First of two parts. N Engl J Med. 2000. 342(4): 256–63.
15. Beppu S, Suzuki S, Matsuda H et al. Rapidity of progression of aortic stenosis in patients with congenital bicuspid aortic valves. Am J Cardiol. 1993. 71(4): 322–7.
16. Levinson GEA, Alpert JS. Aortic Stenosis. 3 ed. Valvular Heart Disease, ed. JS Alpert, JE Dalen, and SH Rahimtoola. Philadelphia: Lippincott Williams & Wilkins 2000: 183–211.
17. Lindroos M, Kupari M, Heikkila J, Tilvis R. Prevalence of aortic valve abnormalities in the elderly: an echocardiographic study of a random population sample. J Am Coll Cardiol. 1993; 21(5): 1220–5.
18. Rajamannan NM, Gersh B, and Bonow RO. Calcific aortic stenosis: from bench to the bedside – emerging clinical and cellular concepts. Heart 2003; 89(7): 801–5.
19. Fox CS, Vasan RS, Parise H et al. Mitral annular calcification predicts cardiovascular morbidity and mortality: the Framingham Heart Study. Circulation 2003; 107(11): 1492–6.
20. Jeon DS, Atar S, Brasch AV et al. Association of mitral annulus calcification, aortic valve sclerosis and aortic root calcification with abnormal myocardial perfusion single photon emission tomography in subjects age < or = 65 years old. J Am Coll Cardiol. 2001; 38(7): 1988–93.
21. Adler Y, Koren A, Fink N et al. Association between mitral annulus calcification and carotid atherosclerotic disease. Stroke 1998; 29(9): 1833–7.
22. Carabello BA, Stewart WJ, Crawford FA Jr. Aortic valve disease. In Textbook of Cardiovascular Medicine. EJ Topol, ed. Lippincott-Raven 1997: 533–55.
23. Morgan-Hughes GJ, Roobottom CA, Marshall AJ. Aortic valve imaging with computed tomography: a review. J Heart Valve Dis. 2002 Sep; 11(5): 604–11.
24. Morgan-Hughes GJ, Owens PE, Roobottom CA, Marshall AJ. Three dimensional volume quantification of aortic valve calcification using multislice computed tomography. Heart 2003 Oct; 89(10): 1191–4.
25. Liu F, Coursey CA, Grahame-Clarke C et al. Aortic valve calcification as an incidental finding at CT of the elderly: severity and location as predictors of aortic stenosis Am J Roentgenol. 2006 Feb; 186(2): 342–9.

26. Koos R, Mahnken AH, Sinha AM, et al. Aortic valve calcification as a marker for aortic stenosis severity: assessment on 16-MDCT. AJR Am J Roentgenol. 2004 Dec; 183(6): 1813–8.

27. Koos R, Kuhl HP, Muhlenbruch G et al. Prevalence and Clinical Importance of Aortic Valve Calcification Detected Incidentally on CT Scans: Comparison with Echocardiography. Radiology 2006, Aug 14.

28. Rosenhek R, Binder T, Porenta G et al. Predictors of outcome in severe, asymptomatic aortic stenosis. N Engl J Med. 2000 Aug 31; 343(9): 611–7.

29. Feuchtner GM, Dichtl W, Friedrich GJ et al. Multislice computed tomography for detection of patients with aortic valve stenosis and quantification of severity. J Am Coll Cardiol. 2006 Apr 4; 47(7): 1410–7.

30. Alkadhi H, Wildermuth S, Plass A et al. Aortic stenosis: comparative evaluation of 16-detector row CT and echocardiography. Radiology 2006 Jul; 240(1): 47–55.

31. Jacobs JE, Srichai M, Kim D, Hecht E, Kronzon I. Quadricuspid aortic valve: Imaging findings on multidetector helical CT with echocardiographic correlation. J Comput Assist Tomogr. 2006 Jul-Aug; 30(4): 569–71.

32. Morgan-Hughes GJ, Owens PE, Roobottom CA, Marshall AJ. Dilatation of the aorta in pure, severe, bicuspid aortic valve stenosis. Am Heart J. 2004 Apr; 147(4): 736–40.

33. Liu PS, Sutton MG, Litt HI. Diffuse supravalvular aortic stenosis: comprehensive imaging with ECG-gated CT angiography. Int J Cardiovasc Imaging. 2006, Jul 5.

34. Sebastia C, Quiroga S, Boye R et al. Aortic stenosis: spectrum of diseases depicted at multisection CT. Radiographics 2003 Oct; 23 Spec No: S79–91.

35. Carabello BA. Progress in mitral and aortic regurgitation. Prog Cardiovasc Dis. 2001; 43(6): 457–75.

36. Rahimtoola SH. Aortic regurgitation. Atlas of Heart Disease, ed. E. Braunwald. Vol. 11. 1997, Philadelphia: Current Medicine, 7–9.

37. Feuchtner GM, Dichtl W, Schachner T et al. Diagnostic performance of MDCT for detecting aortic valve regurgitation. AJR Am J Roentgenol. 2006 Jun; 186(6): 1676–81.

38. ACC/AHA guidelines for the management of patients with valvular heart disease. A report of the American College of Cardiology/American Heart Association. Task Force on Practice Guidelines (Committee on Management of Patients with Valvular Heart Disease). J Am Coll Cardiol 1998; 32(5): 1486–588.

39. Lung B, Gohlke-Barwolf C, Tomos P et al. Recommendations on the management of the asymptomatic patient with valvular heart disease. Eur Heart J. 2002; 23(16): 1252–66.

40. Filgner CL, Reichenbach DD, Otto CM. Pathology and etiology of valvular heart disease, 2 ed. Valvular Heart Disease, ed. CM Otto. Philadelphia: WB Saunders 2004: 30–3.

41. Alpert JS, Sabik J, Cosgrove DM III. Mitral Valve Disease. In Textbook of Cardiovascular Medicine. EJ Topol, ed., Lippincott-Raven 1997; 503–32.

42. Grover-McKay M, Weiss RM, Vandenberg BF et al. Assessment of cardiac volumes and left ventricular mass by cine computed tomography before and after mitral balloon commissurotomy. Am Heart J. 1994 Sep; 128(3): 533–9.

43. White ML, Grover-McKay M, Weiss RM, Vandenberg BF et al. Prediction of change in mitral valve area after mitral balloon commissurotomy using cine computed tomography. Invest Radiol. 1994 Sep; 29(9): 827–33.

44. Willmann JK, Kobza R, Roos JE et al. ECG-gated multidetector row CT for assessment of mitral valve disease: initial experience. Eur Radiol. 2002 Nov; 12(11): 2662–9.

45. Alkadhi H, Bettex DA, Wildermuth S et al. Dynamic cine imaging of the mitral valve with 16-MDCT: a feasibility study. AJR Am J Roentgenol. 2005 Sep; 185(3): 636–46.

46. Carabello BA. Progress in mitral and aortic regurgitation. Prog Cardiovasc Dis. 2001; 43(6): 457–75.

47. Mann JM, Davies MJ. The pathology of the mitral valve, 2 ed. Mitral Valve Disease, ed. FC Wells and LM Shapiro. London: Butterworths 1996: 16–27.

48. Morgan-Hughes G, Zacharkiw L, Roobottom C, Marshall AJ. Images in cardiovascular medicine. Tumor-like calcification of the mitral annulus: diagnosis with multislice computed tomography. Circulation 2003 Jan 21; 107(2): 355–6.

49. Barber JE, Ratliff NB, Cosgrove DM III, Griffin BP, Verseley I. Myxomatous mitral valve chordae. I: Mechanical properties. J Heart Valve Dis. 2001; 10(3): 320–4.

50. Otsuji Y, Handschumacher MD, Schwammenthal E et al. Insights from three-dimensional echocardiography into the mechanism of functional mitral regurgitation: direct in vivo demonstration of altered leaflet tethering geometry. Circulation 1997; 96(6): 1999–2008.

51. Alkadhi H, Wildermuth S, Bettex DA et al. Mitral regurgitation: quantification with 16-detector row CT – initial experience. Radiology 2006 Feb; 238(2): 454–63.

52. Lembcke A, Wiese TH, Enzweiler CN et al. Quantification of mitral valve regurgitation by left ventricular volume and flow measurements using electron beam computed tomography: comparison with magnetic resonance imaging. J Comput Assist Tomogr. 2003 May-Jun; 27(3): 385–91.

53. Lembcke A, Borges AC, Dushe S et al. Assessment of mitral valve regurgitation at electron-beam CT: comparison with Doppler echocardiography. Radiology 2005 Jul; 236(1): 47–55.

54. Lembcke A, Borges AC, Dohmen PM et al. Quantification of functional mitral valve regurgitation in patients with congestive heart failure: comparison of electron-beam computed tomography with cardiac catheterization. Invest Radiol. 2004 Dec; 39(12): 728–39.

55. Ewy GA. Tricuspid Valve Disease, 3 ed. Valvular Heart Disease, ed. JS Alpert, JE Dalen, SH Rahimtoola. Philadelphia: Lippincott, Williams & Wilkins 2000: 377–92.

56. Otto CM. Right sided valve disease, 2 ed. Valvular Heart Disease, ed. CM Otto. Philadelphia: WB Saunders 2004: 415–36.

57. Groves AM, Win T, Charman SC et al. Semi-quantitative assessment of tricuspid regurgitation on contrast-enhanced multidetector CT. Clin Radiol. 2004 Aug; 59(8): 715–9.

58. Yeh BM, Kurzman P, Foster E et al. Clinical relevance of retrograde inferior vena cava or hepatic vein opacification during contrast-enhanced CT. AJR Am J Roentgenol. 2004 Nov; 183(5): 1227–32.

59. Fox DJ, Khattar RS. Carcinoid heart disease: presentation, diagnosis, and management. Heart 2004; 90(10): 1224–8.

60. Veitch AM, Morgan-Hughes GJ, Roobottom CA. Carcinoid heart disease as shown by 64-slice CT coronary angiography. Eur Heart J. 2006; 27(19): 2271.

61. Mylonakis E, Calderwood SB. Infective endocarditis in adults. N Engl J Med. 2001; 345(18): 1318–30.

62. Mahesh B, Angelini G, Caputo M, Jin XY, Bryan A. Prosthetic valve endocarditis. Ann Thorac Surg. 2005; 80(3): 1151–8.

63. Cribier A, Eltchaninoff H, Tron C et al. Treatment of calcific aortic stenosis with the percutaneous heart valve: mid-term follow-up from the initial feasibility studies: the French experience. J Am Coll Cardiol. 2006 Mar 21; 47(6): 1214–23.

64. Meier B. The Current and Future State of Interventional Cardiology: A Critical Appraisal. Cardiology 2006 Apr 27; 106(3): 174–189.

65. Feldman T, Herrmann HC, St Goar F. Percutaneous treatment of valvular heart disease: catheter-based aortic valve replacement and mitral valve repair therapies. Am J Geriatr Cardiol. 2006 Sep-Oct; 15(5): 291–301.

20

Multislice Computed Tomography Evaluation of Congenital Heart Disease

Robert C. Gilkeson, Kenneth G. Zahka, and Ernest S. Siwik

Traditional evaluation of congenital heart disease was first performed with conventional angiography.[1] While the information enabled with catheter angiography is important in the evaluation of patients with CHD, it remains an invasive procedure requiring sedation and significant radiation. The development of echocardiography enabled real time evaluation with excellent anatomic detail and functional information. It is widely available, portable and is performed without ionizing radiation. Echocardiography has become the primary diagnostic method of choice in the evaluation of patients with CHD.[2] This technique enables non-invasive evaluation of anatomy, myocardial and valvular function.

The advent of Magnetic Resonance Imaging (MRI) and its continued advances provide evaluation of myocardial and valvular function with improved three-dimensional evaluation.[3] Recent literature has established MRI as the gold standard for evaluation of ventricular function. Continuing advances in MR angiography and ultrafast MR techniques now enable evaluation of vascular anatomy with spatial resolution now approaching conventional angiography.[4]

Significant advances in CT imaging of congenital heart disease were first performed with EBCT.[5] Faster imaging times with EBCT enabled superior spatial and anatomic information when compared to conventional single slice CT. ECG gating technology further provided functional information not possible with conventional CT technology.[6]

While effective, the limited availability and prohibitive cost of EBCT technology has limited its widespread clinical utility.

Multislice CT provides excellent three-dimensional evaluation of cardiovascular anatomy in patients with CHD.[7] Recent studies have demonstrated that retrospective ECG gating enables functional evaluation similar to conventional echocardiography.[8] While MSCT requires ionizing radiation, the marked reduction in imaging times can often avoid the sedation sometimes needed in echocardiography and usually required with MRI.

Current multislice CT technology offers an important complement to traditional imaging techniques in the evaluation of CHD. There are relative diagnostic 'blind spots' in echocardiography.[9] Transthoracic echocardiography can be limited in the comprehensive evaluation of the right ventricle, particularly important in the patient with congenital heart disease. The transverse and descending aortic arch is often suboptimally visualized with echocardiography, important information in patients with suspected aortic arch anomalies. Evaluation of branch and distal pulmonary arteries are limited in echocardiography as is the assessment of the pulmonary veins and venous drainage. In patients with right heart enlargement, anomalous pulmonary drainage must be assessed. The anatomic limitations of echocardiography are particular strengths of the three-dimensional evaluation with MSCT.

While transesophageal echocardiography is a more sensitive evaluation of intracardiac pathology, there are important complications to be considered in patients with congenital heart disease. Patients with congenital heart disease and associated esophageal anomalies have a greater risk of esophageal perforation and injury undergoing TEE. In patients with congenital heart disease, the tracheobronchial tree is often affected. Vascular rings, pulmonary artery enlargement and anomalous vascular relationships will compromise the central airways.[10] In the congenital heart patient that presents with shortness of breath, compromise of the tracheobronchial tree is important to consider.[11,12] Performing TEE in patients with aortic arch anomalies and vascular rings can compromise the pediatric airway.[13] While echocardiography will often delineate the important vascular relationships in patients with congenital heart disease, CT is an important non-invasive imaging modality in the anatomic delineation of vascular and airway relationships.

It is similarly important to recognize both the advantages and limitations in the use of CT in the assessment of patients with congenital heart disease. Continued advances in multislice CT technology offer significantly decreased imaging times when compared to echocardiography and MRI. This advantage in imaging times significantly decreases the need for sedation. Studies in early single slice helical CT sited sedation rates of 30%, a significant improvement when compared to MRI.[14,15] Evaluation of the pediatric patient with multislice CT has described a sedation rate of 6%.[16]

In the CT evaluation of young children and infants with congenital heart disease, radiation dose issues are particularly important to consider. Close consultation with our pediatric cardiology colleagues is necessary to determine the optimal imaging study for the patient. While conventional cardiovascular CT imaging is generally performed at 120 kV in adults, diagnostic cardiovascular imaging in children can be performed at 80 kV. Recent studies with this technique have described both significant decreases in radiation dose while maintaining excellent visualization of pertinent cardiovascular pathology.[17] In infants, 50 mAs is chosen, while children 6–12 are imaged at 65 M mAs.

Imaging protocols in children utilize non-ionic iodinated contrast material (300–320 mg I/ml) administered with volumes of 2 ml/kg. In imaging the very small infant, contrast with limited access will often be injected via an indwelling umbilical venous catheter. Before injection of the catheter, close inspection of the scout is important to establish the position of the catheter. Occasionally, the UVC tip can be located in the ductus venosus. In this setting, the

catheter will be carefully repositioned in the more proximal IVC to avoid the contrast injection within the hepatic parenchyma that can occur when the catheter is within the ductus venosus. In infants, contrast material is usually hand injected. With hand injection, the scan is empirically begun after 50% of the contrast material is injected. In very small infants, we have found that an indwelling NG can produce significant artifacts that can particularly limit three-dimensional reconstruction. We will request temporary NG tube removal, if clinically feasible.

In children with antecubital IV access, contrast can be power injected at 2 cc/sec. Depiction of cardiovascular pathology requires optimal contrast opacification of cardiovascular structures. Close consultation with our pediatric cardiologists and cardiac surgeons precedes all cardiac CT evaluations. Bolus tracking techniques are performed to optimize maximal contrast opacification in the most anatomically important vascular structures. Bolus tracking is performed with placement of the tracking device placed in the most important vascular structures to be assessed. Imaging of children with congenital heart disease is optimally performed with 64-slice scanning, though most pertinent information can often be obtained with 16 and 4-slice technology. In the infant, slice collimation is performed at 1 mm slice thickness with 0.5 mm reconstructions. In children, 2 mm slice thickness with 1 mm slice reconstructions are obtained. The significant dose increases in radiation dose with retrospective ECG gating necessitates judicious use of the technique. ECG gating is performed when precise coronary anatomy is needed and definitive aortic valve imaging is required.[18] In children, coronary artery evaluation is performed primarily for evaluation of coronary artery anomalies, not stenosis or plaque characterization. Due to these imaging requirements, mAs is lowered to 175–200 mAs. The advent of dose synchronization with the ECG signal enables periodic decrease in radiation dose during the systolic phase of the cardiac cycle, reserving the maximal dose during the diastolic phase when coronary artery motion is optimally visualized.[19]

As there have been significant hardware developments in MSCT technology, similar software advancements have continually improved the three-dimensional reconstruction of cardiovascular anatomy in patients with CHD. All vendor workstations offer rapid post-processing of complex congenital lesions, often enabling anatomic depictions historically reserved for invasive angiography. More importantly, the multiplanar, three-dimensional nature of these reconstructions present complex anatomy in imaging planes familiar to the pediatric cardiologist. This enhanced visualization has become the most significant factor in the acceptance and increasing use of MSCT in the patient with CHD.

In evaluation of the patient with CHD, primary review of the axial images remains important for accurate diagnosis. The majority of imaging review is performed utilizing multiplanar reconstruction (MPR) imaging. MPR enables visualization of atrioventricular septal defects in imaging planes analogous to echocardiography. Maximal intensity projection (MIP) imaging is instrumental in evaluation of the great vessels. The flexibility offered with variable slab thickness MIP is particularly important in the evaluation of aortic arch and pulmonary artery anomalies.[20] Volume rendering is most often utilized in presurgical evaluation.[21] When compared to catheter angiography, the three-dimensional relationships of vascular anatomy and the chest wall are significantly enhanced with MSCT.[22]

Continued advances in surgical therapies have enabled the patient with congenital heart disease to survive into adulthood.[23] While this chapter will present a number of examples of infants and children with congenital heart disease, it is increasingly important to understand the imaging manifestations of the adult patient with corrected/palliated congenital heart disease.[24] We are all currently experiencing the explosion of the use of MSCT in the emergency room. In many centers, MSCT has become an increasing method of triage in the patient with a wide range of cardiorespiratory symptoms.[25] In our experience, this phenomenon has resulted in the increasing diagnoses of the adult with previously unrecognized congenital heart disease. This chapter will present a number of these examples to help in the recognition of this important patient population.

I EVALUATION OF CONGENITAL DISEASES OF THE AORTA

The accurate and non-invasive diagnosis of thoracic aortic disease has been a particular benefit to MSCT imaging.[26] The rapid acquisition of images and three-dimensional capabilities of MSCT enables sophisticated depiction of congenital aortic disease in the youngest patients. The common association of congenital thoracic aortic anomalies and tracheobronchial pathology establish MSCT as a particularly powerful imaging modality in congenital aortic disease.[27]

It is important to recognize common congenital variants of aortic arch anatomy. While commonly asymptomatic, their recognition is important particularly in patients undergoing

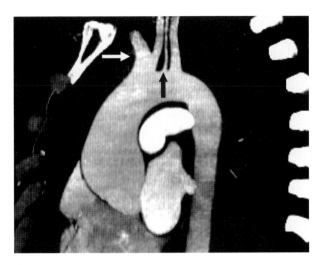

Figure 20.1   17-year-old with Marfans disease for aortic aneurysm evaluation. Sagittal oblique MPR demonstrates bovine aortic arch (white arrow) and direct origin of the left vertebral artery (black arrow).

neurovascular procedures and aortic surgery. The bovine aortic arch is seen in 25% of patients, representing a common origin of the brachiocephalic and left common carotid artery. Direct origin of the left vertebral is identified in 1% of patients. Probably due to the improved visualization of multiplanar imaging, we have seen an increased association of these two congenital variants (Figure 20.1). Recognition of these common variants is particularly important in preventing neurologic complications in patients undergoing complex aortic and aortic arch reconstruction surgery.[28]

The most important congenital aortic anomalies include double aortic arch, left aortic arch and aberrant right subclavian, and right aortic arch with aberrant left subclavian. The anatomy of these anomalies may predispose children to tracheal and esophageal compression, resulting in tracheal and esophageal compression.[29] The double aortic arch represents a persistence of the embryologic double aortic arch, and is the most common cause of a symptomatic vascular ring.[30] The right arch is characteristically larger and superior to the left aortic. The presence of symptoms is often due to the relative atresia of the left aortic arch. Stridor will present in patients with associated tracheomalacia (Figure 20.2). Double aortic arch may first present in adults, often the result of an abnormal mediastinal contour on chest radiographs. While uncommon, recognition of this anomaly in the older population is important to avoid misinterpretation of the double aortic arch as adenopathy or a mediastinal mass.

The left aortic arch and aberrant right subclavian is seen in 1% of patients. The aberrant subclavian often arises from

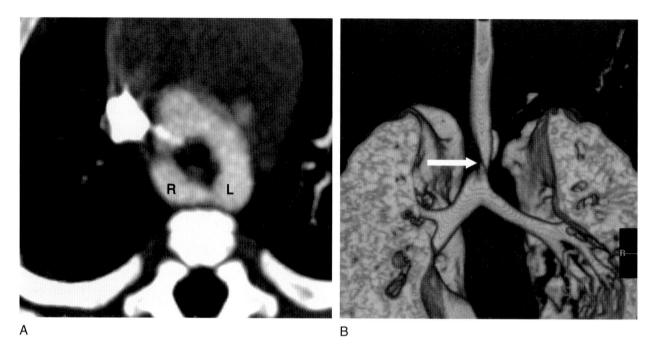

A   B

Figure 20.2   2-week-old male with stridor. A. Axial MIP images demonstrate double aortic arch (R = right aortic arch, L = left aortic arch). B. Coronal reconstruction of the airway shows focal narrowing of the trachea at the level of the right aortic arch (arrow).

the diverticulum of Kommerell, representing the embryonic remnant of the right aortic arch. The presence of symptoms of stridor or dysphagia will correspond to the relative size of the associated diverticulum of Kommerell.[31] While commonly seen in the pediatric population, it is important to recognize this entity in the adult population. It has been well recognized that the aberrant right subclavian is prone to advanced atherosclerotic disease and increased incidence of aneurysmal disease (Figure 20.3). Distal embolization of atherosclerotic plaque has been described in this population.

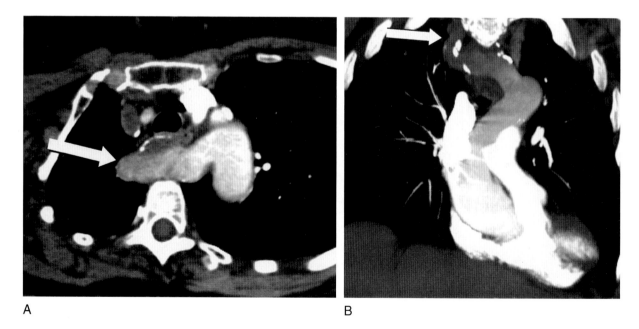

A   B

Figure 20.3   57-year-old woman presents with dyspnea. A. Axial MIP demonstrates aneurysmal aberrant right subclavian artery crossing posterior to the trachea and esophagus (arrow). B. Coronal MIP better defines the full course of the aberrant, atherosclerotic right subclavian artery.

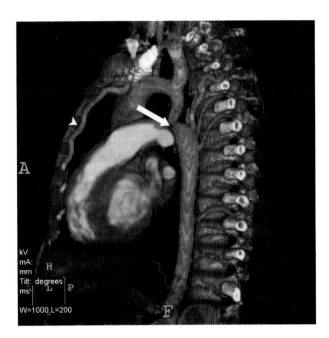

Figure 20.4 11-year-old male presents with hypertension and murmur. Volume rendered sagittal oblique image confirms focal coarctation of the aorta (arrow). Note prominent collateral vessels including internal mammary artery.

In the adult population undergoing cardiac surgery, identification of this anomaly is particularly important. Cardiopulmonary bypass is often performed via axillary artery cannulation and retrograde perfusion to the brain via the brachiocephalic artery. In patients with left aortic and aberrant right subclavian artery, axillary cannulation will only perfuse the right subclavian via the descending aorta, markedly increasing the risk of operative stroke if this anomaly is not recognized.

Coarctation of the aorta is a diagnosis traditionally made with catheter angiography. The ability of MRI to define the anatomy of the coarctation while quantifying flow velocity and pressure gradients has made this an increasingly powerful tool. MSCT is currently able to both quickly and non-invasively define the anatomic extent of the coarctation while depicting the presence of collateral flow from internal mammary and intercostal artery is important in evaluation of this congenital anomaly[32,33] (Figure 20.4). While well defined in the pediatric population, aortic coarctation is an important entity to consider in adults presenting in acute aortic syndromes (Figure 20.5).

Williams syndrome is a rare but well classified syndrome of supravalvular aortic stenosis (Figure 20.6), elfin facies and hypercalcemia. Evaluation of patients with Williams syndrome will often present with a diffuse arteriopathy involving the peripheral pulmonary arteries, thoracoabdominal coarctation and visceral arterial involvement. The speed and comprehensive anatomic coverage enables MSCT to become a powerful and comprehensive tool in evaluation of these patients.[34]

An increasing literature has described reports of congenital valvular disease with MSCT. The integration of ECG gating

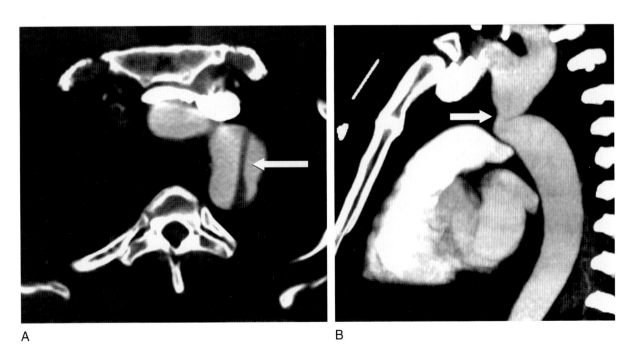

A   B

Figure 20.5 22-year-old male presents with chest pain. A. Axial MIP demonstrates aortic dissection involving the aortic arch (arrow). B. Sagittal oblique MIP image demonstrates focal aortic coarctation (arrow) distal to the arch dissection.

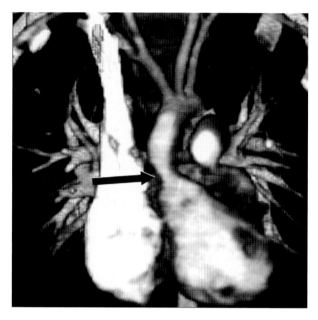

Figure 20.6 3-year-old with Williams syndrome. Coronal volume rendered image reveals focal supravalvular stenosis (arrow).

significantly improves assessment of aortic valve disease.[35] MSCT can define aortic valve calcification, leaflet architecture and accurate assessment of valve area. The most common congenital valvular lesion is the bicuspid aortic valve, found in 1–2% of patients.[36] While bicuspid aortic valve is often first diagnosed with echocardiography, MSCT imaging capabilities allows accurate diagnosis of the patient with bicuspid aortic valve (Figure 20.7). While less defined in the literature, congenital lesions of the subvalvular apparatus can be diagnosed with MSCT (Figure 20.8).

2 EVALUATION OF CONGENITAL DISEASE OF PULMONARY ARTERIES AND VEINS

From the advent of spiral CT, assessment of a wide variety of congenital pulmonary artery lesions have been described. The increased imaging speed and capacity for three-dimensional reconstruction allow accurate assessment of the most complex congenital pulmonary artery lesions. In arteriovenous malformations, MSCT defines the angioarchitecture important to the diagnosis of pulmonary AVMs.[37,38] In the small child, this is particularly helpful for the non-invasive preprocedural evaluation of AVMs (Figure 20.9).

Pulmonary artery atresia and stenosis is seen in a wide variety of congenital lesions. While echocardiography can assess the central pulmonary arteries, visualization of the branch and peripheral pulmonary arteries are limited. MSCT can accurately and non-invasively visualize the peripheral pulmonary arteries in the child often assessed with catheter angiography. While Tetralogy of Fallot is the congenital heart most commonly associated with pulmonary artery atresia, a wide variety of congenital pulmonary /stenoses can present in

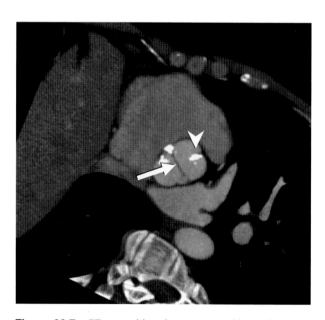

Figure 20.7 57-year-old male presents with aortic stenosis. Sagittal oblique MIP image demonstrates bicuspid aortic valve (arrow) with associated calcification (arrowhead).

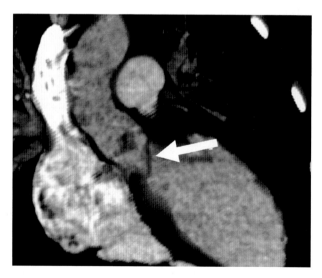

Figure 20.8 24-year-old presents with chest pain and left ventricular hypertrophy on EKG. Coronal volume rendered image reveals linear soft tissue within the aortic outflow tract consistent with subaortic web (arrow).

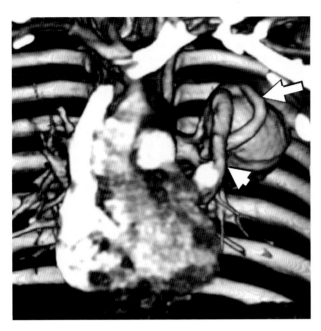

Figure 20.9 2-month-old with left upper mass on chest radiograph. Coronal volume rendered image demonstrates large arteriovenous malformation with feeding artery (arrow) and draining vein (arrowhead).

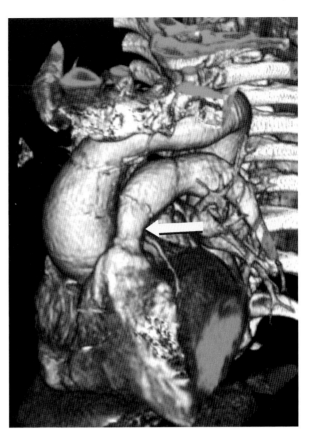

Figure 20.10 24-year-old S/P Ross procedure and pulmonary homograft repair presents with exercise intolerance. Oblique coronal volume rendered image defines focal stenosis of the right ventricular outflow tract (arrow).

the palliated adult with corrected CHD (Figure 20.10). Unsuspected congenital pulmonary artery anomalies can be diagnosed in adults undergoing CT angiography evaluation for pulmonary embolus (Figure 20.11).

MSCT provides particular advantages in the assessment of the systemic and pulmonary veins. Echocardiography can be particularly limited in assessment of pulmonary venous anatomy and venous drainage patterns. Pulmonary vein stenosis/atresia can present with infiltrates and unusual patterns of pulmonary edema. While these atretic pulmonary veins are incompletely evaluated with echocardiography, MSCT can identify the atretic veins and systemic collateral arterial supply associated with these disorders (Figure 20.12).

Congenital anomalies of pulmonary venous drainage are reported in 04–0.9% of patients.[39] Anomalies of pulmonary venous drainage are often suspected when echocardiography demonstrates enlarged right-sided cardiac structures, when the pulmonary veins are poorly visualized. Partial anomalous pulmonary venous return (PAPVR) is more common in males than females[40] while reports describe the prevalence of anomalous venous drainage of right-sided pulmonary veins to the SVC and right atrium,[41] recent reports describe the most common anomalous drainage pattern as the left upper lobe pulmonary vein draining into the left vertical vein[42] (Figure 20.13). In evaluation of patients with partial anomalous venous return of the right upper lobe, it is particularly important to assess for sinus venosus

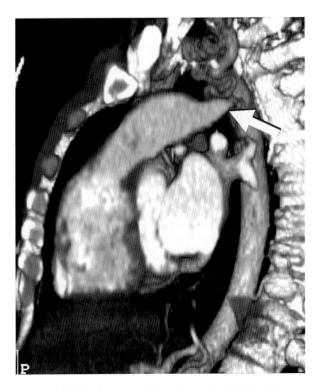

Figure 20.11 27-year-old male evaluated for dyspnea and suspected pulmonary embolism. Sagittal oblique volume rendered image demonstrates distal atresia of the left pulmonary artery (arrow).

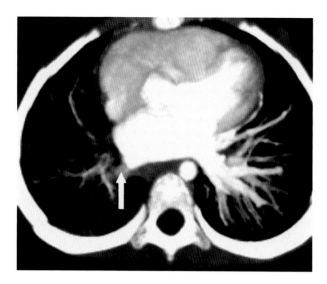

Figure 20.12 2-month-old presents with right-sided edema on chest radiographs. Echocardiography could not identify right-sided pulmonary veins. Axial MIP image illustrates atresia of right-sided pulmonary veins (arrow).

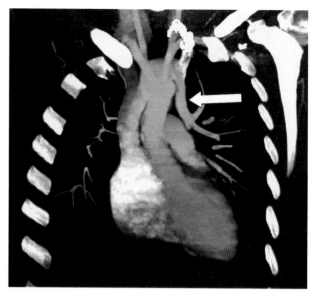

Figure 20.13 22-year-old male presents with right ventricular enlargement on echocardiogram. Coronal MIP image demonstrates anomalous left upper lobe pulmonary venous drainage via a vertical vein to left brachiocepahalic vein (arrow).

defects, an atrial septal defect located in the superior aspect of the atrial septum[43] (Figure 20.14).

3 EVALUATION OF CONGENITAL DISEASE OF THE CARDIAC CHAMBERS AND CORONARY ARTERIES

While echocardiography is preferred in the evaluation of atrioventricular defects, MSCT can depict important atrioventricular septal defects. The ever improving spatial resolution of MSCT can detect ventriculoseptal defects in the smallest patient. Recent reports suggest that while the intracardiac shunt can be clearly defined, in some cases directionality of flow can also be assessed.[44] The increased utilization of MSCT in evaluation of chest pain and coronary artery disease has resulted in increased detection of previously undiagnosed atrioventricular septal defects. We have recently seen a significant number of patients with previously undiagnosed atrial septal defects presenting with chest pain and pulmonary artery hypertension (Figure 20.15).

Though rare, the congenital cardiomyopathies have been well described. Arrhythmogenic right ventricular dysplasia (ARVD) and Uhls disease primarily involve the right ventricle. These cardiomyopathies present with clinical signs of right heart failure, and imaging studies demonstrate marked enlargement of right-sided cardiac structures.[45] The right ventricle is markedly dilated, and fatty infiltration of the right

ventricle in ARVD is classically reported.[46] While echocardiography is the traditional method of evaluation, reports have described the use of MSCT in evaluation of these cardiomyopathies.[47] Isolated non-compaction of the ventricular myocardium is a rare cardiomyopathy that usually affects the

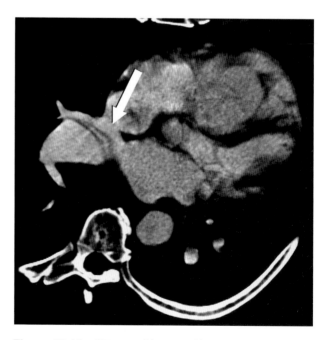

Figure 20.14 67-year-old man with shortness of breath following surgery for colon cancer. No prior history of congenital heart disease. Axial oblique MIP image demonstrate atrial septal defect in the superior aspect of the interatrial septum (arrow) consistent with sinus venosus ASD.

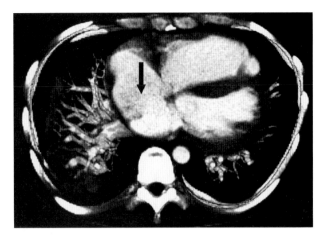

Figure 20.15 57-year-old woman presents for evaluation of pulmonary artery hypertension. No prior history of congenital heart disease. Axial MIP images demonstrate large ASD with no identifiable atrial septal tissue (arrow). Note changes of pulmonary artery hypertension.

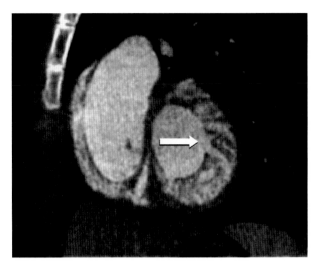

Figure 20.16 9-year-old with prior history of Non-Compaction Syndrome diagnosed at birth. Short axis MIP view of the heart illustrates prominent trabecular network of non-compacted myocardial tissue (arrow).

left ventricle. The disorder is felt to result from a failure of normal endomyocardial embryogenesis. Imaging studies demonstrate prominent trabecular meshwork with deep intratrabecular processes.[48,49] The improved spatial resolution of MSCT enables an accurate depiction of this rare cardiomyopathy (Figure 20.16).

4 CONGENITAL DISEASE OF THE CORONARY ARTERIES

While more common in the congenital heart disease population, isolated coronary artery anomalies are rare.[50] In autopsy series it is seen in 0.3–0.5% of patients, while coronary artery anomalies are seen in 0.3–1.3% in patients undergoing cardiac catheterization.[51] While the majority of coronary anomalies are benign and incidental findings[52] it is important to accurately identify those anomalies associated with ischemia and sudden cardiac death. Autopsy studies have described incidence rates of sudden cardiac death in 70–80% of patients with these anomalies.[53]

In the CT assessment of anomalous coronary arteries, it is important to review the normal anatomy of the coronary arteries and their origins from the appropriate aortic sinuses. Relating the aortic valve to a clockface, the normal right coronary artery origin exits the right aortic sinus between 10 to 1 o'clock. The left coronary artery exits the left coronary sinus at between 2 and 5 o'clock. In the pediatric population, coronary artery anomalies are often first identified during echocardiographic evaluation. An anomalous coronary artery

is first suspected when the coronary artery is not visualized in the expected coronary sinus. While the origins of the anomalous coronary arteries can be then identified, echocardiographic evaluation of the distal course of these vessels is limited. The accurate delineation of these anomalous vessels is essential to future management, and multislice CT enables a non-invasive diagnostic alternative.

The most important of these anomalies is the anomalous coronary artery arising from the opposite sinus of Valsalva: the left coronary artery arising from right aortic sinus, and the right coronary artery arising from the left aortic sinus. Further, it is important to identify the complete course of these anomalous vessels. The anomalous coronary artery that travels between the aorta and pulmonary artery is associated with significant morbidity and mortality.

A number of theories have been proposed to explain the etiology of ischemia and sudden cardiac death in these patients. These interarterial coronary arteries may have a significant intramural component before exiting the aorta. This intramural course results in a slit-like orifice and compromised blood flow that may be particularly important in the child and young athlete[54] (Figure 20.17). The interarterial coronary artery may take an acute angle as it returns to its appropriate atrioventricular groove. This acute angle may compromise blood flow and place myocardial tissue at risk.[55] Dynamic compression of the interarterial coronary artery between the aorta and pulmonary artery is also hypothesized to be a source of compression and symptoms of chest pain and clinical signs of coronary ischemia (Figure 20.18). It is also recognized that the interarterial anomalous

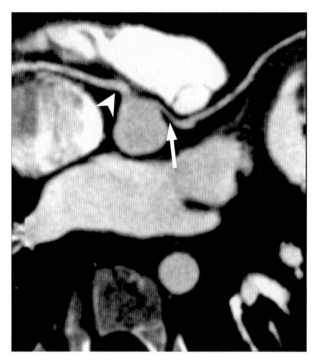

Figure 20.17 6- year-old with syncopal episode. Axial MP demonstrates anomalous origin of left coronary artery from right aortic sinus. Note narrowing of intramural portion (arrow) before exiting to interventricular groove.

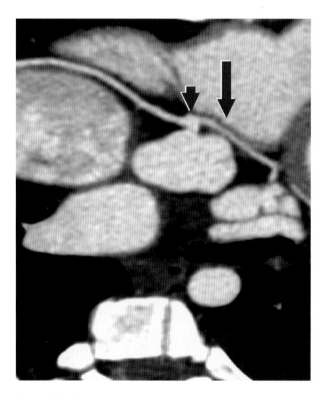

Figure 20.18 12-year-old with suspicion of anomalous left coronary artery on echocardiogram. Axial MIP demonstrates the right and left coronary artery share a common infundibulum arising from the right aortic sinus. Note interarterial course of left coronary artery as it returns to interventricular groove (arrow).

coronary artery my also take an intramyocardial course as it courses distally, an additional risk factor for ischemia and death.[56] Often superior delineation of these anomalies has established MSCT as the imaging method of choice when coronary anomalies are suspected in our pediatric patients.

This chapter has presented the wide variety of imaging manifestations of congenital heart disease. Imaging advances in MSCT have expanded indications for the evaluation of CHD from the youngest infant to the previously undiagnosed adult. A comprehensive CHD imaging service, with the close collaboration of radiologists, pediatric cardiologists and surgeons, will continue to define the important role of MSCT in the evaluation and treatment of our patients with congenital heart disease.

REFERENCES

1. Amplatz K, Moller JH. Radiology of congenital heart disease. Anne S. Patterson, ed., Mosby yearbook, 1993.
2. Seward JB. Biplane and multiplane transesophageal echocardiology: evaluation of congenital heart disease. Am J Card Imaging 1995 Apr; 9(2): 129–36.
3. Boxt LM. Magnetic resonance and computed tomographic evaluation of congenital heart disease. J Magn Reson Imaging 2004 Jun; 19(6): 827–47.
4. Ley S, Zaporozhan J, Arnold R et al. Preoperative assessment and follow-up of congenital abnormalities of the pulmonary arteries using CT and MRI. Eur Radiol. 2007 Jan; 17(1): 151–62. Epub 2006 Jun 24.
5. Boyd DP. Computed tomography: physics and instrumentation. Acad Radiol. 1995 Sep; 2 Suppl 2: S138–40.
6. McCollough CH, Morin RL. The technical design and performance of ultrafast computed tomography. Radiol Clin North Am. 1994 May; 23(3): 521–36.
7. Bean MJ, Pannu H, Fishman EK. Three-dimensional computed tomographic imaging of complex congenital cardiovascular abnormalities. J Comput Assist Tomogr. 2005 Nov–Dec; 29(6): 721–4.
8. Dewey M, Muller M, Eddicks S et al. Evaluation of Global and Regional Left Ventricular Function with 16-Slice Computed Tomography, Biplane Cineventriculography, and Two-Dimensional Transthoracic Echocardiography: Comparison with Magnetic Resonance Imaging. JACC Vol 48, No. 10, 2006; Nov 21, 2006: 2034–44.
9. Ayres NA, Miller-Hance W, Fyfe DA et al. Pediatric Council of the American Society of the Echocardiography. Indications and guidelines for performance of transesophageal echocardiography in the patient with pediatric acquired or congenital heart disease; report from the task force and the Pediatric Council of the American Society of Echocardiography. J Am Soc Echocardiogr. 2005 Jan; 18(1): 91–8.
10. Hopkins KL, Patrick LE, Simoneaux SF et al. Pediatric great vessel anomalies: initial clinical experience with spiral CT angiography. Radiology 1996 Sep; 200(3): 811–15.
11. Katz M, Konen E, Rozenman J, Szeinberg A, Itzchak Y. Spiral CT and 3D image reconstruction of vascular rings and

associated tracheobronchial anomalies. J Comput Assist Tomogr. 1995 Jul–Aug; 19(4): 564–8.

12. Choo KS, Lee HD, Ban JE et al. Evaluation of obstructive airway lesions in complex congenital heart disease using composite volume-rendered images from multislice CT. Pediatr Radiol. 2006 Mar; 36(3): 219–23. Epub 2006 Jan 4.

13. Kharasch ED, Sivarajan M. Gastroesophageal perforation after intraoperative transesophageal echocardiography. Anesthesiology 1996 Aug; 85(2): 426–8.

14. Kaste SC, Young CW, Holmes TP, Baker DK. Effect of helical CT on the frequency of sedation in pediatric patients. AJR Am J Roentgenol. 1997 Apr; 168(4): 1001–3.

15. White KS. Reduced need for sedation in patients undergoing helical CT of the chest and abdomen. Pediatr Radiol. 1995; 25(5): 344–6.

16. Pappas JN, Donnelly LF, Frush DP. Reduced frequency of sedation of young children with multisection helical CT. Radiology 2000 Jun; 215(3): 897–9.

17. Frush DP, Yoshizumi T. Conventional and CT angiography in children: dosimetry and dose comparisons. Pediatr Radiol. 2006 Sep; 36(Supplement 14): 154–8.

18. Abbara, S, Penn AJ, Maurovich-Horvat P et al. Feasibility and optimization of aortic valve planimetry with MDCT. AJR Am J Roentgenol. 2007 Fed; 188(2): 356–60.

19. Jakobs TF, Becker CR, Ohnesorge B et al. Multislice helical CT of the heart with retrospective ECG gating: Reduction of radiation exposure by ECG-controlled tube current modulation. Eur Radiol 12: 1081–6, 2002 May. Epub 2002 Feb 21.

20. Fishman EK, Lawler LP. CT angiography: principles, technique and study optimization using 16-slice multidetector CT with isotropic datasets and 3D volume visualization. Crit Rev Comput Tomogr. 2004; 45(5–6): 355–88.

21. Gilkeson RC, Markowitz AH, Ciancibello L. Multisection CT evaluation of the reoperative cardiac surgery patient. Radiographics 2003 Oct; 23 Spec No. S3–17.

22. Gasparovic H, Rybicki FJ, Millstine J et al. Three dimensional computed tomographic imaging in planning the surgical approach for redo cardiac surgery after coronary revascularization. Eur J Cardiothorac Surg 2005 Aug; 28(2): 244–9.

23. Samyn MM. A review of the complementary information available with cardiac magnetic resonance imaging and multislice computed tomography (CT) during the study of congenital heart disease. Int J Cardiovasc Imaging 2004 Dec; 20(6): 569–78.

24. Siegel MJ. Multiplanar and three-dimensional multi-detector row CT of thoracic vessels and airways in the pediatric population. Radiology 2003 Dec; 229(3): 641–50. Epub 2003 Oct 16.

25. White CS, Jeudy J, Read K et al. Aortic valve bypass for aortic stenosis: imaging appearances on multidetector CT. Int J Cardiovasc Imaging 2006 Jul 20; [Epub ahead of print].

26. Eichhorn J, Fink C, Delorme S, Ulmer H. Rings, slings and other vascular abnormalities. Ultrafast computed tomography and magnetic resonance angiography in pediatric cardiology. Z Kardiol. 2004 Mar; 93(3): 201–8.

27. Choo KS, Lee HD, Ban JE et al. Evaluation of obstructive airway lesions in complex congenital heart disease using composite volume-rendered images from multislice CT. Pediatr Radiol. 2006 Mar; 36(3): 219–23. Epub 2006 Jan 4.

28. Mauney MM, Cassada DC, Kaza AK, Long SM, Kern JA. Management of innominate artery injury in the setting of

bovine arch anomaly. Ann Thorac Surg. 2001 Dec; 72(6): 2134–6.

29. Berdon WE. Rings, slings, and other things: vascular compression of the infant trachea updated from the midcentury to the millennium–the legacy of Robert E Gross, MD, and Edward BD Neuhauser, MD. Radiology 2000 Sep; 216(3): 624–32.

30. Juraszek AL, Guleserian KJ. Common Aortic Arch Anomalies: Diagnosis and Management. Curr Treat Options Cardiovasc Med. 2006 Sep; 8(5): 414–18.

31. Alper F, Akgun M, Kantarci M et al. Demonstration of vascular abnormalities compressing esophagus by MDCT: special focus on dysphagia lusoria. Eur J Radiol. 2006 Jul; 59(1): 82–7. Epub 2006 Mar 2.

32. Becker C et al. Spiral CT angiography and 3D reconstruction in patients with aortic coarctation. Eur Radiol 1997; 7: 1473–7.

33. Goo HW, Park IS, Ko JK et al. CT of congenital heart disease: normal anatomy and typical pathologic conditions. Radiographics 2003 Oct; 23 Spec No. S147–65.

34. Goo HW, Park IS, Ko JK et al. Computed tomography for the diagnosis of congenital heart disease in pediatric and adult patients. Int J Cardiovasc Imaging 2005 Apr–Jun; 21(2–3): 347–65; discussion 367.

35. Willmann JK, Weishaupt D, Lachat M et al. Electrocardiographically gated multi-detector row CT for assessment of valvular morphology and calcification in aortic stenosis. Radiology 2002 Oct; 225(1): 120–8.

36. Williams DS. Hereditary hemorrhagic telangiectasia. J Insur Med. 2006; 38(3): 230–2.

37. Hofmann LV, Kuszyk BS, Mitchell SE, Horton KM, Fishman EK. Angioarchitecture of pulmonary arteriovenous malformations: characterization using volume-rendered 3-D CT angiography. Cardiovasc Intervent Radiol. 2000 Mar-Apr; 23(2): 165–70.

38. Lawler LP, Fishman EK. Arteriovenous malformations and systemic lung supply: evaluation by multidetector CT and three-dimensional volume rendering. AJR Am J Roentgenol. 2002 Feb; 178(2): 493–5.

39. Van Meter C Jr, LeBlanc JG, Culpepper WS 3rd, Ochsner JL. Partial anomalous pulmonary venous return. Circulation 1990 Nov; 82(5 Suppl): IV 195–8.

40. Snellen HA, van Ingen HC, Hoefsmit EC. Patterns of anomalous pulmonary venous drainage. Circulation 1968 Jul; 38(1): 45–63.

41. Brody H. Drainage of the pulmonary veins into the right side of the heart. Arch Pathol. 1942; 33: 221–40.

42. Haramati LB, Moche IE, Rivera VT et al. Computed tomography of partial anomalous pulmonary venous connection in adults. J Comput Assist Tomogr. 2003 Sep–Oct; 27(5): 743–9.

43. Toyoshima M, Sato A, Fukumoto Y et al. Partial anomalous pulmonary venous return showing anomalous venous return to the azygos vein. Intern Med. 1992 Sep; 31(9): 1112–16.

44. Funabashi N, Asano M, Sekine T, Nakayama T, Komuro I. Direction, location, and size of shunt flow in congenital heart disease evaluated by ECG-gated multislice computed tomography. Int J Cardiol. 2005 Nov 4 [Epub ahead of print].

45. Tandri H, Bomma C, Calkins H, Bluemke DA. Magnetic resonance and computed tomography imaging of arrhythmogenic right ventricular dysplasia. J Magn Reson Imaging 2004 Jun: 19(6): 848–58.

46. Wu YW, Tadamura E, Kanao S et al. Structural and functional assessment of arrhythmogenic right ventricular

dysplasia/cardiomyopathy by multi-slice computed tomography: Comparison with cardiovascular magnetic resonance. Int J Cardiol. 2006 Nov 10 [Epub ahead of print].

47. Cheng JF, Mohammed TL, Griffith BP, White CS. CT of Uhl's anomaly in an adult. Int J Cardiovasc Imaging 2005 Dec; 21(6): 663–6.

48. Koh YY, Seo YU, Woo JJ, Chang KS, Hong SP. Familial isolated noncompaction of the ventricular myocardium in asymptomatic phase. Yonsei Med J. 2004 Oct 31; 45(5): 931–5.

49. Chin Tk, Perloff JK, Williams RG, Jue K, Mohrmann R. Isolated noncompaction of left ventricular myocardium. A study of eight cases. Circulation 1990 Aug; 82(2): 507–13.

50. Deibler AR, Kuzo RS, Vohringer M et al. Imaging of congenital coronary anomalies with multislice computed tomography. Mayo Clin Proc. 2004 Aug; 79(8): 1017–23.

51. Alexander RW, Griffith GC. Anomalies of the coronary arteries and their clinical significance. Circulation 1956 Nov; 14(5): 800–5.

52. Yamanaka O, Hobbs RE. Coronary artery anomalies in 126,595 patients undergoing coronary arteriography. Cathet Cardiovasc Diagn. 1990 Sep; 21(1): 28–40.

53. Frescura C, Basso C, Thiene G et al. Anomalous origin of coronary arteries and risk of sudden death: a study based on an autopsy population of congenital heart disease. Hum Pathol. 1998 Jul; 29(7): 689–95.

54. Bonnet D, Cormier V, Villain E, Bonhoeffer P, Kachaner J. Progressive left main coronary artery obstruction leading to myocardial infarction in a child with Williams syndrome. Eur J Pediatr. 1997 Oct; 156(10): 751–3.

55. Roberts WC, Siegel RJ, Zipes DP. Origin of the right coronary artery from the left sinus of valsalva and its functional sequences: analysis of 10 necropsy patients. Am J Cardiol. 1982 Mar; 49(4): 863–8.

56. Frescura C, Basso C, Thiene G et al. Anomalous origin of coronary arteries and risk of sudden death: a study based on an autopsy population of congenital heart disease. Hum Pathol. 1998 Jul; 29(7): 689–95.

21

Computed Tomographic Imaging of the Cardiac and Pulmonary Veins: Role in Electrophysiology

Kalpathi L. Venkatachalam and Peter A. Brady

1 INTRODUCTION

Diagnosis and management of complex heart rhythm disorders, in particular atrial fibrillation (AF), continues to evolve. Understanding of the mechanisms of arrhythmias, along with advances in catheter ablative technology and advanced mapping techniques, facilitates execution of electrophysiologic procedures which, in experienced centers, can be carried out with high efficacy and low complication rates.

Evolution in electrophysiologic and ablative procedures has been possible in large part because of advances in cardiac imaging technology, which have a role both in the diagnosis of cardiac disorders that may be the substrate for arrhythmias as well as in providing anatomic data crucial to the planning, execution, and follow-up of arrhythmia procedures.

Imaging modalities most useful in the management of heart rhythm disorders include echocardiography

(transthoracic, transesophageal and intra-cardiac), MRI and multi-gated CT. Each of these imaging techniques has inherent benefits and limitations.

The purpose of this chapter is to describe the utility of multi-detector cardiac computed tomography (MDCT) in diagnosis and treatment of heart rhythm disorders (Table 21.1). Since MDCT is most commonly used in the management of patients with atrial fibrillation, this rhythm will be used as the basis for understanding the applications and benefits of MDCT in diagnosis, treatment (catheter ablation) and follow-up of patients with heart rhythm disorders.

1.1 Atrial fibrillation

Atrial fibrillation is a disorganized atrial rhythm believed to initiate from rapidly-firing foci within the thoracic veins.

Table 21.1 Cardiac CT imaging in electrophysiology

Diagnosis	Peri-operative evaluation
Arrhythmogenic right ventricular dysplasia/cardiomyopathy (ARVD/C) Pulmonary vein anatomy Intracardiac mass/thrombus	Left atrial and pulmonary vein topography (electro-anatomic mapping) Anatomy and post-operative substrate including conduit function in congenital heart disease Coronary sinus anatomy for planned cardiac resynchronization therapy

Impulses from these veins are believed to capture the atria in a rapid and irregular way, resulting in symptoms and the electrocardiographic signature of AF.

Endocardial catheter based techniques that use radiofrequency energy delivered via steerable catheters placed within the left atrium aim, in most cases, to electrically isolate the thoracic veins from the left atrium. Although differences exist in the precise techniques used to isolate electrical activity arising from the pulmonary and other thoracic veins, whether circumferential lesions at the veno-atrial junction or encircling lesions remote from the vein orifice, the success rate of AF ablation in eradicating symptomatic episodes of AF in experienced centers is high.[4,12]

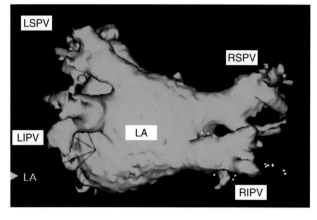

Figure 21.1   3D CT (posterior view) of the normal anatomic relationship between pulmonary veins and left atrium.

2 PLANNING CATHETER ABLATION OF ATRIAL FIBRILLATION: ANATOMIC CONSIDERATIONS

2.1 Pre-operative MDCT

Pre-operative MDCT allows precise anatomic imaging of the heart and thoracic veins and is important, since successful planning of catheter ablation of AF is facilitated by detailed information regarding the number and topology of pulmonary veins, left atrial size and the relationship of the left atrium to other thoracic structures such as the esophagus. In addition, MDCT may reveal the presence of inflammatory or malignant extra-cardiac tumors that may rarely be the cause of AF or atrial septal anomalies, including fibromas or lipomatous atrial septa that might make transseptal puncture more challenging. Detailed anatomic knowledge of normal structural relationships within the thorax is essential prior to AF ablation.

2.2 Normal pulmonary vein anatomy and the relationship of thoracic structures to the left atrium

In most cases 4 pulmonary veins empty into the left atrium (two left sided veins – superior and inferior, and two right sided veins – superior and inferior).[1,2,5] The most common anatomic relationship between these veins is illustrated in Figures 21.1–21.3.

2.3 Normal anatomic relationship between left atrium and esophagus

In the majority of individuals the esophagus course immediately posterior to the left atrium separated by approximately 2–5 mm of soft tissue. The importance of this close anatomic relationship is that prolonged ablation within the left atrium posteriorly, particularly if higher power and temperature settings are used, may risk damage to the esophagus which can have important and possibly fatal consequences. The relationship between the left atrium and the esophagus is shown in Figure 21.4.

2.4 Anatomic variants of pulmonary veins

Although the most common anatomic configuration of the pulmonary veins is two left and two right sided pulmonary veins that each connect to the left atrium via separate ostia, variation is not uncommon. Prior knowledge of the correct number and topology is important since undetected anatomic variation may increase the complexity of ablation and impact procedural success.

The most common anatomic variant of the pulmonary veins is the presence of a common antrum or 'outlet' connecting upper and lower veins. Next frequent are separate ostia for the right middle pulmonary vein into the left atrium, multiple accessory pulmonary veins or a single pulmonary vein. Anomalous pulmonary venous connections

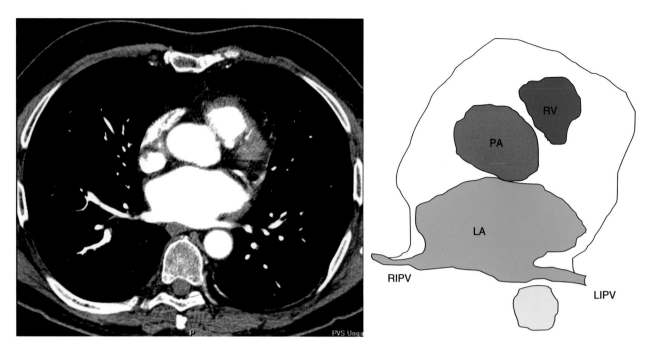

Figure 21.2 Normal anatomic relationship (coronal view) between inferior (lower) pulmonary veins (right and left). RIPV, right inferior pulmonary vein; LIPV, left inferior pulmonary vein.

(e.g. pulmonary veins that drain into the right atrium) and persistent left superior vena cava (with or without occlusion of the coronary sinus) are important to be aware of as they necessitate significant change in ablative approach. Cortriatriatum, which involves septation of the left atrial cavity, is another rare but important anatomic variation in pulmonary vein and left atrial anatomy that impacts AF ablation and is also easily identified by MDCT.

Examples of anatomic variants of pulmonary veins are illustrated in Figures 21.5 – 21.9.

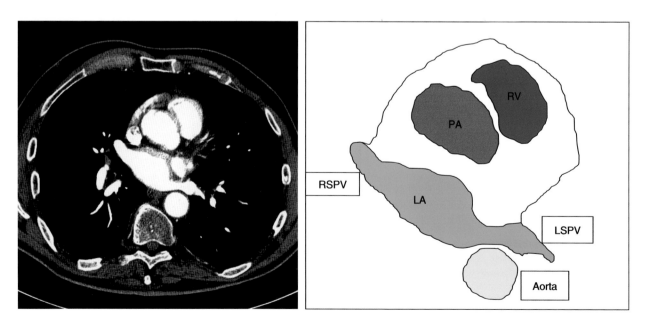

Figure 21.3 Normal anatomic relationship (coronal view) between superior (upper) pulmonary veins (right and left). Note: right ventricle and pulmonary trunk (anterior) and proximity of the esophagus and descending aorta to ostia of the left sided veins. LSPV, left superior pulmonary vein; RSPV, right superior pulmonary vein; PA, pulmonary artery; RV, right ventricle.

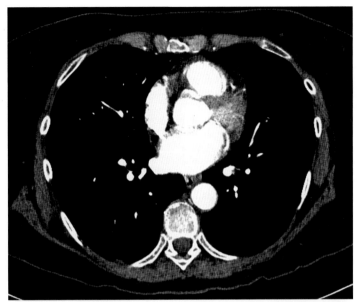

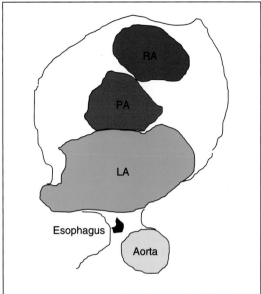

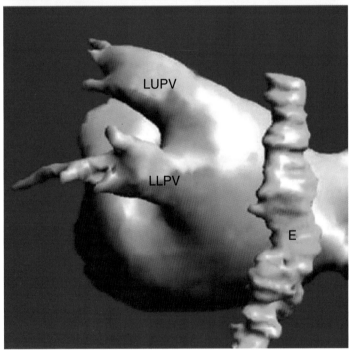

Figure 21.4 MDCT (top left) and line drawing (top right) showing relationship between esophagus and posterior left atrium. Also shown (bottom left) is a 3D-CT reconstruction of the posterior left atrium demonstrating its proximity to the esophagus.[19]

Variation in ablative strategy based upon anatomic differences in pulmonary veins might include use of wider area circumferential lesions that isolate both upper and lower veins within a common antrum or separate ostial lesions in cases where single or discrete ostia between individual veins and the left atrium exist.

Pre-procedural MDCT also provides for comparison with a post-procedural MDCT (typically performed 3 months following AF ablation) to assess for evidence of pulmonary vein stenosis resulting from ablation close to or within the pulmonary vein.

3 LEFT ATRIAL SIZE

Increased left atrial size is a determinant of outcome in patients with AF and may serve as a substrate for sustained re-entrant atrial arrhythmias. Therefore, accurate quantification of LA size is useful in determining possible need for linear ablative lesions within the left atrium. In addition, changes in left atrial size following ablation (reverse atrial remodeling) may have implications for long-term success and can be readily quantified with MDCT[6,7] (Figure 21.10).

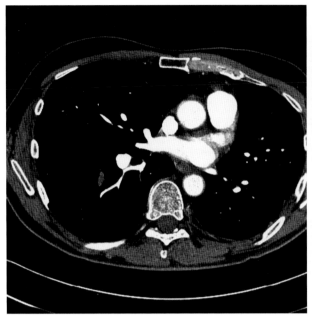

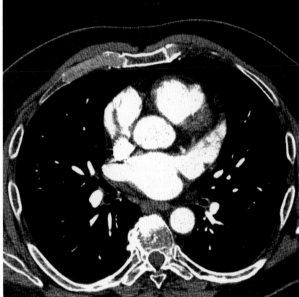

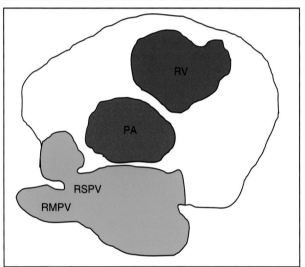

Figure 21.5 MDCT illustrating a common antrum between the RSPV and RMPV. This may require the use of a larger mapping catheter during ablation to confirm loss of pulmonary vein potentials. RMPV, right middle pulmonary vein; PA, pulmonary artery; RV, right ventricle.

3.1 Use of MDCT in cardiac resynchronization therapy

Cardiac resynchronization therapy (CRT) has emerged as an important therapeutic modality in select patients with drug-refractory heart failure. Resynchronization of ventricular contraction can be achieved via an endocardial approach utilizing the coronary sinus (CS) to allow left ventricular pacing in most cases. Since variation in CS anatomy is common, one application of MDCT is to facilitate the procedure by visualization of suitable coronary veins for lead placement prior to implantation (Figure 21.11).[17] Unfortunately CT provides no physiologic information regarding myocardial properties of the target site including pacing and sensing parameters or proximity of the phrenic nerve that may lead to diaphragmatic capture.

4 INTRA-OPERATIVE MDCT AS A GUIDE TO AF ABLATION

Advances in the complexity of arrhythmias that are amenable to catheter ablation has followed in large part the availability of advanced three-dimensional mapping systems that allow accurate identification of the source of an arrhythmia (in cases of a focal mechanism) or in identification of potential circuits using activation mapping techniques or by using a voltage map to identify myocardial scar. More recently, integration of the 'electrical' map with a three-dimensional rendering of the 'anatomy' derived from CT has been possible. These two datasets can then be 'merged' to give an electro-anatomic map of the desired chamber for use during the procedure. Examples of

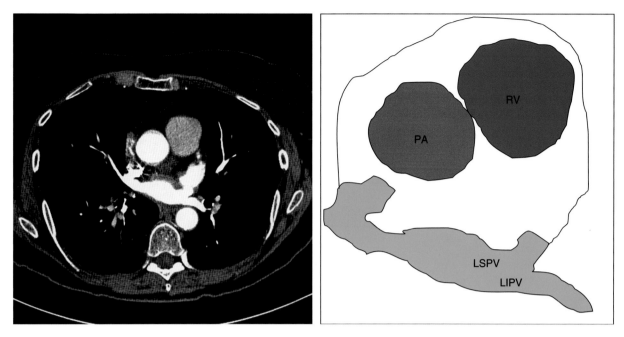

Figure 21.6   Common antrum between the LSPV and LIPV.

commonly used 'electro-anatomic' mapping systems include Carto(®) mapping (Biosense Webster) and NavX(®) (St Jude) (Figures 21.12 and 21.13). An additional advantage of these mapping tools is reduced need for fluoroscopy during the ablation procedure.

4.1 Cardiac CT in congenital heart disease

Arrhythmias are common in patients with congenital heart disease in both uncorrected and corrected (surgical) patients

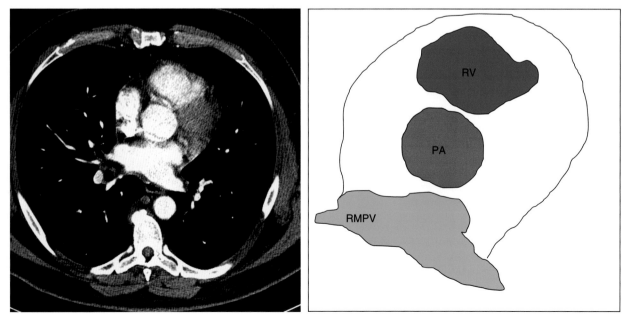

Figure 21.7   Separate ostium of right middle PV.

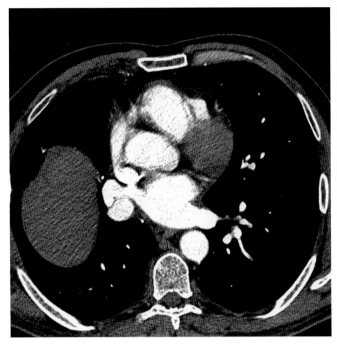

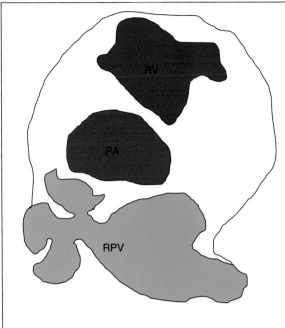

Figure 21.8 Single right pulmonary vein.

with the majority of arrhythmias arising in patients with Ebstein's anomaly of the tricuspid valve and following Mustard, Senning and Fontan procedures. Patients late after repair of Tetralogy of Fallot are predisposed to ventricular arrhythmias. In the majority of cases, observed arrhythmias are re-entrant atrial arrhythmias that utilize scar or suture lines or both as a part of the circuit. Although the usefulness of CT in the management of patients with congenital heart disease continues to evolve, it does provide anatomic detail of both the atria and ventricles as well as location of surgical

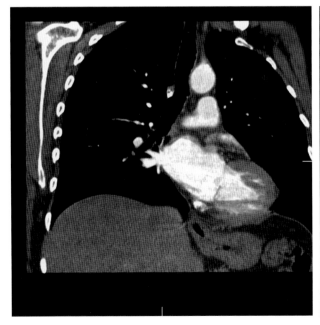

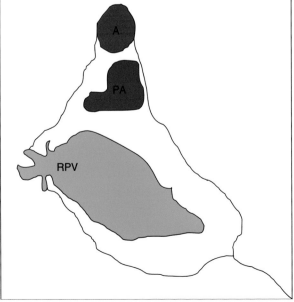

Figure 21.9 Multiple right sided pulmonary veins.

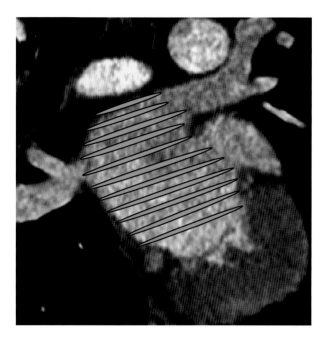

Figure 21.10 Simpson's Rule for LA size (coronal view). Addition of individual area of each ellipse (in two dimensions) allows LA volume measurement that is then normalized to body surface area giving a left atrial volume index (normal 16–28 mL/m²).

conduits, facilitating appropriate planning of ablative intervention. In addition, electro-anatomic merging of CT data with mapping data is useful (Figure 21.14).

4.2 MDCT in ischemic VT ablation

Knowledge of scar location is crucial in planning the ablation of ventricular tachycardia (VT) in patients with ischemic heart disease. A rough idea for VT exit site can be obtained from the 12-lead electrocardiogram during VT. The presence of an implantable defibrillator (present in most patients with ischemic VT) precludes the use of an MRI scan to delineate myocardial scar. However, MDCT may allow precise localization of the myocardial scar responsible for the re-entrant circuit. Correlating this information with electro-anatomical mapping allows for accurate targeting of ablation sites.[18] See Figure 21.15.

4.3 MDCT and diagnosis of complications of catheter ablation

CT is most useful in diagnosis and management of complications in patients with atrial fibrillation, in particular pulmonary vein stenosis and atrial-esophageal fistula.

5 PULMONARY VEIN STENOSIS AFTER AF ABLATION

Thermal injury to the pulmonary veins results in pulmonary vein stenosis in around 1–3% of patients undergoing AF ablation, even in experienced centers, and relates to temperature, anatomic/tissue characteristics as well as operator experience. Significant (greater than 50–70% stenosis) of a pulmonary vein is a potentially serious and difficult-to-manage complication of AF ablation that is associated with significant morbidity. Thus, avoidance of pulmonary stenosis is desirable. Common symptoms of pulmonary vein stenosis/occlusion include: dyspnea, cough, hemoptysis and pleuritic chest pain. In most cases, severity of symptoms relates to both the severity of stenosis and number of affected veins, with few or no symptoms occurring in patients with

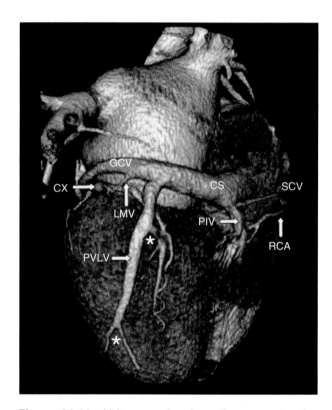

Figure 21.11 Volume-rendered cardiac reconstruction (posterolateral view). This image illustrates the most common anatomic configuration of the coronary sinus and tributaries. In most cases, the posterior interventricular vein (PIV) or middle cardiac vein (MCV) is the first tributary running in the posterior interventricular groove while the second is the posterior vein of the left ventricle (PVLV) that typically has several side branches (asterisks) followed by the left marginal vein (LMV). The great cardiac vein (GCV) continues as anterior cardiac vein in the anterior interventricular groove. Note also the proximity of the circumflex coronary artery (CX) and right coronary artery (RCA).[17]

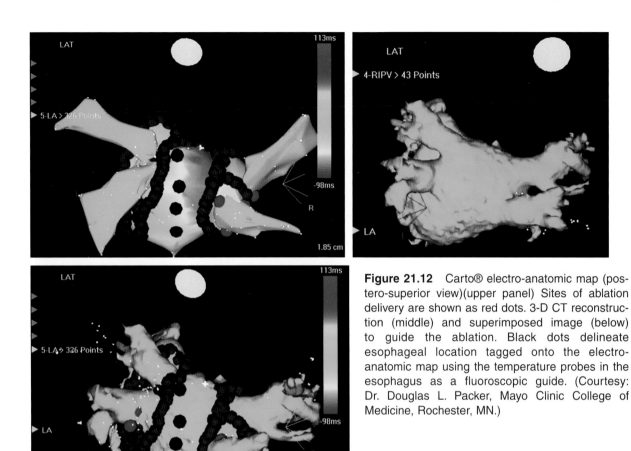

Figure 21.12 Carto® electro-anatomic map (postero-superior view)(upper panel) Sites of ablation delivery are shown as red dots. 3-D CT reconstruction (middle) and superimposed image (below) to guide the ablation. Black dots delineate esophageal location tagged onto the electro-anatomic map using the temperature probes in the esophagus as a fluoroscopic guide. (Courtesy: Dr. Douglas L. Packer, Mayo Clinic College of Medicine, Rochester, MN.)

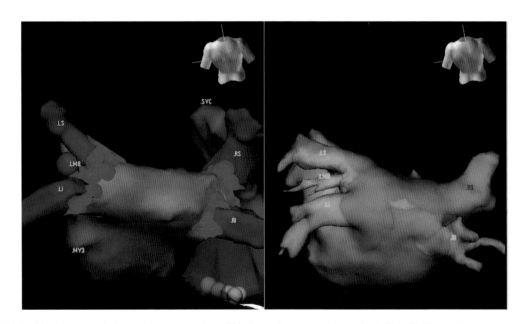

Figure 21.13 NavX map of the pulmonary veins. Ablation sites are shown (red dots (left)) and superimposed on the 3D CT image. Three dimensional CT reconstructions prior to merge with electrical map (right).

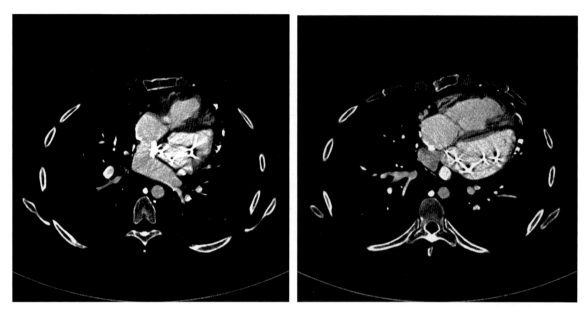

Figure 21.14 CT image (coronal section) of D-TGA following Mustard procedure (creation of intra-atrial baffle) in which left atrium drains into morphologic RV (systemic ventricle)(left panel). Right panel illustrates connection between right atrium and non-systemic LV via the Mustard baffle. Also note artifact due to multiple pacemaker leads within the left (non-systemic) ventricle.

less than moderate stenosis of only 1 or 2 pulmonary veins. Hemoptysis may be present if pulmonary infarction occurs.[13] Typically, symptoms evolve over 1–3 months following the ablation procedure and may initially be attributed to pulmonary etiology unless the index of suspicion is high.

In our practice, routine MDCT is obtained at 3 months following AF ablation unless symptoms arise sooner and allows rapid and effective diagnosis of pulmonary vein stenosis (Figure 21.16).

Appropriate management of symptomatic pulmonary vein stenosis is challenging and may necessitate balloon dilatation (on multiple occasions) or stent placement as appropriate. These procedures are performed in most cases via transseptal catheterization using fluoroscopic

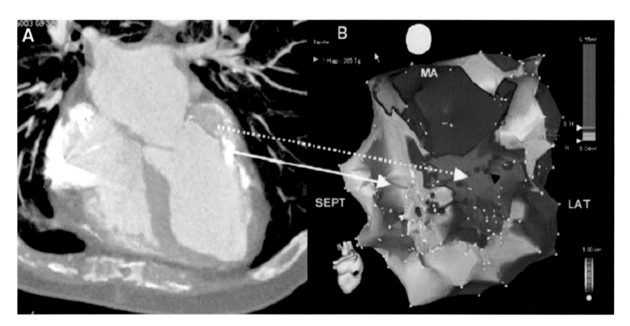

Figure 21.15 Cardiac CT showing myocardial scar (inferolateral wall) close to mitral annulus (bold arrow) with 'viable' submitral isthmus (dotted arrow). Voltage map (right) delineates scar using color coded voltages matched to CT.[18]

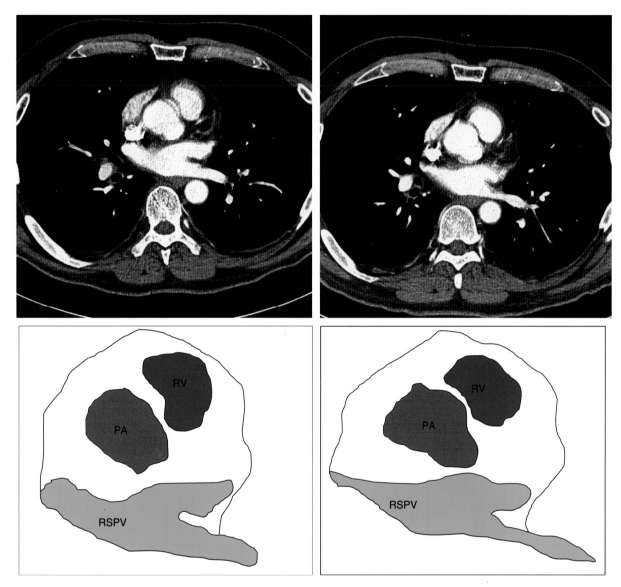

Figure 21.16   RSPV ostium prior to (left panel) and following (right panel) the pulmonary vein isolation procedure demonstrating stenosis at the ostium of the vein as it enters the left atrium.

and intracardiac echocardiographic guidance (Figures 21.17 and 21.18).[13]

5.1 Atrial-esophageal fistula

One recently described complication of AF ablation is development of an atrial-esophageal fistula.[14,20,21]

5.1.1 Clinical presentation

Typically, patients present with a febrile illness or chest pain along with neurological deficits and subsequent hemodynamic collapse.

Although rare, it is thought to be more common following wider-area ablation and creation of linear lesions within the left atrium and with use of high temperature and power.

CT imaging of the left atrial-esophageal interface can help to establish the diagnosis (Figure 21.19). Prompt recognition of this potentially life-threatening complication is essential.

During the ablative procedure, precise location of the esophagus and avoidance of thermal injury is important. In some cases pre-procedural barium swallow is used to outline the course of the esophagus in relation to the left atrial wall. In addition, intra-operative monitoring of esophageal temperature via a probe placed in the esophagus may be used. Tagging of the esophagus during construction of the left

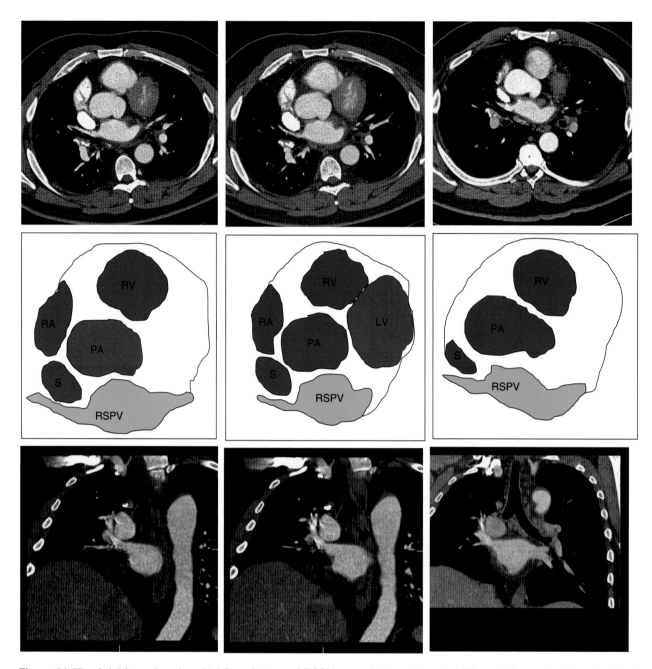

Figure 21.17   Axial (upper) and sagittal (lower) views of RSPV pre-ablation (left panels). The middle panels show significant RSPV stenosis post-ablation. The panels on the right show the same vessel after balloon dilatation of the RSPV was performed.

atrial electro-anatomic map allows the operator to avoid placing high thermal lesions in close proximity to the esophagus (Figure 21.12).

5.1.2 Treatment

In addition to general supportive care, temporary esophageal stenting with antibiotics may prevent progression and allow healing to occur.[22]

5.2 CT measurement

Comparing the pulmonary vein ostial diameters to the baseline values in a particular patient by CT is the established approach to diagnosing pulmonary vein stenosis. While making these measurements, it is important to obtain an image of the entire venous ostium in a single slice. This requires the carina between the superior and inferior veins to be visualized entirely. Oblique CT views can easily establish the plane of the orifice. Accurate measurements also

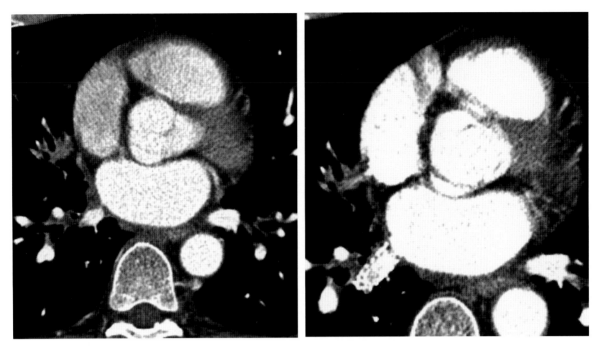

Figure 21.18 RIPV with severe stenosis (left) and with bare-metal stent in place (right).

require orthogonal display of the long axis of each vein. Figure 21.20 shows the measurement planes for the various pulmonary veins.

5.3 Limitations of MDCT

One limitation of CT is the impact of abnormal heart rhythms on image quality and volume measurements.

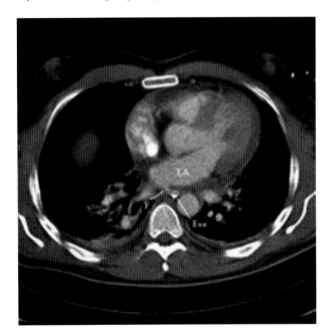

Figure 21.19 Atrial-esophageal fistula **(arrow)** following wide-area circumferential ablation for atrial fibrillation.[20] **LA, left atrium.**

Specifically, irregular arrhythmias such as atrial fibrillation and flutter or frequent premature atrial or ventricular complexes will prevent consistent gating and lead to image degradation. Similarly, cardiac volume can also vary significantly with rhythm disturbances with apparent change in cardiac volumes affecting accurate acquisition and registration of electro-anatomical images. These limitations can be overcome using ECG gating image acquisition that allows signal averaging and improved image signal/noise ratios.

Respiratory phase also affects image quality and volume measurement since, during normal inspiration, the left atrium moves both inferiorly and anteriorly with respect to the aorta and may impair image registration. This can be avoided by acquiring images near end-expiration.[16] Whether gated MDCT will improve sensitivity for detection of thrombus within the left atrium or its appendage (and thereby avoid the need for a transesophageal echocardiogram prior to AF ablation) is unknown.

5.4 Imaging protocol for PVI (pre/post)

A 2-phase protocol is used with an MDCT scanner. In the first phase, a range-finding scan is undertaken at 10-mm intervals to determine the superior and inferior borders of the heart.

A complete image set is then obtained after injection of 125 mL of contrast medium, yielding images at 1.25 mm. This allows a 0.6 mm axial image interval when reconstructed. For analysis, commercial analysis software may be used. The axial images are then reformatted for assessment of each pulmonary vein from axial, coronal, sagittal and oblique images.[13]

On the day before the procedure:

• MDCT (chest) with course, number, anatomy and dimensions of the pulmonary veins is performed.

• The same protocol is used three months post-procedure for comparison.

6 UTILITY OF CT IN ARRHYTHMIA DIAGNOSIS

Although diagnosis of heart rhythm disorders is primarily an electrical one, anatomic substrates for arrhythmias need to be excluded in some cases. A typical example of an

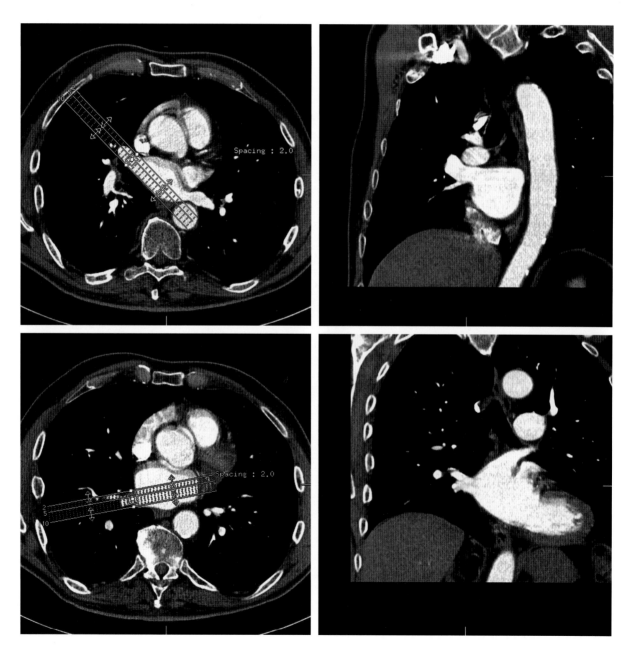

Figure 21.20   CT showing measurement of ostial diameter, axial (left), sagittal (right) (top–bottom RSPV, RIPV, LSPV, LIPV). Oblique cuts with views of the carina allow accurate and reproducible measurement of the ostium.

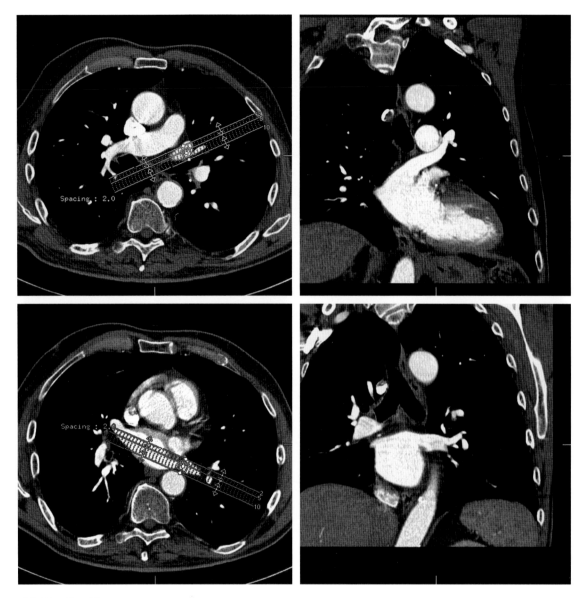

Figure 21.20 Cont'd

'anatomic' arrhythmic condition is arrhythmogenic right ventricular dysplasia/cardiomyopathy.

6.1 Arrhythmogenic Right Ventricular Cardiomyopathy (ARVC)

ARVC is a relatively uncommon cardiomyopathy that predominantly affects the right ventricular myocardium. It is characterized by fatty infiltration of the myocardium that leads to progressive replacement of ventricular myocardium with fat causing dilatation and reduced right ventricular function. In advanced stages this process may also affect left ventricular myocardium.

These myocardial architectural changes provide the substrate for re-entrant ventricular arrhythmias and present typically with palpitations, pre-syncope or sudden cardiac death. An important differential diagnosis of ARVC is (idiopathic) right ventricular outflow tract VT. In this condition, the ventricular myocardium is essentially normal and without evidence of a cardiomyopathic process. In contrast to ARVC, idiopathic right ventricular outflow tract VT has a benign prognosis. Thus, accurate distinction between these conditions is essential.

Characteristic CT features of ARVC include the presence of outpouching, prominent trabeculation and dilation of the right ventricle with later development of reduced systolic function, which are absent in patients with idiopathic RVOT VT (Figure 21.21).

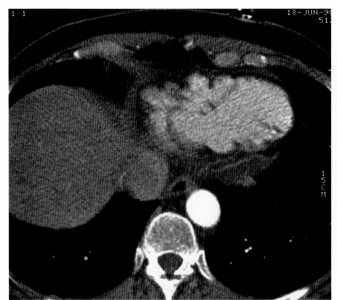

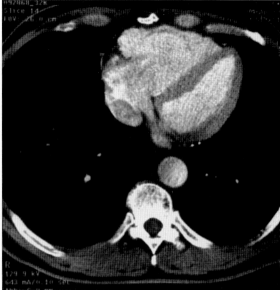

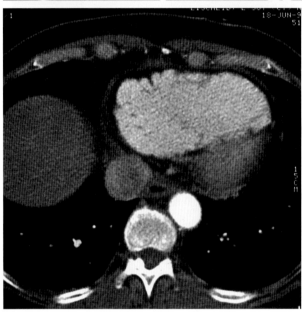

Figure 21.21 Coronal CT demonstrating trabeculation and outpouching, along with dilatation of the right ventricle characteristic of ARVC.

Magnetic resonance imaging (MRI) also allows multiplanar evaluation of the right ventricle (RV), enabling accurate morphologic and functional assessment without geometric assumptions. Since intra-myocardial fat accumulation is a hallmark of ARVC, MRI has excellent tissue characterization capability and is therefore an alternative modality to CT.[11,15]

REFERENCES

1. Giuliani E et al. Mayo Clinic Practice of Cardiology. Mosby 1996.
2. Lemola K et al. Topographic analysis of the coronary sinus and major cardiac veins by computed tomography. Heart Rhythm 2005; 2; 694–9.
3. Mao S et al. Coronary venous imaging with electron beam computed tomographic angiography: Three-dimensional mapping and relationship with coronary arteries. Am Heart J 2005; 150: 315–22.
4. Pappone C et al. Atrial Fibrillation Ablation: State of the Art. Am J Cardiol 2005; 96[suppl]: 59L–64L.
5. Schwartzmann D et al. Characterization of Left Atrium and Distal Pulmonary Vein Morphology using Multidimensional Computed Tomography. J Am Coll Cardiol 2003; 41(8): 1349–57.
6. Beukema WP et al. Successful Radiofrequency Ablation in Patients With Previous Atrial Fibrillation Results in a Significant Decrease in left Atrial Size. Circulation 2005; 112: 2089–95.
7. Wozakowska-Kaplon B. Changes in left atrial size in patients with persistent atrial fibrillation: a prospective echocardiographic study with a 5-year follow-up period. Int J Card 2004; 101: 47–52.

8. Lobel RM et al. Multidetector computed tomography guidance in complex cardiac ablations. Coron Artery Dis 2006; 17: 125–30.

9. Cronin P et al. MDCT of the left atrium and pulmonary veins in planning radiofrequency ablation for atrial fibrillation: a how-to guide. Am J Roentgenol 2004; 183: 767–78.

10. Wood MA et al. A comparison of pulmonary vein ostial anatomy by computerized tomography, echocardiography and venography in patients with atrial fibrillation having radiofrequency catheter ablation. J Am Coll Cardiol 2003; 93: 49–53.

11. Hendel RC et al. ACCF/ACR/SCCT/SCMR/ACNC/NASCI/SCAI/SIR 2006 Appropriateness Criteria for Cardiac Computed Tomography and Cardiac Magnetic Resonance Imaging.

12. Pappone C et al. A randomized trial of circumferential pulmonary vein ablation versus antiarrhythmic drug therapy in paroxysmal atrial fibrillation: the APAF Study. J Am Coll Cardiol 2006; 48(11): 2340–7.

13. Packer DL et al. Clinical presentation, investigation, and management of pulmonary vein stenosis complicating ablation for atrial fibrillation. Circulation 2005; 111(5): 546–54.

14. Pappone C et al. Atrio-esophageal fistula as a complication of percutaneous transcatheter ablation of atrial fibrillation. Circulation 2004; 109(22): 2724–6.

15. Fogel MA et al. Usefulness of Magnetic Resonance Imaging for the Diagnosis of Right Ventricular Dysplasia in Children. Am J Cardiol 2006; 97: 1232–7.

16. Malchano ZS et al. Integration of Cardiac CT/MR Imaging with Three-Dimensional Electroanatomical Mapping to Guide Catheter Manipulation in the Left Atrium: Implications for Catheter Ablation of Atrial Fibrillation. J Cardiovasc Electrophysiol 2006; 17: 1221–9.

17. Van de Veire NR. et al. Non-invasive visualization of the cardiac venous system in coronary artery disease patients using 64-slice computed tomography. J Am Coll Cardiol 2006; 48(9): 1832–8.

18. Bello D et al. Catheter ablation of ventricular tachycardia guided by contrast-enhanced cardiac computed tomography. Heart Rhythm 2004; (4): 490–2.

19. Orlov et al. Three-dimensional rotational angiography of the left atrium and esophagus – A virtual computed tomography scan in the electrophysiology lab? Heart Rhythm 2007; (4): 37–43.

20. Schley et al. Atrio-oesophageal fistula following circumferential pulmonary vein ablation: verification of diagnosis with multislice computed tomography. Europace 2006 Mar; 8(3): 189–90.

21. Scanavacca et al. Left atrial-esophageal fistula following radiofrequency catheter ablation of atrial fibrillation. J Cardiovasc Electrophysiol. 2004 Aug; 15(8): 960–2.

22. Bunch et al. Temporary esophageal stenting allows healing of esophageal perforations following atrial fibrillation ablation procedures. J Cardiovasc Electrophysiol. 2006 Apr; 17(4): 435–9.

22

Extracardiac Findings on Cardiac Computed Tomographic Imaging

Karen M. Horton and Elliot K. Fishman

1 INTRODUCTION

Gated non-contrast CT imaging of the heart for the detection and quantification of coronary artery calcium has been shown to be valuable in determining individual risk of a future significant cardiac event.[1–3] Studies also suggest that calcium scoring may be more useful than other well accepted conventional risk factors. In addition to non-contrast coronary scans, recent advancements in MDCT scanners and 3D cardiac imaging software have resulted in increased acceptance of coronary MDCT angiography as part of a diagnostic work-up in a symptomatic patient.[4,5] Given the potential usefulness of MDCT as both a screening and diagnostic study, it is certain that both non contrast cardiac CT and CTA of the coronary arteries will be performed with increased frequency in coming years.

Cardiac CT scans (both non contrast calcium scoring exams and coronary CTA exams) involve irradiating the entire mid-thorax. Therefore, other structures (lungs, heart, aorta, bones, chest wall, etc.) are visible on the scan, depending on the field of view. This chapter will discuss the prevalence and clinical significance of non-cardiac findings on cardiac CT scans. The controversy surrounding the responsibility of the interpreting physician to report these abnormalities will be discussed.

2 SCAN TECHNIQUE

When performing a cardiac CT, whether it be a non contrast gated CT for coronary artery scoring or a full contrast enhanced CT angiogram of the coronary arteries, these studies consist of a CT through the mid thorax. Typically, the scan begins at the level of the carina and extends through the base of the heart. Therefore, the entire mid thorax is irradiated. Depending on the field of view of the reconstruction, the volume of visible thoracic structures will vary (Figure 22.1). For example, in a recent study by Haller et al. the authors calculated the volume of the thorax visible on a cardiac CT in comparison with a standard full chest CT.[6] The authors reconstructed the data twice. For the focused study, a smaller field of view was utilized, usually including the region from the carina to the base of the heart. This field of view is typically between 26–30 cm.[2] In addition, the authors created a separate reconstruction using the maximum field of view, which is dependent on the patient's size. By opening up the field of view this would include the entire mid thorax and chest wall. The authors then compared the volume of the thorax visible on both fields of view compared with a standard full chest CT. The authors concluded that when a smaller focused field of view is utilized that approximately 35.5% of the chest volume is visible in the reconstructed field of view.[6] When the maximum field of view is utilized then 70.3% of the chest volume

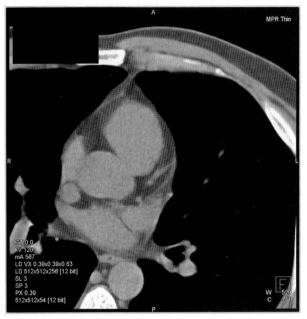

A

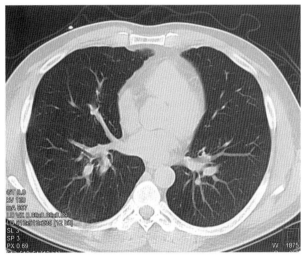

B

Figure 22.1 (A) Noncontrast cardiac CT performed for coronary calcium scoring. Example of small field of view (20 cm²). (B) Noncontrast cardiac CT performed for coronary calcium scoring. Example of larger field of view (32 cm²) to include the entire thorax.

was visible on the cardiac CT examination when compared to a full CT of the chest.[6]

Therefore, this study by Haller quantifies the amount of potential information visible on the cardiac CT scan depending on how the study is reconstructed. The technologist can reconstruct the study in both a small and larger field of view without additional radiation to the patient. A prominent cardiologist, John Rumberger, discussed this in a recent editorial where he acknowledges that a significant portion of the chest is irradiated during a cardiac CT.[7]

Rumberger also notes that these CT scans are diagnostic and in fact high resolution thin section images of the same technical quality as a standard chest CT. Therefore, according to Rumberger, the interpreting physician has an obligation to review the entire scan, as all irradiated areas can potentially harbor pathology.[7]

Investigators are beginning to recommend that when performing a cardiac CT scan, the study should be done in both a small focus field of view as well as a maximum field of view to allow identification of all potential abnormalities. Also, researchers note that the studies should be reviewed in soft tissues windows, bone windows and lung windows in order to maximize the possibility of detecting abnormalities.[8] Changing the window width and window level is as easy the as push of a button and does not require any additional reconstructions or reformations.

3 PREVELANCE OF NONCARDIAC FINDINGS

As stated above, a dedicated cardiac CT is actually a CT scan through the entire mid thorax and therefore these studies contain information about the heart, great vessels, pericardium, lungs, chest wall, spine, and in some cases upper abdomen, in addition to information about the coronary arteries (Figures 22.2–22.4).

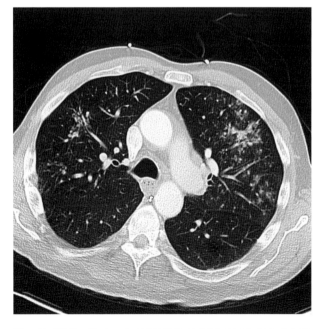

Figure 22.2 Example of incidental bilateral pneumonia found on a CTA of the coronary arteries in a patient with chest pain.

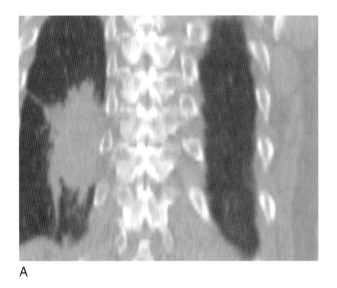

A

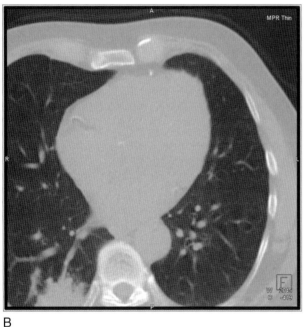

B

Figure 22.3 (A & B) Example of incidental right lower lobe lung cancer found on a noncontrast cardiac CT performed for coronary calcium scoring.

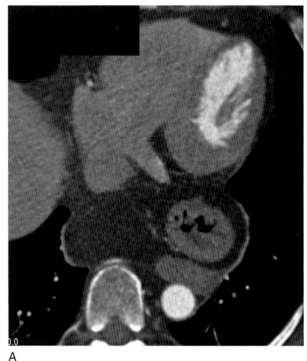

A

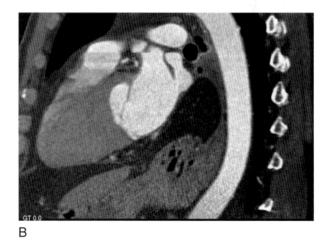

B

Figure 22.4 (A & B) Example of incidental hiatal hernia as well as a large amount of herniated fat in a patient undergoing a cardiac CTA exam.

The first large study which addresses the prevalence of extra cardiac abnormalities on cardiac CT was published by Hunold in 2001.[9] These investigators reviewed a total 812 consecutive patients who underwent electron-beam computed tomography. Five hundred and eighty-three of the patients received IV contrast. Investigators only reviewed the mediastinal windows for extracardiac pathology and used a relatively small field of view (26 cm[2]). A total of 2055 noncoronary pathologic findings were observed in 953 patients.[9] The authors found lung abnormalities in 28%, abdominal abnormalities in 2%, mediastinal pathology in 4%, and spine abnormalities in 5%. These abnormalities included a large number of minor relatively insignificant findings such as scars, granulomata, atelectasis, etc. Nodules were only found in 1.1% of patients in that study.[9] However, remember that no lung windows were reviewed. Therefore, the actual number of lung nodules in that cohort is unknown. Even though that study had some limitations, it brings to the forefront that potentially significant abnormalities may be visualized outside of the heart on various cardiac CT studies.

The following year, in 2002 we published a study in Circulation describing the prevalence of significant non-cardiac findings on electron-beam computed tomography scans performed for coronary artery calcium scoring.[8] In that study, 1326 consecutive patients underwent coronary artery calcium screening with electron-beam computed tomography. A 35 cm^2 field of view was utilized. These studies were reviewed by one of two board certified CT radiologists. Review included bone windows, mediastinal windows, and lung windows on all patients. Of the 1326 patients, 103 (7.8%) had significant extra cardiac pathology which required either clinical or imaging follow-up.[8] This included 53 patients with non-calcified lung nodules less than 1 cm in size, and 12 patients with lung nodules greater than 1 cm in size as well as 24 patients with infiltrates, 7 patients with indeterminate liver lesions, 2 patients with sclerotic bone lesions, 2 patients with breast abnormalities, 1 patient with polycystic liver disease, and 1 patient with esophageal thickening, as well as 1 patient with ascites.[8] At the time of publication, only 1 of the patients with a lung nodule had undergone surgery. In that patient a 9 mm nodule was removed from the right middle lobe and was shown at pathology to be a 9 mm bronchoalveolar carcinoma. Since that time, we are aware of 1 additional patient in whom lung cancer has been diagnosed after following a lung nodule detected on a cardiac scan. In that study, as the authors, we concluded that it should be the responsibility and obligation of the physician interpreting the cardiac CT scan to review the entire study including the lungs and the bones.

A similar study was also published in 2004 by Schragin in which the clinic files of 1366 patients who underwent electron beam scanning over a 12 year period were reviewed.[10] Those reports contained both a description of the cardiac and non-cardiac findings by a board certified radiologist. The authors went on to match the patients with the national death index. Two hundred and seventy-eight patients (20.5%) had 1 or more non-cardiac findings on the scan.[10] Fifty-seven patients (4.2%) received recommendations for diagnostic CT follow-up. 46 of these 57 were for pulmonary nodule follow-up. After cross-indexing their patients with the national death index, 1 death was noted in a patient from metastatic renal cell cancer who was found to have a lung mass on the coronary scoring study.[10]

Another more recent study confirming the importance of non-cardiac findings on coronary examinations was published in 2006 in The Journal of American College of Cardiology.[11] Onuma et al. reviewed the cardiac MDCT scans in 503 patients. In those patients, a cardiologist assessed the heart while a radiologist reviewed the other organs. Those investigators found 346 new non-cardiac findings identified in 292 patients (58.1%) a total of 114 (22.7%) had clinically significant findings, including 4 cases of malignancy (0.8%).[11] Two cases of lung cancer were found

and 2 cases of breast cancer. The authors concluded that it is essential that the CT study be reviewed by a radiologist whether or not a cardiologist interprets the coronary portion of the exam.[11]

The final study, which also supports the high prevalence of non-cardiac findings on coronary CT studies, was published by Haller et al. in 2006.[6] In this study 166 patients with suspected coronary artery disease were examined with contrast enhanced MDCT. These images were reviewed for extra cardiac findings and were classified as none, minor, or major with respect to the impact on patient management and treatment. Extra-cardiac findings were detected in 41 patients (24.7%); these were classified as minor in 19.9% and major in 4.8%. Among the major findings noted by the authors, which had an immediate impact on patient management, was the presence of bronchial carcinoma as well as pulmonary emboli.[6]

Therefore, the landmark studies described above all agree that important pathology will be overlooked unless the entire study is reviewed. Many of the findings will be insignificant such as scars, granulomata, etc. but, in a small percentage of patients, a significant extra cardiac finding will be visible and can have potentially devastating consequences for the patient. In each of the published studies where malignancies were diagnosed, the most common were lung cancer and breast cancer. Other important life threatening conditions such as pulmonary emboli were also diagnosed on the contrast enhanced exams. Also, Onuma makes a point that review of the extra cardiac structures may indeed explain the patient's symptoms in those found not to have significant coronary disease.[11] In that study, 32 of 201 patients in whom coronary disease was ruled out, the non-cardiac findings on the CT were considered sufficient to explain the patient's symptoms.[11]

Despite the evidence cited above, there are still physicians who oppose reviewing the extracardiac structures for pathology. A study by Budoff et al. in 2006 describes potential limitations of reviewing the extracardiac anatomy.[12] First he acknowledges that in this patient population there is a high rate of nodule detection. Second, he is concerned with the cost of following these nodules, the radiation dose to the patient, as well as the potential risk of biopsy, etc. Third, he is concerned with potential increased cancer risk in patients undergoing follow-up CT scans. Finally, Budoff is concerned about unnecessary anxiety for both the patients and physician regarding the follow-up of insignificant findings. He concludes that 'the weight of the evidence suggests that it is most prudent to not specifically reconstruct and re-read CTA scans for lung nodules'.[12]

3.1 Discussion

As described above, when performing a cardiac CT the entire mid thorax is irradiated and therefore the structures included in that region can have potential pathology. Over the years, there has been significant controversy regarding the obligation of the interpreting physician to evaluate all the irradiated anatomy. This probably stems from the fact that both cardiologists and radiologists are involved in reviewing these studies. Dr. Rumberger wrote a very nice editorial in The Journal of The American College of Cardiology in 2006 were he specifically addresses this issue.[7] First, he makes the point that as physicians we have a medical legal responsibility to review the entire study as 'failure to diagnose' remains one of the most common issues in malpractice. Also, as noted above in a study by Onuma, 32 of 201 patients in whom the coronary artery disease was ruled out, the non-cardiac findings on the CT were sufficient to explain the symptoms.[11] Therefore, as physicians, our main duty is to try to explain the patient's symptoms, even if no coronary artery disease is present on the study. Next, Rumberger describes the medical moral responsibility the physician has to review the entire study. As radiologists, we were always taught that we were responsible to review the entire study. It makes no sense to limit our interpretation specifically to the organ of question. For example, when an abdominal CT scan is performed to evaluate the pancreas, it is still the radiologist's responsibility to evaluate the adjacent organs for potential pathology. In that example, when we perform a pancreatic CT, we often can use a focus field of view centering on the pancreas, but we also reconstruct the study with a larger field of view so we can visualize all the entire abdominal organs. The CT scan performed for cardiac imaging is a diagnostic CT scan with high resolution thin section imaging which is adequate to visualize these structures. It has been noted that, even in low-dose studies considered 'non-diagnostic' for other exam inations, SPECT/CT investigators have found potentially significant abnormal findings in the CT portion of these exams even though a very low technique (2.5-mA) was utilized.[13]

Rumberger also acknowledges the medical-economic impact of screening studies.[13] Screening CT scans in general, whether it be lung cancer screening, virtual colonoscopy, whole body screening, or cardiac CT scanning, are increasing every year. Incidental findings on CT scans, both screening and diagnostic, are relatively common. Incidental findings can lead to additional clinical and radiographic follow-up which in some cases may not be unnecessary. Some opponents to CT screening suggest that this may result in significant economic impact due to follow-up of insignificant incidental findings. However, as Rumberger acknowledges, the medical community as well as the radiological community need to publish guidelines on how to follow-up incidental findings.[13]

Given all the information described above, we feel it is the obligation of the interpreting physician to evaluate the entire CT scan. This will require reconstruction of both a small focus field of view as well as a larger field of view to include the entire mid thorax. Therefore, in most cases, this will require a qualified radiologist to review the entire examination, even if a cardiologist has interpreted the coronary artery portion of the study.

In addition to detecting these important non-cardiac abnormalities, clearly the radiologist and the clinician need a strategy to follow unsuspected findings on screening studies. Budoff addresses these concerns in his article.[12] Although we agree with many of the his conclusions, we do not believe that these potential abnormalities should be ignored. It is our opinion that the entire study be reviewed and all abnormalities be reported. In order to minimize the impact of unnecessary follow-up, cost, radiation dose and patient anxiety, the radiological and medical community in general needs to decide the appropriate way to handle these findings.

First of all, it is important to select appropriate patient for both screening and diagnostic cardiac scans. Selections of subjects for screening in particular should be based on prior determination of risk factors. As described in a study by Obuchowski et al., images from screening studies should be interpreted with a high sensitivity but positive findings on screening exams should be handled with a level of surveillance appropriate for risk.[14] This is especially important when unsuspected incidental findings are seen. Clearly, a reasonable strategy for follow-up of these abnormalities needs to be addressed. For example, in an article on whole body screening studies published by Furtado et al. in Radiology in 2005, those investigators reviewed 1192 consecutive patients undergoing whole body screening. In that study, the radiologist recommended at least one additional follow-up in 37% of patients.[15] This seems like a very high percentage of supposedly normal patients which required additional radiological follow-up. For example, in that study, lung nodules were the most common findings in which the radiologist recommended follow-up. However, when reviewing their reports, there was no strategy for follow-up. The follow-up of nodules ranged between 1 month to 12 months with no relationship to nodule size.[15]

It is clear that the radiologic community needs to come up with reasonable guidelines to handle these incidental non-cardiac abnormalities. An example of this can be seen in an article published by MacMahon et al. in Radiology 2005.[16] These were guidelines for management of small pulmonary nodules detected on CT scans quoting a statement from the Fleischner Society. In that article, the contributors reviewed the current data on lung nodules. They determined that lung nodules are common and seen in 51% of smokers over the age of 50. The authors acknowledge that our ability to detect small lung nodules has improved with each new generation scanner. Therefore, the old recommendations based on older CT scans and chest x-rays are not appropriate for following nodules detected on scans today. These authors describe new guidelines that can be used by the interpreting physician to follow unsuspected lung nodules. The authors took into account data on lung nodule detection rate, data from the lung cancer screening trials, data based on nodule size, growth rate and relative risk. The management approach in allows the interpreting physician to recommend reasonable follow-up for these small nodules based on patient risk and nodule size.[16] For example, a 3 mm nodule detected incidentally in a low risk patient would not require additional radiographic follow-up. A 3 mm nodule detected in a high-risk patient would require a 12 month follow-up scan. If the nodule were stable at that time, no additional follow-up would be needed. This is a logical and reasonable way to approach incidental nodule detection on cardiac scans.

4 IMPRESSION

Cardiac CT scans are being performed with increased frequency. When performing both screening noncontrast CT scans of the heart as well as contrast enhanced coronary artery CT angiography studies, the entire mid thorax is irradiated. Many studies have been published by both radiologists and cardiologists, describing the importance of reviewing the extra-cardiac structures in order to diagnose important pathology. New strategies for follow-up of incidentally detected pathology (i.e. lung nodules) have recently been published which offer a reasonable approach.

REFERENCES

1. Arad Y, Goodman KJ, Roth M, Newstein D, Guerci AD. Coronary calcification, coronary disease risk factors, C-reactive protein, and atherosclerotic cardiovascular disease events: the St. Francis Heart Study. J Am Coll Cardiol 2005; 46(1): 158–65.
2. Greenland P, LaBree L, Azen SP, Doherty TM, Detrano RC. Coronary artery calcium score combined with Framingham score for risk prediction in asymptomatic individuals. Jama 2004; 291(2): 210–15.
3. LaMonte MJ, FitzGerald SJ, Church TS et al. Coronary artery calcium score and coronary heart disease events in a large cohort of asymptomatic men and women. Am J Epidemiol 2005; 162(5): 421–9.
4. Moshage WE, Achenbach S, Seese B, Bachmann K, Kirchgeorg M. Coronary artery stenoses: three-dimensional imaging with electrocardiographically triggered, contrast agent-enhanced, electron-beam CT. Radiology 1995; 196(3): 707–14.
5. Schmermund A, Rensing BJ, Sheedy PF, Bell MR, Rumberger JA. Intravenous electron-beam computed tomographic coronary angiography for segmental analysis of coronary artery stenoses. J Am Coll Cardiol 1998; 31(7): 1547–54.
6. Haller S, Kaiser C, Buser P, Bongartz G, Bremerich J. Coronary artery imaging with contrast-enhanced MDCT: extracardiac findings. AJR Am J Roentgenol 2006; 187(1): 105–10.
7. Rumberger JA. Noncardiac abnormalities in diagnostic cardiac computed tomography: within normal limits or we never looked! J Am Coll Cardiol 2006; 48(2): 407–8.
8. Horton KM, Post WS, Blumenthal RS, Fishman EK. Prevalence of significant noncardiac findings on electron-beam computed tomography coronary artery calcium screening examinations. Circulation 2002; 106(5): 532–4.
9. Hunold P, Schmermund A, Seibel RM, Gronemeyer DH, Erbel R. Prevalence and clinical significance of accidental findings in electron-beam tomographic scans for coronary artery calcification. Eur Heart J 2001; 22(18): 1748–58.
10. Schragin JG, Weissfeld JL, Edmundowicz D, Strollo DC, Fuhrman CR. Non-cardiac findings on coronary electron beam computed tomography scanning. J Thorac Imaging 2004; 19(2): 82–6.
11. Onuma Y, Tanabe K, Nakazawa G et al. Noncardiac findings in cardiac imaging with multidetector computed tomography. J Am Coll Cardiol 2006; 48(2): 402–6.
12. Budoff MJ, Fischer H, Gopal A. Incidental findings with cardiac CT evaluation: should we read beyond the heart? Catheter Cardiovasc Interv 2006; 68(6): 965–73.
13. Goetze S, Pannu HK, Wahl RL. Clinically significant abnormal findings on the "nondiagnostic" CT portion of low-amperage-CT attenuation-corrected myocardial perfusion SPECT/CT studies. J Nucl Med 2006; 47(8): 1312–18.
14. Obuchowski NA, Graham RJ, Baker ME, Powell KA. Ten criteria for effective screening: their application to multislice CT screening for pulmonary and colorectal cancers. AJR Am J Roentgenol 2001; 176(6): 1357–62.
15. Furtado CD, Aguirre DA, Sirlin CB et al. Whole-body CT screening: spectrum of findings and recommendations in 1192 patients. Radiology 2005; 237(2): 385–94.
16. MacMahon H, Austin JH, Gamsu G et al. Guidelines for management of small pulmonary nodules detected on CT scans: a statement from the Fleischner Society. Radiology 2005; 237(2): 395–400.

23

Computed Tomographic Angiography: Technical Considerations

Jacobo Kirsch, Eric E. Williamson, and Dominik Fleischmann

1 MDCT ANGIOGRAPHY – TECHNOLOGY DEVELOPMENT

The basic concept of computing a cross-sectional image from multiple x-ray projections to create images of an anatomic structure has remained the fundamental principle of computed tomography (CT) since its origin in 1971. The evolution of this powerful tool has been spearheaded by hardware and software advances that allow for rapid, robust acquisition of scan data and prompt, flexible workstation display.

1.1 Early development of CT

In the early 1980s, CT imaging consisted of step-and-shoot axial scanning, acquiring anatomic data in single slices. Each of these anatomic slices was obtained during a single breath-hold while the patient table stayed motionless. This scan technique resulted in discontinuous images with the potential for misregistration between contiguous slices, and was therefore not well adapted to imaging the vascular system. Two major developments, spiral (helical) scanning and multi-detector row CT, provided the impetus for the development and rapid advance of clinical CT angiography.

1.2 Spiral/helical scanning

The introduction of slip-ring technology triggered the development of spiral scanners in the early 1990s, which allowed continuous imaging as the patient moved through the CT gantry. Spiral CT for the first time transformed CT into a true three-dimensional, volumetric imaging technique. In addition, comparable large anatomic volumes such as the chest or the abdomen could be completed within a single breath-hold.[1] In addition to improving spatial resolution along the z-axis, this method of scanning eliminated misregistration artifacts between adjacent slices. The ability to interpolate overlapping axial images at arbitrary positions along the z-axis permitted improved generation of multiplanar reformations. In 1993, Rubin et al. demonstrated its potential for evaluation of vascular structures in a series of 15 patients imaged with a single-slice spiral CT scanner and rapid contrast medium injection optimized to visualize the abdominal aorta and its main branches.[2] This new technology, based on slip-ring technology, used an x-ray source and its opposing detector array rotating around the patient while the scanner table was being translated through it in the z-axis (third generation). All single slice scanners used a fan-shaped x-ray beam with only one detector row in the z-axis (Figure 23.1).

Although revolutionary for the time, such scanners still had relatively slow gantry rotation speed (in the range of 1s/360dgr) that, coupled with the use of available single row detector elements, limited the anatomic coverage possible per patient breath-hold. The trade-off between spatial resolution (section thickness) and volume coverage often translated into asymmetric (anisotropic) voxels which limited the utility of 3-dimensional reformations of the scan data. Still, volumetric acquisition using spiral scanning

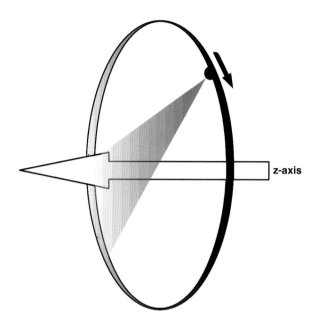

Figure 23.1   Spiral scanning: The table is fed through the bore of the CT as its gantry continuously rotates acquiring a volume set in a helical/spiral fashion.

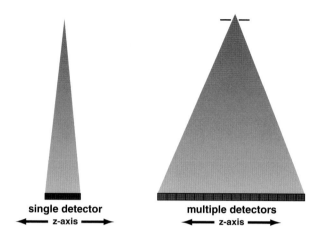

Figure 23.2   Detectors configuration: In the MDCT scanner, the greater number of detector rows in the z-direction helps to increment coverage and enhance scanning speed.

techniques laid the groundwork for the explosion in CT angiography applications that was to come.

1.3 Multi-detector CT

Not until the development of 4-slice multidetector-row computed tomography (MDCT) scanners in the late 1990s and the availability of 8- and 16-slice MDCT scanners in the early 2000s, did the speed of scanning and range of z-axis coverage expand sufficiently to enable breath-hold image acquisition in multiple phases of contrast enhancement and single-phase imaging over extended anatomic regions. At the same time, improvements in gantry rotation speed further increased the scan coverage area, making imaging of the entire inflow and runoff vessels feasible during a single acquisition.[3]

While single-detector CT comprised a single row with a linear array of multiple detector elements, MDCT utilizes multiple adjacent rows of parallel detector elements creating a 2-dimensional matrix of elements that allows the acquisition of at least 4 sections per x-ray tube rotation (Figure 23.2). It should be noted that the number of sections or 'slices' acquired per gantry rotation is not determined by the number of rows of detector elements, but rather by the number of 'channels' of data reconstructed from exposure of the detector array.

Three types of detector arrays are used for MDCT: matrix array, adaptive array and hybrid array. *Matrix detectors* consist of multiple rows identical in width (Figure 23.3). When the CT acquisition is performed, various collimation settings are available, based on the configuration of detector elements used. For example, an 8-row CT scanner might utilize an array of 16 rows of 1.25 mm detector elements. In such a system, selecting the eight innermost detector rows

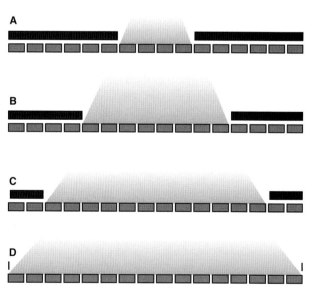

Figure 23.3   Matrix detector: Multiple rows of same-width detectors are aligned and by using different collimations, the slice thickness can be adjusted according to the clinical need. In example A, only the inner 4 detectors are being used, which results in 4 slices of 1.25 mm thickness each. If the collimation is extended to include all 16 rows, they can be combined into 4 slices of 5 mm thickness each, as in example D.

would allow eight channels of data to be acquired at 1.25 mm collimation. Signal from adjacent detector elements can also be combined to produce thicker channels. For instance, selecting all 16 detector rows could produce eight channels of data at 2.5 mm collimation. The advantage of combining detector rows to produce wider slices is the associated increase in z-axis coverage per gantry rotation. The disadvantage of such a scheme is a compromise in z-axis resolution.

Adaptive array and *hybrid array* detectors utilize detector rows that increment in size from the center to the periphery (Figure 23.4). In each of these systems, the detector elements in the center of the array are narrower, permitting higher resolution images to be obtained over a smaller coverage area. The detector elements at the periphery of the array are wider, which allows a larger amount of x-rays to contact them due to the decrease in the perpendicular septa separating the detectors. The difference between adaptive and hybrid detector arrays is that adaptive arrays have multiple,

variable-thickness rows of detector elements, while hybrid arrays have only two different thickness elements. As with a matrix detector array, variable collimation widths can be achieved by combining the information obtained with multiple contiguous rows of detectors. Depending on the manufacturer and scanner model, there are multiple variations to the organization and sizes of the matrix elements.

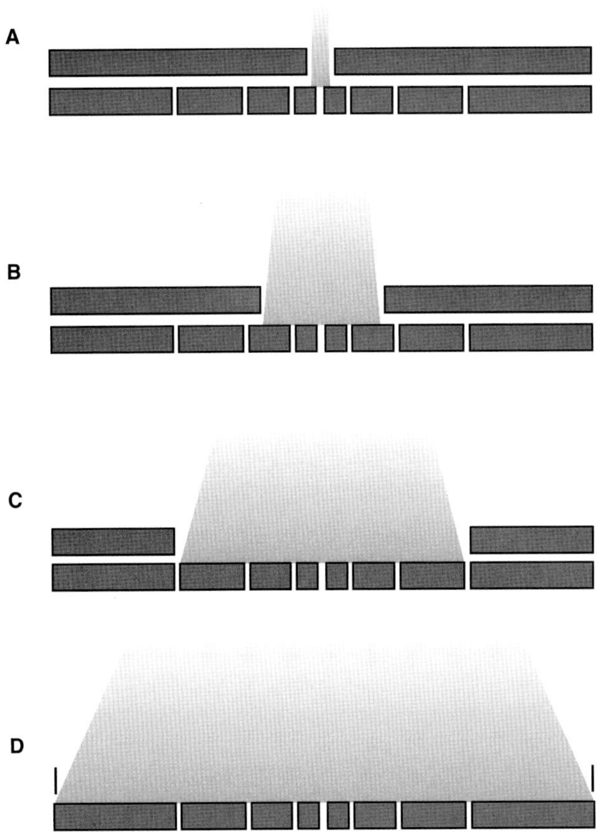

2 IMAGE ACQUISITION & DISPLAY TECHNIQUES

As CT angiography and the equipment we use to perform it have evolved, the techniques that we employ to take advantage of these advances have also changed. Accurate performance of CTA requires understanding of technical factors, including contrast media kinetics, basic scan parameters, and various post-processing techniques.

2.1 Contrast administration

Strong opacification of the vasculature is critical for diagnostic-quality CT angiography. As CT technology has evolved to allow scanning of extended coverage areas in shorter time intervals, appropriate delivery of intravenous contrast medium has become increasingly complicated and contrast medium injection protocols are continually evolving. For example, imaging of both inflow and runoff vessels in a single contrast medium injection requires careful planning to ensure optimal opacification of the vascular territory of interest.

The goal contrast medium administration for CT angiography is to achieve adequate uniform arterial enhancement throughout the vascular territory of interest for the entire duration of the CT acquisition. Although patient-dependent variables such as cardiac output and patient body habitus have an effect on arterial enhancement in CT angiography, many important variables that help determine image quality are under the control of the operator.[4] These operator controlled variables include: scan timing, contrast volume and injection rate, contrast medium concentration, and saline flush.

Figure 23.4 Adaptive array detector: In contrast to the matrix detector, in this type, the rows increment in width form the center to the periphery. The concept is similar as they can be combined as the collimation is widened. However, the lesser amount of septa in this detector allows for more x-rays to contact them.

2.1.1 Timing Options

There are three main options for scan timing in relation to contrast injection: fixed time delay, timing bolus or bolus tracking. Using a *fixed time delay* involves initiating the CT scan at a predefined interval after the contrast injection is started. Although fixed time delay can be used successfully for many routine thoracic and abdominal CT protocols, especially if the patient has no underlying cardiovascular disorder, for cardiovascular CT studies the scan delay should be individualized for every patient.[5] We recommend using an individualized scan delay, acquired either by timing bolus or automated bolus tracking, for all CT angiography studies to ensure optimal arterial opacification.

A *test bolus* is a straightforward method to determine the time interval between the beginning of an injection and the arrival of contrast medium in the arterial territory of interest (contrast medium transit time, t_{CMT}). A patient's t_{CMT} is then used to determine the scan delay for CT angiography. This method involves the injection of a small volume of contrast medium (usually 15–20 mL), followed by repetitive low-dose CT scanning at a single table position, usually at the anatomic region to be scanned. A region of interest (ROI) is placed in an artery in the scan field (typically the aorta) and the enhancement is recorded over time. A graph of this relationship is used to calculate the time to peak enhancement, which is used to determine the scan delay.[6] The test bolus technique is the most robust method of determining the t_{CMT} and subsequently the scan delay; however, it has the drawback of increasing the amount of contrast medium injected without adding to the enhancement of the images used for diagnosis.

Automated *bolus tracking* (triggering technique) is a slightly more sophisticated method for determining scan delay. Bolus tracking uses multiple low-dose scans acquired at a single table position, similar to the test bolus technique; however, the entire bolus of contrast is administered and scan initiation is triggered 'real-time' once arterial enhancement at the anatomic region of interest reaches a certain threshold.[7] Depending on the manufacturer, the CT acquisition can be manually triggered or automatically initiated once the Hounsfield units in the ROI reach some predefined threshold level. The bolus tracking technique is effective and conserves contrast media; however, if the ROI is placed incorrectly, if the patient moves, or if there are venous inflow problems, the scan can fail to initiate correctly. There is an important difference between automated bolus triggering and test-bolus techniques in the fact that automated bolus triggering inherently increases the scanning delay relative to the true tCMT. This is due to technical reasons, since monitoring of bolus arrival is not truly real time, and once the scan initiation is triggered, additional time is needed for table repositioning and for providing a breath-hold command.

While this slight increase of the scanning delay improves initial arterial enhancement, it's main limitation is that the user is often unaware of this fact, and of its magnitude (which may vary substantially between scanner models, and scanning protocols). The inherent increase of the scanning delay (relative to the true tCMT) caused by automated bolus triggering is easily compensated for by slightly increasing the injection duration accordingly.

2.1.2 Early arterial contrast medium dynamics

Arterial enhancement is directly proportional to the number of iodine molecules present in the vascular territory to be imaged. Since routine 'first pass' CT angiography is performed using an intravenous injection, the arterial iodine concentration can be controlled by varying the concentration, amount and rate of this intravenous iodine injection. Before arriving in the arterial system, the contrast bolus must pass through the venous system, the right side of the heart, the pulmonary circulation and left side of the heart. This results in a broadening on the bolus (with an asymmetric 'tail') The iodinated contrast material used for CT angiography has an extracellular bio-distribution and after reaching the systemic circulation it rapidly redistributes or 're-circulates' and re-enters the right heart via the systemic veins. This redistribution occurs promptly enough through certain organs, particularly the brain and kidneys, that the re-circulated contrast has an additive effect on bolus broadening and thus downstream arterial enhancement.[4] Thus, first pass (with it's bolus broadening) and recirculation effects combine to determine the contrast media kinetics of CT angiography. While injection protocols have traditionally been described using contrast medium volumes and flow rates (due to the fact that these parameters are keyed into the power injector), this is poorly suited for CTA. Injection parameters for CTA are best described and understood as injection rate (iodine administration rate or flux) and injection duration, since these two parameters control time-depending arterial enhancement. Contrast medium volume is a derived parameter.

The effect of the injection rate of iodinated contrast medium (for a given iodine concentration) on arterial enhancement is straightforward: The iodine flux (mg iodine/s) is directly proportional to the arterial enhancement. Thus, increasing the injection flow rate or increasing the iodine concentration of the contrast agent both translate into proportionally greater arterial opacification. The effect of the injection duration is less intuitive and more difficult to understand. A bolus injection of contrast can be best understood as a series of small 'test' injections administered one after another (Figure 23.5). Due to bolus broadening and recirculation effects, such a series of injections produces an upward sloping plateau of enhancement with an overall duration proportional to the duration of the intravenous injection. Peak arterial enhancement is dependent not only on the rate, but also on the duration of the contrast injection. The key to effective CT angiography is to match the scan acquisition to this 'plateau' phase of enhancement; however, since the curve rises over time, enhancement during the CT acquisition can become non-uniform. Non-uniform enhancement becomes more obvious in CTA studies with comparably long scan and injection times (20–30s or more). This non-uniformity can be addressed by the use of biphasic injection protocols (Figure 23.6). Biphasic contrast injection protocols utilize an initial high injection rate (typically 6–8 mL/sec) to rapidly increase the arterial iodine concentration. This initial rapid bolus injection is followed by a longer,

slower injection (typically 3–5 mL/sec) to maintain the plateau phase of arterial enhancement. Biphasic injections are useful in long acquisitions, such as gated chest with non-gated abdomen pelvis studies, or lower extremity CTA.[8]

Whether a monophasic or biphasic injection protocol is used, the contrast injection duration is typically matched to the duration of the CT scan acquisition to optimize arterial enhancement without wasting contrast. Typically, an additional time factor is added to the injection duration to account for the time it takes to initiate the CT scan (see bolus triggering, above). Typical injection rates for CT angiography are set between 4 to 6 mL/sec. Thus, for a twelve second scan of the abdominal aorta, the amount of contrast might be described as (5 mL/sec × 12 sec) + (5 mL/sec × 5 sec) for a total of 85 mL of contrast.

Although the traditional 'injection duration equals scan duration' approach works quite well for extended scan ranges and long scan durations, the recent development of faster CT scanners has caused acquisition times to become

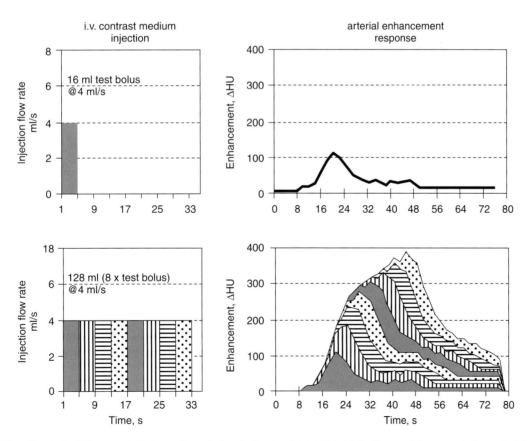

Figure 23.5   Simple 'additive model' shows the relation between the contrast injection and the cumulative arterial enhancement. (a) The arterial enhancement curve after the intravenous injection of a 16 mL test-bolus. (b) The cumulative arterial enhancement following the intravenous injection of a full 128 mL bolus. Due to the asymmetric shape of the test enhancement curve and due to recirculation effects (the 'tail' in the test enhancement), arterial enhancement (the 'time integral of 8 test boluses') increases continuously over time. There is no enhancement plateau. (Adapted from Reference 5 with permission.)

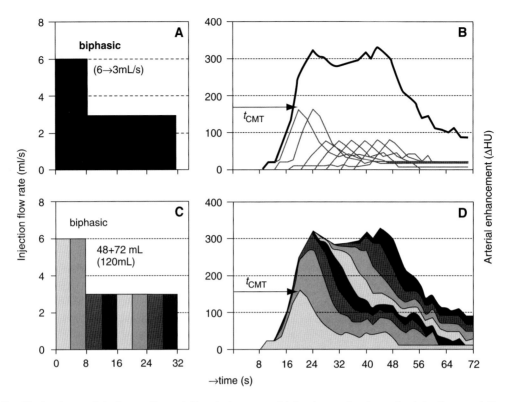

Figure 23.6 Bi-phasic model shows the relation between a biphasic contrast media injection and the cumulative enhancement. (a) The arterial enhancement curve after the intravenous injection of a 6 mL test-bolus followed by a 3 mL by second phase. (b) The cumulative arterial enhancement following the intravenous injection of a full 120 mL contrast dose in 2 phases: 48 mL bolus injection followed by an additional 72 mL of contrast at 3 mL/s. Due to the asymmetric shape of the test enhancement curve and due to recirculation effects (the 'tail' in the test enhancement), arterial enhancement (the 'time integral of 8 test boluses') increases continuously over time creating an enhancement plateau.

shorter. For a given contrast injection rate, decreasing the injection duration will also decrease the peak enhancement. This becomes important because such a decrease in enhancement can be a limiting factor for acquiring diagnostic quality arterial images. Usually, the goal is for CT angiography to obtain enhancement of at least 200 Hounsfield units (HU) for the aorta, and approximately 300 HU for the pulmonary arteries or aortic side branches (arch branch vessels, bronchial, renal, celiac and mesenteric arteries) to be visualized.[7]

Several strategies can be employed to increase arterial enhancement appropriate for modern MDCT systems. As mentioned earlier, increasing the iodine flux directly translates into stronger arterial enhancement. For example, when the iodine concentration is increased from 300 mg I/mL to 370 mg I/mL, and the injection flow rate is increased from 4 mL/s to 6 mL/s, this results in almost double the iodine flux (1.2 g I/s vs 2.2 g I/s). However, injection rates are limited by cannula size and patient tolerance. For limited coverage ranges and very short scan times, injection rates cannot be

raised high enough to produce adequate enhancement. An alternative to increasing the injection rate is to again use a contrast agent with a higher concentration of iodine and using a longer injection duration (relative to the scan time).[4] A proportionately longer scanning delay can be built into the scan protocol such that scan initiation occurs at some predetermined time after the contrast bolus arrives. This type of protocol allows adequate opacification to build up without using excessive injection flow rates.

Flushing the venous system with saline immediately after the contrast injection serves a dual purpose as it can reduce contrast volumes by conserving approximately 15 mL of contrast which would otherwise remain in the arm veins, and at the same time reduce perivenous streak artifacts in the chest by removing dense contrast material from the brachiocephalic veins, the superior vena cava, and right heart. Although a saline flush can be performed manually or by layering the saline solution in the same syringe as the contrast media, new dual barrel power injectors are the most convenient and practical way to flush the veins.

2.2 Scan parameters

One of the most basic and at times confusing aspects of multi-detector CT angiography is the terminology used to describe the way a CT scan is acquired and reconstructed. The purpose of this section is to define basic CT scan parameters and to discuss the principles of their use. In multi-detector CT, it is important to distinguish scan acquisition parameters from scan reconstruction parameters. Scan acquisition parameters determine the way a CT scanner acquires the projection data, while scan reconstruction parameters describe the way the CT scanner assembles the projection data into transverse CT images (Table 23.1).

2.2.1 Scan acquisition

The two most important scan acquisition parameters are *slice collimation* (SC) and *table feed per rotation* (TF), both of which are expressed in millimeters. The relation between these two parameters provides the common definition of *pitch* (P), so that $P = TF/(N \times SC)$, where N is the number of detector rows. Thus, for a 16-row MDCT system performing a CT angiogram with slice collimation of 0.75 mm and a pitch of 1.0, the table feed per rotation would equal 12 mm. This number is important, because, along with the *gantry rotation speed* and the scan *coverage area*, it determines the time required to complete the CT acquisition (*scan duration*). As previously discussed, the scan duration is a major determinant of contrast injection duration, as well as determining the length of time the patient needs to hold his breath. So in the example above, if the gantry rotation speed is 0.5 seconds and the coverage area is 280 mm (a reasonable estimate for an abdominal CT angiogram), the CT acquisition will take 14 seconds to complete.

2.2.2 Scan reconstruction

Once the raw projection data is acquired, it is 're-organized' and re-constructed into axial slices by mathematical technique. These axial images are described by their *slice width* (SW) and *reconstruction interval* (RI) in millimeters. Slice width describes the thickness of the reconstructed slices and the reconstruction interval defines the distance between axial slices. The RI is usually chosen smaller than the SW, resulting in an overlap of the slices. For example, a dataset used to evaluate the size of an abdominal aortic aneurysm might be reconstructed with a width of 1.5 mm (SW) without any overlap (RI also equals 1.5 mm), while an examination of smaller structures such as the renal arteries might require thinner sections reconstructed with a slight overlap, for instance, SW = 1.25 and RI = 0.8.

Reconstructions can be performed in any of a number of widths and intervals, as long as the slice collimation used in the CT acquisition is less than or equal to the reconstructed slice width. For this reason, CT angiography typically is performed with narrow collimation and reconstructed in thin slices to form a *secondary raw dataset*. This dataset can then be used to reconstruct images in various perspectives without loss of image data. These reconstructions can be performed in multiple different planes, can be overlapped,

Table 23.1 Acquisition parameters for peripheral CTA, for a scanning range of 105–130 cm (Note that depending on the detector configuration and table increment, acquisition times vary substantially)

Scanner gantry rotation time in seconds	Collimation (mm)	TI (mm)	STh (mm)	RI (mm)	Scanning time (s)	Slices
4-detector						
0.8-s scanner	4 × 2.5	15	2.5	1.5	56–70	<900
0.5-s scanner	4 × 2.5	15	3.0	1.5	35–43	<900
0.5-s scanner	4 × 1.7	7	1.5–2.0	1.0	75–93	<3100
8-detector						
0.5-s scanner	8 × 1.25	16.75	1.25	0.8	31–39	<1625
16-detector						
0.5-s scanner	16 × 1.5	33	2.0	0.75	16–20	<1700
0.5-s scanner	16 × 0.75	18	1.0	0.5	29–36	<2600
64-detector						
0.5-s scanner*	64 × 0.6	15	2.0	1.2	15–18	<1800

TI, table increment per 360° gantry rotation; *STh*, section thickness; *RI*, reconstruction interval.
*Faster gantry rotation speeds can be acquired, such as 0.33 sec. However, these are exclusively used for cardiac imaging.

projected as 3-dimensional images, or created at different slice thicknesses, depending on the specific clinical question to be answered.

The most obvious advantages of this type of acquisition and reconstruction, other than the speed with which it can be acquired, is the capacity to avoid misregistration from one slice to the next associated with different breath-holds used during conventional axial scanning. The ability to project data in multiple planes without distortion of anatomic structures has obvious clinical benefits. The major disadvantage of thin-section, volumetric CT acquisition and reconstruction of multiple datasets is the tremendous increase in data that results and the associated strain placed on systems used for image storage and retrieval. A typical CT angiogram of the chest, abdomen, pelvis, and lower extremities can produce well over 1,000 axial images. Such an explosion of imaging data has also created challenges for image display and interpretation. These challenges require innovative solutions, including new methods of image post-processing.

2.3 Post-processing techniques

Today's state-of-the art workstations offer several postprocessing techniques to evaluate and interpret CT angiography. The type of technique chosen will depend on the specific clinical question that needs to be answered. However, reviewing the axial data set should still represent the starting point of any examination, not only to assess the vascular structures, but the extra-vascular ones as well.

2.3.1 Multiplanar reformations (MPR)

Cross-sectional views are extremely helpful to assess the vessel lumen. Images in any of the standard planes (axial, coronal, and sagittal) are easily obtained with most postprocessing software. The addition of oblique planes can reveal information that would be extremely difficult to obtain otherwise. A specific type of oblique MPR is the *curved planar reformation* (CPR) which involves manual or semi-automated extraction of a centerline of the vessel to be examined and then viewing the vessel in longitudinal cross-section around this centerline. The advantage of this technique is that the entire length of the defined vessel can be evaluated without obscuration by overlying structures, notably vessel wall calcifications or stents. The disadvantage is the inherent reliance on an accurate centerline. Any deviation from the true center of the vessel of interest can

produce an apparent stenosis within a normal-caliber vessel. Also, this technique can be time-consuming and in some instances the lack of extravascular landmarks for localizing findings precisely can become an issue. A potential solution to this problem is the generation of so-called multi-path CPRs. Multi-path CPRs simultaneously display longitudinal cross sections through the entire peripheral arterial tree at arbitrary viewing angles, thus restoring spatial perception[9,10] (Figure 23.7).

2.3.2 Thick MPR

The same technique that allows us to obtain reconstructions in different planes can be applied to specific volumes of the data set. By varying the slice width and reconstruction interval, data from multiple contiguous slices of imaging data can be reconstructed in thick 'slabs' (Figure 23.7). This image data can be then manipulated during interpretation (windowing, changing the thickness of the slab of information) to allow us to focus on a particular area of interest. The advantage of this technique is that anatomic landmarks can be better preserved and a wealth of data can be depicted with very few images. The disadvantage is that overlapping structures can obscure findings, making precise diagnosis of abnormalities difficult.

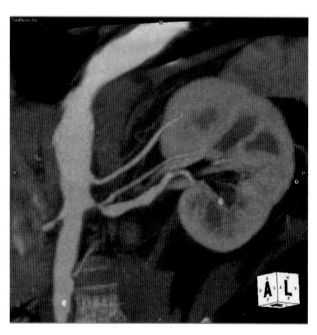

Figure 23.7   MPR: Oblique MPR through the aorta, left renal artery and left kidney shows narrow stenosis as the origin of the artery.

2.3.3 Maximum intensity projection (MIP)

Maximum intensity projection images display a volume of image data, much like thick MPR images. The difference is that the MIP technique preferentially displays the structure within the image volume that has the maximum density (Figure 23.8). MIP images provide the most 'angiography-like' display of the vasculature and are ideal for communicating findings to referring services. As with thick MPR, the main disadvantage is the potential of obscuring the region of interest by overlying structures, particularly hyperdense structures such as the spine and the long bones of the extremities, and obscuration of the vessel lumen by calcified plaque and stents.

2.3.4 Volume rendering (VR)

Unlike other three-dimensional reconstruction techniques, volume rendered images utilize the contributions of each voxel within the image dataset to be reconstructed. When examining these volumes of data, the anatomic region of interest can be exposed using clip planes to cut away overlapping structures or by altering the overall image opacity so that underlying structures become visible. The advantage of VR images is that large volumes of image data can be visualized simultaneously and anatomic landmarks are preserved (Figure 23.9). At their best, such images can produce gorgeous examples of what can be achieved with the technology. Unfortunately, since every pixel in the dataset contributes to the image, VR images require more computer processing power than other techniques. Additionally, such images are somewhat limited when attempting to evaluate the vessel lumen, notably in the presence of vessel calcifications and stents.

3 CLINICAL PERSPECTIVES – CURRENT & FUTURE APPLICATIONS

3.1 Body/cardiac/neuro

Since being introduced, multidetector-row CT has been rapidly spreading across the radiology departments and taking over new roles while replacing older technologies and different modalities. Routine examinations of the chest, abdomen, and pelvis, as well as peripheral, intracranial, and coronary vessels are commonly performed. Additionally, it is now used in different phases of contrast administration (un-enhanced, arterial, venous, etc.) and physiologic states (systole, diastole) allowing for a much more comprehensive examination.[7,11,12]

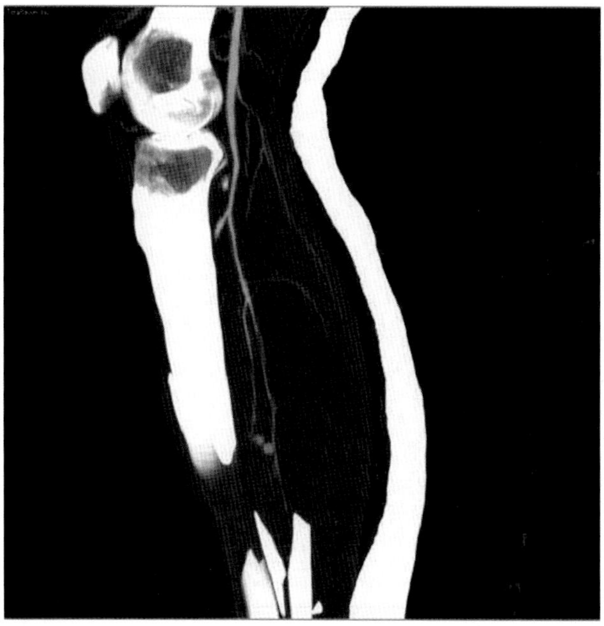

Figure 23.8 MIP: Para-sagittal MIP of a right lower extremity post-trauma demonstrates in the same plane a comminuted fracture of the tibia and its relation to the lower extremity arteries. Two small pseudoaneurysms are in close proximity to the fracture segments.

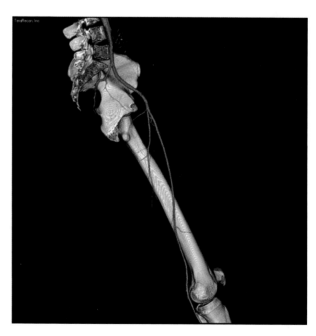

Figure 23.9 VRT: Lateral VRT reconstruction of the left thigh shows in detail the relation between the femur and lower extremity arteries.

Historically, the limitations provided by the trade-off between scan length and spatial resolution along the z-axis in the earlier scanners translated into very region specific examinations, i.e. renal arteries CTA. Therefore the initiation of CT angiography relied on separate areas of interest with very specific scan parameters according to the size of the imaged vessels and their span. Nowadays, the entire body can be imaged in one acquisition, and protocols are converging to only a few basic techniques.

3.2 Future perspectives

In patients for whom a low dose of iodinated contrast is desired, intra-arterial injections of contrast via catheters placed in the interventional suite before imaging could be an option. Some attempts have already been performed with good image quality. However, even though this is a feasible technique utilizing low injection rates and low iodinated contrast volumes, catheter modifications are probably going to be required to obtain consistent and homogeneous opacification of the vessels, especially in their segments most proximal to the catheter where mixing with non-opacified blood will be suboptimal.

An exciting frontier in CT angiography lies with the recently introduced dual-source computed tomography (DSCT) system. This type of scanner is equipped with two X-ray tubes and two corresponding detectors, mounted on a rotating gantry with an angular offset of 90°. This new technology allows both X-ray tubes to be operated at different kV and mA settings, allowing the acquisition of dual-energy data. A potential application of dual energy CT is the separation of bones and iodine-filled vessels in CT angiographic examinations by subtraction of voxels as determined by their Hounsfield attenuation values.

The introduction of CT fluoroscopy made real-time CT imaging available for procedure guidance.[13] This capability has evolved even further with new developments in C-arm CT (Angiographic CT) that allow to obtain images while a procedure is being performed in similar fashion as an angio-suite would. This technology is designed to overcome the limited topographic orientation associated with cross-sectional CT fluoroscopy. However, it is still somewhat limited by a much slower rotational speed of the C-arm and the need for special 'metal-free' beds or carts that would obscure the images; however its portability is opening new doors to the way we perform interventions.

REFERENCES

1. Fuchs T, Kachelriess M, Kalender WA. Technical advances in multi-slice spiral CT. Eur J Radiol. 2000; 36: 69–73.
2. Rubin GD, Dake MD, Napel SA, McDonnell CH, Jeffrey RB Jr. Three-dimensional spiral CT angiography of the abdomen: initial clinical experience. Radiology 1993 Jan; 186(1): 147–52.
3. Rubin GD, Schmidt AJ, Logan LJ et al. Multi-detector row CT angiography of lower extremity arterial inflow and runoff: initial experience, Radiology 2001; 221: 146–58.
4. Fleischmann D. Use of high-concentration contrast media in multiple-detector-row CT: principles and rationale. Eur Radiol. 2003 Dec; 13 Suppl 5: M14–20.
5. Fleischmann D. Present and future trends in multiple detector-row CT applications: CT angiography. Eur Radiol. 2002 Jul; 12 Suppl 2: S11–5.
6. Hittmair K, Fleischmann D. Accuracy of predicting and controlling time-dependent aortic enhancement from a test bolus injection. J Comput Assist Tomogr. 2001 Mar–Apr; 25(2): 287–94.
7. Prokop M. Multislice CT angiography. Eur J Radiol. 2000 Nov; 36(2): 86–96.
8. Fleischmann D, Rubin GD, Bankier AA, Hittmair K. Improved uniformity of aortic enhancement with customized contrast medium injection protocols at CT angiography. Radiology 2000 Feb; 214(2): 363–71.
9. Kanitsar A, Fleischmann D, Wegenkittl R, Felkel P, Groeller E. CPR – curved planar reformation. In: IEEE Visualization. Boston: IEEE Computer Society, 2002; 37–44.
10. Roos JE, Fleischmann D, Koechl A et al. Multi-path curved planar reformation (mpCPR) of the peripheral arterial tree in CT angiography (CTA). Radiology 2007, 10.1148/radiol. 2441060976).
11. Napoli A, Fleischmann D, Chan FP et al. Computed tomography angiography: state-of-the-art imaging using multidetector-row technology. J Comput Assist Tomogr. 2004 Jul–Aug; 28 Suppl 1: S32–45.
12. Fleischmann D, Hallett RL, Rubin GD. CT angiography of peripheral arterial disease. J Vasc Interv Radiol. 2006 Jan; 17(1): 3–26.
13. Daly B, Templeton PA. Real-time CT fluoroscopy: evolution of an interventional tool. Radiology 1999; 211: 309–15.

24

Computed Tomographic Angiography of the Thoracic Aorta

Brad Thompson and Edwin J.R. van Beek

1 INTRODUCTION

Diseases that affect the thoracic aorta are commonly associated with high rates of mortality, with many requiring some form of immediate surgical intervention. Understandably, there is a critical need for establishing an immediate and accurate clinical diagnosis of suspected aortic disease at the time of presentation. There are several modalities that can be used in the radiographic evaluation of the thoracic aorta, namely angiography, magnetic resonance imaging (MR), and computed tomography (CT). Deciding which one to use, however, largely depends on a host of factors dependent upon the scenario and clinical suspicion as well as availability, convenience, patient stability, and of course total exam time. For example, angiography, long considered to be the gold standard in aortic imaging, appears to be best suited in the setting of trauma, but is invasive, potentially inconvenient, and lengthy, which may delay definitive treatment. Being able to provide multiplanar images of the thoracic aorta and do so without ionizing radiation, MR imaging is probably best suited for surveillance exams of known and stable aortic diseases. However, lengthy exam times, susceptibility to undesirable artifacts and difficult patient monitoring during the exam make MR less attractive in the acute setting. In view of these shortcomings, computed tomography, by virtue of its unique and distinct technical advantages, has emerged as *the* ideal modality in the radiographic assessment of the thoracic aorta, especially in emergent clinical settings. With the development of expanded scanner configurations, and shorter image acquisition speeds,

multi-detector CT (MDCT) is a fast and convenient modality able to provide rapid and reproducible high spatial resolution images of the entire aorta, usually within one breath hold. Slice acquisitions as thin as 1–2 mm provide the ability to create 2D, 3D and angiographic reconstructions that rival traditional angiography in representation and image quality. EKG gating of images has improved image quality by removing troublesome motion artifacts that have been associated with slower scanners. Furthermore, additional developments such as dose modulation and partial reconstruction algorithms have respectively decreased radiation exposures and scan times considerably. Finally, by providing a complete assessment of the cardiopulmonary and musculoskeletal system, CT may identify either unsuspected findings or alternative diseases that may explain the clinical presentation. This chapter will briefly discuss multi-slice CT protocols relating to aortic imaging and review disease processes of the thoracic aorta that can be readily diagnosed with multi-slice CT.

2 TECHNICAL CONSIDERATIONS

The technical issues relating to imaging of the thoracic aorta with MDCT primarily involve the speed of image acquisition, anatomical coverage, and slice thickness. With rapid expansion of helical scanner platforms from four to 64 channel detector configurations, Z-axis coverage continues to shorten, and coupled with progressively faster scanners,

Table 24.1   Routine 16-slice CT angiographic protocol for thoracic aorta imaging

Thoracic aorta protocol	16 slice scanner
kV	120
mA	130
Kernal	B30f
Slice thickness (mm)	1.5
Table feed (mm)	1.5
Collimation	0.75
Scan time (msec)	500

Table 24.2   Routine i.v. contrast injection protocol for 16-slice thoracic aortography

IV contrast protocol	16 slice helical scanner
Concentration	300 mg I/ml
Dose	100–120 cc
Rate of infusion	3–5 cc/sec (20 gauge IV)
Delay	20–30 sec
Saline flush	Desirable

the time required to cover the entire thoracic aorta with MDCT can now be easily accomplished within one breath-hold. This concomitantly has had beneficial repercussions relating to contrast doses which are correspondingly smaller. Table 24.1 lists a typical helical CT protocol for a 16-slice scanner for the thoracic aorta.

Usual imaging protocols for aortic disease should be tailored to include the entire thorax and upper abdomen in order to evaluate for unsuspected findings, as in cases of trauma where there may be associated fractures, hemothorax and/or pneumothorax, and solid organ injury. Radiographic evaluation should also include assessment of branch vessels, especially the great vessels to the head and neck in cases of aortic dissection.

2.1 Intravenous contrast considerations

In patients with suspected aortic disease, excellent contrast enhancement of the entire aorta and branch vessels is requisite, requiring careful consideration to dose, infusion rates and timing. Obviously without contrast, the sensitivity for the determination of leak, dissection, and thrombosis is limited. Similarly, use of iodinated non-ionic contrast material enables radiologists to create CT angiograms which may be necessary as part of preoperative planning. Table 24.2 provides general guidelines for contrast administration. In order to optimize the contrast enhancement of the thoracic aorta, initiation of scanning has to be synchronized with the arterial phase of the bolus of contrast material. With older CT scanners, technologists could generally be assured of an arterial location of contrast after approximately one-half of the total dose was injected. This protocol was predicated upon doses of 150 ml of contrast and risked suboptimal aortic enhancement, especially in patients with poor cardiac output, left heart obstructive disease (aortic/mitral valve stenosis)

or pulmonary hypertension. With multi-slice scanners, the determination of optimal contrast enhancement is straightforward, and can be accomplished using bolus tracking software included with most scanners, whereby time–density curves can be generated that accurately depict time of peak enhancement. Using this technique, a test bolus of 10 ml of contrast material is injected and preliminary single level scans centered at the aortic arch enable the technologist to visually inspect the transit of contrast as it moves through the thoracic aorta. Once the peak bolus is reached in the target area, scanning can be initiated manually. Alternatively, placing a region of interest within the ascending aorta, a time–density curve can be generated that graphically calculates the time to peak enhancement of the thoracic aorta. Some scanners are equipped with automatic start-scan functions that initiate scanning once a prescribed CT density has been achieved at the target region of interest. Injection of contrast material in the right arm and use of a saline flush (chaser) help to decrease undesirable streak artifacts originating from high concentrations of IV contrast in the central venous circulation. With further expansion of multi-slice scanner configurations, which provide greater Z-axis coverage, total contrast volume requirements for aortic imaging continue to decrease. This phenomenon thereby reduces not only cost but has expanded the applicability of CT in patients with borderline renal function. Patients with normal renal function can tolerate 150 ml of contrast. Pediatric doses are usually limited to 2–3 ml of 300 mgI/kg. An important consideration for total dose administration, however, relates to the scan duration required to cover a prescribed anatomical area. In larger patients and in cases where scan coverage may need to include the abdominal aorta (dissection) larger total doses of contrast material may be required. The following equation can be used to determine total dose:

Contrast volume (ml) = Flow rate (ml/s) × scan duration (s).

Optimal enhancement of the thoracic aorta and branch vessels generally require CT attenuation values of 300 Hounsfield Units (HU). In larger patients, achieving this level of enhancement may require faster infusion rates on the order of 5 ml/s.

3 CLINICAL APPLICATIONS

The widely accepted application of MDCT in the evaluation of thoracic aortic disease primarily relates to its rapid speed, and reproducible high-resolution images. As such, thinner slice collimation scans which are readily performed by MDCT enable superior multi-planar and angiographic representations of the aorta and branch vessels which are desirable as part of pre-operative planning. In acute chest pain syndromes, especially in the setting of trauma, dissection, aneurysms, intramural hematoma, such thin slice helical acquisitions enable volumetric reconstructions to be performed rapidly that can be invaluable in defining vascular anatomy, and extent of disease. Furthermore, the versatility of CT in aortic imaging is further enhanced by its ability to demonstrate incipient complications, such as aortic rupture in cases of trauma, vascular occlusion with or without solid organ infarction, and can provide alternative diagnoses that may result in acute chest pain such as pericarditis or pulmonary embolism.

4 NORMAL ANATOMY

The thoracic aorta is composed of three layers, the intima (endothelial lining), the media (containing smooth muscle, elastic and collagen fibers) and the adventitia (containing vasa vasorum, nerves, lymphatics and elastic and collagen fibers).

The root of the aorta is surrounded by the four heart chambers in the valve plane. The sinus of Valsalva just above the valve level contains the origins for the left and right coronary arteries. Immediately above the sinus is the anatomic sinutubular ridge, which is important for surgical planning. It subsequently follows an oblique course from anterior coursing to the right initially, followed by an arch from right anterior to left posterior, where it descends anterolateral to the thoracic spine through the diaphragmatic hiatus into the retroperitoneal space. At the level of the arch, in approximately 75% of subjects it gives off 3 branches: the right innominate artery, the left common carotid artery and the left subclavian artery. In approximately 20% of subjects, the innominate and the left common carotid arteries have a common ostium, while the left vertebral artery arises separately in 6% of subjects.[1] Just past the left subclavian artery, the ligamentum arteriosus (the

remnant of the ductus arteriosus) attaches medially into the arch. Diameters of the thoracic aorta have been determined using CT studies.[2,3] Although there is a significant range, the rule of thumb is that the mid ascending aorta should not exceed 3.5 cm, while the descending aorta should not exceed 2.5 cm in diameter.

5 ADULT PRESENTATIONS OF CONGENITAL DISEASES

In approximately 1% of the population, a host of variations of the normal thoracic aortic branching pattern exist, and these tend to be completely asymptomatic and of no clinical significance. An aberrant right subclavian artery or an aberrant left subclavian artery with a right arch can produce dysphagia, while a double aortic arch can result in a tight vascular right involving the esophagus as well as the trachea. Although many of these variations will be detected early in life, some tend to become symptomatic only in later life with dilatation and elongation of arteries. Aberrant subclavian arteries are more prone to developing aneurysms.

CT has proven extremely valuable in diagnosing these variants. MRI has also been applied successfully, and in many situations is the imaging method of choice. Invasive catheter angiography has been completely replaced by these two methods.

5.1 Coarctation

Coarctation is congenital narrowing in the region of the isthmus, which often goes undetected until adulthood. There is a male:female ratio of 4:1, and it is commonly associated with bicuspid aortic valve (up to 50%) and Turner syndrome.

The site of stenosis influences later development. If the stenosis is proximal to the ductus arteriosus, symptoms will develop early due to a lack of collateral formation in utero. If the stenosis is at the level of the duct or beyond, collateral circulation will develop and patients will present in adult life. Mortality is significant in patients who survive into adult life, but remain undetected, and is predominantly related to heart failure, aortic rupture, and secondary hypertension complications in the upper body (cerebral aneurysms).

The main findings at chest radiography include left ventricular hypertrophy, signs of heart failure and bilateral rib notching of ribs 3–9 (if the coarctation is proximal to the left subclavian artery, only right sided rib notching is present). Computed tomography will demonstrate aortic caliber

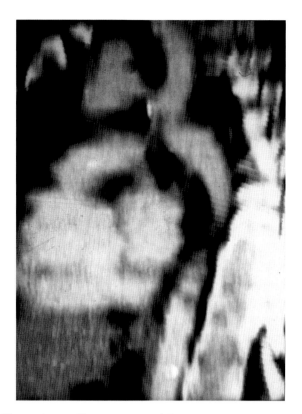

Figure 24.1 Electron beam CT angiogram, demonstrating acute caliber change inferior to the aortic arch.

change (Figure 24.1), collateral circulation, flow abnormalities into the left subclavian artery and hypertrophy of intercostals vessels with rib notching. Many patients with coarctation will have surgery at a young age and will have CT (or MRI) as part of follow-up,[4] although newer methods of treatment include interventional radiological techniques such as stenting and angioplasty.[5]

5.2 Aortic stenosis

Aortic stenosis may arise at three levels (valvular, subvalvular and supra-valvular), but only the *valvular stenosis* is likely to present in adults. This form of aortic stenosis occurs in 1–2% of the population, mainly in relation to bicuspid valves either in isolation or together with coarctation. The bicuspid valve leads to changes in blood flow, with resultant premature aging leading to fibrosis and calcification.[6,7] Most patients will present in the 4th–6th decades of life due to signs of heart failure, angina pectoris, decreased exercise tolerance and even sudden death. The PA chest radiograph may be normal or show premature dilatation (similar to unfolding) of the ascending aorta (Figure 24.2a).

The CT findings (Figures 24.2b and 24.2c) include calcification of the aortic annulus and aortic valve, post-stenotic dilatation of the ascending aorta, left ventricular

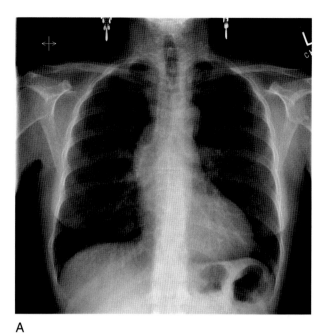

A

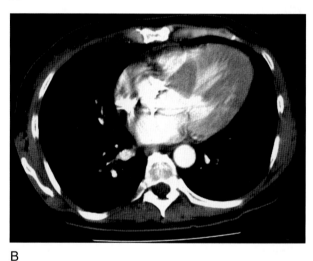

B

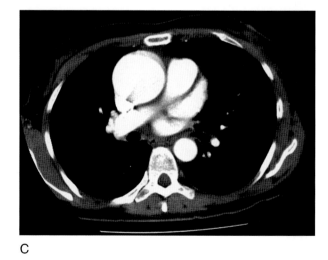

C

Figure 24.2 A. CXR in 49-year old main with syncope. Distended ascending aorta. B. CT at valvular level demonstrating extensive leaflet calcifications in bicuspid valve. C. CT at ascending aorta level demonstrating post-stenotic aneurysm.

hypertrophy and, later in the disease process, signs of heart failure with dilatation of the left-sided heart chambers and pulmonary venous congestion.[8]

6 AORTIC ANEURYSMS

Aneurysms may be divided in true aneurysms (which comprise all three layers of the aortic wall) and false aneurysms (which are contained ruptures that are bound by peri-adventitial tissues and sometimes a partially intact adventitital layer).

A classification of aortic aneurysms was proposed in order to have more uniform reporting.[9] A modification for thoracic aortic aneurysms is summarized in Table 24.3.

6.1 Primary connective tissue disorders

6.1.1 Marfan disease

Marfan's disease was first described in 1896 by the French physician Antoine Marfan (1858–1942), and was later identified as an autosomal dominant disorder, located on chromosome 15, with a variable expression (70% are transmitted, 30% consist of spontaneous mutations). The prevalence is approximately 5 per 10,000, and results in inadequate strength and metabolism of collagen fibers. The disease has a number of presentations, including increased height, pectus excavatum or carinatum, scoliosis, luxation of the lens (leading to cataract) and spontaneous pneumothorax.[10] Cardiovascular diseases caused by media degeneration with wall weakening affect approximately 90% of patients; the main associations are dilatation of the ascending aorta (with resultant aortic valve insufficiency), dissection of the entire aorta and aneurysms of the coronary arteries occurring at a young age (Figure 24.3). Less common findings include mitral valve prolaps, dilatation of the pulmonary artery,

mitral annulus calcification and dilatation or dissection of the descending aorta, all occurring before the age of 40 years. The diagnosis of Marfan's disease is largely clinical from the outset. However, management is heavily reliant on imaging and screening for large vessel complications using echocardiography, MR angiography and CT angiography.[11] The early diagnosis of aortic dilatation has made a dramatic impact on the survival of these patients, and early surgery is commonplace. At a later age, the follow-up usually focuses on detection of recurrent disease involving the descending aorta, the coronary arteries and the heart valves; both echocardiography and CT angiography are commonly employed.

6.1.2 Ehlers Danlos syndrome

Ehlers Danlos syndrome (EDS) comprises a group of more than 10 genetic disorders with inability to synthesize mature collagen and connective tissue, leading to loss of support and resultant increased elasticity and fragility. The actual genetic defects have been demonstrated in many (but not all) of these disorders.[12] The prevalence of EDS is approximately 1:400,000. The clinical features depend on the type, but prematurity, joint hyper mobility, spontaneous pneumothorax, heart valve disorders (mitral valve prolapse), ocular fragility, skin bruising and in the most severe type, EDS type IV, large artery dissection and rupture.[13] This complication is almost always unexpected and lethal, and until until recently only three survivors have been described.[14] In all these cases, CT is capable of demonstrating the underlying thoracic abnormalities as well as the complications of these syndromes.

6.1.3 Post-stenotic dilatation

Post-stenotic development of thoracic aortic aneurysm is particularly prevalent in patients with valvular stenosis,

Table 24.3 Classification of thoracic aortic aneurysm (modified from[14])

Primary connective tissue disorders	Marfan, Ehlers-Danlos
Mechanical	Post-stenotic
Miscellaneous	Tuberous sclerosis, Turner syndrome
Pseudo-aneurysm	Trauma, dissection, anastomotic
Arteritis-related	Takayasu, Behcet
Infectious (mycotic)	Bacterial, fungal, spirochetal
Degenerative	Non specific (arteriosclerosis), inflammatory
Graft failure	

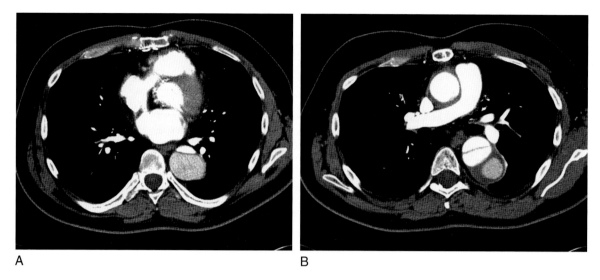

A   B

Figure 24.3   A. Patient with known Marfan's disease, post aortic root repair. B. A large dissection is shown in the descending aorta, with concomitant aneurysm formation.

which occurs with ageing (Figure 24.2). Factors including elevated lateral wall pressures and shear stress with turbulent flow result in progressive dilatation of the aorta.

6.1.4 Miscellaneous causes of thoracic aortic aneurysm

Tuberous sclerosis is an autosomal dominant disease, with its major impact on the central nervous system. It has been associated with both thoracic and abdominal aortic aneurysm, partly explained by increased fragmentation of elastic fibers and also related to hypertension.[15]

Turner syndrome, the result of karyotype 45 XO, can exhibit extensive large artery abnormalities, including thoracic aortic aneurysm, due to increased wall stiffness. Patients treated with high doses of growth hormone have been shown to respond with improved distensibility and decreased aneurysm development and growth.[16]

6.1.5 Traumatic aortic tears and pseudo-aneurysm

Rupture of the wall of the aorta may lead to a hematoma that is contained by peri-adventitial tissues. This will result in a growing mass-like lesion, representing the expanding hematoma (Figure 24.4).

Multiple injuries are common in trauma, and multi-slice CT, by virtue of its ability to provide a rapid global radiographic assessment of the chest and cardiopulmonary

system, is now considered the modality of choice in the evaluation of trauma patients. The accessibility of scanners to most trauma departments, coupled with faster scan times and quick throughput, have made MDCT ideal in the evaluation of acute trauma patients.

Blunt chest trauma is associated with substantial mortality. Among the long list of potential chest injuries, aortic injury accounts for 3%.[17] Aortic tears (intimal disruption) are most commonly encountered in injury relating from rapid deceleration, as are experienced with high speed motor vehicle collisions or long distance falls. Tears from such mechanism can occur anywhere along the thoracic

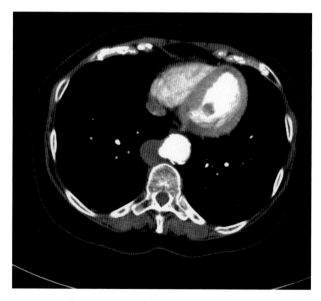

Figure 24.4   Elderly patient with penetrating aortic ulcer and formation of pseudo-aneurysm.

aorta and the overall mortality rate of traumatic aortic injury is 80–90%.[18] Approximately 20–25% of all on-scene fatalities occur from acute ascending aortic injury, resulting in death from rapid exsanguinations.[19] Tears in this location account for 5–10% of all cases.[18] The vast majority of aortic tears (90%) occur at the aortic isthmus near the ligamentum arteriosum (Figure 24.5). Anatomically this location corresponds to the transition point where the aorta becomes fixed in location, allowing the more mobile unfixed transverse segment (arch) to flex during deceleration. Tears in this location are most commonly encountered clinically since these patients are most likely to reach a hospital.[17,20] Immediate diagnosis is crucial, however, since with each passing hour following the injury, the mortality rate increases by 1%.[18] Rapid recognition and management of aortic tears is critical, since survival rates approach 60–70% with surgical intervention.[17]

Recognition of acute aortic trauma by CT is generally straightforward and relates to detection of direct or indirect signs of injury. Key to the diagnosis is the presence of an intimal flap, commonly in the region of the aortic isthmus, that resembles a short segment dissection (Figure 24.5). The presence of a pseudoaneurysm in this same region is additional evidence of acute aortic injury. The sensitivity of CT compared with conventional aortography for the identification of aortic tears is 100%.[21,22] Obvious extravasation

of contrast also serves as direct evidence of aortic injury. In many cases the presence of para-aortic or mediastinal hematoma serves as indirect evidence of aortic injury. Although the existence of blood in the mediastinum can originate from alternative sources such as venous hemorrhage or spinal fractures, this finding alone should always raise the suspicion for aortic injury, particularly if the mechanism of rapid deceleration is known and the majority of the mediastinal blood is centered around the arch and descending aorta. The presence of mediastinal blood has a specificity of 87% and a sensitivity of 99.3% for predicting aortic injury.[23] However some investigators have reported that a normal thoracic aorta by MDCT alone is sufficient evidence to exclude aortic injury even in the presence of mediastinal hematoma.[24,25] Even if no intimal irregularities suggest an intimal tear, the presence of mediastinal blood generally warrants further evaluation with angiography as confirmatory proof of aortic integrity. Conversely, the negative predictive value of a normal chest CT (i.e. no direct or indirect signs) for aortic injury in the setting of acute trauma is 100%.[22,26,27,28,29] In circumstances where there is an equivocal mediastinal widening on admission chest radiographs, or when the suspicion of aortic injury is low, exclusion of mediastinal blood by MDCT essentially obviates the need for further diagnostic imaging with aortography.

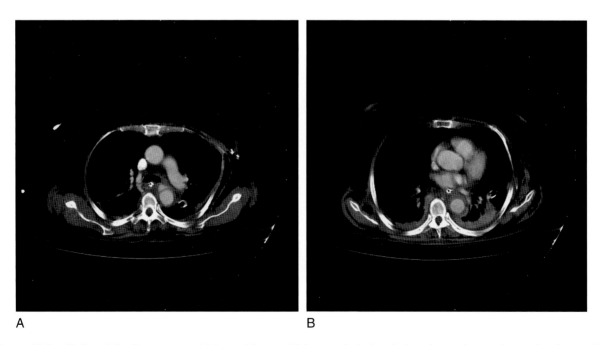

A   B

Figure 24.5 Patient following motor vehicle accident at high speed. A. Just below the arch, anterior to the descending aorta, a traumatic dissection has developed with fluid in the mediastinum. B. Below the level of the tear, fluid is seen surrounding the descending aorta.

Furthermore, screening of trauma patients with abnormal chest films by CT may provide alternative reasons for mediastinal widening such as mediastinal lipomatosis, adenopathy, and paraspinal hematomas secondary to vertebral body fractures.

6.2 Arteritis of the aorta

6.2.1 Takayasu's arteritis

Takayasu's arteritis is a primary arteritis of the aorta, its main branch arteries and the pulmonary artery, which occurs ten-fold more common in women than in men. Although the traditional association is with Asian women, other races are also affected. The early findings are usually subtle with mild wall thickening. As the disease progresses, stenosis, post-stenotic dilatation, aneurysms and acute thrombosis and/or occlusion will occur (hence the term 'pulse-less disease'), which become evident at any angiographic diagnostic imaging test (angiography, CT and MRI are all employed in the management of this disorder). Collateral circulation may become dominant, and rib notching has been described.[30,31]

6.3 Behçet disease

This systemic disorder, which is a vasculitis of unknown origin, primarily affects young adults between 20 and 40 years of age. Men are twice more affected than women, and it is more common among Mediterranean, Middle-Eastern and Japanese populations with a world-wide distribution.[32,33]

The main clinical presentations are urogenital ulceration, erythema nodosum, thrombophlebitis and ocular disease,[34] but significantly, aneurysms (both of the aorta, the coronary arteries and the pulmonary vessels) are common and may have a fatal outcome due to major hemorrhage.

Both CT and MRI will demonstrate aneurysm of the major thoracic vessels, thrombophlebitis (with resultant pulmonary embolism), lymphadenopathy, pleural effusions and evidence of hemorrhage anywhere in the chest.

6.4 Infective aneurysm

Although traditionally described as syphilitic aneurysm, the most commonly found organisms today are Staphylococcus aureus, although Salmonella, Chlamydia and less frequently fungal infections (particularly in immunocompromised patients) have also been described. Penetrating injuries and endocarditis with systemic embolization are the most frequent underlying etiologies for development of focal infectious arteritis, leading to media necrosis and aneurysm formation.[35] Traditionally, these aneurysms were located in the ascending aorta, but they may occur at any site in the thoracic (and abdominal) aorta and can demonstrate air in the aortic wall (Figure 24.6).

6.5 Degenerative aneurysm

This entity, traditionally described as 'arteriosclerotic aneurysm,' is increasing in prevalence and occurs more frequently with advancing age. Although most commonly encountered in the abdominal aorta, the thoracic aorta is also a recognized site and considered more difficult in management due to complex vascular supply and branches from the thoracic aorta. Several risk factors have been described, including ageing, smoking, abnormal cholesterol metabolism and obesity.

Early in the disease process, the media and adventitia layers of the aorta become infiltrated with lymphocytes, plasma cells and macrophages, while the vaso vasorum may show features of arteritis ultimately leading to media degeneration.[36] Once the media layer starts to degenerate, there is

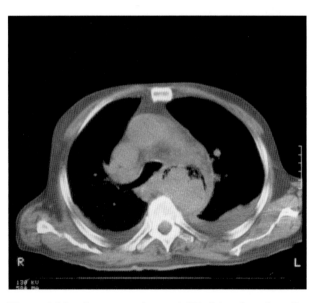

Figure 24.6 Contrast-enhanced CT of the chest in a diabetic patient with low-grade fever and acute onset back pain. There is a focal aneurysm with air in the aortic wall. At surgery, this was found to be a mycotic aneurysm due to Salmonella infection.

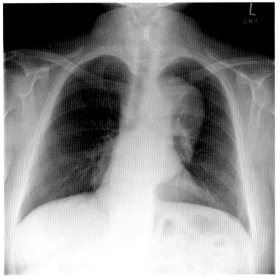

A

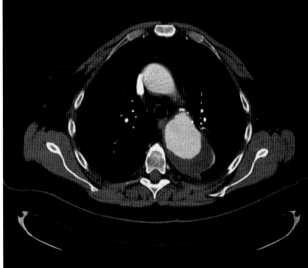

B

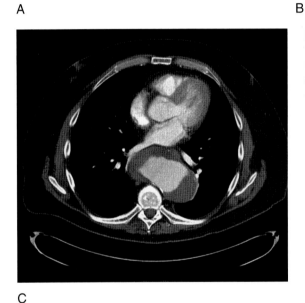

C

Figure 24.7 Patient presenting for routine investigation for vague chest discomfort. A. Chest X-ray demonstrates large aortic aneurysm. B. CT at level of the lower end of the arch shows developing descending aorta aneurysm. C. CT at level of the left atrium shows extensive mural thrombus in aneurysm.

progressive loss of elastic and collagen fibers, and an aneurysm will develop (Figure 24.7).

6.6 Graft aneurysm

Once patients have undergone surgical repair (most commonly with Dacron and polytetrafluoroethylene grafts in current practice, but previously with a host of other compounds), the risk for recurrence of aneurysm is not negligible. There are two main mechanisms for graft aneurysm: (1) development of an aneurysm at the site of anastomosis with the native vessel and (2) failure of the graft itself. More recently, endovascular stent grafts have largely replaced the

surgical repair of thoracic aortic aneurysms and dissections.[37–39] However, although the surgical complication rate is significantly less using the endovascular approach, endovascular grafts are not immune to development of aneurysm development, and follow-up using imaging remains an important component of patient management.

7 AORTIC DISSECTION

Pathologically, aortic dissection is characterized by an acute process related to intimal disruption, resulting in the dissection of blood through the tunica or muscular layer of the aortic wall. The prevalence of aortic dissection has been reported to be 5–10 per million people by autopsy studies, and 27 per million per year by population studies.[20] Usually a disease process of older adults, there are many disease processes associated with acute aortic dissection (Table 24.4). Patients with acute aortic dissection present with severe chest or back pain often mimicking acute myocardial infarction. Approximately 70% of patients are hypertensive.[18] Men are affected three times more often than women.[17] Disparate or unequal pulses or blood pressures in the extremities may also be identified, reflecting impaired branch vessel perfusion due to impeded flow or frank vascular occlusion.

The diagnosis of aortic dissection relies upon the identification of an intraluminal flap which corresponds to the inward displacement of the intima as blood insinuates itself through the tunica media (Figure 24.3). The identification of the intimal flap requires CT scans with IV contrast, though occasionally the identification of inwardly displaced atherosclerotic intimal calcifications within the lumen on noncontrast scans also suggests the diagnosis. The process of dissection creates two separate channels of blood flow, one through the native lumen (true lumen) and a second (false) lumen that reflects blood flow in the newly created channel through the tunica media. In cases where flow is maintained in the false lumen, both lumens show evidence of contrast enhancement, although blood flow within the false lumen is typically slower than that in the true lumen, and as such demonstrates a lesser degree of enhancement. The reported sensitivity and specificity for contrast-enhanced CT for dissection is 94–100% and 87–100% respectively.[17,18]

In the assessment of aortic dissection, the diagnostic goals are several. First the entire extent of the dissection needs to be determined and classified. This usually requires that the entire aorta and iliac vessels be included on the CT acquisition to document the distal extent. Identification of the initiation point is critical as this determines therapy. Second, complications such as aortic leak or frank rupture, and pericardial effusion, should be quickly identified so as to permit rapid surgical intervention. Thirdly, integrity of all branch vessels needs to be determined. This requires exams to be tailored with sufficient Z-axis coverage to cover all major thoracic and intra-abdominal arteries. Similarly, the field of view should be wide enough to permit visual interrogation and documentation of perfusion defects of end organs such as the liver, kidneys and bowel. Extension of the dissection into carotid or vertebral arteries can result in dangerous derangements in cerebral blood flow resulting in stroke. End organ infarction may occur due to occlusion of vessels such as the renal and mesenteric arteries. Identification of branch vessel involvement may also dictate changes in the surgical approach required to repair these vessels. Finally, patency of the false lumen needs to be identified and documented. Since the thickness of the aortic wall is compromised, aneurysm formation of the aorta is much more likely in cases where the flow through the false lumen is maintained compared to those dissections where the false lumen undergoes thrombosis.

The classification of aortic dissection is a key factor determining whether management is medical or surgical. Dissections that involve the ascending thoracic aorta (Stanford type A; Debakey I and II) usually require immediate surgical repair, as these types are linked with incipient life threatening complications such as acute coronary arterial occlusion, pericardial tamponade, and aortic valve insufficiency (Figure 24.8). In 60% of all cases of dissection,

Table 24.4 Diseases implicated in the development of aortic dissection[43]
Cystic medical necrosis
Marfan's Syndrome
Ehlers-Danlos Syndrome
Turner Syndrome
Trauma
Aortic coarctation
Bicuspid aortic valve
Intramural hematoma
Pregnancy
Cocaine use
Penetrating athersclerotic ulcer
Infection/aortitis
Spontaneous

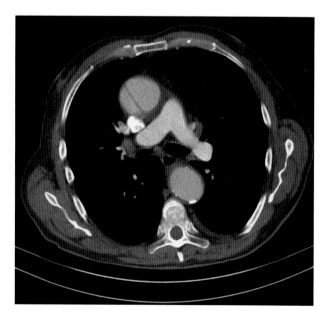

Figure 24.8 Example of a type A dissection, which extends into the ascending aorta.

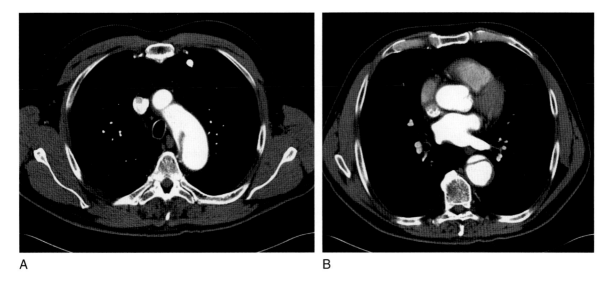

A   B

Figure 24.9 A. Example of a type B dissection, which only involves the descending aorta. B. The intimal flap is seen extending into, but not beyond the aortic arch.

the site of the intimal tear is just above the aortic valve.[20] The one-year survival rate for type A dissections is 30%.[20]

Dissections that involve only the aorta distal to the origin of the left subclavian artery are classified as type B (Stanford) or type III (DeBakey) (Figure 24.9). Since the acute life threatening complications relating to sudden death from pericardial tamponade and coronary artery occlusion are not a consideration with dissections originating with the descending thoracic aorta, type B dissections are generally managed medically with observation, antihypertensive therapy and radiographic surveillance to evaluate for progression and aneurysm formation. Branch vessel involvement, regardless of type, usually requires restorative surgical repair. Similarly, surveillance scans depicting aneurysm development may eventually necessitate surgery.

8 INTRAMURAL HEMATOMA

Intramural hematoma (IMH) represents a localized hemorrhage within the tunica media of the wall of the aorta (Figure 24.10). Constituting 10–20% of acute aortic syndromes,[29] the clinical presentation and demographics of IMH are similar to aortic dissection, occuring most frequently in older adults (median age of 68 years). Approximately 53% of patients with IMH are hypertensive at presentation.[20]

IMH are generally thought to arise from rupture of the vasa vasorum, although IMH can also result from penetrating atherosclerotic ulcers (PAU), or fracture of the intima at an atherosclerotic plaque.[23] The incidence of IMH has been

reported to be 13–27% in clinical series.[20,40] IMH also has been cited as a precursor to eventual aortic dissection in 4–13% of cases[20,41–43] (Figure 24.11).

The CT diagnosis of IMH is established by the identification of a focally thickened hyperattenuated aortic wall segment that reflects the hematoma within the media. These features are best shown on unenhanced sequences, which should be included routinely as part of standard protocols for patients with acute chest or back pain suspected to

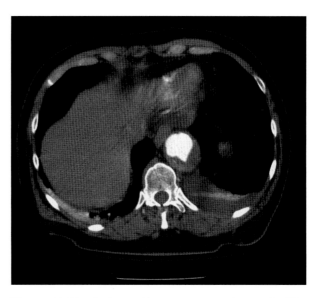

Figure 24.10 Patient with acute onset chest pain. The aorta wall is thickened and there is increased attenuation in the wall of the aorta indicating acute hemorrhage. This is the hallmark of intramural hematoma.

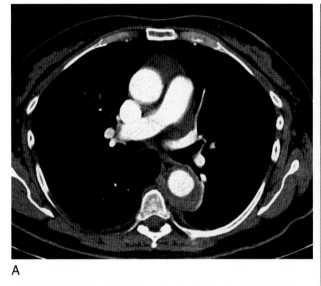

A

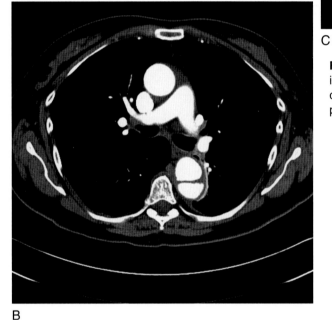

B

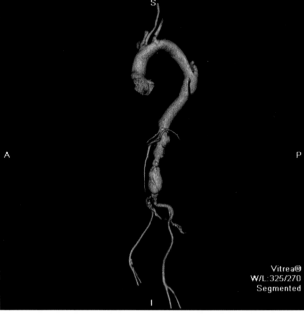

C

Figure 24.11 A. Example of a patient being followed for intramural hematoma. B. The hematoma progressed into a dissection during follow-up. C. 3D reconstruction of complex aortic disease with aneurysm and dissection.

be of aortic origin. The sensitivity for the detection of IMH is often lowered by use of contrast material as the hyperattentuation of the contrast can mask the mural hematoma, rendering its identification more difficult. On contrast-enhanced studies, the mural hematoma should not enhance as might be expected with the false lumen of aortic dissection. The differentiation between IMH and the thrombosed false lumen of aortic dissection is further facilitated by the recognition of the typical spiraling course characteristic of dissection, in contrast to the more eccentrically located IMH, which tends to be shorter along the long axis of the aorta. An identifiable intimal tear is also not characteristic of IMH. Luminal narrowing and inward displacement of intimal calcification are encountered in both IMH and

dissection, and while these findings are important visual clues that aid in the diagnosis, neither can be used alone to differentiate between these two entities.[17,44]

The classification of IMH is identical to aortic dissection: Type A are located in the ascending aorta (48%) and type B in the descending aorta (44%).[23] Similarly, the location dictates treatment options: Type B is usually managed medically, but require routine radiographic surveillance to exclude development of aortic dissection, rupture or eventual aneurysm formation that occurs in up to 30% of patients.[20,40,45,46] The threat of dissection appears to increase in relation to the overall caliber of the aorta, with greatest risk occurring with aortic diameters measuring 5 cm or greater.[43] Because of complications similar to dissection,

IMH in the ascending aorta requires surgical or endovascular repair. Surgery is likewise indicated when associated complications such as rupture or branch vessel occlusion are present regardless of the location. Partial or complete resolution of IMH has been reported in 40–80%.[47] The overall mortality of IMH is reported to be 21%.[20]

9 PENETRATING ATHEROSCLEROTIC ULCER

Penetrating atherosclerotic ulcers (PAU), like IMH and dissection, are typically found in older, hypertensive patients, usually with known pre-existing peripheral vascular disease. Clinical symptoms likewise mimic these two entities, specifically acute chest or back pain. Histologically, PAU is characterized by mushroom or collar-button shaped ulcerated lesions that transgress the intimal surface of the ortic wall, extending into the tunica media (Figure 24.4). If the adventitia is disrupted, PAU can result in the formation of aneurysms, pseudoaneurysms, dissection or frank aortic rupture. The ulcer is typically found in areas of atherosclerotic plaque. In some cases where there is associated hemorrhage within the media, radiographic changes within the wall reflecting an IMH can also be identified. Conversely, IMH may be an initiating event for PAU.[20] The typical locations of PAU are usually concentrated in areas of the aorta where the most advanced atherosclerotic plaque development occurs, namely the descending thoracic aorta and abdominal aorta. Since minimal complicated atherosclerotic plaque development occurs in the ascending aorta due to higher blood flow velocities, lesions proximal to the aortic arch are uncommon. Prognosis of PAU is variable; rupture has been reported in 38% of patients following presentation.[48] In most cases, surgical resection or endovascular therapy is generally warranted, particularly in cases with lesions in the ascending aorta. Lesions that demonstrate growth or leak are likewise candidates for surgical intervention. Surveillance studies of non-complicated lesions reveal eventual growth in 30–50% of penetrating ulcers[20] although some PAU lesions may undergo spontaneous healing.[49]

10 CONCLUDING REMARKS

CT angiography of the thoracic aorta has almost completely replaced traditional catheter-based techniques. The technique is easily applicable, versatile and well-placed to demonstrate the extent of disease processes. The introduction of more advanced scanner technology has further enhanced its diagnostic power and potential.

The only drawbacks are the requirements for intravenous iodinated contrast agents (which may limit the use in patients with pre-existing renal compromise) and the need for ionizing radiation (which is a larger issue in young patients requiring repeated follow-up examinations). These drawbacks are to be considered in weighing up the choice for CT angiography versus MR angiography, as described elsewhere in this book.

REFERENCES

1. Sutton D, Rhys Davies E. Arch aortography and cerebrovascular insufficiency. Clin Radiol 1966; 17: 330–45.
2. Aronberg DJ, Glazer HS, Madsen K, Sagel SS. Normal thoracic aortic diameters by computed tomography. J Comput Assist Tomogr 1984; 8: 247–50.
3. Fitzgerald AW, Donaldson JS, Poznanski AK. Paediatric thoracic aorta: normal measurements determined with CT. Radiology 1987; 165: 667–9.
4. Baum U, Anders K, Ropers D et al. Multi-slice spiral CT imaging after surgical treatment of aortic coarctation. Eur Radiol 2005; 15: 353–5.
5. Macdonald S, Thomas SM, Cleveland TJ, Gaines PA. Angioplasty or stenting in adult coarctation of the aorta? A retrospective single center analysis over a decade. Cardiovasc Intervent Radiol 2003; 26: 357–64.
6. Lippert JA, White CS, Mason AC, Plotnick GD. Calcification of aortic valve detected incidentally on CT scans. Am J Roentgenol 1995; 164: 73–7.
7. Nistri S, Sorbo MD, Main M et al. Aortic dilatation in young men with normally functioning biscuspid aortic valves. Heart 1999; 82: 19–22.
8. Sebastia C, Quiroga S, Boye R et al. Aortic stenosis: spectrum of diseases depicted at multisection CT. Radiographics 2003; 23: S79–S91.
9. Johnston KW, Rutherford RB, Tilson MD et al. Suggested standards for reporting on arterial aneurysms. Subcommittee on Reporting Standards for Arterial Aneurysms, Ad Hoc Committee on Reporting Standards, Society for Vascular Surgery and North American Chapter, International Society for Cardiovascular Surgery. J Vasc Surg 1991; 13: 452–8.
10. Summers KM, West JA, Peterson MM et al. Challenges in the diagnosis of Marfan syndrome. Med J Aust 2006; 184: 627–31.
11. Posniak HV, Olson MC, Demos TC, Benjoya RA, Marsan RE. CT of thoracic aortic aneurysms. Radiographics 1990; 10: 839–55.
12. Mao JR, Bristow J. The Ehlers-Danlos syndrome: on beyond collagens. J Clin Invest 2001; 107: 1063–9.
13. Alkadhi H, Wildermuth S, Desbiolles L et al. Vascular emergencies of the thorax after blunt and iatrogenic trauma: multi-detector row CT and three-dimensional imaging. Radiographics 2004; 24: 1239–55.
14. Dambrin C, Marcheix B, Birsan T, Delisle MB. Survival after spontaneous aortic rupture in a patient with

Ehlers-Danlos syndrome. Eur J Cardiothorac Surg 2005; 28: 650–2.

15. Jost CJ, Gloviczki P, Edwards WD et al. Aortic aneurysms in children and young adults with tuberous sclerosis: report of two cases and review of the literature. J Vasc Surg 2001; 33: 639–42.

16. Van den Berg J, Bannink EM, Wielopolski PA et al. Aortic distensibility and dimensions and the effects of growth hormone treatment in the Turner syndrome. Am J Cardiol 2006; 97: 1644–49.

17. Ledbetter S, Stuk JL, Kaufman JA. Helical CT in the evaluation of emergent thoracic aortic syndromes. Radiol Clin N Am 1999; 37: 575–89.

18. Gotway MB, Dawn SK. Thoracic aorta imaging with multislice CT. Radiol Clin N Am 2003: 41; 521–43.

19. Groskin SA. Selected topics in chest trauma. Radiology 1992; 183: 605–17.

20. Takahashi K, Stanford W. Multidetector CT of the thoracic aorta. Int J Cardiovasc Imaging 2005; 21: 141–53.

21. Parker MS, Matheson TL, Rao AV et al. Making the transition: the role of helical CT in the evaluation of potentially acute thoracic aortic injuries. Am J Roentgenol 2001; 176: 1267–72.

22. Rubin GD. CT angiography of the thoracic aorta. Sem Roentgenol 2003; 38: 115–34.

23. Rubin GD. MDCT imaging of the aorta and peripheral vessels. Eur J Radiol 2003: 45; S42–S49.

24. Gavant ML, Flick P, Menke P, Gold RE. CT aortography of thoracic aortic rupture. AJR 1996: 166; 955–61.

25. Gavant ML, Menke P, Fabian T et al. Blunt traumatic aortic rupture: detection with helical CT of the chest. Radiology 1995: 197; 125–33.

26. Agee CK, Metzler MH, Churchill RJ et al. Computed tomographic evaluation to exclude traumatic aortic disruption. J Trauma 1992: 33; 876–81.

27. Fisher RG, Chasen MG, Lamki N, Diagnosis of injuries of the aorta and brachiocephalic arteries caused by blunt chest trauma: CT vs aortography. AJR 1994: 162; 1047–52.

28. Madayag MA, Kirshenbaum KJ, Nadimpalli SR et al. Thoracic aortic trauma: Role of dynamic CT. Radiology 1991: 179; 853–55.

29. Tatli S, Yucel EK, Lipton MJ. CT and MR imaging of the thoracic aorta: current techniques and clinical applications. Radio Clin N Am 2004: 42; 565–85.

30. Matsunaga N, Hayashi K, Sakamoto I, Ogawa Y, Matsumoto T. Takayasu arteritis: proten radiology manifestations and diagnosis. Radiographics 1997; 17: 579–94.

31. Yamada I, Shibuya H, Matsubara O et al. Pulmonary artery disease in Takayasu's arteritis: angiographic findings. Am J Roentgenol 1992; 159: 263–9.

32. James DG. Behçet's syndrome. N Engl J Med 1979; 301: 431–2.

33. Tunaci A, Berkmen YM, Gokman E. Thoracic involvement in Behçet disease: pathologic, clinical and imaging features. Am J Roentgenol 1995; 164: 51–6.

34. Chajek T, Fainaru M. Behçet disease. Report of 41 cases and a review of the literature. Medicine 1975; 54: 179–96.

35. Munakata M, Hirotani T, Nakamichi T, Takeuchi S. Mycotic aneurysm of the descending aorta with hemoptysis. Ann Thorac Cardiovasc Surg 2004; 10: 314–16.

36. He R, Guo DC, Estrera AL et al. J Thorac Cardiovasc Surg 2006; 131: 671–8.

37. Piffaretti G, Tozzi M, Lomazzi C et al. Complications after endovascular stent-grafting of thoracic aortic diseases. J Cardiothor Surg 2006; 12 (in press).

38. Fattori R, Nienaber CA, Rousseau H et al. Results of endovascular repair of the thoracic aorta with the Talent Thoracic stent graft: the Talent Thoracic retrospective registry. J Thorac Cardiovasc Surg 2006; 132: 332–9.

39. Kaya A, Heijmen RH, Overtoom TT et al. Thoracic stent grafting for acute aortic pathology. Ann Thorac Surg 2006; 82: 565–6.

40. Sawhney NS, DeMaria AN, Blanchard DG. Aortic intramural hematoma. Chest 2001: 120: 1340–6.

41. Nienaber CA, von Kodolitsch Y, Peterson B et al. Intramural hematoma of the thoracic aorta: diagnostic and theurapuetic implications. Circulation 1995; 92: 1465–72.

42. von Kodolitsch Y, Csosz SK, Koschyk DH et al. Intramural hematoma of the aorta: predictors of progression to dissection and rupture. Circulation 2003; 107: 1158–63.

43. Castañer E, Andreu M, Gallardo X, Mata JM, Cabezuelo MA, Pallardo Y. CT in nontraumatic acute thoracic aortic disease: Typical and atypical features and complications. Radiographics 2003: 23; S93–S110.

44. Kazerooni E, Bree RL, Williams DM. Penetrating atherosclerotic ulcers of the descending aorta: evaluation with CT and distinction from aortic dissection. Radiology 1992; 183: 759–65.

45. Sueyoshi E, Matsuoka Y, Sakamoto I et al. Fate of intramural hematoma of the aorta: CT evaluation. J Comput Assist Tomogr 1997; 21: 931–8.

46. Kaji S, Akasaka T, Horibata Y et al. Long-term prognosis of patients with type A aortic intramural hematoma. Circulation 2002; 106 (Suppl 1): 1248–52.

47. Kaji S, Nishigami K, Akasaka T et al. Prediction of progressino or regression of type A intramural hematoma by computed tomography. Circulation 1999; 100 (Suppl 2): 281–6.

48. Tittle SL, Lynch RJ, Cole PE et al. Midterm follow-up of penetrating ulcer and intramural hematoma of the aorta. J Thorac Cardiovasc Surg 2002; 123: 1051–9.

49. Quint LE, Williams DM, Francis IR et al. Ulcerlike lesions of the aorta: imaging features and natural history. Radiology 2001; 218: 719–23.

25

Computed Tomography for Pulmonary Embolism

Philip A. Araoz

1 HISTORY

In the late 80s and early 90s two scanners became available which were fast enough to allow reliable contrast opacification of the great vessels. One was the electron beam CT (EBCT) scanner, which was expensive and not widely available. The other was the single detector helical scanner. As a result, in 1992, a European group published a prospective study in which single detector helical CT was compared to pulmonary angiography as a reference standard for the detection of pulmonary embolism (PE) in 42 patients.[1] Shortly thereafter several groups began publishing small prospective trials using single detector CT or EBCT.

While these early studies were promising, they showed variable sensitivities for detection of PE, often in the low 70s. In particular, single detector helical scanners were inconsistent in detecting subsegmental pulmonary emboli. Thus, by the mid to late 1990s there was debate in the literature as to whether CT (meaning single detector helical CT) could be used as a first line study for detection of pulmonary embolism.

Two things changed this perception. First, several groups wrote papers in which patients with a CT negative for PE were followed clinically (discussed further in the next section). Second, scanner technology improved rapidly. About 1998 the four-detector helical scanner was introduced. Then the eight detector scanner in 2000, 16 detector scanners in 2002, 64 detector scanners in 2004, and as of this writing in 2006 venders are introducing dual source and 256 detector scanners. Studies using catheterization as a gold standard could not be performed fast enough, and in any

case practicing clinicians had already widely accepted four-detector CT for PE strongly enough that most institutions now consider it unethical to perform catheter pulmonary angiography on a patient with a negative CT.[2] Thus for PE, as with aortic dissection, review papers will occasionally cite papers from the early/mid 1990s and call into question the sensitivity of CT for detection of PE,[3] because studies using catheter angiography as a reference standard have not been performed on modern scanners and never will. The studies of CT for PE which examined consecutive patients and used pulmonary angiography as a reference standard are summarized in Table 25.1.[1,4–12]

2 DIAGNOSTIC ACCURACY OF CT FOR PULMONARY EMBOLISM

If multi-detector CT (MDCT) scans can no longer be compared to catheter pulmonary angiography, how can we judge the accuracy of MDCT?

2.1 MDCT vs catheter pulmonary angiography

We can judge the accuracy of multidetector CT based on the two studies in which multidetector CT was compared to catheter angiography. Qanadli performed 2 detector CT with 5 mm collimation on 157 patients who underwent

Table 25.1   Prospective studies of CT for pulmonary embolism using catheter pulmonary angiography as a reference standard

Author	Year	N	Scanner	Slice thickness (mm)	Smallest vessel	Sens	Spec	PPV	NPV
Remy-Jardin	1992	42	Single detector helical	5	Segment	100	96	95	100
Blum	1994	10	Single detector helical	5	Segment	100	100	100	100
Teigen	1995	60	EBCT	3	Segment	65	97	94	82
Goodman	1995	20	Single detector helical	5	Subsegmental	64	89	88	67
Remy-Jardin	1996	75	Single detector helical	5	Segmental	91	78	85	86
Christiansen	1997	70	Single detector helical	3 or 5	Segmental	89	96	89	96
Drucker	1998	47	Single detector helical	NR	Segmental	53	97	89	82
Qanadli	2000	157	2 detector helical	2.5	Subsegmental	90	94	90	94
Velmahos	2001	22	Single detector helical	3	Subsegmental	45	82	71	60
Ruiz*	2003	66	Single detector helical	3	Subsegmental	91/88	82/86	75/82	94/91
Winer-Muram	2004	93	4 detector helical	3.2	Subsegmental	100	89	69	90

N – number of patients.
Sens – sensitivity.
Spec – specificity.
PPV – positive predictive value.
NPV – negative predictive value.
* The study by Ruiz had two observers and the numbers in each cell are for observer 1 and 2.

catheter pulmonary angiography.[10] They studied vessels to the subsegmental level (i.e. fifth order arteries) and found a sensitivity of 90% and a specificity of 94%. Winer-Muran performed 4 detector CT with 3.2 mm collimation in 93 patients who underwent catheter pulmonary angiography. They also studied vessels to the subsegmental level and found a sensitivity of 100% and specificity of 89%.[13] These results are promising, especially the high sensitivity.

2.2 MDCT vs a combined reference standard

We can also judge the accuracy of multidetector CT from management studies which did not use catheter angiography as a gold standard. The largest such study was the recent Propsective Investigation of Pulmonary Embolism Diagnosis II (PIOPED II) trial. In this study 824 patients had multidetector CT prospectively compared to a composite reference standard in which a patient was considered to have PE if they had one of the following: a high probability ventilation-perfusion scan, a positive catheter pulmonary angiogram, deep venous thrombosis (DVT) detected at lower extremity venous ultrasound.[2] They found that multidetector CT still had a fair sensitivity (83%) and a very good specificity (96%). While the 83% sensitivity was disappointing, the study had limitations. Most of the patients (84% of them)

were scanned on 4 detector scanners, which as of this writing are at least 3 generations from being state of the art. The use of a composite reference, especially DVT, can be criticized as there is no certainty that patients with DVT necessarily have PE.

2.3 Clinical outcome of patients with CT negative for PE

However, if the concern about CT, even multidetector CT, is suboptimal sensitivity (i.e. possible false negative results) then the strongest line of evidence in favor of using it as a first line test is the large body of literature regarding the outcomes of patients with negative CT for PE. Quiroz recently published a review of studies in which patients with a single detector helical CT was negative for PE were followed clinically.[14] Articles from their review are summarized in Table 25.2.[15–27] Using subsequent PE or DVT as the reference standard, they found negative likelihood ratio (false negative divided by true negative rate) of single detector helical CT was 0.07, and the negative predictive value was 99.1%. In a separate meta-analysis Moore estimated that the 3 month rate of subsequent thromboembolism in patients with a CT negative for PE who did not receive thromboembolism was 1.4% and the rate of fatal PE was 0.51%.[28] These rates of subsequent thrombembolic

Table 25.2 Number of false negative CTs for PE using clinical outcome as the reference standard

Author	Year	N	Subsequent PE	Subsequent DVT
Donato	2003	300	1	0
Feretti	1997	125	1	4
Garg	1999	82	0	0
Goodman	2000	285	0	0
Gottsater	2001	244	0	5
Kavanagh	2004	85	0	0
Krestan	2004	325	2	8
Lombard	2003	41	0	0
Lomis	1999	121	0	3
Nilsson	2002	449	0	3
Ost	2001	81	0	0
Remy-Jardin	2002	208	0	10
Swensen	2002	1010	0	11

N – number of patients treated with anticoagulation followed for clinical events.
PE – pulmonary embolism.
DVT – Deep venous thrombosis.
Table is modified from Table 1 from Quiroz.

events are comparable to that of the general population, indicating that if small PEs are going undetected by single detector CT, they do not appear to be clinically significant. It is unknown whether even lower rates of subsequent events could be achieved with current generation multidetector CT scanners.

3 TECHNIQUE

The most important factors for a successful CT for PE are minimal motion and good contrast opacification of the pulmonary arteries.

3.1 Motion

Minimizing motion is the single most important part of the CT scan. In a retrospective review of 237 technically inadequate CTs for PE, Jones found motion to be the most common reason for an inadequate examination (74%).[29] For an adequate study, patients must hold their breath for the duration of the scan, which may be difficult in the population referred for suspicion of PE. On a single detector scanner, scanning in a single breath-hold typically requires limiting the anatomic coverage, usually from the aortic arch to the diaphragm. Scanners with four detectors or greater can usually cover the entire chest in a single breath-hold.

3.2 Contrast

The second most important part of the CT scan is to maximize contrast opacification of the pulmonary arteries. In the same study of inadequate CTs for PE, Jones found poor contrast bolus to be the second most common cause of inadequate examinations (40%).[29]

Achieving good contrast in the pulmonary arteries starts with injection of a tight bolus of contrast. At our institution we inject at a *rate* of 4 mL/sec with a power injector, preferably through an 18 g or larger antecubital IV.

The *volume* should be sufficient for continuous injection before scanning (until the peak bolus arrives in the pulmonary artery), and then throughout the scan. The delay from start of injection to arrival of the bolus varies from patient to patient, but is typically 10–15 seconds. Duration of the scan varies greatly between generations of CT scanners, from 20–30 seconds for single detector scanners to less than 8 seconds for dual-source or 256 detector scanners.

Thus for a 256 detector CT scanner, a PE study could, in theory, be performed with as little as 5.75 mL of contrast. (15 second delay + 8 second scan = 23 seconds of contrast injection required. Twenty-three seconds of contrast injection divided by 4 mL/sec injection rate equals 5.75 mL of contrast required). However, in general using such low volumes leaves little room for error and provides little opacification to the aorta and other structures of interest.

At our institution PE studies are typically performed (as of this writing) on 16 and 64 detector scanners. Regardless of scanner type we use 120 mL of contrast, which provides a much longer bolus than needed. To take advantage of this long bolus, we frequently trigger our bolus off of the ascending aorta, so that the pulmonary arteries, heart, and aorta are all well opacified.

Once the injection rate, the IV, and the contrast dose have been selected, the next step is *identifying the peak* bolus in the pulmonary artery. This is typically done with either bolus timing or bolus tracking software. With bolus timing, a region-of-interest (ROI) is placed over the main pulmonary artery and a bolus of contrast (typically about 20 mL) is then injected. The time to peak opacification is recorded and this delay is used to determine when to start scanning. With bolus triggering, an ROI is placed over the pulmonary artery and the full contrast dose is injected. When a pre-set density is detected within the ROI, scanning is automatically triggered. The goal is to achieve a scan for which the pulmonary arteries have opacification of at least 200 HU. At our institution the preset density for triggering the scan is 150 HU, with the idea being that in the second or two it takes for scanning to begin, and the duration of the scan itself, the contrast in the pulmonary artery will increase to the minimum 200 HU needed. This works well on 16 detector scanners or slower, but on 64 detector scanners or faster, better results may be achieved by raising the bolus triggering threshold from 150 HU to 200 HU, though this has not been studied.

3.3 Other parameters

The technique used at our institution for 16 and 64 detector scanners are summarized in Table 25.3. The most important variable listed is collimation (slice thickness). A review of Table 25.1 shows that in most studies of CT for PE, slice thickness was usually 3 mm or 5 mm. With 16 and 64 detector scanners, slice thicknesses of 1–1.5 mm are possible while

maintaining acceptable levels of noise. A few studies have been performed in which the subjective visualization of subsegmental arteries with thinner collimation (down to 1.25 mm slice thickness) was compared to thicker (usually 3 mm) collimation, and they have found that thinner collimation leads to better visualization of subsegmental pulmonary arterial branches.[30-33] Direct comparison of thicker (3–5 mm) and thinner (1–2 mm) collimation CT for detection of PE has not been performed. On a practical note, in obese patients, collimation of 1.5 mm or less can lead to enough noise as to degrade visualization of small (segmental and smaller) vessels, in which case reconstruction at 2.5 mm or 3 mm is often helpful.

4 ACUTE PE – INTERPRETATION

4.1 Non-PE/incidental findings

When reviewing a CT for PE, like any CT, the entire scan must be evaluated. In 11–70% of cases a cause other than PE will be identified as the source of symptoms.[34] Unsuspected, asymptomatic disease will also be detected. In a retrospective study of 1106 CT PE studies, Kino found unsuspected lung cancers in 5 patients.[35] In a small study of 163 patients, Hasegawa found 16 patients with tracheomalacia detected at CT.[36]

Likewise, when reviewing CTs done for non-vascular purposes, the scan should be reviewed for PE. Retrospective studies of CTs done for indications other than PE have shown PEs incidentally detected in 4% of all in-patients,[37] 2.6% to 4% of all oncology patients[38–39] and an impressive 24% of trauma patients with moderately to severe injuries.[40] Image review of non-contrast CTs should also include inspection of the pulmonary arteries because there have been case reports of PEs detected on non-contrast CTs.[41]

Table 25.3 Sample PE protocols for 16 and 64 detector CT scanners

Scanner	16 detector	64 detector
Rotation time (sec)	0.5	0.5
Detector configuration	16×1.5	24×1.2
Pitch	1.0	0.5
Feed (mm/rot)	24	14
kVp	120	120
Slice thickness (mm)	1.0–1.5	1.0–1.5
Recon increment	1.0–1.5	1.0–1.5
FOV (mm)	300	200

4.2 Image display/review

Though review of hard copy images is becoming increasingly rare, it bares stating that images should be reviewed by paging through images on a workstation and not reviewing hard copy images. Workstation paging has been shown to improve detection of PE[42] and minimizes interpretive errors that occur from not continuously following the pulmonary arteries (such as mistaking a pulmonary vein for a pulmonary artery or mistaking a lymph node for a PE).

Optimal window setting has not been established, but the traditional mediastinal window setting (width 400, level 30) may be too narrow and low considering that optimal opacification of the pulmonary arteries is greater than 200 and typically will be greater than 300. Bae has suggested a window level of about half the mean pulmonary artery attenuation (150–200) and a wide width (700).[43]

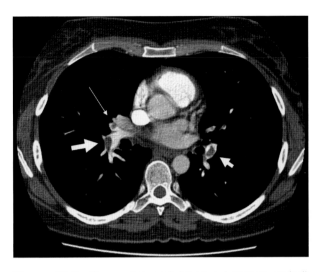

Figure 25.2 Segmental and lobar pulmonary emboli. 4 detector CT in a 42-year-old woman shows emboli in the right middle lobe segmental pulmonary artery (thin arrow), and in the right lower lobe (longer thick arrow) and left lower lobe (shorter thick arrow) lobar pulmonary arteries.

4.3 CT findings of acute PE

Studies of MDCT for PE have most often used the presence of a low attenuation filling defect as the criteria for a PE.[12,13] Qanadli also used complete occlusion by a thrombus in a normal or enlarged vessel.[10] Several articles have also required that the clot be seen on 2 contiguous slices,[44,45] which is our clinical practice and anecdotally appears to reduce false positive findings. Examples of positive CT scans are shown in Figures 25.1–25.3. Indirect findings for acute PE have been reported and include a wedge shaped consolidation in the periphery (a pulmonary infarct) or oligemia of an affected segment but these findings without direct visualization of PE are not enough to interpret a scan as positive for PE.

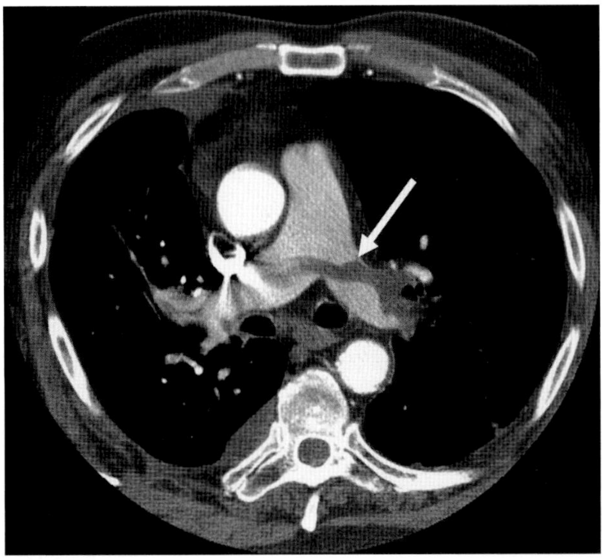

4.4 False positive findings

Early studies performed on single detector scanners with 5 mm collimation and interpreted on hard copies have reported a variety of false positive findings that should not be confused with PE on modern, multi-detector scanners. For example, in 1992 Remy-Jardin reported hilar lymph nodes as their most frequent source of false positive CT for PE.[1]

With only two studies available comparing MDCT to pulmonary angiography, it is difficult to make definitive statements about the sources for false positive findings for PE in the modern era. In a study of 93 patients scanned on a 4-detector scanner, Winer-Muram found 8 false positives, mostly segmental and subsegmental levels, which appear to have been caused by poor contrast opacification at CT (Figure 25.4).[13] Winer-Muram did not specify whether a filling defect had to appear on two consecutive images. If not, this could have contributed to their false positive rate. In a study of 147 patients and using a very early 2-detector scanner Qanadli found three false positives, also apparently due to poor contrast opacification in small vessels.

Figure 25.1 Saddle pulmonary embolism. 4 detector CT in a 68-year-old man shows a large PE (arrow) saddling the bifurcation of the main pulmonary artery.

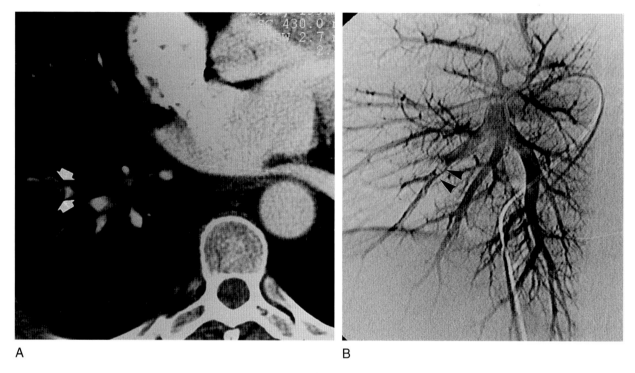

A   B

Figure 25.3 Subsegmental pulmonary emboli confirmed with catheter angiography. (a) Subsegmental pulmonary emboli are shown on 2-detector helical CT (arrowheads) in a 54-year-old woman. (b) Selective left anterior oblique catheter angiogram in the right-lower-lobe artery shows subsegmental clots (arrowheads). Taken from Figure 2 of Qanadli.

4.5 False negative findings

In the two studies comparing MDCT to cath, only one false negative CT was reported.[10,13] That example (reported by Qanadli)[10] a single subsegmental embolus was missed at CT (Figure 25.5). In a technically adequate study, the most likely sources of false negative scans are likely to be from isolated subsegmental PEs. However, experience with single detector helical CT, summarized in Table 25.2, suggests that these patients have no increased likelihood of future thromboembolic events and that lack of detection of these small emboli are likely not clinically significant.

4.6 Suboptimal/uninterpretable examinations

As mentioned in the discussion on technique, motion and poor contrast opacification are the main causes of inadequate examinations. At our institution, the interpreting physician checks CTs for PE before the patient leaves the department, usually while the patient is still on the scanning table. This check is for image quality and also to detect PEs and refer the patient (especially an outpatient) for immediate treatment. For suboptimal examinations due to motion

or contrast we will typically re-inject the patient with contrast and repeat the examination.

There are also causes of suboptimal findings inherent to the patient. The most common one (especially in inpatients) is atelectasis or consolidation, typically in the lower lobes which causes crowding of the peripheral pulmonary arteries. In our institution we attempt to follow the vessels into the consolidation, which is possible with thin collimation of modern scanners. Likewise it may be difficult to follow the small pulmonary arteries in patients with emphysema or otherwise distorted lung architecture, but it is generally possible.

4.7 Rare mimic – pulmonary artery sarcoma

Very rarely a neoplasm, typically a primary pulmonary artery sarcoma, may mimic a pulmonary embolism. In these cases patients may report gradual onset and long duration of symptoms (perhaps months) and may have symptoms more often associated with malignancy than with PE (such as weight loss), though shortness of breath and chest pain are still the most common presenting symptoms.[46] At CT pulmonary artery sarcomas are usually large, often occluding the left or right main pulmonary artery (Figure 25.6).

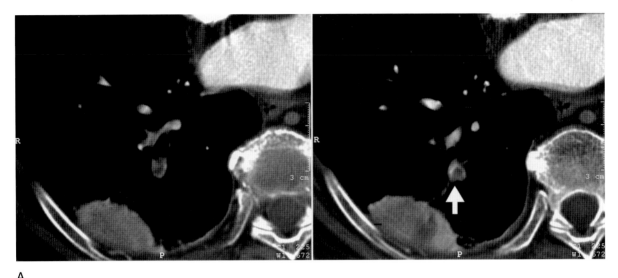

A

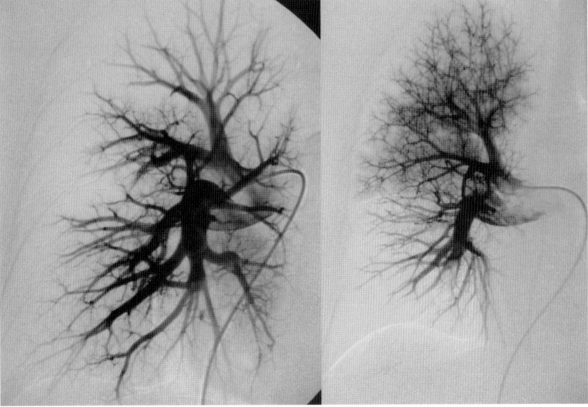

B

Figure 25.4 False positive CT for PE. (a) Four detector CT images from a 76-year-old woman shows a right lower lobe segmental and subsegmental filling defect (arrow) (b) Catheter pulmonary angiogram oblique (left image) and posteroanterior (right image) are normal. Taken from Figure 2 of Winer-Muram.

Enhancement or extension outside the vessel lumen, if seen, can be used to suggest a malignancy.[47] If not, lack of resolution (or growth) on follow up are suggestive. Magnetic resonance imaging,[48] or positron emission tomography[49] may be used to characterize a mass in questionable cases.

5 CHRONIC PE

It is important to distinguish acute PE, which is treated with anticoagulation, from chronic PE, which is not. It is not known how many patients with acute PE go on to develop

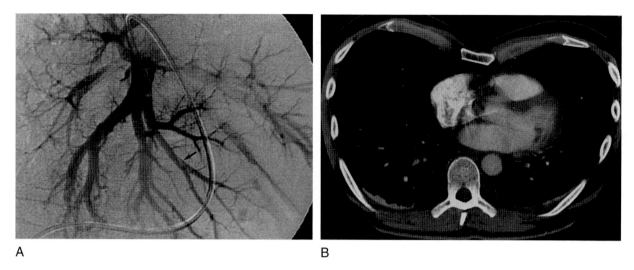

A   B

Figure 25.5   False negative CT for PE. (a) Selective right anterior oblique arteriogram in the left lower lobe artery performed in a 52-year-old man shows a pulmonary embolism (arrow) in the medial subsegmental branch of the anterior basal pulmonary artery. (b) 4 detector CT finding has suboptimal contrast, but was considered negative. Taken from Figure 3 of Qanadli.

chronic PE, though a prospective study of 314 patients with acute PE found that 1% went on to develop chronic pulmonary hypertension.[50] It is also not known how long PE must be present to develop imaging features associated with chronic PE, though one review paper has suggested that

more than 50% of patients with acute PE still have acute-appearing PE visible after 6 months.[51]

Most of what is known about chronic PE is from patients who present late in the disease with signs and symptoms related to pulmonary hypertension.[52] Pathologic and

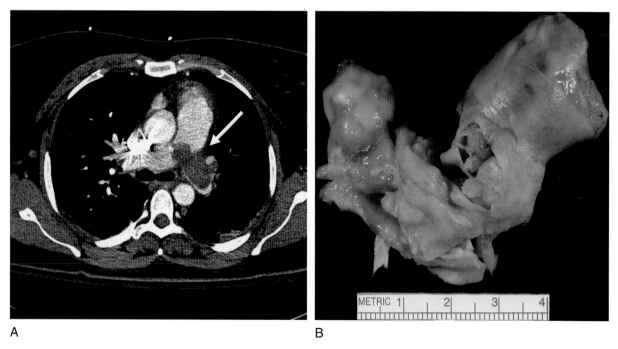

A   B

Figure 25.6   Primary pulmonary artery sarcoma. (a) 16 detector CT performed in a 40-year-old woman with 3 month history of progressive dyspnea on exertion shows a lobulated filling defect in the left pulmonary artery (arrow). The filling defect did not decrease in size with intrapulmonary arterial thrombolytic therapy, which raised the suspicion for a pulmonary artery sarcoma. The patient went to surgery for resection of the mass which was shown to be a high grade spindle cell primary pulmonary artery sarcoma. (b) Gross photograph of the tumor.

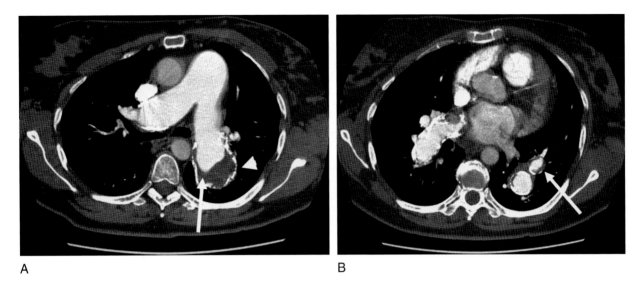

A   B

Figure 25.7 Chronic pulmonary emboli – laminar thrombus. 8 detector CT taken in a 54-year-old female at (a) the level of the pulmonary artery bifurcation and (b) a more inferior level shows chronic pulmonary emboli with laminar clot adherent to the walls of the pulmonary artery (arrows). The arterial walls are also calcified (arrowhead).

imaging studies in patients with this type of advanced disease show that chronic emboli persist through varying degrees of adhering to the walls and recanalization, which leads to several appearances. Chronic emboli that maintain a large attachment to the wall appear as long, laminar structures along the wall of a pulmonary artery and may have calcification (Figure 25.6).[53] Chronic emboli that recanalize centrally may appear as webs or bands (Figure 25.8). These are findings that have well established correlation at catheter angiography.[54]

Patients with chronic PE will often have mosaic perfusion in the lungs, findings seen more often with vascular causes than other causes of pulmonary hypertension (Figure 25.9).[55] Mosaic perfusion by itself, without visible

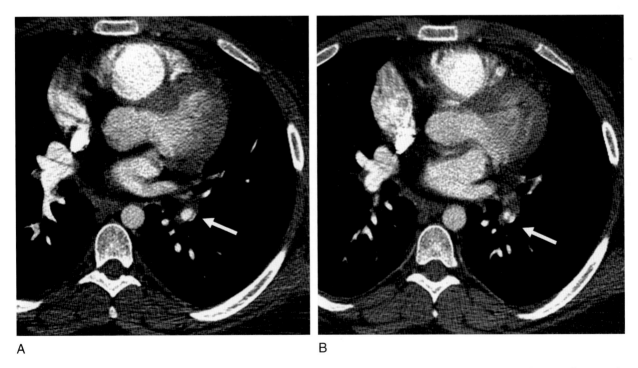

A   B

Figure 25.8 Chronic pulmonary emboli – webs and bands. 16 detector CT taken in a 26-year-old female. Consecutive images (a) and (b) show a discrete web in the left lower lobe pulmonary artery (arrows).

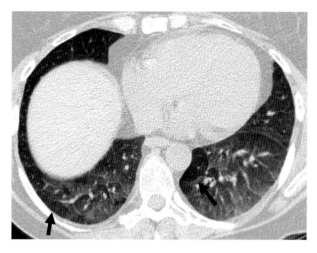

Figure 25.9 Mosaic perfusion. Expiratory, high resolution 8 detector CT in a 54-year-old female. In the lungs there are sharply demarcated areas of low attenuation (mosaic perfusion) indicating small vessel disease.

emboli, should raise the possibility of small vessel disease, including small chronic PE.

6 PROGNOSIS

In hemodynamically stable patients, acute PE is treated with anticoagulation, but in patients with cardiogenic shock, more aggressive treatment with thrombolytics has been shown to decrease mortality.[56] There has therefore been interest in identifying which (if any) patients not in florid cardiogenic shock might also benefit from thrombolytics, that is hemodynamically stable patients with some other finding that labels them high risk.

6.1 Echocardiography

Since the mid to late 1990s there has been interest in using echocardiographically-detected right heart dysfunction as a prognostic factor in acute PE. The studies examining an association between echocardiography right heart variables and mortality in acute PE are listed in Table 25.4. The evidence is compelling for an association. Six of the ten studies were prospective, and seven of the ten show a significant association of right heart strain with death (either all-cause or PE-specific).

However, there are limitations. The studies suffer from variable inclusion criteria. Five of the ten included patients without direct evidence for PE,[57–61] including patients with clinical suspicion only. In one of the ten, no inclusion criteria

were given at all.[62] Only two of the studies were performed on the population of interest (i.e. hemodynamically stable patients).[62,63] In the remaining studies, no multivariable analysis was performed to show if echocardiographic findings add to prognostic information above clinical variables. Also, none of the studies address whether thrombolytics improve prognosis in the patients with echocardiographic right heart strain.

6.2 CT

In spite of the limitations of the echocardiographic studies, their positive findings have sparked interest in finding CT variables with prognostic information in acute PE (Table 25.5). The CT literature has the advantage that all patients have direct confirmation of their PEs (by CT of course) and therefore have more uniform patient populations. These studies also have the advantage of being able to directly evaluate the prognostic impact of the clot burden as well as right heart function. The disadvantage is that most of the studies are retrospective and, to date, none have used ECG gating to allow for direct visualization of wall motion, making the right heart evaluation limited compared to echocardiography.

The results of the CT studies are mixed, particularly regarding the prognostic impact of clot burden. Of the ten studies listed in Table 25.5, only three show an association between clot burden and death.[64–66] These studies were small, each with 120 patients or fewer. The largest study of 1,092 patients showed that for one of their two observers, increased clot burden had a small but significant *decreased* risk of death.[67] The authors explained this by noting that autopsy studies show that most patients who die from PE die within an hour of onset of symptoms[68–72] and suggested that patients with large PE who survive long enough to undergo imaging may be healthier than average. Thus there are definitely conflicting data about whether clot burden is predictive of death in PE.

On the other hand, of the seven studies that examined signs of right heart strain all but one showed some association between right heart findings and mortality. ECG gating was not used in any of these studies. Some authors have suggested gating the CT to allow for wall motion analysis and right and left ventricle ejection fraction measurement to allow for additional prognostic information.[73]

In sum, early studies with echocardiography and CT suggest that signs of right heart strain are associated with mortality in PE; however, to date there has been limited evidence that these findings add prognostic information

Table 25.4 Studies of echocardiography predicting mortality in acute PE

Author	Year	Design	N	Method of PE diagnosis	Patient selection	Criteria for RV strain	Overall mortality	PE mortality	Follow up	P*
Goldhaber	1993	RCT	101	VQ, PA gram	Consecutive	RV hypokinesis	2%	2%	In-hospital	NS
Ribiero	1997	PC	126	VQ, PA gram	Consecutive	RV hypokinesis	8%	NR	In-hospital	0.002
Kasper	1997	PC	317	PA gram, VQ, echo or clinical suspicion	Consecutive	RV dilatation or tricuspid regurgitation or pulmonary hypertension	9%	4%	In-hospital	0.001
Goldhaber	1999	Registry	1135	VQ, PA gram, or intermediate VQ with DVT	Consecutive	RV hypokinesis	17%**	8%**	3 months	p<0.5 for all-cause mortality
Grifoni	2000	PC	209	VQ, CT, autopsy	Hemodynamically stable	Two of RV dilatation, paradoxical septal motion, or pulmonary hypertension	8%	6%	In-hospital	NS
Jerjes-Sanchez	2001	PC	40	VQ, echo, DVT	Hemodynamically unstable	RV hypokinesis	13%	10%	In-hospital	P<0.001
Kucher	2005	Registry	1035	NR	Hemodynamically stable	RV hypokinesis	12%	NR	30 day	p<0.01
Sukhija	2005	Retro	190	CT	Consecutive	RV dilatation Paradoxical septal motion Pulmonary artery hypertension	33%	NR	In-hospital	P<0.001
Binder	2005	PC	124	VQ, CT, or hypotension and echo	Consecutive	RV dilatation with right atrial hypertension	6%	NR	In-hospital	NS
Scridon	2005	Retro	141	CT, VQ, PA gram, intermediate VQ and DVT, autopsy, echo	Consecutive	RV dilatation with elevated troponin	20%	NR	30 day	p<0.05

RCT – randomized controlled trial.
PC – prospective cohort.
VQ – ventilation perfusion scan.
PAgram – catheter pulmonary angiogram.
DVT – deep venous thrombosis identified on lower extremity ultrasound.
NR – not reported.
NS – not significant.
RV – right ventricle.
Echo – echocardiography.
Retro – Retrospective.
OR – odds ratio.
HR – hazard ratio.
*p is for PE specific mortality if reported, otherwise total mortality.
** The overall and specific mortality cited for Goldhaber's study is for the entire cohort of 2110 patients, not the subset of 1135 who went on to echocardiography.

Table 25.5 Studies of CT predicting mortality in acute PE

Author	Year	N	Design	Scanner	Patient selection	Clot burden†	RV/LV ratio†	Septal bowing†	Overall mortality rate	PE specific mortality	F/U length
Araoz	2003	173	Retro	Single or 4 detector helical	Consecutive	NS	NS	NS	5%	2%	In-hospital
Schoepf	2004	431	Retro	4 detector or 16 detector helical	Consecutive	NR	P = 0.018*	NR	13%	NR	30 days
Wu	2004	59	Retro	4 detector helical	Consecutive	P = 0.002	NR	NR	10%	NR	12 d average
Van de Meer	2005	120	Retro	Single detector helical	Prospective cohort **	P = 0.01	P = 0.04	P = 0.20	15%	6%	3 month
Engelke	2005	89	Retro	4 or 16 detector helical	Consecutive	NS	NR	NR	9%	7%	30 day
Ghuysen	2005	82	Retro	Single detector helical	Consecutive	NS	P = 0.002	NR	15%	NR	In-hospital
Ghaye	2006	82	Retro	Single detector helical	ICU admits	NS	P = 0.011	NR	15%	NR	14 day
Araoz	2007	1092	Retro	EBCT, single, 4, 16 detector helical	Consecutive	NS***	NS	NS/0.05****	9%	5%	In-hospital or 30 day
Ghuysen	2006	82	Retro	Single detector helical	ED patients	NS	P = 0.002	NR	15%	NR	In-hospital
Egelke	2006	96	Retro	4 detector helical	Consecutive	P = 0.043	NR	NR	34%	NR*****	8 9 months mean

NS – not significant.
NR – not reported.
Retro – retrospective.
EBCT – electron beam CT.
ICU – intensive care unit.
F/U – follow up.
ED – emergency department.
* Shcoepf found an association between RV/LV ration and death for CT scans reconstructed in the four-chamber view only, not axial images.
**Van de Meer used prospective cohort of 510 from Advances in New Technologies Evaluating the Localization of PE (ANTELOPE) study.
***Araoz 2006 found that for one of their observers, increased clot burden was associated with a very small but significant decreased risk of PE related death.
****Araoz 2006 had two observers. Septal bowing was associated with death for one observer but not the other.
*****Engleke 2006 did not report the PE specific mortality for the full follow-up, but the 14 day PE related mortality was 3%.
†P values are for association with either overall mortality or PE specific mortality, which ever was reported by the study. For Araoz 2003, NS refers to both overall and PE specific mortality. For Engelke, NS refers to overall mortality. Araoz 2007 studied PE specific mortality.

above clinical variables and no information that treating patients with right heart strain decreases mortality.

7 COMBINING PE WITH AORTA AND CORONARIES

There has been interest in combing CT for PE with CT for aortic dissection and CT for the coronaries into one chest pain examination. Preliminary studies investigating this have shown that such an examination is feasible.[74] The attraction of this type of examination is the potential for very rapid triage in an emergency department. The current limitation is the coronary CT, as CT for the coronaries is much less established than CT for PE or for dissection and to date still requires controlled heart rates for optimal examinations. If a combined PE/dissection/coronary CT were to become widely available, the optimal patient population and the cost effectiveness of such an examination would have to be carefully studied. The introduction of CT for PE alone has resulted in a increase in CT use in the ER and an overall decrease in the rate of positive findings.[75] A general CT for chest pain could potentially be cost saving by shortening emergency department stays, but could lead to an explosion of CT use in lower risk populations than are currently being studied. This raises the possibility of increased costs including the costs of workup of false positive and incidental findings.

8 SUMMARY

CT is a well established technique for diagnosis of pulmonary embolism. CT technology has advanced so rapidly and been so widely accepted that it is no longer possible to perform studies comparing CT to pulmonary angiography as a gold standard. Based on studies using single detector helical scanners there have been some lingering concerns that CT lacks sensitivity for small emboli; however, studies showing good outcome in patients with CT negative for PE suggest that any emboli missed are not clinically significant. Physicians interpreting CT for PE should be aware of the high rate of non-PE related findings, sources of false positive and false negative findings, and should be familiar with the findings of chronic pulmonary emboli. Studies using echocardiography and CT suggest that right heart strain may impart a worse prognosis in PE, but to date specific treatment recommendations cannot be made on imaging alone. In the future, CT for PE, for aortic dissection, and for coronary artery disease may be combined into a single examination.

REFERENCES

1. Remy-Jardin, M et al., Central pulmonary thromboembolism: diagnosis with spiral volumetric CT with the single-breath-hold technique – comparison with pulmonary angiography. Radiology 1992; 185(2): 381–7.
2. Stein, PD et al. Multidetector computed tomography for acute pulmonary embolism. N Engl J Med 2006; 354(22): 2317–27.
3. Rahimtoola, A and Bergin, JD Acute pulmonary embolism: an update on diagnosis and management. Curr Probl Cardiol 2005; 30(2): 61–114.
4. Blum, AG et al. Spiral-computed tomography versus pulmonary angiography in the diagnosis of acute massive pulmonary embolism. Am J Cardiol 1994; 74(1): 96–8.
5. Teigen, CL et al. Pulmonary embolism: diagnosis with contrast-enhanced electron-beam CT and comparison with pulmonary angiography. Radiology 1995; 194(2): 313–19.
6. Goodman, LR et al. Detection of pulmonary embolism in patients with unresolved clinical and scintigraphic diagnosis: helical CT versus angiography. AJR Am J Roentgenol 1995; 164(6): 1369–74.
7. Remy-Jardin, M et al. Diagnosis of pulmonary embolism with spiral CT: comparison with pulmonary angiography and scintigraphy. Radiology 1996; 200(3): 699–706.
8. Christiansen, F. Diagnostic imaging of acute pulmonary embolism. Acta Radiol Suppl 1997; 410: 1–33.
9. Drucker, EA et al. Acute pulmonary embolism: assessment of helical CT for diagnosis. Radiology 1998; 209(1): 235–41.
10. Qanadli, SD et al. Pulmonary embolism detection: prospective evaluation of dual-section helical CT versus selective pulmonary arteriography in 157 patients. Radiology 2000; 217(2): 447–55.
11. Velmahos, GC et al. Spiral computed tomography for the diagnosis of pulmonary embolism in critically ill surgical patients: a comparison with pulmonary angiography. Arch Surg 2001; 136(5): 505–11.
12. Ruiz, Y et al. Prospective comparison of helical CT with angiography in pulmonary embolism: global and selective vascular territory analysis. Interobserver agreement. Eur Radiol 2003; 13(4): 823–9.
13. Winer-Muram, HT et al. Suspected acute pulmonary embolism: evaluation with multi-detector row CT versus digital subtraction pulmonary arteriography. Radiology 2004; 233(3): 806–15.
14. Quiroz, R et al. Clinical validity of a negative computed tomography scan in patients with suspected pulmonary embolism: a systematic review. Jama 2005; 293(16): 2012–17.
15. Donato, AA et al. Clinical outcomes in patients with suspected acute pulmonary embolism and negative helical computed tomographic results in whom anticoagulation was withheld. Arch Intern Med 2003; 163(17): 2033–8.
16. Ferretti, GR et al. Acute pulmonary embolism: role of helical CT in 164 patients with intermediate probability at ventilation-perfusion scintigraphy and normal results at duplex US of the legs. Radiology 1997; 205(2): 453–8.
17. Garg, K et al. Clinical validity of helical CT being interpreted as negative for pulmonary embolism: implications for patient treatment. AJR Am J Roentgenol 1999; 172(6): 1627–31.
18. Goodman, LR et al. Subsequent pulmonary embolism: risk after a negative helical CT pulmonary angiogram – prospective comparison with scintigraphy. Radiology 2000; 215(2): 535–42.

19. Gottsater, A et al. Clinically suspected pulmonary embolism: is it safe to withhold anticoagulation after a negative spiral CT? Eur Radiol 2001; 11(1): p. 65–72.

20. Kavanagh, EC et al. Risk of pulmonary embolism after negative MDCT pulmonary angiography findings. AJR Am J Roentgenol 2004; 182(2): 499–504.

21. Krestan, CR et al. Value of negative spiral CT angiography in patients with suspected acute PE: analysis of PE occurrence and outcome. Eur Radiol 2004; 14(1): 93–8.

22. Lombard, J, Bhatia, R and Sala, E. Spiral computed tomographic pulmonary angiography for investigating suspected pulmonary embolism: clinical outcomes. Can Assoc Radiol J 2003; 54(3): 147–51.

23. Lomis, NN et al. Clinical outcomes of patients after a negative spiral CT pulmonary arteriogram in the evaluation of acute pulmonary embolism. J Vasc Interv Radiol 1999; 10(6): 707–12.

24. Nilsson, T et al. Negative spiral CT in acute pulmonary embolism. Acta Radiol 2002; 43(5): 486–91.

25. Ost, D et al. The negative predictive value of spiral computed tomography for the diagnosis of pulmonary embolism in patients with nondiagnostic ventilation-perfusion scans. Am J Med 2001; 110(1): 16–21.

26. Remy-Jardin, M et al. CT angiography of pulmonary embolism in patients with underlying respiratory disease: impact of multislice CT on image quality and negative predictive value. Eur Radiol 2002; 12(8): 1971–8.

27. Swensen, SJ et al. Outcomes after withholding anticoagulation from patients with suspected acute pulmonary embolism and negative computed tomographic findings: a cohort study. Mayo Clin Proc 2002; 77(2): 130–8.

28. Moores, LK et al. Meta-analysis: outcomes in patients with suspected pulmonary embolism managed with computed tomographic pulmonary angiography. Ann Intern Med 2004; 141(11): p. 866–74.

29. Jones, SE and Wittram, C. The indeterminate CT pulmonary angiogram: imaging characteristics and patient clinical outcome. Radiology 2005; 237(1): 329–37.

30. Patel, S, Kazerooni, EA and Cascade, PN. Pulmonary embolism: optimization of small pulmonary artery visualization at multi-detector row CT. Radiology 2003; 227(2): 455–60.

31. Heuschmid, M et al. Detection of pulmonary embolism using 16-slice multidetector-row computed tomography: evaluation of different image reconstruction parameters. J Comput Assist Tomogr 2006; 30(1): 77–82.

32. Raptopoulos, V et al. Multi-detector row spiral CT pulmonary angiography: comparison with single-detector row spiral CT. Radiology 2001; 221(3): 606–13.

33. Ghaye, B et al. Peripheral pulmonary arteries: how far in the lung does multi-detector row spiral CT allow analysis? Radiology 2001; 219(3): 629–36.

34. Patel, S and Kazerooni, EA. Helical CT for the evaluation of acute pulmonary embolism. AJR Am J Roentgenol 2005; 185(1): 135–49.

35. Kino, A et al. Lung cancer detected in patients presenting to the Emergency Department studies for suspected pulmonary embolism on computed tomography pulmonary angiography. Eur J Radiol 2006; 58(1): 119–23.

36. Hasegawa, I et al., Tracheomalacia incidentally detected on CT pulmonary angiography of patients with suspected pulmonary embolism. AJR Am J Roentgenol 2003; 181(6): 1505–9.

37. Storto, ML et al. Incidental detection of pulmonary emboli on routine MDCT of the chest. AJR Am J Roentgenol 2005; 184(1): 264–7.

38. Sebastian, AJ and Paddon, AJ Clinically unsuspected pulmonary embolism – an important secondary finding in oncology CT. Clin Radiol 2006; 61(1): 81–5.

39. Gladish, GW et al. Incidental pulmonary emboli in oncology patients: prevalence, CT evaluation, and natural history. Radiology 2006; 240(1): 246–55.

40. Schultz, DJ et al. Incidence of asymptomatic pulmonary embolism in moderately to severely injured trauma patients. J Trauma 2004; 56(4): 727–31; discussion 731–3.

41. Kanne, JP et al. Six cases of acute central pulmonary embolism revealed on unenhanced multidetector CT of the chest. AJR Am J Roentgenol 2003; 180(6): 1661–4.

42. Gosselin, MV, et al., Unsuspected pulmonary embolism: prospective detection on routine helical CT scans. Radiology 1998; 208(1): 209–15.

43. Bae, KT et al. CT depiction of pulmonary emboli: display window settings. Radiology, 2005; 236(2): 677–84.

44. Revel, MP et al. Diagnosing pulmonary embolism with four-detector row helical CT: prospective evaluation of 216 outpatients and inpatients. Radiology 2005; 234(1): 265–73.

45. van Belle, A et al. Effectiveness of managing suspected pulmonary embolism using an algorithm combining clinical probability, D-dimer testing, and computed tomography. Jama 2006; 295(2): 172–9.

46. Parish, JM et al. Pulmonary artery sarcoma. Clinical features. Chest 1996; 110(6): 1480–8.

47. Cox, JE et al. Pulmonary artery sarcomas: a review of clinical and radiologic features. J Comput Assist Tomogr 1997; 21(5): 750–5.

48. Weinreb, JC et al. Pulmonary artery sarcoma: evaluation using Gd-DTPA. J Comput Assist Tomogr 1990; 14(4): 647–9.

49. Kim, JH et al. Primary leiomyosarcoma of the pulmonary artery: a diagnostic dilemma. Clin Imaging 2003; 27(3): 206–11.

50. Pengo, V et al. Incidence of chronic thromboembolic pulmonary hypertension after pulmonary embolism. N Engl J Med 2004; 350(22): 2257–64.

51. Nijkeuter, M et al. Resolution of thromboemboli in patients with acute pulmonary embolism: a systematic review. Chest 2006; 129(1): 192–7.

52. Reddy, GP, Gotway, MB and Araoz, PA. Imaging of chronic thromboembolic pulmonary hypertension. Semin Roentgenol 2005; 40(1): 41–7.

53. Bergin, CJ et al. Chronic thromboembolism: diagnosis with helical CT and MR imaging with angiographic and surgical correlation. Radiology 1997; 204(3): p. 695–702.

54. Auger, WR et al. Chronic major-vessel thromboembolic pulmonary artery obstruction: appearance at angiography. Radiology, 1992; 182(2): 393–8.

55. Sherrick, AD, SJ Swensen, and TE Hartman. Mosaic pattern of lung attenuation on CT scans: frequency among patients with pulmonary artery hypertension of different causes. AJR Am J Roentgenol 1997; 169(1): 79–82.

56. Jerjes-Sanchez, C et al. Streptokinase and Heparin versus Heparin Alone in Massive Pulmonary Embolism: A Randomized Controlled Trial. J Thromb Thrombolysis 1995; 2(3): 227–9.

57. Kasper, W et al. Prognostic significance of right ventricular afterload stress detected by echocardiography in patients with

clinically suspected pulmonary embolism. Heart 1997; 77(4): 346–9.

58. Goldhaber, SZ et al. Acute pulmonary embolism: clinical outcomes in the International Cooperative Pulmonary Embolism Registry (ICOPER). Lancet 1999; 353(9162): 1386–9.

59. Jerjes-Sanchez, C et al. High dose and short-term streptokinase infusion in patients with pulmonary embolism: prospective with seven-year follow-up trial. J Thromb Thrombolysis 2001; 12(3): 237–47.

60. Binder, L et al. N-terminal pro-brain natriuretic peptide or troponin testing followed by echocardiography for risk stratification of acute pulmonary embolism. Circulation 2005; 112(11): 1573–9.

61. Scridon, T et al. Prognostic significance of troponin elevation and right ventricular enlargement in acute pulmonary embolism. Am J Cardiol 2005; 96(2): 303–5.

62. Kucher, N et al. Prognostic role of echocardiography among patients with acute pulmonary embolism and a systolic arterial pressure of 90 mm Hg or higher. Arch Intern Med 2005; 165(15): 1777–81.

63. Grifoni, S et al. Short-term clinical outcome of patients with acute pulmonary embolism, normal blood pressure, and echocardiographic right ventricular dysfunction. Circulation 2000; 101(24): 2817–22.

64. Wu, AS et al. CT Pulmonary Angiography: Quantification of Pulmonary Embolus as a Predictor of Patient Outcome – Initial Experience. Radiology 2004; 230(3): 831–5. Epub 2004 Jan 22.

65. van der Meer, RW et al. Right Ventricular Dysfunction and Pulmonary Obstruction Index at Helical CT: Prediction of Clinical Outcome during 3-month Follow-up in Patients with Acute Pulmonary Embolism. Radiology 2005; 235(3): 798–803.

66. Engelke, C, Rummeny, EJ and Marten, K. Acute pulmonary embolism on MDCT of the chest: prediction of cor pulmonale

and short-term patient survival from morphologic embolus burden. AJR Am J Roentgenol 2006; 186(5): 1265–71.

67. Araoz PA, Gotway MB, Harrington JR, Harmsen WS, Mandrekar JN. Pulmonary embolism: prognostic CT findings Radiology 2007 Mar; 242(3): 889–97.

68. Turnier, E et al. Massive pulmonary embolism. Am J Surg, 1973; 125(5): 611–22.

69. Hermann, RE, Davis JH, Holden, WD. Pulmonary embolism: A clinical and pathologic study with emphasis on the effect of prophylactic therapy with anticoagulants. Am J Surg 1961; 102: 19–28.

70. Gifford Jr, RW. and Groves, LK. Limitations in the feasibility of pulmonary embolectomy: A clinicopathologic study of 101 cases of massive pulmonary embolism. Circulation, 1969; 39: 523–30.

71. Donaldson, GA, Williams, C, Scannell, JG, Shaw, RS. A reappraisal of the application of the trendelenburg operation to massive fatal pulmonary embolism. N Engl J Med 1963; 268(4): 171–4.

72. Coon, WW, Coller, FA, Clinicopathologic correlation in thromboembolism. Surgery, gynecology, and obstetrics 1959; 109(3): 259–69.

73. Coche, E et al. Evaluation of biventricular ejection fraction with ECG-gated 16-slice CT: preliminary findings in acute pulmonary embolism in comparison with radionuclide ventriculography. Eur Radiol 2005; 15(7): 1432–40.

74. White, CS et al. Chest pain evaluation in the emergency department: can MDCT provide a comprehensive evaluation? AJR Am J Roentgenol 2005; 185(2): 533–40.

75. Prologo, JD et al. CT pulmonary angiography: a comparative analysis of the utilization patterns in emergency department and hospitalized patients between 1998 and 2003. AJR Am J Roentgenol 2004; 183(4): 1093–6.

26

Computed Tomographic Angiography of the Abdominal Aorta and Iliac Arteries

Eric M. Walser

1 CT ANGIOGRAPHY OF THE ABDOMINAL AORTA AND ILIAC ARTERIES

Technical developments in computed tomography allow fast acquisition of vascular images since the scan time can now be completed during the arterial transit time of a bolus intravenous administration of contrast. The newer, 16 and 64-slice CT scanners have essentially replaced diagnostic angiography for the large and medium sized vessels. This chapter reviews imaging of the abdominal aorta and iliac arteries by multidetector CT (MDCT). This shift in imaging modalities is of great interest to both the physician and the patient, as it allows outpatient imaging of the heart and the vessels with much decreased risk as compared to standard angiography. Additionally, a single IV contrast injection permits three-dimensional, multiplanar, and even endoluminal representation of the vessels and also allows evaluation of the surrounding structures as well as the vessel lumen (Figures 26.1, 26.2). During standard catheter-based angiography only 2-dimensional intraluminal anatomy is visible per individual contrast injection, which is a significant limitation.

2 TECHNOLOGICAL ADVANCEMENTS IN COMPUTED TOMOGRAPHY

Spiral or, more accurately, multi-detector CT (MDCT) is the result of recent developments in CT image acquisition and reconstruction which allow large scan volumes to be scanned quickly with very thin slices. This capability allows for imaging vascular structures during their brief opacification by intravenously-injected contrast material. The growth of CT for vascular indications is a testament to the clinical utility of CT angiography, with a 235% increase in vascular exams from 1991–2002.[1] Simply stated, the technical leap responsible for MDCT was the creation of a cone-shaped x-ray beam striking multiple detector groups and creating image data over a volume, rather than a fan-shaped beam creating image data for one thin axial section per rotation. The larger x-ray beam in MDCT 'spirals' through the z-axis (the length of a human body) in one motion, rather than moving 'step-by-step' or one slice at a time as in conventional CT. The associated complex imaging algorithms involved in MDCT allow the user to define the axial slice thickness after

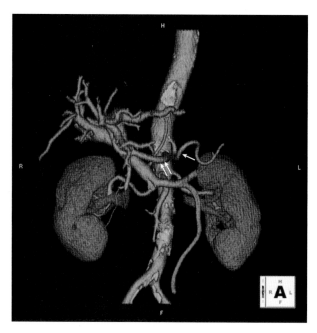

Figure 26.1 CT angiogram of the abdominal aorta shows relationship of mesenteric and portal venous system with the abdominal aorta and its branches. Notice the variant anatomy of separate origins of the splenic artery (arrow) and common hepatic artery (double arrow) from the aorta.

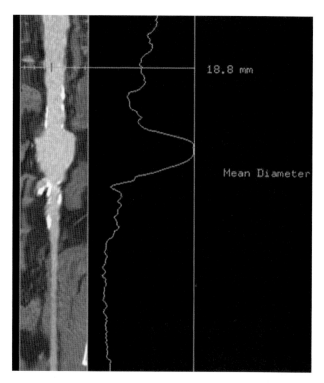

Figure 26.3 Curved coronal reconstruction of the aorta and iliac artery along the center-line of intraluminal contrast. This reconstruction allows measurement of luminal diameters along the course of a vessel regardless of tortuosity.

acquisition and to display 3-dimensional vascular images as well as images reconstructed in any plane imaginable, including customized curved planes or planes along the center line of vascular flow (useful for evaluating vascular disease morphology

and planning for endovascular procedures) (Figure 26.3). The ability to view vessels in multiple projections and orientations is extremely useful in evaluating the abdominal aorta and pelvic arteries due to their complex 3-dimensional arrangements, which is accentuated by tortuosity and dilation in the setting of aneurysmal disease. The obvious advantages of MDCT include rapid image acquisition and post-processing flexibility, better temporal resolution and less image noise. A significant drawback of MDCT is the increased radiation dose to the patient as opposed to conventional CT. The latest MDCT technology will produce high-detail CT angiography from the neck to the feet in about 1 minute.[2]

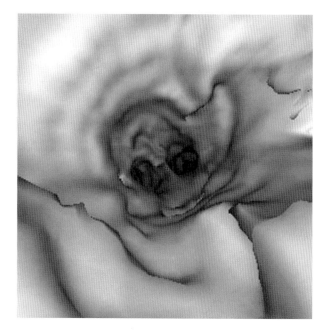

Figure 26.2 Endoluminal (navigator) view of the inside of the abdominal aorta, looking inferiorly at the distal abdominal aortic bifurcation. This is created by a software program using the cross sectional images from MDCT.

3 CT ANGIOGRAPHY VERSUS MR ANGIOGRAPHY?

As MRA requires no iodinated contrast material and allows imaging in multiple different planes of acquisition, it is a reasonable alternative or replacement imaging technique for the aorta and iliac arteries. MRA is also not affected by calcification as severely as is CT. Heavily calcified arteries may still induce artifact by MRA, but luminal narrowings and irregularities are better seen by MRA when atherosclerotic calcification is present. Due to the lack of radiation and iodinated contrast, MRA is the default method for patients unable to receive contrast or radiation due to renal dysfunction, severe contrast allergy or pregnancy. Recent reports of nephrogenic systemic fibrosis after gadolinium administration in patients with renal dysfunction has tempered use of MR contrast in patients with significant renal disease. Additional disadvantages of MR include less spatial resolution than CT. Also, MR is very sensitive to the presence of metal, and clips or stents can severely distort MRA and lead to false diagnoses. CT is less sensitive to these small metallic objects but images may be degraded by streak artifact from large metallic objects such as hip prostheses. CT angiography, especially when done with the newer and faster scanners, allows very high-resolution axial imaging. Complex vessel morphology, as seen in dissections, irregular aneurysms and vascular tortuosity, is better delineated by CT. This is because of artifacts produced by MR imaging in areas where blood flow is turbulent within an acquisition slab. While indications for CT angiography often overlap those for MR angiography, there is some bias for CT angiography in cases requiring a higher degree of detail (Figure 26.4). In the event of iodinated contrast allergy, CTA can also be done with the intravenous injection of gadolinium (60–80 ccs). Although gadolinium provides less intense enhancement, diagnostic images can usually be obtained (Figure 26.5). Additionally, if the surrounding anatomy is important to evaluate, CT angiography provides

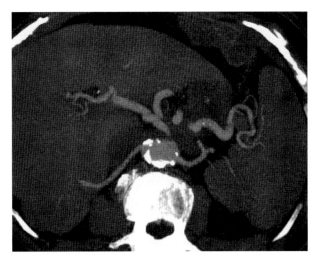

Figure 26.5 CTA of the renal arteries using intravenous injection of 80 ccs gadolinium at 5 ccs/sec. The aorta and branch arteries are well seen despite the reduced attenuation provided by gadolinium.

better resolution images of solid organs. Due to its high spatial resolution, CT angiography is well suited for the evaluation of aneurysms and dissecting hematomas involving the abdominal aorta. The status of the branch arteries and the exact morphology of the aneurysm or dissection itself are very important to surgical or endovascular planning and CT provides the best imaging for this application. The reason for this imaging preference is the improved resolution of the walls of the artery and the thin dissection flap or ulceration. CT angiography allows a very accurate assessment of the diameters and lengths of blood vessels and the entry and re-entry points of arterial dissection. CT imaging is particularly important due to the ever increasing indications for endovascular stent repair of aneurysms and dissection in both the thoracic and abdominal aorta. Placement of these devices requires very exact measurements of the vessel diameters, angulations, and lengths in order to pick the appropriate device for aneurysm or dissection exclusion. Patients with pacemakers or some older cardiac valve prostheses are limited to CTA as these remain contraindications for MR. MRA and CTA are both useful for evaluating abdominal masses which may be vascular in nature such as mycotic aneurysms or traumatic pseudoaneurysms. For imaging neoplasia, CTA and MRA both allow precise evaluation of tumor anatomy and vascular supply although MR has some advantage in characterizing tissue components (i.e. fat or hemorrhage).

4 TECHNIQUE OF CTA

Depending on the intensity of the exam, the CTA is tailored appropriately. Standard principles of cross-sectional imaging

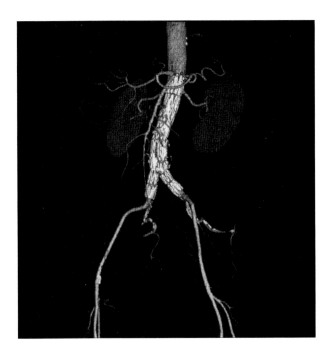

Figure 26.4 CTA of the abdominal aorta after stent-graft placement. The exact position of the endograft and the status of the major branches are seen with clarity.

to facilitate reformatting images in three dimensions include thin sections (2–5 mm) and rapid bolus administration of contrast at 4–5 cc/sec. Whereas solid organ imaging during the peak of parenchymal enhancement is a function of total iodine dose, vascular imaging is dependent on iodine flux, which is, in turn, dependent on iodine concentration and the flow rate of injection.[3] Therefore, the best vascular images result from rapid injections of concentrated iodine contrast material (typically 150 ccs of 300 mg Iodine/ml contrast at 5 ml/sec). Large-bore venous access is required to perform CTA (18-gauge at the least).

Fortunately, new peripherally inserted central catheters (PICC lines) and implanted venous access devices (ports) that can withstand such rapid injections are now available and manufactured and labeled specifically for this purpose. Arterial phase imaging is performed using a test bolus of a small amount of contrast to evaluate the time to start imaging acquisition at that point when contrast is visible in the aorta. Automatic software programs are also available that begin image acquisition as soon as the contrast material starts to arrive in the aorta.

If venous phase imaging is needed, a second series of images are obtained after the arterial phase. The delayed phase imaging is also useful to evaluate the solid organs for mass lesions and for delayed endoleaks in patients who have undergone stent-graft implantation. Standard software is becoming increasingly user friendly and, after image acquisition, 3-D and multiplanar reconstructions of vascular anatomy are easily done. However, one should be aware that image processing introduces artifacts and errors of its own, and source data images should always be reviewed in conjunction with reformatted images. CTA tends to overestimate calcified stenoses but underestimate luminal narrowing by non-calcific plaque – an important point to keep in mind when correlating a patient's clinical presentation and their imaging findings.[4,5] Abnormal CTA should be followed with angiography and possible intervention; however, rare cases will invariably turn out to be false positive. This situation usually involves obese or uncooperative patients or patients with tortuous vessels, where increased noise, motion, or turbulent flow, respectively, create image artifacts.

5 THE NORMAL ABDOMINAL AORTA AND ILIAC ARTERIES

CT angiography of the abdominal aorta and major pelvic arteries is rarely normal but normal arteries are occasionally encountered in young patients undergoing a trauma evaluation. The abdominal aorta is about 13 cm in length and is typically 2 cm in diameter at the crura of the diaphragm, tapering to a smaller caliber below the takeoffs of the celiac, superior mesenteric and renal arteries.[6] The wall of the aorta is normally thin (2–3 mm) and smooth. Fibrous atheromas typically become evident in the posterior wall of the infrarenal aorta after the age of 40 and become increasingly calcified with age. With advanced atherosclerosis, the internal surface of the aorta may become 'shaggy' with multiple large plaques, some of which have obvious ulceration. A particular manifestation of progressive atherosclerosis is a large posterior plaque at the junction of the thoracic and abdominal aorta ('coral-reef' lesion). These lesions rarely limit flow sufficiently to cause chronic lower extremity ischemia, but are prone to act as a nidus for clot formation with distal embolization and acute ischemia (Figure 26.6). The celiac axis and superior and inferior mesenteric arteries are easily seen by CTA. It is quite common (in 50% of patients) for the celiac axis to show significant narrowing and downward displacement at its origin, due to compression from the diaphragmatic crus.[7] This is usually an asymptomatic and incidental finding. Another finding with rare clinical significance is stenosis or occlusion of the inferior mesenteric artery, which is seen frequently in patients over the age of 50 years. Multiple renal arteries are seen unilaterally in about 30% of patients and bilaterally in 12%.[8] The common iliac arteries vary widely in length although very short common iliac arteries are rare.[8] This length variability is important when sizing patients for bifurcated stent grafts in the aorta so that the internal iliac arteries are not inadvertently occluded by the device. Anatomic variants such as circumaortic or retroaortic left renal veins, multiple renal arteries (common) and persistent sciatic arteries (very rare) are well-imaged by CTA and are important when planning open or endovascular repair of aortic pathology.

6 ABDOMINAL AORTIC ANEURYSMS AND DISSECTIONS

CTA is well-suited for the evaluation of patients with abdominal aortic aneurysms (AAA) or dissecting aortic hematomas (DAH) and is utilized most frequently for these indications. In patients with aneurysms considered for stent-graft repair, CTA is preferred due to its improved resolution. Although the anatomic requirements rendering a patient eligible for abdominal aortic stent-grafting continue to evolve, the critical areas remain the diameter of the

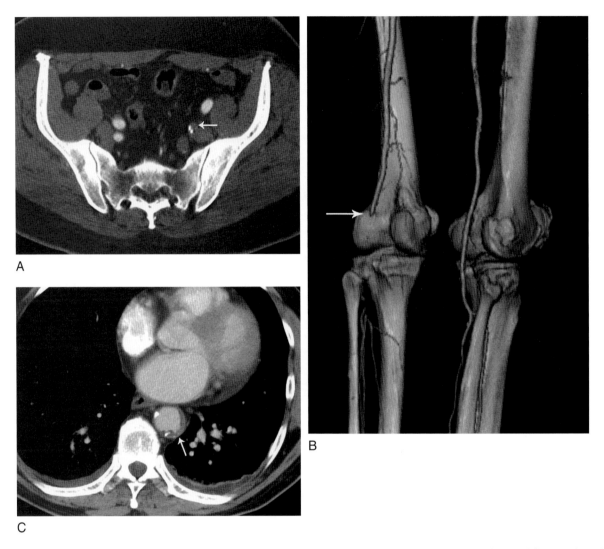

Figure 26.6 CTA of the pelvis and lower extremities shows left internal iliac and popliteal arterial emboli (arrows in a, b). CTA through the chest and abdomen showed atheroma (arrow in c) throughout which was likely responsible for the distal embolization.

proximal and distal stent landing sites and of the arterial access path (the external iliac and common femoral arteries). Although stent grafts with suprarenal fixation allow for the endovascular repair of AAA with a short proximal neck, a fairly straight infrarenal aortic segment with a length of at least 15 mm and diameter of less than about 28 mm is still required for adequate proximal fixation (Figure 26.7) and common iliac artery diameters over 20 mm pose problems with creating an adequate seal at the distal attachment sites for the bifurcated limbs. These diameter, angulation and length limitations vary somewhat between available devices and may become more liberal as new stent graft designs come to market. Aneurysmal common iliac arteries can usually be dealt with by extending the stent graft limb into the narrower external iliac artery

after proximal coil embolization of the internal iliac artery to prevent future endoleaks from retrograde internal iliac artery flow. However, significant perirenal or suprarenal aortic aneurysm extension remains an indication for open AAA repair until fenestrated stent grafts become available for general use (see Figure 26.7). The presence of significant external iliac and/or common femoral arterial occlusive disease or severe tortuosity can make insertion of the stent-graft delivery device impossible, or worse, lead to iliac perforation or dissection during the attempted passage of an 18-26 french device through an artery incapable of accommodating it (Figure 26.8). Therefore, pre-procedure CTA is mandatory to insure an external iliac artery diameter of at least 7–8 mm with tortuosity not to exceed about 90–120 degree angulations throughout its course. Although one can 'cheat' these

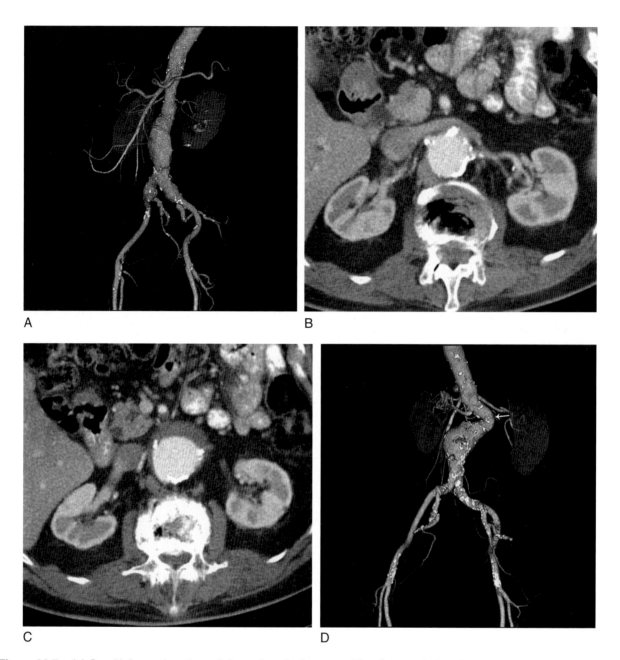

Figure 26.7   (a) Good infrarenal aortic neck for endograft placement. The diameter is less than 30 mm and there is no significant tortuosity. (b,c) Transverse CTA images 3 mm apart show near immediate aortic dilation (c) just below the renal arteries. Aneurysms involving the renal arteries or within 15 mm of the lowest renal artery cannot be repaired with available stent grafts and require open aneurysmoraphy. (d) severely angulated infrarenal aortic aneurysmal neck (arrow) is also a contraindication to endovascular stent graft placement.

guidelines for non-calcified iliac arteries, heavily calcified vessels are less forgiving in this regard. In patients with unacceptable access arteries in the pelvis, an alternative is to create a 'chimney' of prosthetic material anastomosed to the common iliac artery via a retroperitoneal incision. After insertion of a stent-graft through this conduit, the distal end is anastomosed to the femoral artery at the groin (Figure 26.9). Severe but unilateral iliac aneurysmal or occlusive disease can also be completely bypassed by the insertion of an aorto-uniiliac stent-graft on the opposite side with occlusion of the proximal common iliac artery on the unsalvageable side and placement of a crossed femoral artery bypass (Figure 26.10). Further considerations in pre-stent-graft CTA include the presence of supernumery renal arteries, visceral artery stenoses and internal iliac artery patency. Since many patients with aortic aneurysms are chronic smokers, the solid organs and lung bases should be carefully examined for the presence of mass lesions. We have

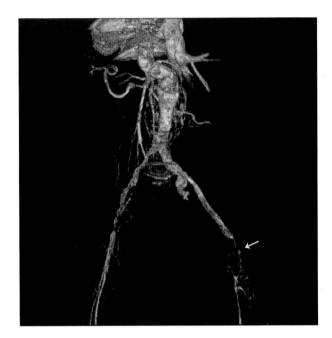

Figure 26.8 Patient with AAA and severe iliac occlusive disease, worse on the right, and severe narrowing in the left external iliac and common femoral arteries (arrow). Such severe atherosclerotic stenoses preclude passage of available stent graft delivery devices.

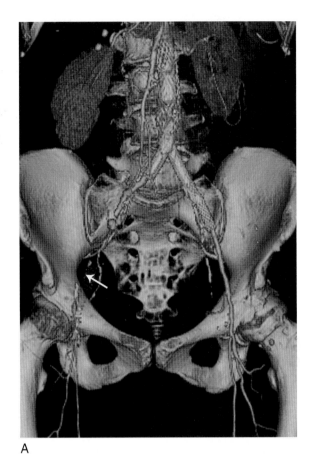

A

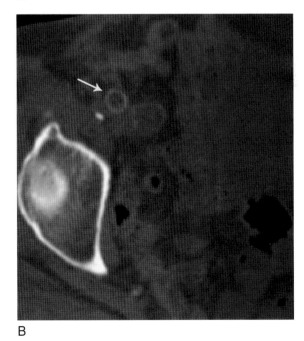

B

Figure 26.9 Severe iliac artery disease on the right (arrow in a) necessitated placement of a stent graft device through a PTFE 'chimney' sewn to the right common iliac artery via a retroperitoneal incision. The distal part of this graft was then anastomosed to the right common femoral artery. Unfortunately, this PTFE graft ultimately occluded (arrow in b).

discovered renal and bronchogenic carcinomas on several occasions during the initial evaluation and follow up of patients with AAA (Figure 26.11). The indication for repair of AAA is a diameter over 5 cm with ultrasound or CT follow up every 6 months to a year in those patients with smaller aneurysms. However, some physicians advocate earlier repair in women (4 cm AAA diameter) and there are ongoing trials evaluating the effects of early AAA repair (4.5–5.0 cm) so that the 5 cm threshold has some exceptions.[9–11] Some patients also undergo repair at smaller AAA diameters due to inflammatory or painful aneurysms or rapid enlargement (over 5 mm in 6 months) or, of course, hemorrhage. After endovascular aneurysm exclusion, periodic CTA is required to monitor aneurysm sac diameter and evaluate for endoleaks which arise in a significant number of patients (15–20%).[12] Although MRA is acceptable follow up in certain patients who cannot receive iodinated contrast, this modality is hampered by artifacts caused by the metallic composition of many current devices. CT angiography documents the contraction of the aneurysm sac indicating successful treatment and monitors for endoleaks, which appear as contrast pools filling the persistent or enlarging aneurysm sac. On follow up CTA, it is important that early and delayed (2–3 minute) scans are performed, as endoleaks around the stent graft are frequently visible only late after contrast injection. Additionally, a CT scan before IV contrast

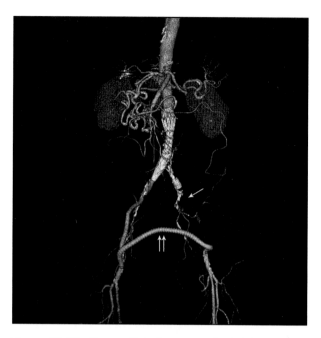

Figure 26.10   Severe iliac disease on the left (arrow) was bypassed by placing an aorto-uniiliac device on the right. The stent graft occluded the left iliac artery necessitating placement of a crossed femoral bypass (double arrow) to maintain flow to the left leg.

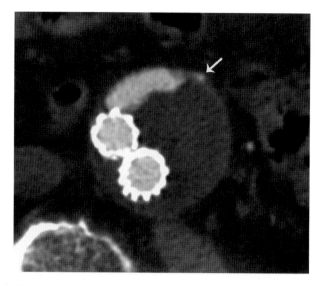

Figure 26.12   Type 2 endoleak. Retrograde arterial flow causes pooling of contrast in the anterior aneurysm sac. The source of this endoleak is the inferior mesenteric artery (arrow points to the ostium of the inferior mesenteric artery).

administration is advisable to avoid interpreting calcifications or hyperdense thrombus as an endoleak on the enhanced study. The most common type of endoleak is the type II endoleak from retrograde flow in a lumbar artery or the inferior mesenteric artery (Figure 26.12). Type I endoleaks occur when arterial blood flows around the stent attachment sites (1a from the proximal attachment site and 1b from the distal (limb) attachment sites), and are less common than type 2 leaks due to the fact that most attachment site leaks are recognized and treated at the time of stent-graft placement. Type 3 endoleaks occur at the junction points of modular devices and type 4 endoleaks are usually transient phenomena after graft placement and are visible as contrast 'weeping' through porous graft material. The timing and location of contrast appearance in the sac usually allows confident diagnosis of the type of endoleak. Type 2 endoleaks typically appear on the delayed scan only and can often be traced to the offending lumbar or other artery, whereas type 1 leaks are visible originating from the attachment sites immediately during the arterial phase of the study (Figure 26.13). The routine CTA follow up schedule for stent graft patients is one month post procedure and then 6–12 months thereafter, with more frequent CTAs obtained in those patients with endoleaks or who show lack of aneurysm sac shrinkage. The troubling theory of 'endotension' may explain why some patients (2%) have persistently dilated or enlarging aneurysm sacs despite adequate stent graft placement and no apparent endoleaks.[13] This phenomenon may arise from endoleaks that are undetectable with our current imaging techniques or may be a consequence of

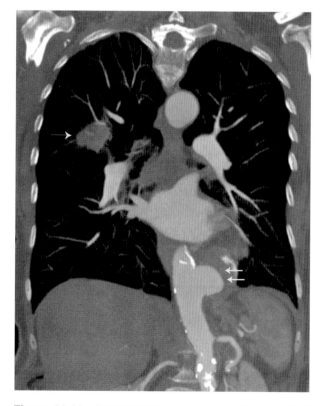

Figure 26.11   Bronchogenic cancer (arrow) in the right upper lung seen during CTA for evaluation of a penetrating ulcer in the lower thoracic aorta (double arrow).

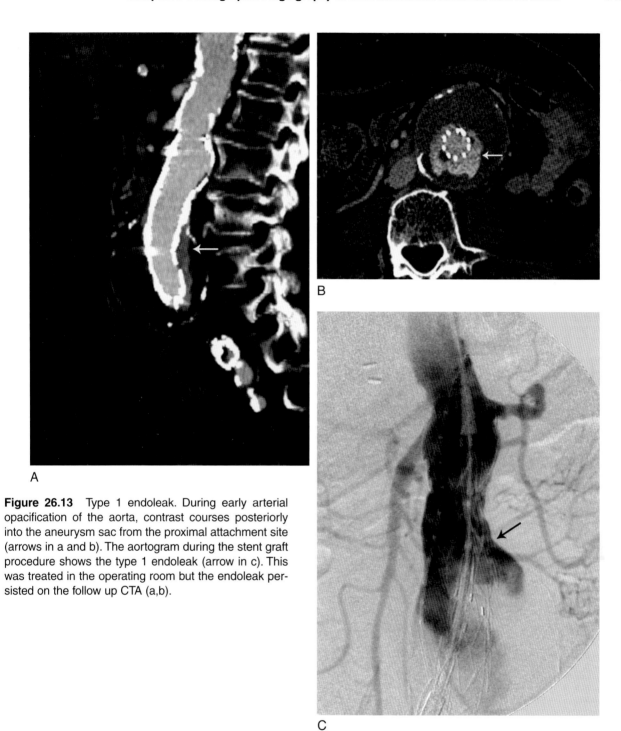

Figure 26.13 Type 1 endoleak. During early arterial opacification of the aorta, contrast courses posteriorly into the aneurysm sac from the proximal attachment site (arrows in a and b). The aortogram during the stent graft procedure shows the type 1 endoleak (arrow in c). This was treated in the operating room but the endoleak persisted on the follow up CTA (a,b).

continued arterial pressure propagation through intact stent-graft material.[14–16] Whatever the cause, these patients and patients with enlarging sacs from documented endoleaks are reliably diagnosed and followed by CTA with referral for percutaneous endoleak embolization or conversion to open AAA repair in those patients deemed at risk of rupture. Patients with stable or shrinking sacs and a type II endoleak are usually followed since a significant proportion (30–50%)

will regress spontaneously.[17,18] Branch vessel or iliac artery occlusions can rarely complicate endovascular stent grafts and can be easily seen and characterized by CTA. Lower extremity or visceral ischemia less than 30 days after stent-graft repair of AAA often indicates error during the initial procedure, which can usually be explained with CT imaging if the interpreting physician has familiarity with the construction and implantation procedure for the stent graft device in

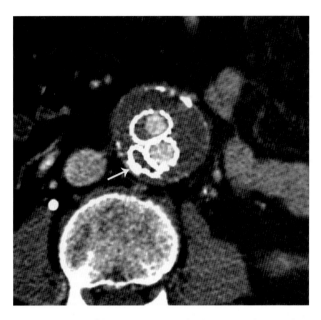

Figure 26.14   CTA post endograft placement in a patient with left leg ischemia. The left limb of the graft (arrow) was inadvertently placed outside of the limb extension of the graft body, resulting in an endoleak and reduced perfusion of the left leg.

question (Figure 26.14). Groin complications after stent grafting include seromas, pseudoaneurysm formation, or infection and all are easily diagnosed during CTA surveillance.

After open AAA repair, CTA follow up is not routinely performed and is limited to those patients with specific problems after surgery. Endoleaks after open AAA repair

are rare due to the fact that the lumbar arteries are oversewn at the time of aortic prosthetic implantation. A few cases exist, however (Figure 26.15). More commonly, CTA is used to evaluate for aortoenteric fistula and gastrointestinal hemorrhage or for extension of aneurysmal disease to the iliac arteries or suprarenal or thoracic aorta which occurs in 5–15% of patients[19,20] (Figure 26.16). Ischemic complications to the lower extremity occur in about 3% of cases and are also easily detected with CTA.[21]

DAH is almost always a distal extension of a type B thoracic aortic dissection, arising from arterial mediolysis or necrosis secondary to hypertensive vasculopathy or secondary to congenital causes such as Marfan's disease. Although isolated DAH in the abdominal aorta can occur, it is often secondary to trauma or iatrogenic injury from retrograde femoral artery catheterization. We have seen the occasional occurrence of asymptomatic infrarenal aortic 'webs' in patients with a remote history of trauma but more significant lesions such as penetrating atherosclerotic ulcers or focal abdominal aortic dissections can be diagnosed and characterized with CTA (Figures 26.17, 26.18). Stent graft or open repair of such focal lesions is generally more straightforward than that of a traditional AAA since the aorta is affected over a short distance and treatment may involve the use of a simple covered tube graft rather than a bifurcated one. In the evaluation of the abdominal component of a thoracic DAH, the crucial evaluation points are branch vessel involvement, the distal extent of dissection and the maximum diameter of the dissected aorta (Figure 26.19). Indications for treatment

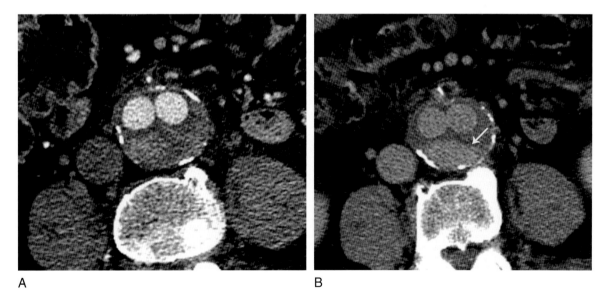

A   B

Figure 26.15   (a) Follow up CTA in a patient who had a remote history of open repair of AAA and now has back pain. There is a faint blush of contrast posteriorly in the aneurysm sac on early images. Delayed CTA (b) shows more prominent contrast pooling (arrow) consistent with a slow, type 2 endoleak from unligated lumbar arteries.

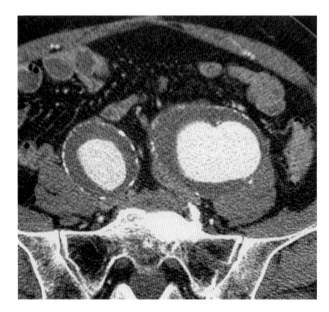

Figure 26.16   Huge iliac aneurysms developed in this patient 5 years after open repair of AAA using a tube graft.

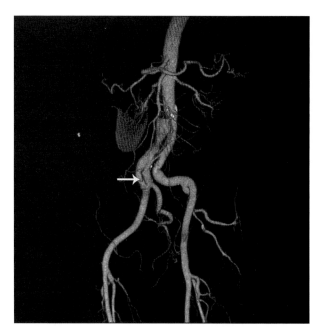

Figure 26.18   Distal aortic focal dissection extending into the right common iliac artery. A flap is visible as the dissection spirals inferiorly (arrow). This patient had remote blunt abdominal trauma also.

include significant ischemic effects due to branch vessel involvement, enlarging aortic diameter or diameter over 5 cm, or the coexistence of ascending thoracic aortic dissection requiring treatment. While stent grafts have been used successfully to treat DAH, most have been placed in the thoracic aorta to exclude the entry site of the false lumen and direct arterial flow into the true lumen. CTA of the pelvis is

helpful in such cases to identify the appropriate iliac artery for catheter and device placement since the dissection may spiral down one iliac artery and not the other.

7 ABDOMINAL AORTIC ATHEROSCLEROSIS

As mentioned earlier, atherosclerotic lesions are nearly universally apparent by CTA in patients at middle-age and above. Symptomatic aortoiliac occlusive disease is initially suspected by symptoms (hip, thigh, leg claudication), and signs (diminished femoral pulse) and non-invasive vascular exams pointing to significant arterial occlusion above the groin. CTA can confirm this diagnosis and clarify the extent and severity of aortoiliac arterial disease, although current practice patterns favor MRA, due to speed, and lack of radiation and iodinated contrast exposure. Percutaneous endovascular treatment is applicable in many patients with focal arterial occlusive disease but CTA or MRA is pivotal in weeding out those patients best served by operative therapy, such as those with extensive aortoiliac disease. Patients found to be poor candidates for percutaneous therapy can then be immediately referred for aortobifemoral or crossed femoral bypass grafting without the need for further invasive studies, such as diagnostic arteriography. If a patient has aortoiliac

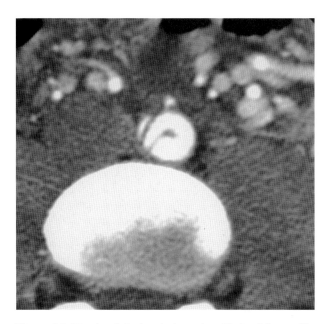

Figure 26.17   Aortic 'cobwebs' consist of intimal flaps without significant flow obstruction in a young male patient with a history of blunt abdominal trauma and splenectomy. These arterial injuries may not require intervention but can act as a nidus for clot formation and subsequent embolization.

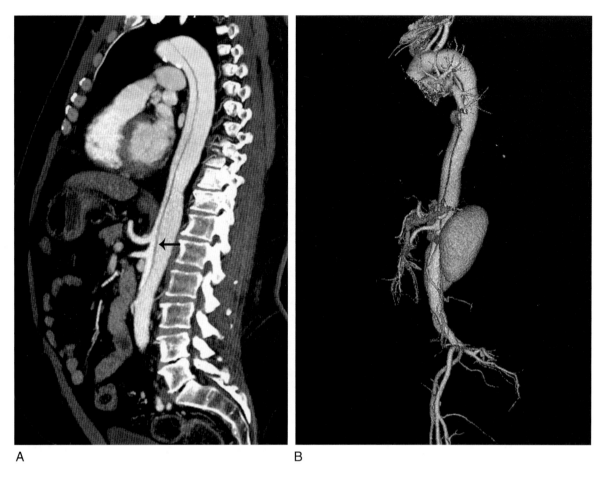

A   B

Figure 26.19 Type b aortic dissection involving the descending thoracic aorta and extending into the abdomen. Notice the celiac axis and superior mesenteric artery arise from the true lumen (arrow) with the intimal flap lying posteriorly within the aortic lumen.

disease amenable to endovascular therapy, CTA is helpful in pre-procedure planning for arterial access and for estimating the size and length of stents or angioplasty balloons needed. In this way, at the time of intervention, limited diagnostic arteriography is required and fluoroscopy and contrast injections are confined to the area of interest, limiting radiation dose to the patient and risk of contrast-induced nephrotoxicity. Hypoplastic aortoiliac syndrome (anatomic) and LeRiche syndrome (clinical) refer to the buttock, thigh and leg claudication and erectile dysfunction that goes with significant occlusive disease centered on the distal abdominal aorta and proximal iliac arteries although all types of aortoiliac occlusive disease are evaluable with CTA (Figure 26.20).[22]

8 ABDOMINAL AORTIC TRAUMA AND INFECTION

Trauma and infection are less frequent indications for CTA but are easily imaged with minor modifications to the

aneurysm/dissection protocols. In general, aortic infection or trauma manifest as mycotic or penetrating-injury pseudoaneurysms, respectively. These arterial lesions are best imaged by CTA and delayed imaging is unnecessary unless one requires evaluation of the abdominal and pelvic venous structures (1–2 minute delay) or the renal collecting system and bladder (5–10 minute delayed imaging). Mycotic aortic pseudoaneurysms typically arise from staphylococcal or pseudomonas infections and are almost always associated with positive blood cultures (Figure 26.21). Associated branch vessel involvement or occlusion are reliably visualized during CTA as well as any associated perivascular abscess formation. Patients with these infected pseudoaneurysms are poor candidates for stent graft insertion due to the infected field and generally undergo aortic resection and retroperitoneal drainage with extra-anatomic arterial bypass creation (such as axillofemoral and crossed femoral bypass). Patients with traumatic vascular injuries are more suitable for endovascular repair if hemodynamically stable and if a suitable device is available 'off the shelf' to implant in an

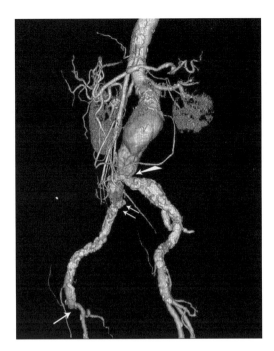

Figure 26.20   CTA in a patient evaluated for AAA repair. Upper large arrow shows a calcific stenosis in the left common iliac artery origin. The right internal iliac artery is occluded (double arrows) and a prosthetic right femoral-popliteal bypass graft is also occluded (lower smaller arrow). The presence of such arterial occlusive disease improves pre-procedure planning in patients who are candidates for endovascular therapy.

expeditious manner. However, for the most part, CTA prepares these injured patients for surgical repair by evaluating the extent and branch vessel involvement of traumatic injuries to the abdominal aorta. In severely injured trauma victims with hypotension, CTA will often show a marked and diffuse constriction of the aorta and its major branches secondary to severe vasospasm. 'Shock aorta,' as this condition is called, is associated with a poor prognosis and need for further fluid resuscitation. Due to the nature of an emergency CTA, hypotension, arterial spasm and frequent motion artifacts, the image quality of these exams is often poor (Figure 26.22).

9 CONGENITAL AND IDIOPATHIC INFLAMMATORY CONDITIONS OF THE ABDOMINAL AORTA

Rarely, idiopathic and congenital aortic disease is manifest by CTA. Usually these conditions are diagnosed in children or young adults and affect the major branches off of the abdominal aorta. Tubular or focal stenoses involving the aorta in

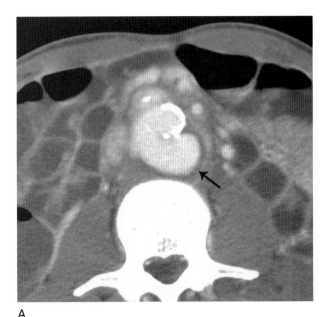

A

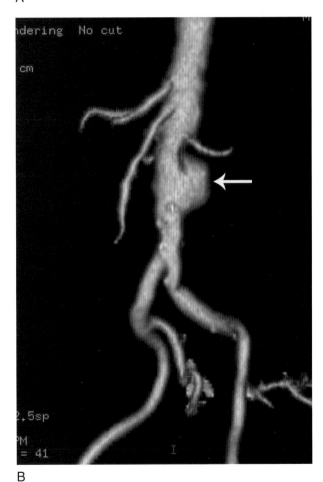

B

Figure 26.21   Volume-rendered CTA of abdominal aorta (a) shows a pseudoaneurysm (arrow) beginning below the renal arteries. The blood cultures were positive for staphylococcus. (b) Volume rendered image of focal pseudoaneurysm (arrow).

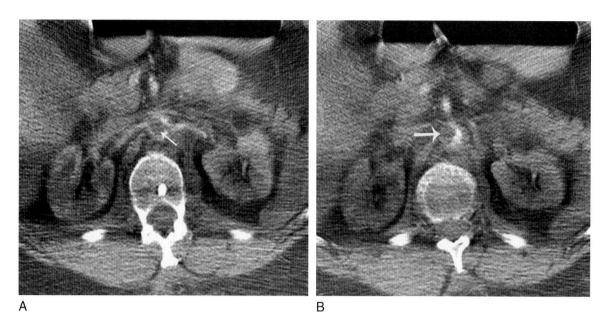

A   B

Figure 26.22   Jet ski accident with massive blunt abdominal injury. CTA is poor quality but shows a filling defect in the aortic lumen extending to the renal arteries (arrows in a,b) with diminished perfusion of both kidneys. At surgery, the aorta was completely transected above the renal arteries with an intimal flap herniating inferiorly.

young patients may indicate disorders such as neurofibromatosis and abdominal aortic coarctation or, rarely, inflammatory vasculitides such as Takayasu arteritis.[23] CTA findings are non specific and include segmental narrowings or occlusions and focal aneurysms. Young patients with DAH or AAA may suffer from a variety of rare conditions with disordered or deficient collagen formation such as progeria, pseudoxanthoma elasticum, Marfan's disease, Ehlers Danlos syndrome, Turner syndrome, or familial

aortic aneurysm syndrome (Figure 26.23). In adulthood, retroperitoneal fibrosis (RPF) can present with wall-enhancement or an encasing mass of the abdominal aorta. RPF is generally discernable from the alternative diagnosis of lymphoma, although this occasionally requires percutaneous biopsy (Figure 26.24). Non-specific aortic wall thickening can be seen in inflammatory aortitis, such as from giant cell arteritis, Cogan's syndrome (young adults with vasculitis, interstitial keratitis and vestibuloauditory dysfunction), or as a

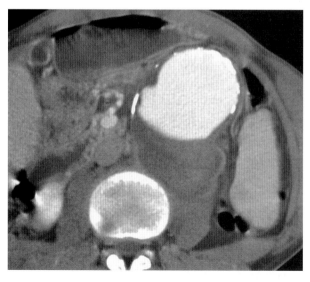

Figure 26.23   Enormous AAA in a 20 year old male patient with familial aneurysm disorder. He suffered a congenital collagen defect and had multiple arterial aneurysms and bronchiectasis.

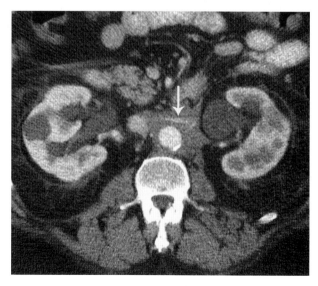

Figure 26.24   Retroperitoneal fibrosis with soft tissue encasing the aorta and narrowing the left renal vein (arrow). There is also bilateral hydronephrosis.

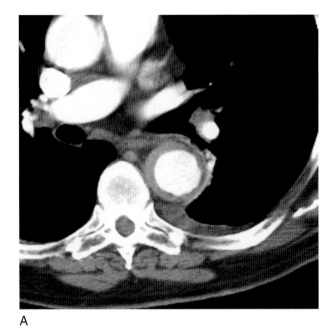

A

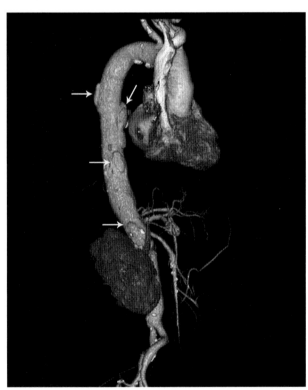

B

Figure 26.25 (a) Diffuse thickening of the descending thoracic aorta in a patient with back pain could represent early intramural hematoma or aortitis. (b) Later, CTA shows the development of multiple penetrating aortic ulcers in the thoracic and abdominal aorta (arrows) indicating a degenerative vascular disorder rather than inflammatory.

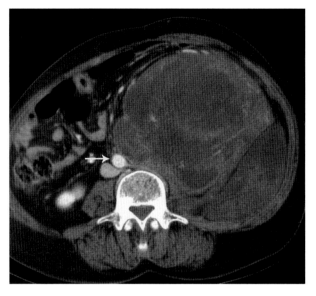

Figure 26.26 Large retroperitoneal sarcoma with displacement but not invasion of the abdominal aorta (arrows). This mass showed arterial enhancement peripherally and transcatheter embolization was done prior to resection.

precursor to penetrating aortic ulceration or dissecting hematoma (Figure 26.25).

10 AORTIC NEOPLASTIC DISEASE

Primary neoplasms of the abdominal aorta are exceedingly rare and most leiyomyosarcomas arising from blood vessels do so from the vena cava. Case reports of primary aortic cancers exist and present as intra and extraluminal masses involving the abdominal aorta. Reported tumors include angiosarcomas and leiyomyosarcomas.[24,25] CTA of the abdomen in the setting of neoplasm usually concerns the evaluation of a very bulky abdominal mass, frequently a sarcoma, in which surgery is contemplated. CTA is effective in evaluating the extent of the mass and its encroachment, encasement or invasion of the aorta or its major branches. Additionally, CTA can assess the vascularity of these large tumors and, if hypervascular, these tumors can undergo preoperative embolization for local control and reduction of resectional bleeding (Figure 26.26).

REFERENCES

1. Fox SH. Emerging developments in multidetector CT. Presented at the Advances in Multidetector CT Meeting, Washington DC, September 13–14, 2003.

2. Westerman BR, Current status of MDCT. Presented at the Advances in Multidetector CT Meeting, Washington, DC, September 13–14, 2003.

3. Herman S, Computed tomography contrast enhancement principles and the use of high-concentration contrast media. J Comput Assist Tomogr 2004; 28: S7–11.

4. Leber AW, Becker A, Knez A et al. Accuracy of 64-slice computed tomography to classify and quantify plaque volumes in the proximal coronary system: a comparative study using intravascular ultrasound. J Am Coll Cardiol 2006; 47(3): 672–7.

5. Malagutti P, Nieman K, Meijboom WB et al. Use of 64-slice CT in symptomatic patients after coronary bypass surgery: evaluation of grafts and coronary arteries. Eur Heart J 2007; 28(15): 1879–85.

6. Woodburne RT. Essentials of human anatomy. New York: Oxford University Press, 1994.

7. Strandness DE, Jr, van Breda A. Vascular diseases: surgical and interventional therapy. New York: Churchill Livingston, 1994.

8. Kadir S. Atlas of normal and variant angiographic anatomy. Philadelphia: Saunders, 1991.

9. Takaqi H, Umemoto T. Prophylactic endovascular repair of small abdominal aortic aneurysm. Eur J Vasc Endovasc Surg 2006; 31(5): 562.

10. Golledge J, Muller J, Coomans D et al. 'The small abdominal aortic aneurysm.' Eur J Vasc Endovasc Surg 2006; 31(3): 237–8.

11. Palamara AE. Regarding: 'The study of endovascular repair of small (<5.5 cm) aneurysms.' J Vasc Surg 2005; 42(4): 822.

12. Hobo R, Buth J, EUROSTAR collaborators. Secondary interventions following endovascular abdominal aortic aneurysm repair using current endografts. A EUROSTAR report. J Vasc Surg 2006; 43(5): 896–902.

13. Du Toit DF, Saaiman JA, Carpenter JP. Endovascular aortic aneurysm repair by a multidisciplinary team: lessons learned and six-year clinical update. Cardiovasc J S Afr 2005; 15(1): 36–47.

14. Meier GH, Parker FM, Godziachvili V et al. Endotension after endovascular aneurysm repair: the Ancure experience. J Vasc Surg 2001; 34(3): 421–6.

15. Gilling-Smith GL, Brennan J, Harris P et al. Endotension after endovascular aneurysm repair: Definition, classification and strategies for surveillance and intervention. J Endovasc Surg 1999; 6: 305–7.

16. White GH, May J, Petrasek P et al. Endotension: an explanation for continued AAA growth after successful endoluminal repair. J Endovasc Surg 1999; 6(4): 308–15.

17. Veith FJ, Baum RA, Ohki T et al. Nature and significance of endoleaks and endotension: summary of opinions expressed at an international conference. J Vasc Surg 2002; 35(5): 1029–35.

18. Baum RA, Carpenter JP, Stavropoulous SW et al. Diagnosis and management of type 2 endoleaks after endovascular aneurysm repair. Tech Vasc Interv Radiol 2001; 4(4): 222–6.

19. Calcagno D, Hallett JW Jr, Ballard DJ et al. Late iliac artery aneurysms and occlusive disease after aortic tube grafts for abdominal aortic aneurysm repair. A 35 year experience. Ann Surg 1991; 214: 733–6.

20. Kalman PG, Rappaport DC, Merchant N et al. The value of late computed tomographic scanning in identification of vascular abnormalities after abdominal aortic aneurysm repair. J Vasc Surg 1999; 29: 442–50.

21. Johnston KW. Multicenter prospective study of nonruptured abdominal aortic aneurysm. Part II. Variables predicting morbidity and mortality. J Vasc Surg 1989; 9: 437–47.

22. Walton BL, Dougherty K, Mortazavi A et al. Percutaneous intervention for the treatment of hypoplastic aortoiliac syndrome. Catheter Cardiovasc Interv 2003; 60(3): 329–34.

23. Hata A, Noda M, Moriwaki R et al. Angiographic findings of Takayasu arteritis: new classification. Int J Cardiol 1996; 54 Suppl: S155–63.

24. Abularrage CJ, Weiswasser JM, White PW et al. Aortic angiosarcoma presenting as distal arterial embolization. Ann Vasc Surg 2005; 19(5): 744–8.

25. Chiche L, Mongredien B, Brocheriou I, Kieffer E. Primary tumors of the thoracoabdominal aorta: surgical treatment of 5 patients and review of the literature. Ann Vasc Surg 2003; 17(4): 354–64.

27

Mesenteric and Renal Computed Tomographic Angiography

Fred M. Moeslein, Eric E. Williamson, and Dominik Fleischmann

I INTRODUCTION

The last decade has witnessed an exciting and at times breathtaking evolution in cross-sectional imaging. The lightning pace of change in MRI and CT has completely revolutionized the way we as practicing radiologists and our referring clinician colleagues evaluate patients for a wide array of pathologies. Multidetector CT has transformed CT imaging from a two-dimensional into a powerful three-dimensional imaging modality. This evolution has brought to the mainstream single breath-hold imaging of the abdomen and pelvis, with sub-millimeter isotropic acquisitions. This change is particularly evident in the field of CT angiography, where the advances in CT technology now allow us to detect subtle changes in second and third order segmental branches in the mesenteric and renal vasculature. The recent advances allow CT angiography not only to rival, but in many cases to replace, diagnostic digital subtraction angiography in the evaluation of arterial and venous pathologies. The vast array of image display tools, including maximum intensity projection (MIP), multiplanar reformations (MPR), and volume-rendering (VR), allow analysis of the huge data sets with relative ease. Further, these powerful display tools allow us to communicate our findings to our referring physicians with a clarity unimagined even a decade ago. Clearly a picture is worth a thousand words!

The following passages lay out a brief synopsis of the many varied applications of CT angiography in the mesenteric and renal circulations. Hopefully the summary of current applications will inspire the reader to expand the breadth of studies currently employed within their own practice or institution.

1.1 ACQUISITION AND RECONSTRUCTION CONSIDERATIONS

Modern MDCT technology continues to evolve at lightning speed. At the time of this writing, 16 and 64 channel units are commonplace, and with the impending roll out of next generation 128, 256 and dual source 64 and 128 channel scanners. Of course older 4 and 8 channel scanners remain in use, but presumably will be phased out in favor of the faster scanners in due course. The rapidly changing playing field makes a discussion of acquisition techniques an undoubtedly dated endeavor, far better covered in the referred literature. However, certain guidelines will undoubtedly persist despite the rapid advances. Faster scan speeds provide several advantages. The newest technology makes single breath hold acquisitions well tolerated even by the most uncooperative patients. Second, the speed of acquisition now allows sub-millimeter collimation, even across broad territories, such as the mesentery or extremities. Isotropic imaging is key to multiplanar reformations, and since the introduction of the 16 channel scanners, sub-millimeter z-axis collimation has become commonplace. Lastly, precontrast imaging should be considered when performing studies in the setting of suspected acute bleeding, dissection, renal calculi or renal masses, as the precontrast images are the most sensitive to hemorrhage and subtle calcification.

The new generation of scanners has brought a torrent of information to the imaging specialist. It is imperative that CTA studies be read with access to a 3D workstation, or preferably on such a workstation. While review of the transverse images often remains the basis for diagnosis, a great deal of essential information is obtained by the creation and review of the 3D reconstructions. At our institution, all CT angiographic studies are evaluated with maximum intensity projection (MIP) images, multiplanar reformatted (MPR) images, and volume-rendered (VR) images. With practice, the real-time interactive creation and review of these reconstructions is rapid and will aid immensely in the accurate diagnosis of mesenteric pathologies.

1.2 Contrast medium administration

Contrast material delivery optimization is crucial to the CTA examination. The newest generation scanners acquire images with such speed that it has become possible to outrun the contrast medium bolus. It therefore has become imperative for each user to optimize scan techniques to match contrast bolus delivery and data acquisition for the specific equipment used. In addition, as scan times shorten it becomes an imperative to individualize scanning delays. This can be accomplished either by test bolus injection, or preferably by bolus tracking protocols. With bolus tracking, scanning of the region of interest begins at a predetermined time following the arrival of contrast material within a target vessel, which then triggers the CTA data acquisition.

The scanning and contrast medium administration protocol will vary depending on the choice of vascular bed or target organ parenchymal enhancement. In general if only a CTA is performed, a short rapid bolus will suffice; however, if end organ parenchymal opacification is desired then a longer contrast injection will be required. These parameters will vary greatly from system to system, based mostly on the number of channels but also with vendor specific technical issues. It will therefore be incumbent upon the individual user to tailor the CTA exams to each scanner.

Special consideration should be given to patients with renal failure and renal insufficiency. In the past, it was common to recommend MRA or gadolinium enhanced CT or angiography for these patients. However, with the recognition that nephrogenic systemic fibrosis may be associated with gadolinium administration in the setting of renal impairment, this practice can no longer be recommended.[1,2] The current recommendation for evaluating the renal arteries in patients with renal impairment is sonographically, if possible, or by angiography with limited contrast administration or with carbon dioxide as a contrast agent. As our understanding of nephrogenic systemic fibrosis advances, there may be new recommendations forthcoming.

2 MESENTERIC CTA

2.1 Clinical applications

2.1.1 Acute mesenteric ischemia

Antonio Beniviene first described acute mesenteric ischemia (AMI) in the fifteenth century. In 1926, Cokkinis wrote: 'occlusion of the mesenteric vessels is apt to be regarded as one of those conditions of which the diagnosis is impossible, the prognosis hopeless, and the treatment almost useless.' Sadly the morbidity and mortality of this grave disease remains little changed in the intervening period. The reported average mortality of AMI still exceeds 60%, which is little changed over the last 50 years.[3,4]

The diagnosis and treatment of AMI remains difficult in large part from the nebulous constellation of presenting signs and symptoms. The classic presentation is abdominal pain out of proportion to the patient's physical findings that persists beyond 2 to 3 hours. Other common presenting symptoms are given in Table 27.1. As the initial diagnosis is often delayed, it is not uncommon for patients to present with an acute abdomen, including distension, rigidity and hypotension secondary to bowel infarction.[5] Numerous etiologies may cause AMI, and these are given in Table 27.2.

Table 27.1 Presenting signs and symptoms of acute mesenteric ischemia

Abdominal pain
Occult fecal blood (in up to 50% of cases)
Melena or hemachezia (in up to 15% of cases)
Leukocytosis (in up to 75% of cases)
Metabolic acidosis (in up to 50% of cases)
Fever
Nausea
Anorexia
Diarrhea

Table 27.2 Etiologies of acute mesenteric ischemia

Arterial occlusion (50%)
    Embolus – usually to the superior mesenteric
        artery
    Thrombotic occlusion
    Aortic aneurysm
    Vasculitis
    Fibromuscular dysplasia
    Trauma
Non-occlusive ischemia (25–30%)
    Systemic hypotension
    Cardiac failure
    Septic shock
    Mesenteric vasoconstriction
Venous occlusion (10–15%)
    Portal hypertension
    Hypercoagulation
    Trauma
    Intraabdominal inflammatory disease
    Surgery
Extra-vascular etiologies (<5%)
    Incarcerated hernia
    Volvulus
    Intussusception
    Adhesive disease

Table 27.3 CT findings associated with acute mesenteric ischemia

Pneumatosis intestinalis
SMA occlusion
Combined celiac and IMA occlusion
Arterial embolism
SMA or portal venous gas
Focal lack of bowel wall enhancement
Free intraperitoneal gas
Superior mesenteric or portal venous thrombosis
Solid organ infarction
Bowel obstruction
Bowel dilatation
Mucosal enhancement
Bowel wall thickening
Mesenteric stranding
Ascites

As Table 27.2 illustrates, the grand majority of etiologies can be diagnosed by CTA. The power of CT in the diagnosis of AMI emerges from the ability to evaluate both the mesenteric vasculature and soft tissues simultaneously.[6–8]

In patients where AMI is suspected, administration of 500–750 mL of a low-attenuation oral contrast agent (e.g., water or methylcellulose) is recommended. This allows evaluation of the bowel wall enhancement and does not interfere with 3D reconstruction of the vascular anatomy.[7] Imaging should be performed in the early arterial phase as well as within the portal venous phase in order to adequately evaluate both the arterial and venous mesenteric structures. The portal venous phase is most often sufficient for evaluating the parenchymal enhancement within the abdominal organs.

There is a wide range of possible findings in AMI (Table 27.3).[9] The most common etiology of AMI is acute embolic occlusion of the SMA (40–50%) (Figure 27.1). SMA emboli tend to lodge at the origin of the middle colic artery and produce an abrupt cut-off of the vessel on CTA.[10] In the setting of acute embolic disease, few if any collateral vessels are detected. In contradistinction, when acute mesenteric thrombosis is the cause of AMI, the occlusion of the SMA tends to occur within the first 2 cm. In these cases, there are often multiple collateral vessels present, which correlate to the classically insidious onset of acute mesenteric

thrombosis. In the setting of mesenteric venous thrombosis, the CT often shows associated bowel wall thickening or dilatation.[9,10]

The findings of AMI in the setting of non-occlusive mesenteric ischemia are less well defined. One report documents normal mesenteric vessels with bowel wall thickening and pneumatosis.[8] A second report detailed abnormally small mesenteric arteries with marked delayed venous filling (greater than 70 seconds following contrast administration).[10] Hopefully the newest generation of scanners coupled with properly attuned clinical acumen will allow more specific and reproducible findings to surface.

2.1.2 Chronic mesenteric ischemia

Chronic mesenteric ischemia (CMI) is almost exclusively caused by severe atherosclerotic disease (>95% of cases) which causes occlusion or severe stenoses of multiple mesenteric vessels (Figure 27.2).[11] Patients classically present with postprandial abdominal pain, weight loss and sitophobia (i.e., food avoidance). It is believed that this clinical triad arises because the diseased mesenteric vasculature is unable to support the increased metabolic demands of motility, secretion and absorption induced by digestion, but remains adequate to support the resting gut. It is generally held that CMI in the setting of atherosclerosis occurs as a result of stenosis or occlusion of at least two of the three main mesenteric vessels. However, there are documented cases of single vessel occlusion, usually of the SMA, leading to CMI.[10]

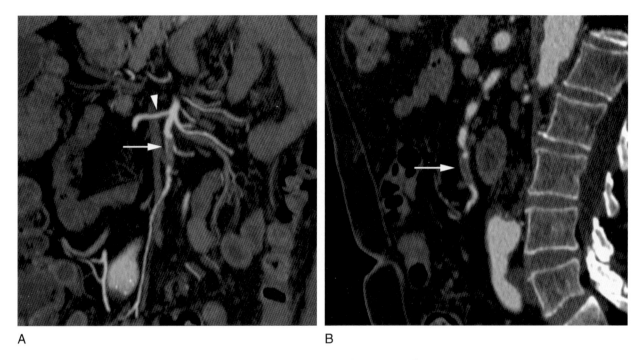

A   B

Figure 27.1 SMA embolism: Coronal (A) and sagittal (B) MPR images of the superior mesenteric artery showing non-occlusive embolism of the mid-distal artery (arrow), beyond the origin of the iliocolic artery (arrowhead).

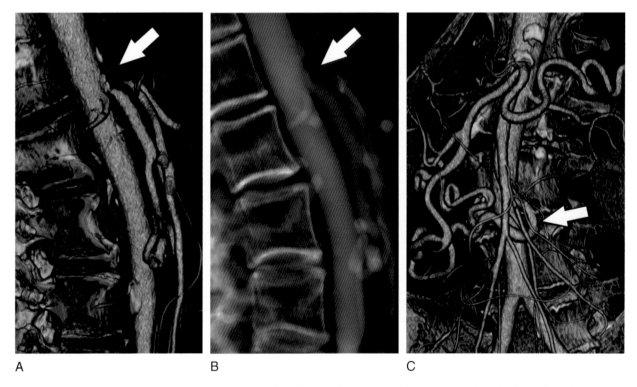

A   B   C

Figure 27.2 Celiac occlusion: Sagittal volume rendered (A) and ray-sum (B) images of a chronically occluded celiac axis (arrow) due to atherosclerosis. The superior mesenteric artery is moderately stenotic at its origin. Coronal volume rendered image (C) shows a prominent collateral vessel arising from the SMA (arrow) which reconstitutes the celiac artery territory.

Non-atherosclerotic causes of CMI are exceedingly rare, but include fibromuscular dysplasia, median arcuate ligament syndrome, vasculitides (e.g., Takayasu arteritis, polyarteritis nodosa, segmental mediolytic arteriopathy) and connective tissue disorders (e.g., Ehlers-Danlos). Even rarer etiologies include abdominal coarctation, neurofibromatosis, post-irradiation arteritis and idiopathic fibrosis.[10]

The CT appearance of fibromuscular dysplasia within the mesenteric vessels mirrors that in the renal arteries (Figure 27.3). Classically, the vessels display a beaded appearance with marked narrowing of the affected vessel in the setting of medial fibrosis, or cylindrical narrowing with prominent aneurismal dilation in the setting of adventitial disease.[10]

External compression of the celiac artery or neural plexus by the crura of the diaphragm causes median arcuate ligament syndrome.[12] The classic angiographic finding is best appreciated on the lateral aortogram as a smooth effacement of the superior aspect of the proximal celiac artery (Figure 27.4). In rare cases, in addition to the celiac artery, this finding may involve the SMA and even renal arteries. CTA not only allows detection of the narrowed vessels but of the offending ligamentous structure. Caution should be exercised during interpretation of studies as this finding can be

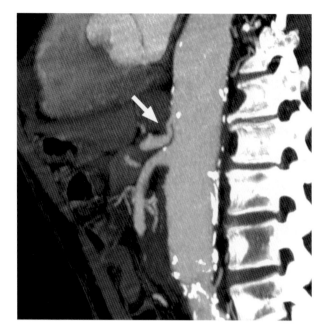

Figure 27.4 Arcuate ligament compression: Lateral oblique thick MPR images show characteristic external compression of the proximal celiac axis by the diaphragmatic crus (arrow). This finding was incidentally noted in an asymptomatic patient.

seen in many asymptomatic patients, and therefore should be correlated with the clinical presentation.

2.1.3 Visceral artery aneurysms

Visceral artery aneurysms were once thought to be rare pathologic entities. However, the increased utilization of cross-sectional imaging has led to the identification of these aneurysms with much greater frequency. Visceral artery aneurysms may involve any of the major visceral vessels and the frequency of this involvement is shown in Table 27.4.[13] Interestingly, the frequency of hepatic and renal arteries aneurysms is increasing, which is believed to

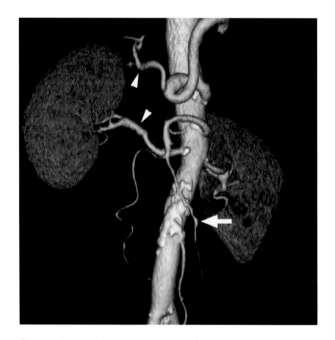

Figure 27.3 Mesenteric FMD: Coronal oblique volume rendered image demonstrates characteristic 'beaded' stenosis and dilatation of the common hepatic artery and right renal artery (arrowheads) as well as stenosis and focal dilatation of the mid superior mesenteric artery (arrow).

Table 27.4 Distribution of visceral artery aneurysms

Artery	Percent of cases
Splenic	60–80%
Hepatic	20%
Gastroduodenal	6%
Superior mesenteric	5.5%
Celiac	4%
Gastric and gastroepiploic	4%
Jejunal and ileocolic	3%
Inferior mesenteric	<1%

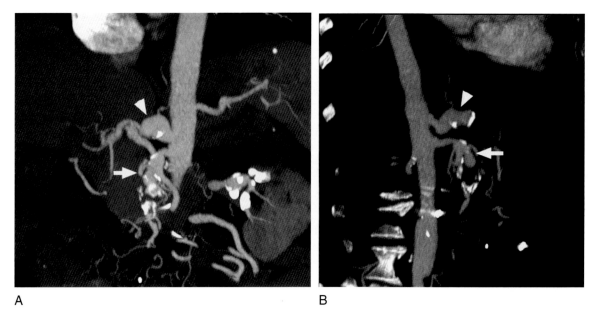

A   B

Figure 27.5 Visceral artery aneurysms: Sagittal oblique MPR (A) and coronal oblique MIP (B) images demonstrate aneurysms of the celiac axis (arrowhead) and superior mesenteric artery (arrow) and multiple visceral branches in this patient with Ehlers-Danlos syndrome.

be secondary to the increased utilization of endovascular procedures.[14]

The role for CTA in the management of this disease process is multifaceted. Obviously the high speed and non-invasive nature of CT makes it an excellent diagnostic tool for detection and surveillance of visceral aneurysms (Figure 27.5). These studies also allow for pretreatment planning, and post-treatment evaluation.

Visceral artery aneurysms are composed of both true aneurysms and pseudoaneurysms, which lack a complete arterial wall. Most visceral aneurysms are degenerative, with loss or fragmentation of the arterial media. Other causes of visceral aneurysms include atherosclerosis, fibromuscular dysplasia and collagen vascular disorders.[15] Pseudoaneurysms often develop as a result of trauma, inflammation, infection or vasculitis (Figure 27.6). Pancreatitis can lead to pseudoaneurysm formation in the splenic, hepatic, gastroduodenal, and pancreaticoduodenal arteries secondary to leakage of pancreatic enzymes.[16]

Both surgical and endovascular options for visceral artery aneurysm treatment are available. Choice of treatment depends in large part on the location of the aneurysm, associated co-morbidities, and local expertise. However, from a treatment planning perspective, it is imperative to exclude the aneurysm from the circulation while maintaining adequate circulatory flow to distal endorgans. The goal of pretreatment imaging is to evaluate the aneurysm size, interval growth, collateral flow, signs of rupture, and location, with particular attention to the relation to branch vessels. Regardless of what methods are employed to treat the aneurysm vigilant post-procedural surveillance is mandatory to exclude reperfusion of the aneurysm.[17]

Splenic artery aneurysms are by far the most common visceral aneurysm. They are four times more common in females than in males. Splenic artery aneurysms also have a strong association with pregnancy, portal hypertension and pancreatitis (Figure 27.7). Most of these aneurysms are small (2–4 cm), asymptomatic, saccular and located in the mid to distal splenic artery. Impending rupture can present with left upper quadrant pain with radiation to the subscapular region. Rupture may be catastrophic, presenting with severe pain, hypotension and often ending in death. In 20–30% of patients, double rupture occurs. The initial rupture is contained within the lesser sac, and subsequently there is free rupture into the peritoneal cavity.[13] Treatment of splenic aneurysms is required in symptomatic patients, following rupture, during pregnancy and in women of childbearing age, as these may rapidly enlarge during a future pregnancy. Furthermore, patients with portal hypertension or liver transplant recipients are candidates for treatment. Finally, rapidly enlarging aneurysms should be considered for treatment. Surgical treatment consists of either artery ligation or aneurysm resection. Endovascular occlusion of the proximal and distal splenic artery, or aneurysm 'trapping', is an excellent

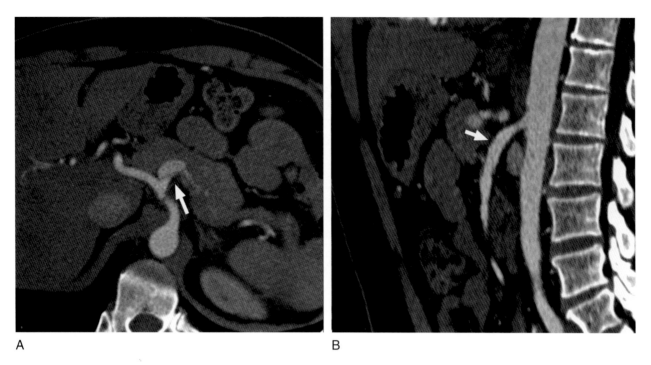

A   B

Figure 27.6   Segmental arterial mediolysis: Axial oblique MPR (A) shows a dissection of the celiac axis extending into the splenic vein (arrow), which is aneurysmally dilated. Sagittal oblique MPR (B) shows a dissection of the superior mesenteric artery (arrow), which is mildly ectatic. Several other visceral dissections and aneurysm formation were also seen in this patient with segmental arterial mediolysis.

minimally invasive alternative for treatment. Post-treatment splenic perfusion occurs via the short gastric and distal pancreatic collaterals.

Hepatic artery aneurysms represent the second to third most common visceral aneurysm. These aneurysms demonstrate a 2:1 male predominance, are most often solitary, and more often located outside the liver

parenchyma. Localization of the hepatic aneurysm suggests the underlying etiology, as extrahepatic aneurysms are most likely the result of degenerative or dysplastic processes. Conversely, intrahepatic aneurysms are usually secondary to trauma, iatrogenic, infection or vasculitis. While hepatic aneurysms may be discovered incidentally, many are symptomatic at presentation secondary to spontaneous rupture.

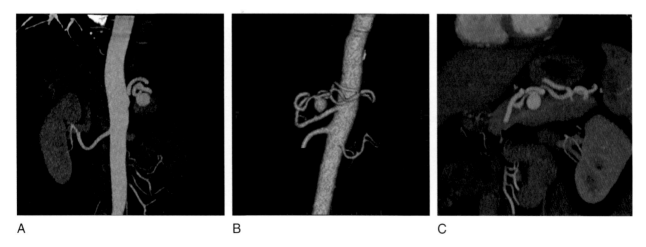

A   B   C

Figure 27.7   Splenic artery aneurysm: Sagittal oblique MPR (A) and volume rendered (B) images demonstrate a saccular aneurysm projecting off the mid splenic artery. Coronal oblique MRP (C) shows how the parenchyma of the pancreas surrounds this aneurysm, which is presumed to be a result of patient's prior pancreatitis.

Quincke's Triad, epigastric pain, hemobilia and obstructive jaundice is present in up to one-third of symptomatic patients. The reported incidence of rupture varies greatly, from 20–80%, and with mortality rates from 20–35%.

Treatment varies by location. Intrahepatic aneurysms, once solely treated by surgical resection, can now be readily treated by endovascular coil occlusion or embolization. Likewise, common hepatic aneurysms can be 'trapped' between distal and proximal coil packs, with distal perfusion supplied via gastroduodenal collateral circulation. Proper hepatic aneurysms were previously treated by surgical ligation and bypass, but recently endovascular treatment utilizing covered stents has gained favor.

2.1.4 Liver transplantation

CT angiography has become invaluable in the preoperative evaluation and planning for liver transplantation. CTA provides valuable information about the hepatic arterial origins and branch pattern, portal vein patency, biliary ductal anatomy, parenchymal integrity, presence or absence of neoplastic lesions, and extrahepatic disease.

The utility of CTA to provide three-dimensional mapping of the arterial and venous systems greatly facilitates preoperative planning in the extremely challenging field of liver related liver donation and identification of subjects with surgical contraindications for harvesting.[18] Of particular importance are the origin and course of the arterial supply to segment IV, the

distance of the segment IV artery to the origin of the right hepatic artery, hepatic and portal vein anatomy, fatty infiltration of the liver parenchyma and potential for insufficient liver volume for paired donor and recipient (Figure 27.8).[19]

In potential transplant recipients, CTA can be invaluable in detection of surgically relevant abnormalities. These include celiac artery stenosis, hepatic artery inflow vessels smaller than 3 mm, splenic artery aneurysms, complete replacement of the hepatic arterial supply to the superior mesenteric artery, and portal vein anomalies.[19]

Furthermore, following transplantation, CTA can be used to evaluate complications including hepatic artery stenosis, pseudoaneurysm or thrombosis, and portal vein thrombosis or stenosis.[18]

2.1.5 Pre and post-oncologic intervention

Primary and metastatic hepatic neoplasms are amenable to a variety of systemic and localized treatments. Multidetector CT plays a vital role in the detection, pretreatment planning, and post-treatment surveillance of these lesions. CTA allows detailed vascular maps for pre-operative planning. Importantly, CTA can show the relationships of the hepatic and portal veins, hepatic arteries and demonstrate tumor invasion of vascular structures.[18]

Transcatheter embolization (TACE) has gained acceptance as a treatment for non-resectable hepatic neoplasms. Triphasic CTA, including non-contrast, late arterial and parenchymal

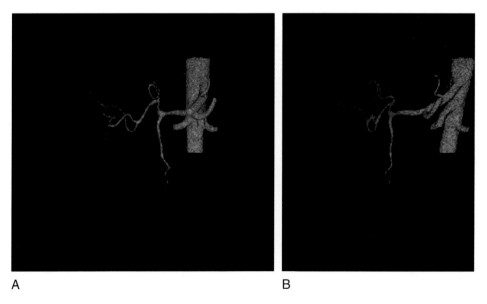

A   B

Figure 27.8   Hepatic donor: Coronal (A) and sagittal oblique (B) volume rendered images of a normal liver for potential donor procedure. Using three-dimensional reformations, liver anatomy can be evaluated and volumetric calculations can be performed.

phase imaging, is performed prior to treatment. This serves as a baseline for treatment planning, and for evaluating treatment success. Following treatment the triphasic CTA is repeated. The non-contrast imaging allows visualization of radioopaque embolic material within the tumor bed and within the hepatic arteries. The arterial phase imaging demonstrates patency of hepatic arterial branches and residual (non-embolized) hypervascular lesions. Lastly, the parenchymal phase imaging allows evaluation of the portal vein patency, and for post-treatment complications such as abscess or necrosis.

3 RENAL CTA

3.1 Clinical applications

3.1.1 Renovascular hypertension

At many institutions, the most common indication for renal CTA is in the evaluation of renovascular hypertension (Figure 27.9). Only 5% of hypertensive patients have an underlying renovascular etiology.[20,21] In those patients with renovascular disease, most are due to atherosclerosis (70%) while fibromuscular dysplasia accounts for another 25%. Given the low incidence of renovascular disease, screening of all hypertensive patients is not practical or justified. Several clinical findings are suggestive of renovascular hypertension, including rapid onset of hypertension, hypertension in a young patient, and sudden deterioration of previously well-controlled hypertension. When present, atherosclerotic renal artery stenosis usually affects the proximal renal artery, most often the ostium.

Conventional teaching is to assess renal artery stenosis by measuring the percent stenosis, just as would be done during catheter angiography (i.e. one minus the ratio of stenotic to normal artery diameters). While this is a simple extrapolation from the two-dimensional world of catheter angiography it may not be the most reproducible or accurate method of analysis. An interesting alternative is cross-sectional area measurements across regions of stenosis. This has been shown to dramatically improve inter-observer variability when compared with simple diameter measurements.[22]

As previously mentioned, the second most common etiology of renovascular disease is fibromuscular dysplasia. Fibromuscular dysplasia (FMD) is a non-inflammatory, non-atherosclerotic vascular disease which most frequently affects women between the ages of 15 and 50 years of age. When present, the distal two-thirds of the main renal artery and its major branch vessels are affected. Fibromuscular dysplasia is classified by the arterial layer, e.g. intima, media or adventitia, which is most involved.[23] The most common form of FMD is medial fibroplasia, accounting for 65–70%

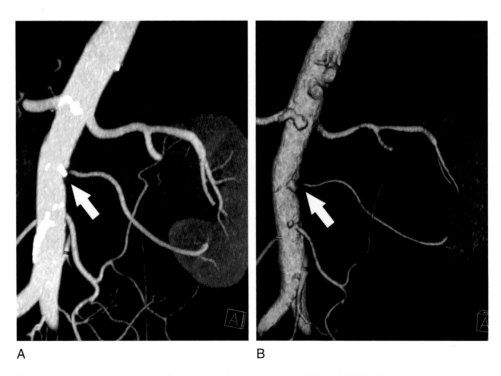

A   B

Figure 27.9   Renal artery stenosis: Coronal oblique volume rendered (A) and MPR (B) images demonstrate osteal stenosis of an inferior accessory left renal artery (arrow).

of cases. It is characterized by the classic 'string of beads' appearance, and may have associated aneurismal dilation present (Figure 27.10). The subadventitial form, which presents with aneurysm formation and by focal stenoses, is the second most common and occurs in 15–20% of cases.[24] Recent work by Sabharwal et al. strongly supports the use of multidetector CTA in the non-invasive evaluation of FMD.[25] The authors used 3D coronal and sagittal MPR, MIP and shaded-surface display reconstructions in the evaluation of the renal vasculature. They found no single reconstruction method was ideal in all situations and report that the three methods are best used in a complimentary manner.[25]

3.1.2 Renal transplantation

End-stage renal disease is increasing at a rate of more than 8% per year. Furthermore, the waiting list for renal transplantation has more than quadrupled in the last 20 years.[26,27] The unrelenting demand for donor organs cannot be sated by cadaveric organs only. Moreover, living donor organs have better graft function and survival when compared to cadaveric grafts.[26] With the move towards living related organ transplantation, and the acceptance of laparoscopic donor nephrectomies, pre-operative imaging has undergone

a significant change as well. The current standard for preoperative imaging is multidetector CT, including CTA, CT venography and CT urography.[28,29]

The left kidney is preferred for laparoscopic living donor nephrectomy because the longer left venous pedicle affords easier removal and implantation.[30] A relative downside to left-sided donor organs is the high frequency of venous variants.[31] Many of these variants, most often lumbar and gonadal veins, anastamose with the renal vein posteriorly, an area which is poorly visualized during laparoscopy. Preoperative imaging that alerts the surgeon to the presence of these variants may help reduce inadvertent ligation or transection of these vessels. This is significant, as transection can lead to significant hemorrhage, sometimes resulting in conversion to an open procedure. Imaging may also detect complex vascular anatomy, leading to the selection of the right kidney for donation in an open procedure. Preoperative imaging may also help detect the less normal kidney, for example, one containing small stones, which is often chosen for donation.[29]

When evaluating studies prior to laparoscopic donor nephectomy, particular attention should be paid to the venous anatomy. Important venous variants detected in a recent series are shown in Table 27.5.[29] Other relevant findings include the number of renal arteries and veins, and the distance from the aorta of the first arterial branch (Figure 27.11).

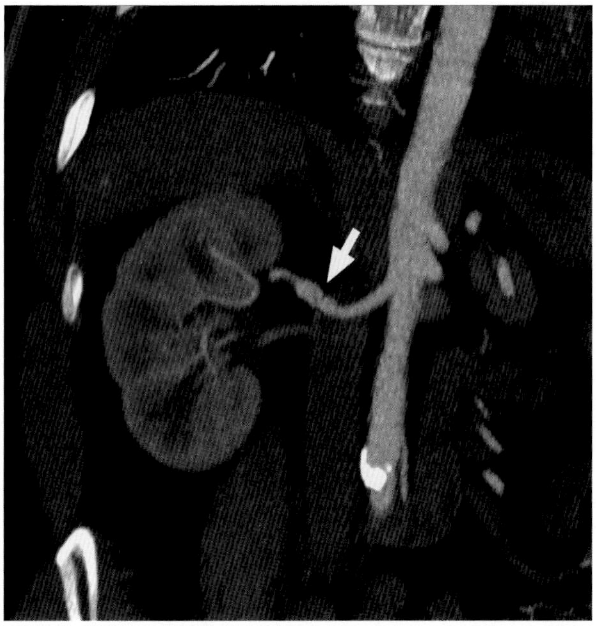

3.1.3 Renal artery aneurysms

Renal CTA is well suited for the evaluation of renal artery aneurysms. These aneurysms are the second most common visceral aneurysm, behind splenic artery aneurysms.[32] Most renal artery aneurysms are asymptomatic. Symptoms may occur in the setting of rupture, embolization to the parenchymal bed or arterial thrombosis. These aneurysms

Figure 27.10 Fibromuscular dysplasia: Coronal oblique MIP image demonstrates characteristic 'beaded' narrowing and dilatation of the mid-distal right main renal artery (arrow), characteristic of fibrous dysplasia.

Table 27.5 Left renal venous anomalies
Major variants
Circumaortic left renal vein
Retroaortic left renal vein
Duplicated inferior vena cava
Minor variants
Prominent gonadal vein
Prominent lumbar vein
Large hemiazygous vein connecting to left renal vein
Splenorenal shunt
Multiple gonadal veins

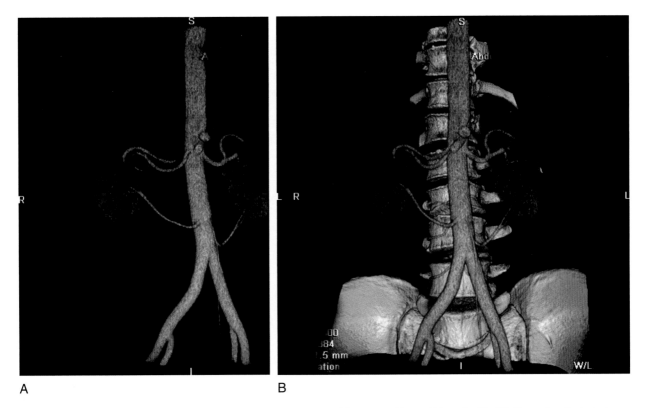

Figure 27.11   Renal donor: Coronal oblique volume rendered images without (A) and with (B) the spine included, performed for potential renal donor procedure, show three right and two left renal arteries.

are associated with hypertension in up to 73% of cases.[33] The pathophysiologic basis for hypertension in the setting of renal artery aneurysm is poorly understood, but may be due to coexisting renal artery stenosis, microembolization from the aneurysm, compression or kinking of the renal artery (leading to functional arterial stenosis) or turbulent flow. Interestingly, improvement in hypertension has been reported following treatment of renal aneurysms.[33] Most renal aneurysms occur at the bifurcation of the main renal artery, and most commonly fibromuscular dysplasia is the underlying etiology. Vasculitides, trauma and degenerative aneurysms are other causes.

Renal CTA plays a vital role in the detection, pretreatment planning, and post-procedural surveillance of renal artery aneurysms. Management is based on patient age, gender, severity of hypertension, pregnancy or anticipation of pregnancy, and anatomic considerations. Young women, especially when anticipating pregnancy, are considered at greatest risk for future rupture. The mortality rate for rupture during pregnancy has been reported at 80%.[34] The surgical literature also supports intervention for aneurysms greater than 2 cm in size, or the setting of rapid aneurysm expansion. Treatment options vary with

anatomic location. Branch vessel aneurysms are most easily treated endovascularly by embolization.[32] Main renal artery aneurysms may be treated surgically by ligation and arterial bypass or nephrectomy.[35] Endovascular management would involve covered stent placement with or without aneurysm embolization.[17]

3.1.4 Renal oncology

Two of the most common renal neoplasms, renal cell carcinoma and angiomyolipomas, are both well evaluated by CTA. Of greatest concern with renal cell carcinoma (RCC) is venous extension, into the renal vein, IVC or beyond. Tumor thrombus is discovered in 4–10% of patients with RCC, and up to half of these patients have extension of thrombus into the intrahepatic IVC or right atrium.[36] The goal of CTA in pretreatment planning is to define the arterial and venous anatomy, extent of vascular involvement by neoplasm, contralateral renal anatomy and disease status. This can usually be accomplished in most cases with arterial phase imaging, followed by one or more delayed phase to evaluate the venous anatomy and possibly the urologic anatomy if partial resection or local ablation is being considered. Arterial phase imaging is crucial for renal mass evaluation as this may detect markedly hypervascular lesions or lesions with marked arterio-venous shunting. These lesions may benefit from preprocedural embolization to decrease bleeding during resection. Additionally, arterial phase imaging will detect contralateral renal artery stenosis, which may be amenable to treatment, thus decreasing the risk of renal insuffiency following tumor resection or nephrectomy.[28] It is important to obtain delayed images with adequate contrast opacification within the venous system in order to assess extent of venous invasion. Precontrast images are also important if the diagnosis of RCC is unresolved prior to obtaining the study. The precontrast imaging allows detection of subtle calcification, and allows accurate determination of tumoral enhancement.

Renal angiomyolipomas (AML) are hamartomatous neoplasms composed of smooth muscle, fat and dysplastic blood vessels in mixed proportions.[37] These benign lesions account for 0.3–3% of renal masses, but have a high propensity for hemorrhage due to the dysplastic vessels within these lesions.[38] Sporadic AMLs occur as solitary lesions, more often in older patients, with a slight female predilection, and account for 70–80% of all AMLs. Conversely, AMLs can also be associated with tuberous sclerosis, and in this setting, tend to be multifocal, larger, bilateral and present at a much earlier age.[39] The risk factors for hemorrhage include size (>4 cm), multifocality and the presence of associated aneurysms. It is important when imaging patients in the setting of renal hemorrhage, or when renal neoplasms are suspected, to obtain precontrast images. Further, in the setting of acute severe hemorrhage, it may not be possible to detect the underlying renal lesion. In these cases, if the patient is stable, repeat imaging after resolution of the hematoma may allow diagnostic evaluation of the lesion.

REFERENCES

1. Boyd AS, Zic JA, Abraham JL. Gadolinium deposition in nephrogenic fibrosing dermopathy. J Am Acad Dermatol 2007; 56(1): 27–30.
2. High WA et al. Gadolinium is detectable within the tissue of patients with nephrogenic systemic fibrosis. J Am Acad Dermatol 2007; 56(1): 21–6.
3. Heys SD, Brittenden J, Crofts TJ. Acute mesenteric ischaemia: the continuing difficulty in early diagnosis. Postgrad Med J 1993; 69(807): 48–51.
4. McKinsey JF, Gewertz BL. Acute mesenteric ischemia. Surg Clin North Am 1997; 77(2): 307–18.
5. Kaleya RN, Boley SJ. Acute mesenteric ischemia: an aggressive diagnostic and therapeutic approach. 1991 Roussel Lecture. Can J Surg 1992; 35(6): 613–23.
6. Horton KM, Fishman EK. 3D CT angiography of the celiac and superior mesenteric arteries with multidetector CT data sets: preliminary observations. Abdom Imaging 2000; 25(5): 523–5.
7. Horton KM, Fishman EK. Multi-detector row CT of mesenteric ischemia: can it be done? Radiographics, 2001; 21(6): 1463–73.
8. Wildermuth S et al. Multislice CT in the pre- and postinterventional evaluation of mesenteric perfusion. Eur Radiol 2005; 15(6): 1203–10.
9. Kirkpatrick ID, Kroeker MA, Greenberg HM. Biphasic CT with mesenteric CT angiography in the evaluation of acute mesenteric ischemia: initial experience. Radiology, 2003; 229(1): 91–8.
10. Shih MC, Hagspiel KD. CTA and MRA in mesenteric ischemia: part 1, Role in diagnosis and differential diagnosis. AJR Am J Roentgenol 2007; 188(2): 452–61.
11. Cognet F et al. Chronic mesenteric ischemia: imaging and percutaneous treatment. Radiographics 2002; 22(4): 863–79; discussion 879–80.
12. Hagspiel KD et al. MR angiography of the mesenteric vasculature. Radiol Clin North Am 2002; 40(4): 867–86.
13. Messina LM, Shanley CJ. Visceral artery aneurysms. Surg Clin North Am 1997; 77(2): 425–42.
14. Shanley CJ, Shah NL, Messina LM. Uncommon splanchnic artery aneurysms: pancreaticoduodenal, gastroduodenal, superior mesenteric, inferior mesenteric, and colic. Ann Vasc Surg 1996; 10(5): 506–15.
15. Hossain A et al. Visceral artery aneurysms: experience in a tertiary-care center. Am Surg 2001; 67(5): 432–7.
16. de Filippi VJ, Vargish T, Block GE. Massive gastrointestinal hemorrhage in pancreatitis secondary to visceral artery aneurysms. Am Surg 1992; 58(10): 618–21.
17. Nosher JL et al. Visceral and renal artery aneurysms: a pictorial essay on endovascular therapy. Radiographics 2006; 26(6): 1687–704; quiz 1687.
18. Guven K, Acunas B. Multidetector computed tomography angiography of the abdomen. Eur J Radiol 2004; 52(1): 44–55.
19. Fleischmann D. Multiple detector-row CT angiography of the renal and mesenteric vessels. Eur J Radiol 2003; 45 Suppl 1: S79–87.
20. Krijnen P et al. A clinical prediction rule for renal artery stenosis. Ann Intern Med 1998; 129(9): 705–11.
21. Safian RD, Textor SC. Renal-artery stenosis. N Engl J Med 2001; 344(6): 431–42.
22. Schoenberg SO et al. High-spatial-resolution MR angiography of renal arteries with integrated parallel acquisitions: comparison with digital subtraction angiography and US. Radiology 2005; 235(2): 687–98.
23. Harrison EG Jr, McCormack LJ. Pathologic classification of renal arterial disease in renovascular hypertension. Mayo Clin Proc 1971; 46(3): 161–7.
24. Stanley JC et al. Arterial fibrodysplasia. Histopathologic character and current etiologic concepts. Arch Surg 1975; 110(5): 561–6.
25. Sabharwal R, Vladica P, Coleman P. Multidetector spiral CT renal angiography in the diagnosis of renal artery fibromuscular dysplasia. Eur J Radiol 2007; 61(3): 520–7.

26. Lind MY, Ijzermans JN, Bonjer HJ. Open vs laparoscopic donor nephrectomy in renal transplantation. BJU Int 2002; 89(2): 162–8.

27. Shaffer D et al. Two hundred one consecutive living-donor nephrectomies. Arch Surg 1998; 133(4): 426–31.

28. Glockner JF, Vrtiska TJ. Renal MR and CT angiography: current concepts. Abdom Imaging 2006.

29. Raman SS et al. Surgically relevant normal and variant renal parenchymal and vascular anatomy in preoperative 16-MDCT evaluation of potential laparoscopic renal donors. AJR Am J Roentgenol 2007; 188(1): 105–14.

30. Jacobs SC et al. Laparoscopic live donor nephrectomy: the University of Maryland 3-year experience. J Urol 2000; 164(5): 1494–9.

31. Satyapal KS et al. Left renal vein variations. Surg Radiol Anat 1999; 21(1): 77–81.

32. Klein GE et al. Endovascular treatment of renal artery aneurysms with conventional non-detachable microcoils and Guglielmi detachable coils. Br J Urol 1997; 79(6): 852–60.

33. Henke PK et al. Renal artery aneurysms: a 35-year clinical experience with 252 aneurysms in 168 patients. Ann Surg 2001; 234(4): 454–62; discussion 462–3.

34. Tham G et al. Renal artery aneurysms. Natural history and prognosis. Ann Surg 1983; 197(3): 348–52.

35. Bruce M, Kuan YM. Endoluminal stent-graft repair of a renal artery aneurysm. J Endovasc Ther 2002; 9(3): 359–62.

36. Kearney GP et al. Results of inferior vena cava resection for renal cell carcinoma. J Urol 1981; 125(6): 769–73.

37. Nelson CP, Sanda MG. Contemporary diagnosis and management of renal angiomyolipoma. J Urol 2002; 168(4 Pt 1): 1315–25.

38. Fujii Y et al. Benign renal tumors detected among healthy adults by abdominal ultrasonography. Eur Urol 1995; 27(2): 124–7.

39. Kang M et al. CT angiography in renal angiomyolipomas. Abdom Imaging 2007.

28

Computed Tomographic Arteriography of the Upper and Lower Extremities

Jeffrey C. Hellinger

I INTRODUCTION

Following the introduction of computed tomographic (CT) angiography in the early 1990s,[1] applications were limited for evaluating the upper and lower extremity vasculature. This was directly related to the length of the complete upper and lower extremity trees and the thin sections required to robustly display the proximal (8–12 mm diameter), mid (5–7 mm diameter), and distal (1.5–4 mm diameter) arteries and veins. Slow scan speeds with single detector-row CT scanners precluded thin section acquisitions in the entire Z-axis of the extremity vascular systems. While CT angiography (CTA) was embraced for aortic, pulmonary, head and neck, mesenteric, and renal peripheral vascular applications, catheter angiography remained the diagnostic modality of choice for the upper and lower extremity vasculature.

Today, however, after nearly two decades of technological advancements, CTA is rapidly becoming a first line angiographic modality for the upper and lower extremities. The greatest influence on this practice change has been multidetector-row CT technology.[2] Submillimeter section thickness and subsecond rotations times are now routinely possible, affording high and isotropic resolution acquisitions with homogenous intravascular enhancement throughout the required 700 to 1400 mm coverage.

Current applications of upper and lower extremity CTA include arterial occlusive disease, vasculitis, trauma, venous occlusive disease, vascular masses, vascular mapping, and dysfunctional hemodialysis fistulas and grafts. Despite the inherent radiation and contrast medium exposures, CTA has important advantages for patients in these clinical settings. CTA is non-invasive, has relatively low cost, is readily available, and is acquired rapidly. Furthermore, CTA is a three-dimensional (3D) acquisition, has excellent spatial detail, and affords simultaneous evaluation of other cardiovascular territories as well as non-cardiovascular systems. These advantages are essential when designing a diagnostic or screening algorithm.

As with all CTA, clinical success of extremity CTA is dependent on technical and interpretative success. From technical and interpretative perspectives, upper and lower extremity CT angiograms remain the most challenging. Synchronizing a large scan acquisition and a single bolus of contrast medium requires the precise selection of acquisition and contrast medium delivery parameters. To minimize radiation exposure and contrast medium dose and to avoid multiple acquisitions, fundamental knowledge of strategies which optimize vessel depiction is paramount. Equally important is the ability to adeptly use various 3D workstation visualization techniques for efficient and effective image display and interpretation. Developing a logical methodology to evaluate the vascular segments and the array of imaged non-vascular anatomical structures is essential.

The purpose of the first section of this chapter is to address these technical considerations and discuss strategies

Table 28.1   Upper extremity CT angiography protocols

Protocol	Coverage	Distance	Application
Aortic arch with runoff	Arterial inflow and outflow	700–1000 mm	Arterial occlusive disease Arterial bypass grafts and stents Vasculitis Trauma Vascular masses Vascular mapping Hemodialysis access
Upper extremity runoff	Targeted arterial outflow	300–600 mm	Trauma Vascular masses Vascular mapping
Indirect venogram	Peripheral and central veins		Veno-occlusive disease
	Targeted	400–700 mm	Vascular mapping
	Complete	700–1000 mm	Venous stents

which afford robust upper and lower extremity CTA. The second section of the chapter will discuss and illustrate clinical applications for upper and lower extremity CTA.

2 EXTREMITY CTA TECHNIQUE

Upper and lower extremity CT angiography can be performed on all currently available multidetector-row CT scanners (4–64 channels). Depending on the clinical indications, three protocols are recommended for imaging the upper (Table 28.1) or lower (Table 28.2) extremity vascular tree: *Aortic Arch* (upper extremity) *or Aortogram* (lower extremity) *with Extremity Runoff; Extremity Runoff; and*

Extremity Indirect CT Venography. Technical considerations for each protocol include patient preparation, image acquisition, contrast medium administration, and image display.

3 PATIENT PREPARATION

Initial patient preparation entails removing all external metallic objects from the anticipated field of view and placing an 18–22 gauge intravenous catheter in an upper extremity vein. For pediatric patients, only 24 gauge catheters may be possible. With upper extremity exams, the catheter is placed in the extremity opposite to the effected side. The final preparation is to position the patient on the CT gantry table with

Table 28.2   Lower extremity CT angiography protocols

Protocol	Coverage	Distance	Application
Abdominal aortogram with runoff	Arterial inflow and outflow	900–1400 mm	Arterial occlusive disease Arterial bypass grafts and stents Vasculitis Trauma Vascular masses Vascular mapping Hemodialysis access
Lower extremity runoff	Arterial outflow	500–800 mm	Trauma Vascular masses Vascular mapping
Indirect venogram	Peripheral and central veins		Veno-occlusive disease
	Targeted	600–900 mm	Vascular mapping
	Complete	900–1400 mm	Venous stents

the extremity as close to isocenter as possible. Pillows, blankets, or both can be utilized to support the patient's body and extremity, while tape can be used to secure positioning of the extremity, including the hand or foot.

Upper extremity patients are positioned supine or prone and head first into the scanner (Figure 28.1). With unilateral

upper extremity exams, isocenter positioning is achieved by extending the upper extremity above the patient's head. The palm is placed ventral when supine and dorsal when prone. The contralateral arm is placed at the patient's side. To optimize isocenter positioning, patients can be rotated into a modified swimmer's position. If the affected extremity can not

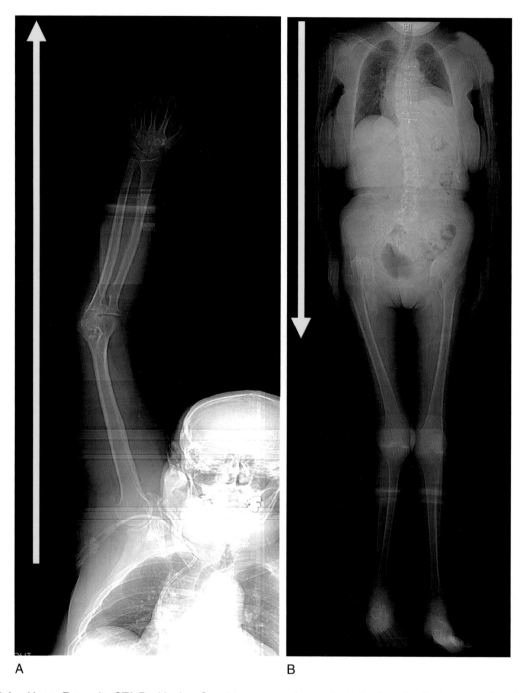

A   B

Figure 28.1   *Upper Extremity CTA Positioning* Scout topograms demonstrate the two standard upper extremity positions for performing upper extremity CT angiography. Depending upon the body habitus and upper extremity mobility, the position of choice is to raise the affected upper extremity above the patient's head (A). The patient's body is placed in a supine, prone, or oblique position and the contralateral upper extremity is placed at the patient's side. Scan direction is caudad-cranial, extending through to the fingers (yellow arrow). If the affected upper extremity can not be raised, it is placed at the patient's side and the contralateral upper extremity is either raised or also placed at the patient's side (B). Scan direction is cranial-caudad (yellow arrow).

be raised above the patient's head, the exam can be performed with the extremity placed along side the patient's body (Figure 28.1). For these cases, the patient's body should be shifted away from the affected extremity. Bilateral upper extremity exams are acquired by scanning each arm either simultaneously (targeted runoff) or by scanning each arm individually (16–64 channel scanners). Bilateral simultaneous upper extremity CT angiograms are best achieved with patients either prone with the arms extended or supine with arms at the patient's side.

Lower extremity patients are positioned supine and feet first into the scanner (Figure 28.2). With unilateral lower extremity exams, the affected lower extremity is placed isocenter by shifting the patient's torso and contralateral lower extremity away from the affected extremity. Bilateral lower extremity CT angiograms are obtained with both extremities placed symmetrically in the gantry isocenter.

4 IMAGE ACQUISITION

4.1 Protocol series

Upper and lower extremity CT angiographic protocols include at least five acquisition series. The first series is the required low dose anterior-posterior scout topogram through the entire regions of interest. For precise coverage and field of view, a lateral view may be required. The second series is an optional non-enhanced acquisition (1.25–5.0 mm thick images). Coverage may be identical to the planned contrast enhanced acquisition or may target a selected region. The objective of the non-enhanced acquisition is to identify high density material. Such material may degrade CTA image quality and interpretation or may itself be obscured by the contrast medium. Vascular calcifications, endovascular stents and stent-grafts, surgical clips, surgical grafts, catheters, bone fragments (i.e. trauma), residual intravenous contrast, active bleeding, and hematomas should be addressed. The third series is a low dose timing acquisition, which is essential for precise synchronization of the image acquisition with either arterial or venous enhancement. Scan timing is determined either with a timing bolus acquisition or bolus tracking software. The fourth series consists of the contrast enhanced angiographic acquisition. Depending on the patient's weight, a tube voltage of 80–120 kV is used along with an amperage of 80–350 mA, unless automated tube current modulation software is utilized. Breath-holding is required only for the portions of

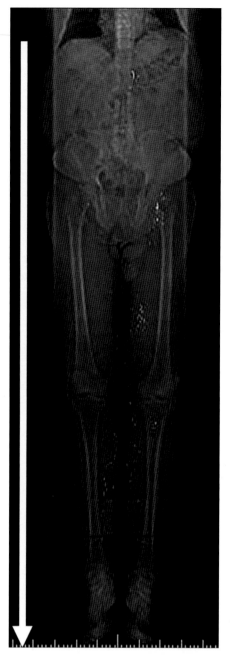

Figure 28.2 *Lower Extremity CTA Positioning* Scout topogram for a lower extremity CT angiogram demonstrates standard lower extremity positioning. Patients are placed supine and feet first into the scanner. Scan direction is cranial-caudad, extending through to the toes (yellow arrow). If imaging is only required through one lower extremity, the affected lower extremity is placed isocenter and the contralateral lower extremity is placed at the periphery of the field of view.

exams which extend through the chest (upper extremity) or abdomen and pelvis (lower extremity). Images are reconstructed with a soft kernel. The fifth series is an optional delayed post-contrast acquisition. The delayed acquisition is useful in assessment of vasculitis, vascular masses, and hemorrhage. It can also be used to acquire a venous phase following an arterial acquisition. Additionally, if the scan acquisition in the fourth series precedes the arrival of contrast medium in the distal extremity, an immediate delayed phase may be helpful to obtain adequately enhanced images through to the hand or foot.

4.2 Extremity CT angiogram

4.2.1 Upper extremity coverage

In the *Aortic Arch with Upper Extremity Runoff* protocol, when the arm is raised, coverage begins at the mid chest to include the aortic arch, and extends in a caudadcranial direction through the fingers, so that the complete inflow and outflow upper extremity vascular tree is evaluated. For an average adult patient, this scan distance may be 700–1000 mm. If the arm is placed at the patient's side, coverage begins at the thoracic inlet and extends through the fingers in a cranialcaudad direction. In the *Upper Extremity Runoff* protocol, outflow segments are targeted. Coverage begins at the shoulder or elbow and extends through to the fingers, in a caudadcranial or cranialcaudad direction, depending on the position of the upper extremity. The scan distance may range between 300 and 600 mm. For both protocols, a delayed acquisition may be programmed to cover the entire vascular tree or only the outflow. If the series is utilized because contrast did not adequately opacify the forearm and hand arteries on the first acquisition, the acquisition begins at the elbow. For the *Upper Extremity Indirect CT Venogram* protocol, central and peripheral veins are evaluated. The arm may be raised or placed at the patient's side, with the acquisition in either a caudadcranial or cranialcaudad direction, respectively. When the arm is raised, coverage begins at the mid chest to include the cavoatrial junction. When the arm is at the patient's side, coverage begins at the thoracic inlet. Depending on the clinical indications, coverage may extend either to the elbow (400–700 mm scan distance) or the hand (700–1000 mm scan distance).

4.2.2 Lower extremity coverage

In the *Abdominal Aortogram with Lower Extremity Runoff* protocol, inflow and outflow arterial segments are imaged. Coverage begins at the diaphragm and extends through to the feet, in a cranialcaudad direction. For an adult patient, the scan distance may be 900–1400 mm. In the *Lower Extremity Runoff* protocol, outflow segments are targeted. Coverage begins just above the hip or the knee and extends through to the toes, in a cranialcaudad direction. The scan distance may range between 500 and 800 mm. For both protocols, a delayed acquisition may be programmed to cover the entire lower extremity vascular tree or only the outflow. If the series is utilized because contrast did not adequately opacify the calf and foot arteries on the first acquisition, coverage begins at the knee and extends to the foot. For the *Lower Extremity Indirect CT Venogram* protocol, peripheral and central veins are evaluated. Targeted coverage (600–900 mm) begins at the popliteal fossa and extends caudadcranially to the suprarenal inferior vena cava. Imaging of the calf veins is not routinely performed.

4.2.3 Acquisition parameters

Table 28.3 lists acquisition (detector configuration, pitch, gantry speed) and reconstruction (slice thickness, reconstruction interval) parameters for upper and lower extremity CT angiograms, using 4-, 8-, 16-, and 64-channel multidetector-row CT scanners. These parameters reflect a balance between the desired spatial resolution, the scan distance, and the scan duration. Parameters for 32- and 40-channel scanners can be adapted from 64-channel scanners.

With 4-channel systems, to scan the complete upper or lower extremity territory in a reasonable duration, a 4 × 2.5 mm detector configuration is required. 2.5 mm images are reconstructed at 1.0–2.0 mm increments, resulting in an effective slice thickness of 3.0 mm. These 'standard resolution' acquisitions are adequate to depict the vascular tree through to the hand or foot. However, when visualization of small palmar or pedal arteries is critical to diagnosis and clinical management, such as in arterial occlusive disease and vasculitis, high resolution imaging with a 4 × 1 mm or 4 × 1.25 mm configuration may be necessary. As the scan duration would be twice as long, the coverage would need to be reduced to minimize venous contamination.

With an 8-channel system, complete extremity vascular trees are imaged with a high resolution technique (8 × 1.25 mm configuration) in a duration comparable to 4 × 2.5 mm acquisitions. Datasets are reconstructed every 0.8 mm into images with a nominal section thickness of 1.25 mm. Coverage can be extended beyond an upper or lower extremity vascular tree by using the fastest gantry speed and maximizing the pitch. To minimize venous contamination, increasing the detector width to 2.5 mm (standard resolution) may be necessary.

Table 28.3 Upper and lower extremity CTA acquisition and reconstruction parameters

MDCT scanner	Mode	Detector configuration (channels × mm)	Pitch	Gantry rotation Time (sec)	Table speed (mm/sec)	Scan time (sec)	Slice thickness (mm)	RI (mm)	Number of images
4-Channel									
GE	SR	4 × 2.5	1.5	0.5	30	30	2.5	1.5	600
Phillips	SR	4 × 2.5	1.5	0.5	30	30	2.5	1.5	600
Siemens	SR	4 × 2.5	1.5	0.5	30	30	2.5	1.5	600
Toshiba	SR	4 × 2.0	1.375	0.5	22	41	2	1.0	900
8-Channel									
GE	HR	8 × 1.25	1.35	0.5	27	33	1.25	0.8	1125
GE	SR	8 × 2.5	1.35	0.5	54	17	2.5	1.5	600
16-Channel									
GE	IR	16 × 0.625	1.375	0.5	28	33	0.625	0.5	1800
Phillips	IR	16 × 0.75	1.25	0.5	30	30	0.75	0.5	1800
Siemens	IR	16 × 0.75	1.2	0.5	29	31	0.75	0.5	1800
Toshiba	IR	16 × 0.5	1.438	0.5	23	39	0.5	0.4	2250
GE	HR	16 × 1.25	1.375	0.5	55	16	1.25	0.8	1125
Phillips	HR	16 × 1.5	1.25	0.5	60	15	1.5	0.8	1125
Siemens	HR	16 × 1.5	1.2	0.5	58	16	1.5	0.8	1125
Toshiba	HR	16 × 1.0	1.438	0.5	46	20	1.0	0.8	1125
64-Channel									
GE	IR	64 × 0.625	0.563	0.7	32	28	0.625	0.5	1800
Siemens	IR	(2) × 32 0.6	0.75	0.5	29	31	0.75	0.5	1800
GE	HR	32 × 1.25	0.938	0.6	63	14	1.25	0.8	1125
Siemens	HR	24 × 1.2	1.2	0.5	69	13	1.5	0.8	1125

Note: Scan times for a distance of 900 mm. SR = Standard resolution; HR = High Resolution; IR = Isotropic resolution; RI = reconstruction interval. Acquisition parameters: detector configuration, pitch, and gantry rotation speed. Reconstruction parameters: slice thickness and reconstruction interval.

With 16-channel systems, isotropic resolution and high resolution modes are utilized. Isotropic exams are acquired with submillimeter collimations (16 × 0.625 mm, 16 × 0.75 mm configurations). These acquisitions further improve visualization of small vessels, such as palmar and pedal arteries. Datasets are generated in a duration similar to 4 × 2.5 mm and 8 × 1.25 mm acquisitions. One of the challenges using this mode is the potential for increased noise and the subsequent need for increasing the amperage, if automated tube current modulation is not utilized. Another challenge is the number of images. Reconstructed at 0.4–0.8 mm increments, up to 3500 images may be generated. A solution to both of these problems is to reconstruct images thicker into 1.0–1.5 mm thick images (high resolution).

For most upper and lower extremity CTA 16-channel applications, the high resolution mode (16 × 1.25 mm or 16 × 1.5 mm configurations) provides adequate detail. However, the table speed is often too fast for contrast medium transit in the upper or lower extremity vascular tree. The result is that the scanner can potentially out-run the bolus. One solution to avoid this pitfall is to slow the acquisition speed by using a lower pitch, by decreasing the gantry rotation speed, or both. A second solution is to slow the scan by acquiring the study with submillimeter collimation. In this instance, the dataset is then reconstructed thicker into 1.0–1.5 mm thick images. A third solution is to lengthen the delay prior to initiating the scan. With a 16-channel system, the increased table speed can be utilized to combine imaging of the extremity vascular trees and other vascular territories in a single acquisition using a high resolution technique.

With a 64-channel system, both isotropic (64 × 0.625 mm, 64 × 0.6 mm configurations) and high resolution (32 × 1.25 mm, 24 × 1.2 mm configurations) modes can also be selected. When using either mode, the table speed is substantially faster than with 16-channel systems. To optimize vascular enhancement through to the digital vessels, it is essential to slow the acquisition speed. Submillimeter collimation, a low pitch, and a slower gantry speed are all options to achieve this goal. With the submillimeter acquisitions, raw data can be reconstructed into high resolution datasets (section thickness 1.0–1.5 mm, reconstruction interval 0.7–0.8 mm), isotropic resolution datasets (section thickness 0.6–0.9 mm, reconstruction interval 0.4–0.7 mm) or both. Automated tube current modulation should be utilized with all isotropic acquisitions to minimize noise and amperage and voltage requirements. Based upon the scan length and duration, an isotropic or a high resolution technique can be prescribed to image not only through the extremity tree, but other vascular territories.

4.3 Exam transfer and storage

Depending on the volume coverage, slice thickness, and reconstruction interval, upper and lower extremity CT angiograms can generate large studies, with up to 2,500 to 3,000 images and 2–3 gigabytes of data. The exam is transferred to and viewed and stored either on a Picture Archiving and Communication System (PACS), a workstation, or both. Solutions to reduce the archived file size include reconstruction of thicker axial images (2.0–2.5 mm) and generation of thin section coronal and sagittal reformations (100–200 images).

5 CONTRAST MEDIUM ADMINISTRATION

Arterial enhancement in upper and lower extremity CT arteriograms should reach at least a minimum of 250–300 Hounsfield Units (HU), while venous enhancement for indirect extremity venograms should be in the range of 120–200 HU. Achieving this enhancement is dependent on synchronizing the acquisition and the delivery of an appropriate amount of iodine. The recommended amount of iodine (iodine dose) is 400–600 mg Iodine per kilogram (1.3–2.0 ml/kg for 300 mg Iodine/ml concentration). For patients who weigh between 60 and 90kg, the iodine should be delivered at a rate (iodine flux) of 1.0–1.5g Iodine per second (3.3–5 ml/sec for 300 mg Iodine/ml concentration). Injection protocols for adult and pediatric upper and lower extremity CT angiograms can achieve these requirements by adjusting the contrast medium concentration (300–370 mg Iodine per milliliter), injection rate (0.7–6ml/second), injection volume (6–150 ml), injection duration, or a combination of these parameters based upon a patient's body weight, the scan distance, and the speed of the scanner.[3]

6 STRATEGIES FOR CONTRAST MEDIUM ADMINISTRATION

6.1 Synchronization

To account for the variable time for contrast medium to travel from the site of intravenous injection to the upper or lower extremity vascular tree, it is necessary to determine the transit time using either a *test-bolus injection* or *automatic bolus triggering*. For complete upper or lower extremity arterial coverage, the aortic arch (upper extremity) or the mid abdominal aorta (lower extremity) serve as reference levels. For targeted extremity runoffs, a proximal outflow artery is used as the reference level. In this instance, automated triggering should be used given the smaller vessel size (3–5 mm).

An indirect extremity CT venogram is obtained after determining the arrival time of contrast to the aortic arch (upper extremity) or the abdominal aorta (lower extremity). An upper extremity venogram is then acquired after an additional 50 second diagnostic delay, while a lower extremity venogram is acquired after a 120–160 second delay.

6.2 Injection parameters

When scanning through complete inflow and outflow territories, an adult upper extremity CT angiogram may cover 700–1000 mm, while a lower extremity CT angiogram may extend over 900 to 1,400 mm. Targeted runoff exams may cover 300–600 mm and 500–800 mm for upper and lower extremity exams, respectively. The key to successful vascular enhancement over these distances is not 'out-running' the contrast bolus. Maintaining optimized enhancement throughout the scan acquisition is best achieved when the CT table speed does not exceed 30 mm/sec.[4] This translates to scan durations of approximately 25–35 seconds and 30–45 seconds for complete upper and lower extremity CT angiograms, and approximately 10–20 seconds and 15–25 seconds for targeted upper and lower extremity CT angiograms, respectively. With this principle in mind, upper and lower extremity injection protocols can be designed based upon slow (≤30mm/second table speed) and fast (>30mm/second) acquisitions.

Slow acquisitions occur with 4 × 2.5 mm, 8 × 1.25 mm, or 16 × 0.625 mm configurations (Table 28.4). In addition, a 64 × 0.6 mm or 64 × 0.625 mm configuration with a low pitch (≤0.8) and slower gantry speed (≥0.5) produces a table speed around 30 mm/sec. With these acquisitions, when the

Table 28.4   Injection protocols for extremity CTA with MDCT table speed ≤30mm/sec

Weight (Kg)	Scan delay (s)	Iodine dose‡ (grams)	Iodine flux (g @ g/s)	300mg I / ml CM Volume (ml)	300mg I / ml CM Biphasic injection (ml @ ml/s)	350mg I / ml CM Volume (ml)	350mg I / ml CM Biphasic injection (ml @ ml/s)	370mg I / ml CM Volume (ml)	370mg I / ml CM Biphasic injection (ml @ ml/s)
51–60	t_{CMT}+2–8*	27.5	5.5 @ 1.1 22 @ 1.0	92	18 @ 3.7 73 @ 3.2	79	16 @ 3.1 63 @ 2.7	74	15 @ 3.0 59 @ 2.6
61–70	t_{CMT}+2–8*	32.5	6.5 @ 1.3 26 @ 1.1	108	22 @ 4.3 87 @ 3.8	93	19 @ 3.7 74 @ 3.2	88	18 @ 3.5 70 @ 3.1
71–80	t_{CMT}+2–8*	37.5	7.5 @ 1.5 30 @ 1.3	125	25 @ 5.0 100 @ 4.3	107	21 @ 4.3 86 @ 3.7	101	20 @ 4.1 81 @ 3.5
81–90	t_{CMT}+2–8*	42.5	8.5 @ 1.7 34 @ 1.5	142	28 @ 5.7 113 @ 4.9	121	24 @ 4.9 97 @ 4.2	115	23 @ 4.6 92 @ 4.0
91–100	t_{CMT}+2–8*	47.5	9.5 @ 1.9 38 @ 1.7	158	32 @ 6.3 127 @ 5.5	136	27 @ 5.4 109 @ 4.7	128	26 @ 5.1 103 @ 4.5
101–110	t_{CMT}+2–8*	52.5	11 @ 2.1 42 @ 1.8	175	35 @ 7.0 140 @ 6.1	150	30 @ 6.0 120 @ 5.2	142	28 @ 5.7 114 @ 4.9
111–120	t_{CMT}+2–8*	57.5	12 @ 2.3 46 @ 2.0	192	38 @ 7.7 153 @ 6.7	164	33 @ 6.6 131 @ 5.7	155	31 @ 6.2 124 @ 5.4

Note: Injection protocols presented are for an average scan distance of 900 mm and a table speed of ≤30 mm/sec. The injection duration is programmed to equal the scan duration. The delay is established by automated triggering or a timing bolus. *When automated triggering is used, the overall scan delay and injection duration are increased by a value equivalent to the inherent delay (i.e. 2–8 sec). The iodine dose (500 mgI/kg) and flux are optimized by adjusting the injection rate and volume. Both vary according to the concentration of the contrast medium. A biphasic injection is utilized, with 20% of the contrast volume administered over the first 5 seconds and 80% administered over the remaining acquisition time. If the injection rate exceeds the tolerable limit for the venous access site, the concentration and/or the injection duration along with the diagnostic delay can be increased. For patients ≤50kg or ≥121kg, the rate and volume are further decreased or increased, respectively. Saline flush is always utilized.

t_{CMT} = contrast medium transit time.

‡ = Average.

CM = Contrast medium.

scan duration is ≥25 seconds, the injection duration is set to equal the scan duration. A biphasic injection protocol is utilized, rather than a uniphasic injection, as the biphasic injection achieves more uniform enhancement for long injection durations (≥25 seconds). The injection rates and volumes for both phases vary according to the body weight and the contrast medium concentration. In the first phase, 20% of the total volume is administered at a higher rate (4–6 ml/s for 60–90 kg patients) over a short duration (i.e. 5 seconds). In the second, the remaining volume is infused at a second, slower injection rate (3–5 ml/s for 60–90 kg patients) for the duration of the examination. If automated triggering is used, the injection duration is extended to account for the inherent delay with this software (2–8 seconds).

When the coverage is targeted to the runoff segments and the table speed ≤ 30 mm/sec, in most acquisitions the injection duration is also set to equal the scan duration. A uniphasic injection is appropriate for the shorter injection duration. An injection rate is derived by determining the patient's appropriate contrast volume for the selected contrast medium concentration and dividing this amount by the injection duration. If the injection rate exceeds the tolerable limit for the accessed vein, the iodine concentration, the injection duration, or both should be increased. If the injection duration is increased, the diagnostic delay should be increased by the same amount.

Fast acquisitions occur with 8 × 2.5 mm, 16 × 1.25 mm, and 16 × 1.5 mm configurations (Table 28.5). With a 64-channel system, a collimation greater than 1.0 (32 × 1.25 mm, 24 × 1.2 mm configurations), a high pitch (>1.0), and a fast gantry speed (<0.5) will routinely result in fast acquisitions. These scan parameters translate into table speeds of 45–70 mm/sec. For upper or lower extremity complete coverage, if the injection duration is set to equal the scan duration, an insufficient iodine dose may be delivered and the scan acquisition may be too fast for the required transit time through the extremity vascular tree. The solution is to use a fixed biphasic injection and increase the scan delay such that the scan and injection durations end simultaneously. For a targeted extremity exam, a fixed uniphasic injection is

Table 28.5   Injection protocols for extremity CTA with MDCT table speed >30mm/sec

Scan time (s)	Scan delay (s)	Iodine dose (grams)	Iodine flux (g @ g/s)	300 mg I / ml CM		350 mg I / ml CM		370 mg I / ml CM	
				Volume (ml)	Biphasic injection (ml @ ml/s)	Volume (ml)	Biphasic injection (ml @ ml/s)	Volume (ml)	Biphasic injection (ml @ ml/s)
30	t_{CMT}	35	7 @ 1.4	117	23 @ 4.7	100	20 @ 4.0	95	19 @ 3.8
			28 @ 1.1		93 @ 3.7		80 @ 3.2		76 @ 3.0
24	t_{CMT}+6*	35	7 @ 1.4	117	23 @ 4.7	100	20 @ 4.0	95	19 @ 3.8
			28 @ 1.1		93 @ 3.7		80 @ 3.2		76 @ 3.0
20	t_{CMT}+10*	35	7 @ 1.4	117	23 @ 4.7	100	20 @ 4.0	95	19 @ 3.8
			28 @ 1.1		93 @ 3.7		80 @ 3.2		76 @ 3.0
16	t_{CMT}+14*	35	7 @ 1.4	117	23 @ 4.7	100	20 @ 4.0	95	19 @ 3.8
			28 @ 1.1		93 @ 3.7		80 @ 3.2		76 @ 3.0
12	t_{CMT}+16*	35	7 @ 1.4	117	23 @ 4.7	100	20 @ 4.0	95	19 @ 3.8
			28 @ 1.1		93 @ 3.7		80 @ 3.2		76 @ 3.0

Note: Injection parameters are for an average scan distance of 900 mm and a table speed of >30 mm. A biphasic protocol with a total injection duration of 30 seconds is required to achieve robust enhancement,. Contrast medium transit time is established with automated triggering or bolus timing. *A diagnostic delay is added to the beginning of the scan duration, so that the delivery of contrast medium and the scan acquisition end together. If automated triggering is used, the diagnostic delay will be reduced by an amount equal to the inherent delay (2–8 seconds). Higher concentration contrast medium affords reduced injection rates and volumes. Saline flush is always used.

selected and the scan delay is similarly increased. To attain the required iodine dose, the injection rate and concentration are varied according to the body weight. If the delay is too long (>15 seconds), unwarranted venous opacification in the inflow and outflow regions may result. In this instance the table speed should be slowed down.

6.3 Saline flush

Saline flush is administered with a dual-chamber injector immediately following the contrast medium infusion. The saline injection improves contrast utilization and reduces perivenous streaks artifacts. Depending on the patient's body size, a small volume (10–50 milliliters) is injected at a rate equal to the contrast medium injection rate. If a biphasic contrast medium protocol is utilized, the saline injection rate defaults to the second injection rate.

7 IMAGE DISPLAY

Interpretation and communication of an upper or lower extremity CTA requires efficient and effective image display. Two (2D) and three dimensional visualization techniques are fundamental and necessitate the use of an advanced 3D workstation. Each technique has advantages and disadvantages, which impact whether a technique is used for vessel overview or analysis. The quality of all post-rocessed images is inherently dependent on acquisition technique and the degree of contrast enhancement.

7.1 Visualization techniques

There are four principle visualization techniques for displaying upper and lower extremity vasculature (Table 28.6): maximum intensity projection (MIP), volume rendering (VR), multiplanar reformations (MPR), and curved planar reformations (CPR). Their interactive use forms the basis for real time interpretation. Generation of protocol-driven static post-processed images aids review of the source images and coronal, sagittal, and oblique reformations. With all techniques, flexible angiographic window and level settings are used. This includes a wide window setting for vascular calcification, high contrast attenuation, or both.

7.1.1 Vessel tree overview

MIP and VR provide angiographic displays of the upper and lower extremity vasculature (Figure 28.3). Either can

Table 28.6   Visualization techniques

	Display	Principle use	Advantages	Disadvantages
MIP	2D	• Angiographic overview	• 'Slice' through dataset in transverse, coronal, sagittal, and oblique projections • Depict small caliber vessels • Depict poorly enhancing vessels • Communicate findings	• Vessel, bone, visceral overlap • Limited stent lumen evaluation • Limited by heavy calcium
VR	3D	• Angiographic overview	• 'Slice' through dataset in transverse, coronal, sagittal, and oblique projections • Structural overview • Spatial perception • Communicate findings	• Opacity-transfer function dependent
MPR	2D	• Vessel analysis • Structure • Flow lumen • Vessel wall	• 'Slice' through dataset in transverse, coronal, sagittal, and oblique projections • Accurate display of stenoses, occlusions, calcification, stents	• Limited spatial perception
CPR	2D	• Vessel analysis • Flow lumen • Vessel wall	• Complete longitudinal vessel cross sectional display • Accurate display of stenoses, occlusions, calcification, stents	• Operator dependent

2D = two dimensional, 3D = three dimensional.

be used to rapidly formulate a structural overview and determine the location of vascular abnormalities. Compared to MIP, VR offers a more comprehensive means to display the upper or lower extremity vasculature and relationships with extravascular structures. Both techniques are dependent on pre-rendering editing to remove bone and other anatomical structures which may obscure visualization of the extremity vasculature. Alternatively, variable sliding thin-slabs or cut-planes can be utilized with interactive rotation, magnification, and window and level settings.

MPRs with coronal, sagittal, and oblique projections provide limited overview of the upper or lower extremity vascular segments. MPR requires stepping through each image and since vessels curve in and out of the planes, standard MPRs can not display an entire vascular segment in one image. The solution is to generate longitudinal cross-sectional 2D CPR static or rotational displays by drawing a center line through the vessel lumen on the axial, coronal, or sagittal images (Figure 28.4). An alternative means to improving the spatial perception of MPR is to apply a thick slab (thick MPR) (Figure 28.4).

7.1.2 Vessel analysis

MPR and CPR technique are more suited for detailed evaluation of vascular segments. Analysis of transverse MPR

cross sections, CPR cross sections, or both is performed through each suspected region of abnormality. These techniques are fundamental for assessing calcified and non-calcified atheromatous plaque, vessel wall thickening, lumen patency, and stent patency. MIP and VR techniques are limited in this evaluation, particularly with diffuse vessel wall calcification. Orthogonal (coronal and sagittal) CPR views are necessary as eccentric lesions may not be accurately depicted in one view alone.

7.2 Source images

Source image review is important for verifying image quality, confirming vascular findings, and assessing non-vascular anatomy. Review of the axial source images is facilitated by generating 2.5–5 mm thick reconstructions. Alternatively coronal and sagittal reformations (1.5–2.0 mm thickness) can be used. The ability to evaluate non-vascular anatomy allows an extremity CTA to be used as complete 'one-stop shop' modality. Relevant non-vascular structures can be assessed with the same bolus of contrast medium. This includes the kidneys and extremity soft tissues and muscles, for signs of ischemia. As the volume coverage includes multiple organ systems, interpretation should also address pathology in unrelated, but, nonetheless depicted organs.

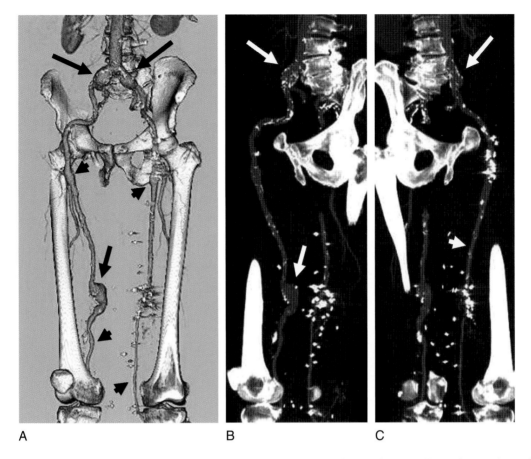

A B C

Figure 28.3 *Angiographic Displays* 64-channel CT angiography was performed for surveillance in a patient with known iliac aneurysms and peripheral atherosclerotic disease, s/p bilateral femoral – popliteal interposition bypass. Volume rendering (A, VR) provides a robust display of the vascular tree, demonstrating bilateral common iliac aneurysms (large arrows) and femoral – popliteal grafts (arrow heads). Note the bilateral proximal graft anastomotic ectasia and the mid right graft aneurysmal formation (small arrow). Maximum intensity projections (MIP) can also be used for angiographic display. MIPs offer the added benefit to localize the extent of vascular calcifications (B). With both VR and MIP, pre-processing editing is often required to remove overlapping structures (i.e. bone, devices). Alternatively, thin-slabs can be applied with VR and MIP. As used in this case, thin-slab MIP through the proximal right lower extremity (B) is targeted to display the right iliac system through the distal graft, again demonstrating the right common iliac aneurysm (large arrow) and the right femoral – popliteal graft aneurysm.

8 CLINICAL APPLICATIONS

8.1 Arterial occlusive disease

8.1.1 Chronic ischemia

The most common cause of chronic ischemia in the extremities is peripheral atherosclerotic disease (PAD). Other causes include radiation arteritis, vasculitis, repetitive compression (i.e. thoracic outlet syndrome), and recurrent thromboembolism. PAD, however, will be the focus of discussion in this section.

Peripheral atherosclerotic disease (PAD) in the lower extremities affects an estimated 12–20 million people.[5,6] PAD occurs with much less frequency in the upper extremity,

but nevertheless can be equally debilitating. Functional activity may be impaired from intermittent claudication. Alternatively, chronic ischemia may lead to threatened limbs with rest pain, non-healing ulcers, and tissue loss. Risk factors for PAD include tobacco use, hypertension, diabetes mellitus, hyperlipidemia, coronary atherosclerotic disease, and carotid atherosclerotic disease.[5,7,8]

CT angiography has proven to be an accurate and reliable modality for PAD evaluation in upper[9] and lower extremity native arteries (Table 28.7)[10–18] stents, and bypass grafts.[19] With regards to native extremity arteries, while CTA is used commonly for assessment of symptomatic patients, CTA can also be applied to screen asymptomatic high risk patients, particularly those who may have an

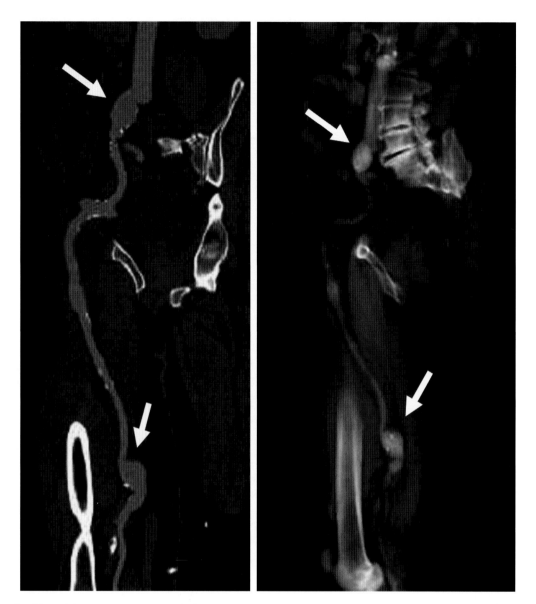

Figure 28.4 *Vessel Analysis* Multiplanar (MPR) and curved planar (CPR) reformations are the principle techniques to analyze the vessel lumen and wall. While MPRs display limited segments of a vascular territory, CPRs are advantageous in that they can display an entire vascular territory of interest in a single two-dimensional image. As illustrated in the same patient from Figure 3, a CPR trace was generated from the distal infra-renal aorta through to the popliteal artery by placing points along the center lumen, confirming no flow limitation and no aneurysm thrombus (A, arrows). An alternative means to improving MPR spatial perception, at the expense structural detail, is to apply a thick MPR (B).

abnormal ankle-brachial index. Earlier diagnosis can guide medical management and endovascular treatments prior to limb ischemia, potentially changing the disease course and improving patient outcome. Similarly, CTA can be used for stent and graft surveillance, prior to patients becoming symptomatic from stent and graft stenoses or occlusions.

CTA PAD evaluation primarily focuses on the arterial lumen and wall (Figure 28.5). Similar information can only be acquired with catheter tongiography by obtaining acquisitions from multiple angles and by using intravascular

ultrasound, both of which add procedural time and expose the patient to potential increased risk. CTA interpretation characterizes atherosclerotic lesions with regards to the number, type (i.e. stenosis, occlusion), location, length, composition, and stenosis percentage. The degree of calcification, the presence of plaque ulcerations and penetrating ulcers, and the nature of eccentric lesions are also addressed. Stents and grafts are evaluated for integrity, patency, neointimal hyperplasia, and in-situ thrombus. In all exams, characterizing and measuring the inflow and outflow distal

Table 28.7 Performance of lower extremity MDCTA

Author	Collimation	TH	N	Sensitivity (%)	Specificity (%)	Accuracy (%)
Ofer[13] 2003	4 × 2.5	3.2				
• >50% stenosis-occlusion			18	91	92	92
Martin[12] 2003	4 × 2.5	5.0	41			
• >75% stenosis				92	97	NA
• occlusion				89	98	NA
Ota[14] 2004	4 × 2.0	2.0	24			
• >50% stenosis				99	99	99
• occlusion				96	98	98
Portugaller[15] 2004	4 × 2.5	2.5	50			
• >70% stenosis-occlusion‡				92	83	86
Catalano[10] 2004	4 × 2.5	3.0	50			
• >50% stenosis-occlusion				96	93	94
Romano[16] 2004	4 × 2.5	3.2	42			
• >50% stenosis-occlusion				93	95	94
Edwards[11] 2005	4 × 2.5	3.2	44			
• >50% stenosis				79/72	93/93	
• occlusion				75/71	82/81	
Willmann[18] 2005	16 × 0.75	0.75	39			
• >50% stenosis-occlusion				96/97	96/97	96/97
Schertler[17] 2005	16 × 0.75	0.75	17			
• >50% stenosis-occlusion				98	95	96

Collimation = No. channels x detector width (mm). TH = slice thickness. N = number of patients. ‡ Cross sectional area reduction

runoff arteries for lesions, stents, and grafts are equally important. Secondary CTA PAD evaluation assesses end organ sequelae which may include skin ulcers, local tissue loss, and generalized muscle atrophy.

All of the CTA findings factor into endovascular and surgical treatment planning, including endovascular access and device selections; surgical approach and graft selections; and technical considerations. With greater pre-procedural knowledge, CTA has the potential to contribute to decreased procedural complications.

8.1.2 Acute ischemia

Acute upper or lower limb ischemia results from arterial occlusion without the development of collateral pathways. Etiologies include: (1) primary thrombosis, (2) arterial thromboembolism, and (3) trauma. Primary native artery thrombosis may result from a ruptured plaque in the setting of chronic PAD or from in-situ aneurysm thrombosis. Extremity arterial emboli arise upstream to the occlusion, either from the heart, atherosclerotic lesions, aneurysms, or regions of intimal irregularity (i.e. chronic repetitive trauma). Stents and grafts can occlude acutely as a result of in-situ thrombosis, emboli, or inflow and outflow flow disturbances.

CTA is also useful for diagnosing acute ischemia and planning the appropriate treatment strategies (Figure 28.6). Typical findings for native arterial acute occlusion are a central arterial filling defect, an abrupt arterial cutoff, or both. Grafts and stents typically show occlusion with a 'cast' of thrombus. Imaging should include the entire vascular tree so that the upstream segments through to the digital arteries are evaluated. Depending on the clinical suspicion for a cardiogenic embolic source, diagnostic assessment can be simplified by combining an ECG-gated cardiac CT angiogram with an extremity CTA. Treatment strategies include catheter directed thrombolysis and surgical thrombectomy.

8.2 Vasculitis

Vasculitis is defined as inflammation of the walls of large, medium, or small vessels. Any organ system may be involved, and most commonly arteries are affected rather than veins. With regards to the extremities, in distinction to atherosclerotic disease, vasculitis occurs more frequently in the upper extremity as opposed to the lower extremity. Patients often present with constitutional symptoms (i.e. fever myalgias, arthralgias, and malaise) and extremity ischemia ranging from pain to ulcerations and gangrene.

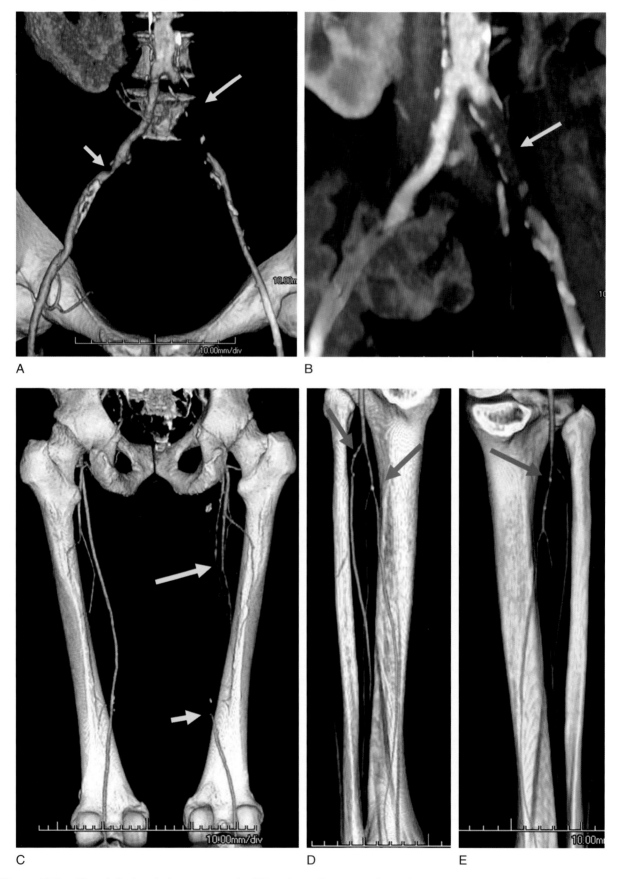

A   B

C   D   E

Figure 28.5 *Chronic Ischemia* Lower extremity CT angiography was performed on a 64-channel multidetector-row scanner, for a patient with worsening left buttock and right thigh claudication. Multi-station runoff images show high grade proximal right external iliac stenosis (A, small arrow), left common iliac occlusion (A, large arrow), and right superficial femoral artery mid segment occlusion (C, arrows), with a three vessel runoff bilaterally (D-E). An oblique MPR (B) through the left iliac system confirms thrombotic occlusion (arrow) as well mixed composition plaque in the imaged distal abdominal aorta and right common iliac artery.

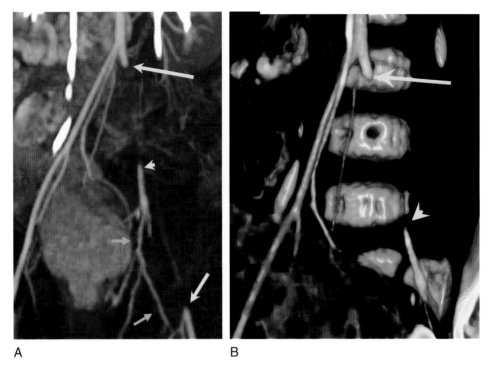

A   B

Figure 28.6 *Acute Ischemia* A 2 year old presents with decreased left pedal pulses following left femoral catheterization. Maximum intensity projection (A) and volume rendered (B) images show long segment occlusion of the left common iliac and external iliac arteries, (long yellow arrow), with left common femoral artery reconstitution (short yellow arrow) via the left internal iliac artery (yellow arrow head) and obturator to medial circumflex artery collateral flow (green arrowheads).

Medium and small vessel involvement can lead to secondary Raynaud's vasospastic phenomenon.

Upper extremity large vessel vasculitides include Takayasu Arteritis and Giant Cell Arteritis. Both may also involve medium size proximal outflow arteries. In the upper and lower extremity, Thromboangiitis Obliterans (Buerger's Disease) and Behçet's disease can involve medium and small size arteries in addition to veins. Small vessel vasculitis is more typically seen in the upper extremity. Etiologies include Rheumatoid arthritis, Sjögrens's syndrome, Wegener's granulomatosis, polyarteritis nodosa, scleroderma, systemic lupus erythematosus, polymyositis, dermatomyositis, and mixed connective tissue disorders.

Following a detailed history and physical examination, evaluation begins with laboratory analysis for elevated cellular inflammatory markers, including erythrocyte sedimentation rate, C-reactive protein, antineutrophilic cytoplasmic antibodies.[20,21] Duplex ultrasound with plesmography is an effective non-invasive means to initially image the extremity vascular morphology and characterize blood flow. While these measures often lead to a working diagnosis of vasculitis, angiography may be required to confirm the diagnosis, define the extent of vasculitis, and exclude concomitant proximal or alternative disease.

CT angiography readily achieves these advanced imaging goals (Figure 28.7). The complete vascular tree is scanned so that coverage affords assessment of the proximal territories as well as the palmar, pedal, and digital vessels. Vascular findings may include smooth short and long segment stenoses, focal stenoses, focal and tandem occlusions, aneurysms, and pseudoaneurysms. Atherosclerotic plaque and embolic sources are typically absent. In Thromboangiitis Obliterans, 'corkscrew' collateral arteries are often present. Recognizing vessel wall thickening with or without adjacent inflammatory changes on the source images is crucial to the specific diagnosis. If palmar, pedal, or digital arteries show poor or absent enhancement during the first pass, an immediate delayed acquisition should be acquired. Venous enhancement on delayed phase with persistent, diffuse poorly enhanced arteries in the hand or foot is indicative of small vessel disease.

8.3 Trauma

Traumatic vascular injuries to the upper and lower extremities can be divided into two groups: (1) exposure injuries and (2) blunt and penetrating trauma. Exposure injuries can

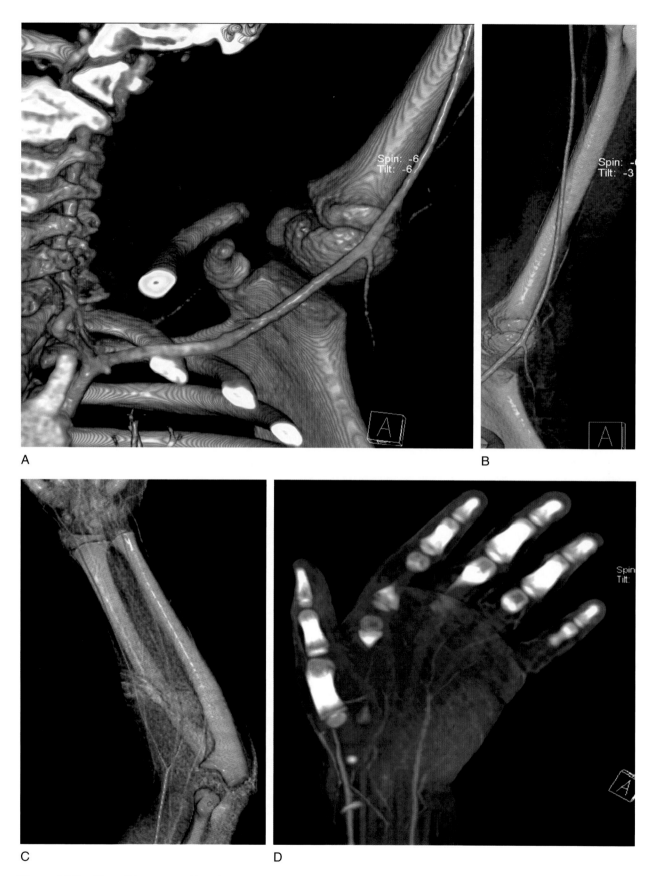

A

B

C

D

Figure 28.7 *Vasculitis* 7 year old male with left 2nd and 3rd digit subacute ischemia. While vasculitis was suspected clinically, upper extremity CT angiography was performed to exclude an alternative etiology. Figures A-C show no inflow stenosis, thoracic compression, or proximal outflow vascular pathology which could cause arterial thromboembolism. Volume rendered (C) and maximum intensity projection (D) images reveal diminutive, poorly enhancing arteries in the distal forearm and hand, consistent with small vessel disease.

be secondary to radiation (radiation arteritis), caustic agents, polyvinylchloride (Acro-osteolysis), electrical current (electrical injuries), and extreme temperatures (thermal injury). Injuries from any of these exposures can result in vascular inflammation and fibrosis. Blunt and penetrating trauma can cause injury to arteries, veins, or both. Blunt extremity vascular injuries are associated with musculoskeletal trauma, repetitive vibration tool exposure, or repetitive work (Hypothenar Hammer Syndrome) or athletic (Thoracic Outlet–Inlet Syndromes) related motions. Penetrating injuries are associated with gun shot wounds and piercing objects – including iatrogenic catheter injuries. While most arterial injuries require endovascular or surgical treatment, most venous injuries can be treated conservatively.

Patients with radiation exposure or repetitive vibration tool, work, or athletic blunt trauma may present with either subacute to chronic ischemia with or without secondary Raynaud's phenomenon. All other trauma patients typically present emergently. In this setting, prompt recognition of extremity arterial injury or uncontrolled venous injury is important for limb survival. Physical examination and targeted Doppler ultrasonography are the core means to initially evaluating these patients. Physical examination should include determination of the ankle or wrist–brachial index. Patients are triaged into three groups: those with definite vascular injury, those with possible vascular injury, and those with proximity injury only.

Signs of definite extremity vascular injury include active hemorrhage, expanding pulsatile hematoma, hemodynamic instability, and limb ischemia. These patients are brought emergently to either the endovascular suite or the operating room for control and repair of the vascular injury. Imaging may be required to provide a vascular map and aid vascular and soft tissue reconstructions.

Patients with possible vascular injury are hemodynamically stable with non-threatened limbs, but may have decreased or absent distal pulses, a bruit, a decreased ankle or wrist brachial index, or a non-pulsatile expanding hematoma. These patients proceed to imaging for evaluation of suspected vascular injury. It is in this group of patients that CT angiography may have the greatest impact, since imaging is used not only for diagnosis, but also for planning of definitive therapy (Figure 28.8).

Proximity injury is defined as a traumatic wound near a vascular structure. Patients are hemodynamically stable, with intact vascular supply and without expanding hematomas. The ankle or wrist brachial index is normal and extremities are viable. These patients are observed for

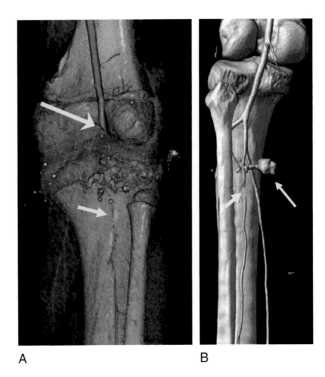

A   B

Figure 28.8 *Trauma* A: An eight year old male sustained a GSW to the left knee. The patient was hemodynamically stable, however distal pulses were diminished. CT angiography demonstrates popliteal artery occlusion (long arrow), with vasospasm present in the reconstituted infrageniculate popliteal artery segment (short arrow). B: A 35 year old female sustained a GSW to the right calf. The patient was hemodynamically stable with a large, non-expanding hematoma. CT angiography demonstrates a focal peroneal artery pseudoaneurysm (large arrow) with focal peroneal occlusion versus vasospasm (short arrow).

delayed signs of vascular injury. Imaging is not initially required.

CT angiography is a useful and effective non-invasive alternative to conventional angiography. In most medical centers, CT scanners are in close proximity to the emergency room, are readily available, and are conducive to managing critical trauma patients. CT also provides a practical complete trauma evaluation in that multiple organ systems are evaluated with one modality.

When the extremity is the only area of injury, targeted *Extremity Runoff* protocols are sufficient. Imaging begins one vascular territory above the injury and continues to the digits. When extremity imaging is combined with other regions of the body, scan coverage is extended. In both situations, a delayed acquisition may be required to further define the vascular injury.

As with conventional angiography, CT angiography readily depicts vascular compression, vasospasm, intimal tears, lacerations, occlusions, pseudoaneurysms, and arterio-venous fistulas. In distinction to catheter angiography, CTA can more reliably define vascular injuries in relation to skeletal fractures and soft tissue injuries, particularly hematomas. Pitfalls include metallic streak artifacts (i.e. hardware, bullets), non-enhancement segments, and early asymmetric venous enhancement. With non-enhanced segments, it is difficult to distinguish vasospasm from traumatic occlusion. With early asymmetric venous enhancement, it is important to distinguish hyperemia from a traumatic arteriovenous fistula.

8.4 Venous occlusive disease

Venous occlusive disease occurs more commonly in the lower extremities as compared to the upper extremities. In both, deep veins are most often involved. Etiologies may be primary or secondary. Primary thrombosis occurs spontaneously or in the setting of intrinsic thrombophilia, extrinsic compression, or both. Causes of thrombophilia include mutations of factor V Leiden and prothrombin and deficiencies of antithrombin, protein C, and protein S.[22] Secondary thrombosis occurs as a result of extrinsic factors which increase the inherent thrombotic state. Common factors include intravenous devices, malignancy, oral contraceptives, surgery, pregnancy, puerperium, and prolonged immobilization.

Patients with venous occlusive disease may present with extremity enlargement, pain, heaviness, and skin discoloration. Physical findings include edema, erythema, and prominent ipsilateral veins with or without a palpable cord. With complete venous outflow obstruction, arterial inflow may be compromised, leading to arterial ischemia with or without gangrene.

Prompt recognition of upper and lower extremity venous thrombosis is critical. Undiagnosed deep venous thrombosis can lead to fatal pulmonary embolism. Diagnostic evaluation focuses on up to four tasks: (1) confirming the presence of thrombus and estimating its burden; (2) determining whether thrombus is occlusive or nonocclusive; (3) assessing the end-organ sequelae, including extremity edema and pulmonary embolism; and (4) identifying primary and secondary risk factors.

Although Duplex ultrasonography is the first line modality to evaluate suspected extremity venous thrombosis, indirect upper and lower extremity CT venography (CTV) provides a comprehensive evaluation of the venous system (Figure 28.9). Key strategies to achieving robust CTV image quality and 3D displays include dosing contrast medium according to the patient's body weight, timing the acquisition to either the late arterial or equilibrium phase, and using a section thickness not greater than 2.0 mm. Acute venous thrombosis manifests on CTV as a central venous filling defect, associated with expanded vein caliber, soft tissue stranding, and edema. Chronic venous thrombosis may appear as mural thickening, webs, or attenuated caliber from recanalization and negative remodeling.

8.5 Vascular masses

Vascular masses in the upper and lower extremity include aneurysms, congenital lesions (i.e. vascular malformations), benign and malignant tumors, and tumor-like conditions. Evaluation begins with an intake of the clinical history, presentation, and physical findings. Imaging options range from conventional radiography and ultrasound to Tc-99m RBC scintigraphy, CT, and MRI.

With CTA, the exam protocol is tailored to the location and the type of suspected or known vascular mass. The primary imaging objectives are to: (1) characterize the location, size, extent, and composition of the mass and (2) map out the vascular supply to the mass (Figure 28.10). Local and distant non-cardiovascular structures are also evaluated, as in the case of vascular tumors. In this instance, local invasion and distant metastasis need to be excluded. Following surgical or endovascular treatment of vascular masses, CTA can also be used to assess for residual and recurrent disease, and assess for post-operative complications.

Targeted *Extremity Runoff* protocols are sufficient for the majority of upper and lower extremity CTA evaluations of vascular masses. Imaging should begin one vascular territory above the mass and continue to the digits. A delayed phase may be required to further define the mass, particularly if the mass is a venous or veno-lymphatic malformation.

8.6 Reconstruction surgery

Options for surgical reconstructions of extremity wounds include direct wound closure, skin grafting, local tissue transfer, and free tissue transfer ('free flap').[23] Depending on the complexity of the wound, the planned surgical reconstruction, and the presence of underlying vascular disease, imaging may be required to map out the arteries and veins.

Imaging is most commonly utilized prior to vascularized tissue transfer reconstructions, whether the extremity is to be the donor or recipient site. Clinically, upper and lower

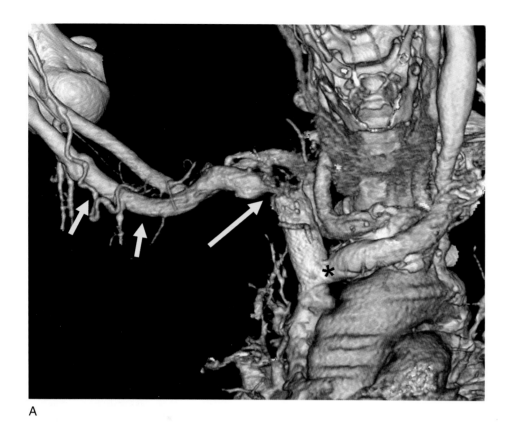

A

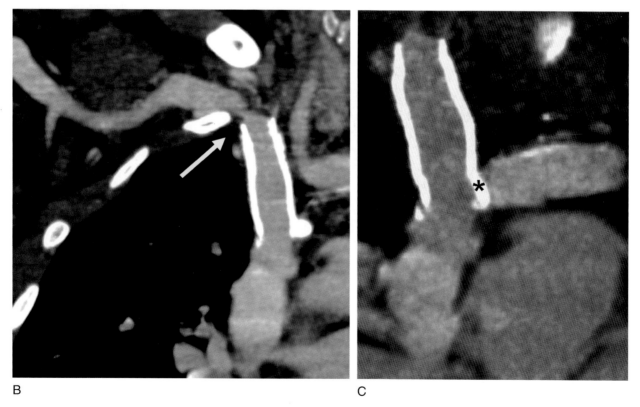

B   C

Figure 28.9 *Indirect CT Venography* Upper extremity CT venography on a 16-channel scanner was performed in a patient with recurrent SVC syndrome. The patient has previously undergone right brachiocephalic vein (BCV) stent placement. VR (A) and targeted MPR (B) images through the right central veins show high grade stenosis of the native right subclavian vein, just proximal to the stent (long arrow) with patent deep veins in the upper arm (A, short arrows). A selective MPR view through the left BCV (C) reveals that the right BCV stent crosses the left BCV origin, obstructing antegrade flow (asterix).

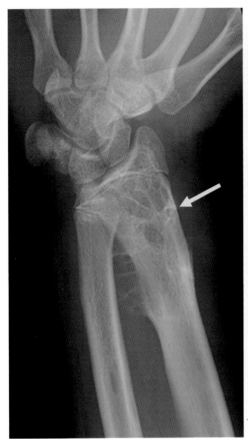

A

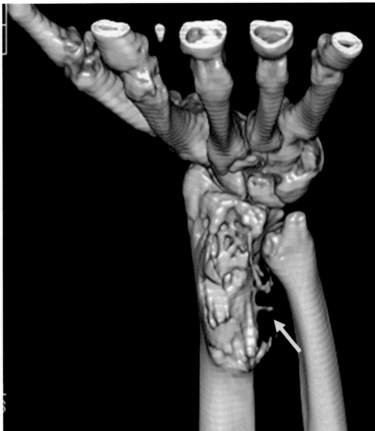

B

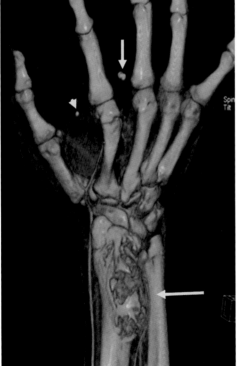

C

Figure 28.10 *Vascular Mass* 16 year old male with a slow flow venous malformation centered at the distal right dorsal forearm. The malformation causes radial erosion and bony overgrowth (A, B; arrows). Primary arterial supply is from the dorsal interosseous artery (C; yellow arrow). A second slow flow venous malformation is present between the 2nd and 3rd metacarpals (short yellow arrow), while a focal phlebolith is present between the first and second metacarpals.

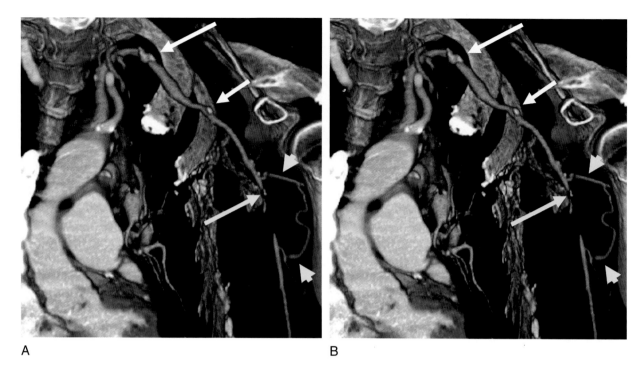

A   B

Figure 28.11   *Vascular Mapping* Left upper extremity CT angiography was performed on a 16-channel scanner to assess candidacy for TRAM (transverse rectus abdominis myocutaneous) flap reconstruction. A select VR image demonstrates diffuse atherosclerotic disease in the left subclavian, axillary, and brachial arteries, with short segment brachial artery occlusion and a well developed collateral artery reconstituting the brachial artery. Given the extent of proximal arterial occlusive disease, the left internal mammary artery and vein (not shown) were used for recipient vascular targets, rather than thoracodorsal targets.

extremity CTA has proven useful to plan surgical procedures, ensure flap viability, and prevent ischemia.[24,25] Objectives are to: (1) assess the patency and caliber of the target arteries and veins; (2) assess the patency of and communication between potential collateral pathways; and (3) screen for normal variant origins, atherosclerotic disease, perivascular fibrosis, radiation arteritis, and other vascular abnormalities (Figure 28.11).

When the upper extremity is considered to be a harvest site, the radius or ulna may be used as composite free flaps. Imaging begins at the subclavian artery level as the radial or ulnar artery may arise aberrantly from as high as the axillary artery. In the lower extremity, the fibula is utilized as a donor free flap. Imaging may begin at the groin or mid thigh, depending on index of suspicion for arterial occlusive disease. For both upper and lower extremities, imaging extends to the digits with assessment of palmar and pedal arches, respectively.

Regarding recipient extremity reconstructions, pedicle or free flaps may be used. CTA coverage is applied in a more targeted fashion such that imaging often begins at one vascular territory above the wound. In most instances, coverage extends through to the digital arteries.

8.7 Hemodialysis access

End-stage renal disease (ESRD) is the non-reversible deterioration of renal function. In the majority of patients, hemodialysis is ultimately necessary. Successful hemodialysis depends upon the performance of the hemodialysis vascular access. Options for vascular access include inserting a temporary or permanent central venous catheter or surgically creating an arteriovenous fistula (AVF) or graft (AVG). Dialysis Outcome Quality Initiative (K-DOQI) and Good Nephrological Practice guidelines recommend autogenous arteriovenous fistula (AVF) as the first choice as AVF have better long term patency rates, fewer complications, and reduced costs.[26] While the majority of access is placed in the upper extremity, lower extremity vasculature can also be used for central lines, AVF, and AVG.

Achieving and maintaining patent vascular access begins with patient history and physical examination. Imaging, however, is an important adjunct and, in this regard, CT angiography is a useful modality. CTA can be performed to map out upper or lower extremity vasculature prior to placing a hemodialysis central line or creating an AVF or AVG. The primary goal of vascular mapping is to define the

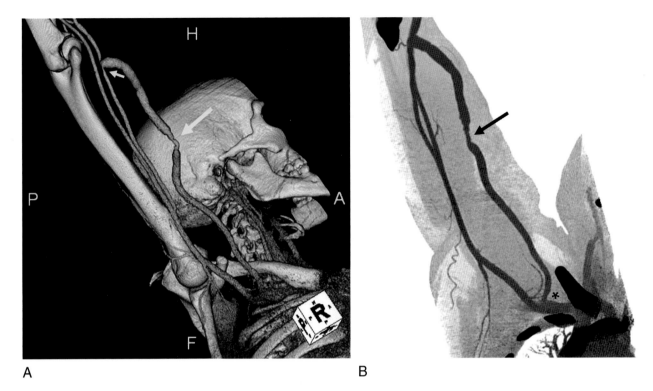

A   B

Figure 28.12 *Hemodialysis Access* Upper extremity CT angiography was performed on a 64-channel scanner to evaluate a right arm arteriovenous fistula (AVF). Venous pressures were elevated. A VR image reveals normal variant high origin of the radial artery off of the brachial artery (A). The hemodialysis AVF is between the radial artery and cephalic vein. As shown on the VR image, there is high grade cephalic vein outflow stenosis (long arrow) as well as mild arterial inflow narrowing (short arrow). An inverted MIP image (B) confirms the stenosis. In addition, it shows the cephalic vein – subclavian vein junction is widely patent.

caliber and patency of inflow and outflow arteries and veins specific to the access site. Recognition of small luminal diameter or arterial and venous stenoses and occlusions guides the decision process for selecting the appropriate vascular access and location. Recognition of venous side branches is also essential, as flow through side branches can contribute to AVF non-maturation.

CTA can also be applied to assess dysfunctional AVF and AVG (Figure 28.12). Inflow and outflow arteries and veins require complete evaluation to exclude flow-limiting stenoses, occlusions, or both. Hemodynamically significant lesions may be found anywhere along the extremity vascular tree, but in most instances are localized in proximity to the access site. AVF should also be assessed for venous outflow side branches. Rarely, AVG and AVF puncture site pseudoaneurysms may be seen. The degree of arterial and venous lesions and in the case of AVF, the presence of side branches will influence decisions for endovascular or surgical treatment.

As iodinated contrast medium is utilized, CTA in ESRD patients should be coordinated with the patient's scheduled hemodialysis. Injection protocols reflect the patient's body weight and the caliber of the accessed vein.

For evaluation of dysfunctional AVG or AVF, targeted non-contrast images are useful to define the location of grafts and surgical clips. Unenhanced images are not routinely required for vascular mapping.

9 CONCLUSION

CT angiography is a comprehensive, robust modality for evaluation of the upper and lower extremity peripheral vascular systems. Its emergence has revolutionized diagnostic algorithms for a wide spectrum of upper and lower extremity vascular disease and continues to facilitate treatment planning while minimizing patient risk. Understanding the core technical principles is essential for clinical success and will help modify current protocols as new technology is developed.

BIBLIOGRAPHY

1. Kalender WA, Seissler W, Klotz E et al. Spiral volumetric CT with single-breath-hold technique, continuous transport,

and continuous scanner rotation. Radiology Jul 1990; 176(1): 181–3.

2. Rubin GD, Shiau MC, Schmidt AJ et al. Computed tomographic angiography: historical perspective and new state-of-the-art using multi detector-row helical computed tomography. J Comput Assist Tomogr. Nov 1999; 23 Suppl 1: S83–90.

3. Fleischmann D. High-concentration contrast media in MDCT angiography: principles and rationale. Eur Radiol. Nov 2003; 13 Suppl 3: N39–43.

4. Fleischmann D, Rubin GD. Quantification of intravenously administered contrast medium transit through the peripheral arteries: implications for CT angiography. Radiology Sep 2005; 236(3): 1076–82.

5. Selvin E, Erlinger TP. Prevalence of and risk factors for peripheral arterial disease in the United States: results from the National Health and Nutrition Examination Survey, 1999-2000. Circulation. Aug 10 2004; 110(6): 738–43.

6. Ostchega Y, Paulose-Ram R, Dillon CF et al. Prevalence of peripheral arterial disease and risk factors in persons aged 60 and older: data from the National Health and Nutrition Examination Survey 1999–2004. J Am Geriatr Soc. Apr 2007; 55(4): 583–9.

7. Ness J, Aronow WS, Newkirk E et al. Prevalence of symptomatic peripheral arterial disease, modifiable risk factors, and appropriate use of drugs in the treatment of peripheral arterial disease in older persons seen in a university general medicine clinic. J Gerontol A Biol Sci Med Sci. Feb 2005; 60(2): 255–7.

8. Bianchi C, Montalvo V, Ou HW et al. Pharmacologic risk factor treatment of peripheral arterial disease is lacking and requires vascular surgeon participation. Ann Vasc Surg. Mar 2007; 21(2): 163–6.

9. Hellinger JC, Napoli A, Schraedley-Desmond P et al. Multidetector row CT angiography of the upper extremity: comparison with digital subtraction angiography (Abstract). Radiologic Society of North America 2004. SSM04–SSM01: 569.

10. Catalano C, Fraioli F, Laghi A et al. Infrarenal aortic and lower-extremity arterial disease: diagnostic performance of multi-detector row CT angiography. Radiology May 2004; 231(2): 555–63.

11. Edwards AJ, Wells IP, Roobottom CA. Multidetector row CT angiography of the lower limb arteries: a prospective comparison of volume-rendered techniques and intra-arterial digital subtraction angiography. Clin Radiol. Jan 2005; 60(1): 85–95.

12. Martin ML, Tay KH, Flak B et al. Multidetector CT angiography of the aortoiliac system and lower extremities: a prospective comparison with digital subtraction angiography. AJR Am J Roentgenol. Apr 2003; 180(4): 1085–91.

13. Ofer A, Nitecki SS, Linn S et al. Multidetector CT angiography of peripheral vascular disease: a prospective comparison with intraarterial digital subtraction angiography. AJR Am J Roentgenol. Mar 2003; 180(3): 719–24.

14. Ota H, Takase K, Igarashi K et al. MDCT compared with digital subtraction angiography for assessment of lower extremity arterial occlusive disease: importance of reviewing cross-sectional images. AJR Am J Roentgenol. Jan 2004; 182(1): 201–9.

15. Portugaller HR, Schoellnast H, Hausegger KA et al. Multislice spiral CT angiography in peripheral arterial occlusive disease: a valuable tool in detecting significant arterial lumen narrowing? Eur Radiol. Sep 2004; 14(9): 1681–7.

16. Romano M, Mainenti PP, Imbriaco M et al. Multidetector row CT angiography of the abdominal aorta and lower extremities in patients with peripheral arterial occlusive disease: diagnostic accuracy and interobserver agreement. Eur J Radiol. Jun 2004; 50(3): 303–8.

17. Schertler T, Wildermuth S, Alkadhi H et al. Sixteen-detector row CT angiography for lower-leg arterial occlusive disease: analysis of section width. Radiology Nov 2005; 237(2): 649–56.

18. Willmann JK, Baumert B, Schertler T et al. Aortoiliac and lower extremity arteries assessed with 16-detector row CT angiography: prospective comparison with digital subtraction angiography. Radiology Sep 2005; 236(3): 1083–93.

19. Willmann JK, Mayer D, Banyai M et al. Evaluation of peripheral arterial bypass grafts with multi-detector row CT angiography: comparison with duplex US and digital subtraction angiography. Radiology Nov 2003; 229(2): 465–74.

20. Falk RJ, Jennette JC. ANCA small-vessel vasculitis. J Am Soc Nephrol. Feb 1997; 8(2): 314–22.

21. Jennette JC, Falk RJ. Small-vessel vasculitis. N Engl J Med. Nov 20 1997; 337(21): 1512–23.

22. Martinelli I, Battaglioli T, Bucciarelli P et al. Risk factors and recurrence rate of primary deep vein thrombosis of the upper extremities. Circulation Aug 3 2004; 110(5): 566–70.

23. Willcox TM, Smith AA. Upper limb free flap reconstruction after tumor resection. Semin Surg Oncol. Oct-Nov 2000; 19(3): 246–54.

24. Chow LC, Napoli A, Klein MB et al. Vascular mapping of the leg with multi-detector row CT angiography prior to free-flap transplantation. Radiology Oct 2005; 237(1): 353–60.

25. Klein MB, Karanas YL, Chow LC et al. Early experience with computed tomographic angiography in microsurgical reconstruction. Plast Reconstr Surg. Aug 2003; 112(2): 498–503.

26. III. NKF-K/DOQI Clinical Practice Guidelines for Vascular Access: update 2000. Am J Kidney Dis. Jan 2001; 37(1 Suppl 1): S137–181.

29

Computed Tomographic Angiography of the Cervical Neurovasculature

Felix E. Diehn and E. Paul Lindell

I INTRODUCTION

Computed tomographic angiography (CTA) is a non-invasive tool for the evaluation of the cervical and cerebral vasculature. The development and application of this technique has occurred later than the competing modalities of digital subtraction angiography (DSA) and magnetic resonance angiography (MRA). While CTA is the relative newcomer, recent advances in CT technology have made it progressively more competitive with these other modalities. The current use of CTA, MRA and DSA in the evaluation of the cervical and cerebral vasculature is in flux, and is driven by the rapid advance in scanner technology. As such CTA needs to be considered in the context of these other examinations. While there is variation in the relative utilization of these modalities among large medical centers, several trends are apparent.

DSA remains the gold standard in vascular imaging of the head and neck. Its spatial resolution remains unrivaled. The dynamic temporal information that can be obtained about collateral flow patterns has not found a sufficient substitute in cross sectional imaging. Furthermore, it suffers from few if any artifacts, which can be problematic for both CTA and MRA. Despite advances including safer contrast material, smaller catheters, and hydrophilic guide wires, DSA remains associated with a small risk of neurologic complications. In a recent prospective study of 2,899 consecutive cerebral DSAs, the incidence of neurological complications was low (1.3% [0.5% permanent, 0.2% reversible, and 0.7% transient]).[1] Similarly, a study of 19,826 consecutive patients undergoing diagnostic cerebral angiography at our institution demonstrated a very low neurological complication rate of 2.63% (2.09% TIA, 0.36% reversible, 0.14% permanent, and 0.05% death related to a neurological condition) (Kaufmann et al, Radiology, in press).[125] However, this finite risk, the relative expense, and the time- and resource-intensiveness of DSA has fostered the development and improvement of noninvasive, cross-sectional imaging methods, including ultrasound (US), MRA, and CTA.

MRA of the neurovasculature has proven to be an excellent test. Anecdotally, MRA of the neurovasculature is currently the test of choice for confirming and measuring significant vascular stenosis suggested by screening US or clinical exam. However, MRA can be limited by the spatial resolution inherent to the commonly used screening examinations and the tendency for interpretation to be performed using approximations of the projectional appearance of DSA.

With the development of helical and multi-detector row CT (MDCT) scanner technology and powerful postprocessing software in the recent years, CT has become more prevalent in clinical practice. These technical advances have resulted in vastly improved spatial and temporal resolution and fostered the development of CTA. Numerous authors have shown CTA to be a cost-effective and minimally invasive alternative to DSA for various neurovascular imaging applications. These applications include evaluation of the cervical neurovasculature, which is the focus of this chapter. Although beyond the scope of the present discussion, CTA has also proved useful for the evaluation of intracranial aneurysms, vascular malformations, cerebral venous pathology, and stroke.

2 TECHNIQUE

CTA is a noninvasive imaging technique capable of producing high quality images of the extracranial and intracranial neurovasculature. Today's helical MDCT scanners allow for rapid, extremely high resolution cross-sectional imaging, with z-axis (craniocaudal) resolutions on the best scanners approximating 0.5 mm. Images are acquired volumetrically with continuous gantry rotation and patient table translation. Commercially available postprocessing software enables the creation of multiplanar 2D and 3D images from the axial source images.

CTA for neuroradiology applications demands high quality image acquisition. In principle, a 3D volume containing the vessels of interest is imaged during their peak enhancement phase. Today's helical MDCT scanners allow imaging of relatively large areas of anatomic coverage with sub-millimeter resolution. Optimal results are dependent on the interplay of multiple factors, which include acquisition parameters, contrast administration and timing, image reconstruction methods, and image postprocessing techniques. A brief discussion of CTA technique and postprocessing as it relates to the cervical neurovasculature follows; the interested reader is referred to several excellent recent reviews.[2-5]

2.1 Image acquisition

Multiple technical parameters must be optimized for successful neurovascular CTA. At present, we perform carotid CTA using 64-slice CT scanners (Sensation 64 system, Siemens, Erlangen, Germany). This MDCT scanner system enables the use of isotropic voxels to the level of 0.4 mm. Such extremely high spatial resolution allows data reconstruction in any plane with minimal partial volume effects.

At our institution, a standard neck CTA protocol consists of the following parameters: caudocranial spiral scan, 0.5 sec rotation, 64 × 0.6 collimation, pitch 0.75, feed 16.3 mm/rotation, 120 kVp, 350 mAs, and 500 mm FOV. Using these parameters, images of the carotid arteries from the aortic arch to the skull base can be obtained in approximately 8 seconds. The fast scan speed allows for exclusive arterial phase acquisitions and results in limited patient motion artifacts, which is particularly helpful in those with decreased mental status.

2.2 Intravenous contrast

A reproducible contrast injection and timing protocol is a prerequisite for high quality neck CTA. In general, high injection rates of highly concentrated contrast material are optimal. MDCT scanners enable faster imaging than single-detector row scanners, with faster injections and lower total volumes of contrast. Using the 64-slice CT scanner systems, we typically inject 100 cc of 350 mg/ml iodinated contrast at 4 cc/sec using a power injector. The right antecubital vein is preferable in order to avoid streak artifact from contrast in the left brachiocephalic vein and superior vena cava. A 30 cc saline bolus 'flush' is administered immediately following the contrast injection to maximize the use of the contrast material and decrease venous streak artifact. We have used volumes as low as 50 cc of contrast and obtained diagnostic studies; however this is only typically performed in light of other limitations, such as renal disease.

When using MDCT, there are two general options for timing the delay between the injection of contrast material and the initiation of the acquisition. Rather than using an empiric delay, both of these methods allow individualization of timing in each patient, thereby minimizing the volume of contrast material and maximizing contrast opacification of the chosen vessels. First, automatic bolus tracking techniques enable real-time detection of the arrival of contrast material. These require only a single injection of contrast material. At our institution, triggering at the level of the aortic arch with a threshold of 50 Hounsfield Units has yielded excellent arterial contrast with little if any confounding venous opacification (see Figure 29.4). In our experience, triggering at the level of the carotid arteries has proved less reliable. Test bolus injections are a second option. These require an additional injection of approximately 15 cc of contrast material to measure the transit time to the internal carotid arteries.

2.3 Image reconstruction

Although we generally acquire images at a collimation of 64 × 0.6 mm, we reconstruct the data to slightly thicker thicknesses of 0.75 mm in order to decrease image noise. Reconstructions are performed with at least 50% overlap to minimize partial volume artifacts and improve 3D postprocessing. In order to maximize precision of stenosis measurements by minimizing blooming artifact associated with calcifications, sharper kernels may yield better edge detection.

2.4 Image postprocessing

There are multiple useful postprocessing techniques commonly employed in CTA which can provide additional information: multiplanar reformation (MPR), maximum intensity projection (MIP), shaded-surface display (SSD), and volume rendering (VR). These can help to increase specificity for detecting pathology and to better display findings to referring physicians. However, the more visually pleasing and easily interpretable techniques are not always as useful or accurate diagnostically. All of these techniques permute the raw image data and frequently both resolution and image information density will suffer. The axial source images are essential to the interpretation of any CTA examination of the neurovasculature. Importantly, these represent the rawest data. They should be reviewed primarily and considered the principal image set for diagnosis. Any finding seen using other postprocessing techniques should be validated using the axial source images.

MPR of the axial source images is the primary diagnostic tool for interpretation of neurovascular CTA, as it has the highest fidelity with the axial source images. MPR is an interactive, technically simple technique that is highly accurate and allows for the creation of views in any plane. MPR images enable precise vessel diameter measurements (see Figure 29.1A, B, and D, and Figure 29.2C). Care should be taken to employ image planes that are perpendicular to the vessel lumen. A useful plane is an oblique sagittal one in the plane of carotid bifurcation. This can readily display a stenosis as well as the normal internal carotid artery beyond the lesion. Since the minimal luminal diameter may be in the right-left direction, oblique coronal MPR can also be helpful. MPR can also be performed as curved planar reformation, which is useful to display tortuous structures. MPRs are generally advantageous compared to MIPs and volume-rendered techniques for luminal and intraluminal information.

MIP images are technically simple and result in a 2D projection of only the highest attenuation of a given scan ray. While MIP images are often more visually pleasing than thin section MPR data, they come at the cost of lost luminal information (see Figure 29.1C and 29.2B). As only the highest attenuation is projected for each pixel, low density luminal thrombus, vessel irregularity from dissection and even stenosis in calcified vessels can be masked. The problem is compounded as MIP images increase in thickness. Despite these limitations MIP images are used as standard views in neurovascular CTA. At our institution, we create 6.5 mm MIP images every 2.5 mm in three orthogonal planes relative to the course of the proximal internal carotid artery. These images are intended more for general overview and not for primary diagnostic interpretation.

SSD is a technique that can provide a 3D surface rendering of a structure of interest. Similar to MIP, this method also results in loss of information (see Figure 29.2A). Thresholds are applied to separate the surface of the object in question. SSD images typically include the contrast-enhanced vessels, calcified plaque, and bone. Manual or automated bone elimination techniques can be applied. Gray-scale shading procedures simulate surface reflections and shadowing from an artificial light source, thereby enhancing depth perception. SSD can provide information about the outer vessel wall and surface characteristics. Unfortunately, using SSD it can be difficult if not impossible to differentiate between intraluminal contrast and calcifications, due to their similar attenuations.

A final type of postprocessing technique is VR. Although this is also a threshold dependent technique, it is generally considered a superior 3D method compared to SSD. This method incorporates all of the raw CTA data. Transfer functions map measured intensities to colors and opacities. User-adjusted display parameters enable separation of different tissue types. Caution is needed as manual adjustment of these parameters can alter vascular lumen measurements. In addition, as a volume technique, VR does not allow for cross sectional evaluation of the lumen. Therefore, we generally do not use VR for measurement of luminal diameters.

3 CAROTID ARTERY ATHEROSCLEROTIC DISEASE

3.1 Rationale

Carotid artery atherosclerotic disease is an important cause of thromboembolic stroke. Several large randomized clinical trials have shown that patients with severe (70–99%) carotid stenoses may benefit from carotid endarterectomy (CEA) by significant reduction in the risk of stroke.[6–10] Moreover, it has been shown that some patients with a moderate (50–69%)

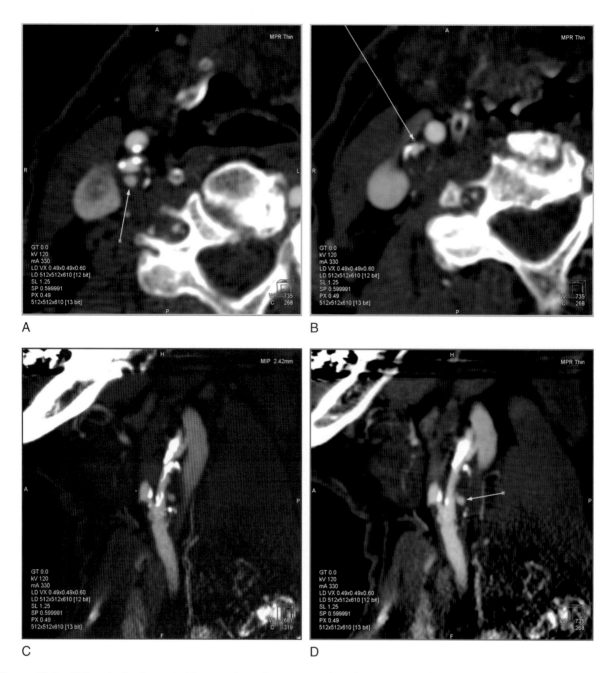

Figure 29.1   This set of reformatted images from the same patient demonstrates the value of multiplanar evaluation in characterizing a complex lesion. In the thicker MIP image (C) it is difficult to identify the true lumen. This highlights the loss of luminal information that results from the inclusion of adjacent calcified plaque in MIP images. Thinner MPR images in multiple planes (A, B, and D) better demonstrate the true lumen and complexity of the lesion. (A) Thin MPR demonstrates a complex right internal carotid artery (ICA) plaque. A contrast-filled ulcer is seen posterior to the narrowed ICA lumen (arrow). (B) Thin MPR at the level of the right ICA bulb demonstrating maximal luminal stenosis with soft plaque posteriorly. (C) Thicker section MIP does not accurately demonstrate the maximal luminal stenosis. The connection to the ulcer is not well seen. (D) Thin section sagittal MPR in the same plane as image C demonstrates the degree of stenosis and overall lesion characteristics with greater fidelity than the MIP image (C).

stenosis may also benefit from surgery.[7,11,12] Because of the correlation between the amount of carotid artery narrowing and the risk of ipsilateral thromboembolic stroke, the measurement of carotid stenosis is crucial to clinical management.

The major randomized CEA clinical trials have determined the percent carotid stenosis using conventional catheter-based angiography, which remains the gold standard.[6,10,13] However, due to the aforementioned relatively increased time, expense and risk of DSA, noninvasive

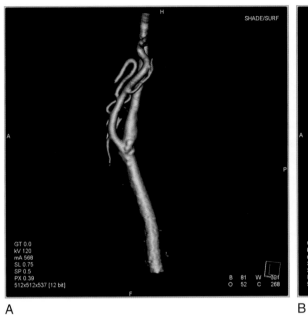

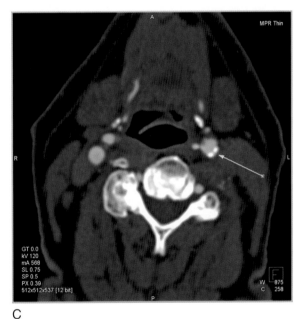

A

B

C

Figure 29.2 Calcified plaque. This set of reformatted images from the same patient highlights the relative value of different postprocessing techniques. (A) The visually pleasing SSD provides surface information but relatively poor luminal information. (B) MIP reconstruction of the same data gives slightly more luminal information but is limited by the prominently calcified plaque. (C) Axial MPR shows the peripheral nature of the calcium and accurate luminal information.

imaging of the carotid arteries is playing an increasingly important role.

3.2 Imaging of carotid artery stenosis

At our and many other institutions, US is typically the initial imaging method of choice for screening of the carotid arteries due to its easy availability, noninvasive nature, cost effectiveness, and speed. However, there is no clear consensus about Doppler criteria for stenosis. A recent review of 13 previously published sets of criteria showed that, although US is excellent at excluding a >70% stenosis (with a sensitivity of up to 98%), it tends to overestimate carotid stenosis.[14] When surgical intervention is considered or when the degree of stenosis by US is equivocal, an additional imaging test is required in many centers to minimize the chance of performing an unnecessary surgery. In patients with renal insufficiency, prior iodinated contrast reaction, or those undergoing a brain MR imaging (MRI) exam, MRA tends to be the preferred choice. However, MDCTA offers advantages of its own compared to MRA. These include generally higher spatial resolution, excellent contrast resolution, lack of flow-related artifacts, comparative ease of acquisition, the possibility of being performed in critically ill patients, speed, 3D capabilities, and a generally increased availability.

The preoperative imaging workup of a patient with carotid stenosis has been and remains controversial. The optimal approach likely takes into account a number of factors, including the clinical question and whether or not the patient is symptomatic. While some are proponents of either MRA, CTA or US for carotid imaging, either generally or in certain clinical situations, others suggest a combination of two of these noninvasive imaging modalities. Meanwhile, even the concept of using noninvasive imaging alone to assess carotid stenosis is not universally accepted, particularly in certain situations – for example, when there is discordance between the results on noninvasive modalities or for moderate stenosis. Some authors emphasize that each individual center should determine its own accuracies for the noninvasive imaging modalities compared with DSA, as well as its own risks of angiography and CEA.[15,16]

At our institution, MRA, CTA and DSA are used for confirmation of US findings. The choice of modality is governed by individual patient situation and need. Typically if intracranial imaging is desired, MRA is performed. When US and MRA/CTA are discordant and when endovascular intervention is contemplated as primary therapy, DSA is utilized.

3.3 Validation studies of CTA

Although the exact role of CTA in carotid imaging has yet to be defined, CTA is a valid imaging alternative to MRA. Both, however, are less accurate than DSA. Since some of the initial reports demonstrating that the carotid artery could be visualized with contrast-enhanced CT in the early 1980s,[17–19] multiple studies have demonstrated high accuracy of CTA for the detection of carotid artery atherosclerotic disease (see Figure 29.2). This has been confirmed in several recent systematic reviews.[20–22] One of these pooled the results of 28 studies limited by the use of only single-slice CT scanners; the pooled sensitivity and specificity for detection of a severe (70–99%) stenosis were 85% and 93%, respectively.[21] As suggested in this review, one problem

with almost all of the included studies is that the analyses often included the asymptomatic contralateral carotid artery, which is likely to cause overestimation of specificity.[21,23,24] A similar review included primarily studies that used single detector row CT scanners, with only 2 of the 43 studies considered employing early dual-detector row technology.[22] This showed a sensitivity of 95% and specificity of 98% for detecting severe stenosis.

A recent comparison of 4-channel MDCTA in 35 symptomatic carotid arteries showed high sensitivity (95%) and specificity (93%) of CTA in the detection of carotid stenosis (>50%) when compared to DSA.[25] All 5 occlusions were detected. In an even more recent comparison between 8-channel MDCTA and DSA in 37 patients,[26] the sensitivity and specificity for severe stenosis when source/MIP images were used were 75% and 96%; for moderate (50–69%) stenosis, the sensitivity and specificity were 88% and 82%, respectively. All four occlusions were detected. It is generally expected that the advent of more advanced MDCT, with the concomitant decrease in section thickness, will further improve upon these results, although data to support this are lacking to date.

In a recent meta-analysis comparing noninvasive imaging with DSA, contrast-enhanced MRA outperformed its counterparts: sensitivities/specificities for a 70–99% carotid stenosis were 94% and 93% for contrast-enhanced MRA, 88% and 84% for MRA, 89% and 84% for US, and 77% and 95% for CTA.[20] Similar to the aforementioned meta-analyses, this review did not include any studies using MDCT. Another recent review of three prospective, blinded studies using contrast-enhanced MRA and three such studies using CTA showed the sensitivity and specificity of MRA for carotid stenosis to be 93–94% and 85–100%, respectively; sensitivity and specificity of CTA were 73–100% and 92–98%, respectively.[27] Some comparative studies suggest that CTA may tend to underestimate carotid stenosis compared to DSA, time of flight (TOF) MRA, or contrast-enhanced MRA (CEMRA),[28–32] while others suggest that CTA may comparatively overestimate stenoses.[33–35] Meanwhile, MRA may also overestimate.[32,36–47]

Despite the better results of MRA in some studies, the inherent advantages of CTA should be considered when deciding on a confirmatory imaging study in any given patient. Berg et al. reported that CTA provided better image quality than 3D TOF MRA.[48] CTA is generally more available, faster, easier, and less expensive to perform. Like MRA, CTA enables imaging from the aortic arch to circle of Willis and offers the capability of detecting tandem stenoses, for which US is limited. Unlike MRA, CTA does not suffer from flow related artifacts, but rather relies on visualization of contrast within the lumen. Claustrophobic patients tend to do better in CT than MR scanners because of the generally larger and shorter bore.

3.4 Factors affecting accuracy of CTA

Despite the encouraging results of CTA in carotid disease, the results of comparison studies can be confounded by several factors. It must be emphasized that the relative accuracies and true sensitivities and specificities of all of the commonly used noninvasive modalities for carotid stenosis remain unknown. In fact, DSA has an intrinsic standard deviation estimated at 8%, suggesting that even this gold standard likely misclassifies a small percentage of carotid stenoses.[49] The North American Symptomatic Carotid Endarterectomy Trial (NASCET) method of measuring percent stenosis, which uses the ratio of luminal diameter at the maximal point of carotid stenosis to the normal distal internal carotid diameter, is the standard for measuring stenoses on DSA. Meticulous attention to detail when making NASCET measurements is critical, but even experienced neuroradiologists have an inherent degree of inter-observer disagreement, estimated at roughly ±7% in one carefully conducted study using conventional angiographic images.[50] In addition, DSA has been shown to generally underestimate carotid stenosis compared to rotational angiography or histopathology,[51–55] due to the limited number of imaging planes and the asymmetric nature of a large proportion of carotid stenoses. Rotational angiography appears to increase the accuracy of conventional angiography in detecting the true, smallest diameter of a stenosis.[52,53] One must also consider that, as technology continues to advance, particularly in CT and MR, results of previously published studies may become outdated relatively rapidly.

While scanner technology impacts diagnostic accuracy, the postprocessing technique used has also been shown to influence the grading of carotid stenoses, both for CT and MR. There is disagreement in the literature regarding the accuracy and relative superiority of the different postprocessing methods. Using a 16-section CT scanner to study 50 patients with symptomatic internal carotid artery stenoses, Lell et al. showed that time-of-flight MRA (evaluated with MPR) and CTA had the highest concordance for stenosis grading.[30] In a study of 89 analyzable carotid arteries using a 16-channel MDCT, Hacklaender et al. evaluated multiple CTA postprocessing techniques (axial source images, sagittal MIP, and sagittal MPR) and their correlation with MRA

using different standard measurement methods, including NASCET.[34] The CTA axial source images using the NASCET method of measuring stenosis agreed most closely to MRA. MIP images tended to be more imprecise. Silvennoinen et al. also found axial source images to be the most reliable in comparison of CTA and DSA, as have other investigators,[56–58] with MIP images proving helpful in certain cases, such as when the vessel had a horizontal or tortuous course or the segment of stenosis was very short.[26] The accuracy of CTA was not improved by the use of semi-automated vessel analysis software in both of these recent studies.[26,34] 3D SSD images have also been shown to be useful when viewed in conjunction with axial source images.[59] Some authors prefer MIPs over MPRs in addition to axial source images; specifically, two groups recently advocated the use of sliding-thin-slab MIPs which preserve the cross-sectional nature of the data.[60,61] In a study using vessel phantoms, Addis et al. showed that axial, MIP, MPR, SSD, and VR display techniques all accurately display vessels and stenoses greater than 4 mm, while VR was more accurate than the others for very small diameters.[62]

CTA window and level settings have also been shown to affect measurement accuracy of carotid stenosis in several studies. One recent study used phantoms of variable levels of stenoses. The authors found an inherent mathematical relationship between the contrast material attenuation coefficient and the optimal window and level settings for both axial and MIP images, with resultant reduction in measurement variability.[63]

Intrinsic characteristics of the patients' vessels can also affect the accuracy of CTA for grading carotid stenosis. For instance, calcified plaque can make stenosis grading difficult, if not impossible, on MIP images, underscoring the importance of viewing the axial source images as well as the utility of MPR images. Heavily calcified plaque, particularly when on both sides of the vessel lumen, can cause a 'blooming' artifact and thereby result in overestimation of a stenosis. However, this artifact is often mitigated with the newer MDCT scanners.[64] Calcifications, ulcerations, and adjacent vessels all can be problematic, particularly for automated analysis methods.[65] A severe stenosis can be associated with poststenotic collapse (see Figure 29.3B), which can render percent stenosis calculations inaccurate.[26,66]

3.5 Carotid artery occlusions

The evaluation of carotid artery atherosclerotic disease by CTA is not limited to measuring stenosis. With regard to

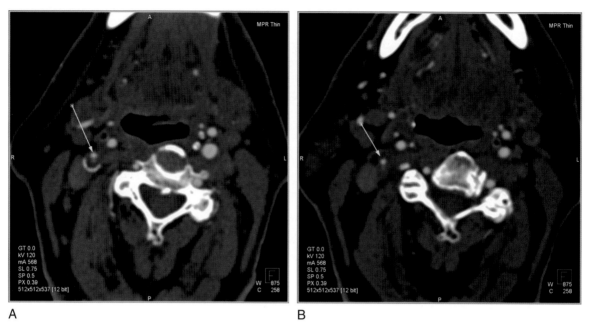

Figure 29.3   Two thin MPR images from the same patient with a high grade right ICA stenosis. (A) The lumen (arrow) is markedly narrowed by a heterogeneous plaque. Posterior to the lumen is a small ~2 mm area of intermediate attenuation compatible with thrombus. This is surrounded by a lower attenuation tissue suggestive of lipid-laden plaque, which is calcified peripherally. (B) An image more cephalad demonstrates that this near occlusion is associated with poststenotic collapse ('distal slimming').

total carotid artery occlusions, the accuracy of CTA has also been reported to be very high in multiple studies, often at or near 100% sensitivity and specificity (see Figure 29.4). In fact, the pooled sensitivity and specificity for detection of a carotid occlusion by CTA in a recent meta-analysis was 97% and 99%, respectively.[21] Meanwhile, US is not able to distinguish between near-total and total occlusion, particularly in cases of heavy plaque calcification.

Near-occlusion stenoses (a.k.a. pseudo-occlusion, hairline residual lumen, string sign) of the carotid artery can also be diagnosed using CTA with a high degree of accuracy (see Figure 29.3A).[67–70] The differentiation between total occlusion and near occlusion has been considered clinically important because the former are usually treated medically, while the latter may benefit from surgery. Initial results from the NASCET, European Carotid Surgery Trial (ECST) and Veterans Affairs trial were conflicting with regard to the benefit of CEA in patients with near-occlusion stenoses.[7,11,12,71,72] Follow-up analysis of patients in the NASCET and ECST, however, suggests that patients with near occlusion may benefit from CEA, although the benefit is muted compared to patients who have severe stenosis without near occlusion.[66]

3.6 Plaque morphology

The rate of stroke ipsilateral to severe carotid stenosis is relatively low. Plaque morphology is increasingly being recognized as an independent risk factor for stroke, with considerable effort being made to identify and image 'vulnerable' plaque features. Plaques which are at increased risk of disruption appear to be associated with a higher risk of ischemic events due to increased embolization and/or occlusion. Typically, such features of vulnerability include, but are not limited to, a large necrotic core, an intraplaque hemorrhage, a lipid-rich core, and an unstable fibrous cap. There is no consensus on the optimal imaging strategy of carotid plaque morphology.[73] Various authors have proposed CTA as a tool for analyzing plaque morphology. Both CT and MRI appear to be capable of correlating plaque component appearance to lipoid, fibroid, calcified or hemorrhagic components (see Figure 29.3).[74–78] The results of more recent studies suggest that single-detector row CTA does not appear to be able to reliably predict plaque histology based on attenuation.[73,79] However, a retrospective study in which primarily MDCT was performed showed that CTA can evaluate for low plaque soft tissue attenuation, which may be a potential marker for ischemic

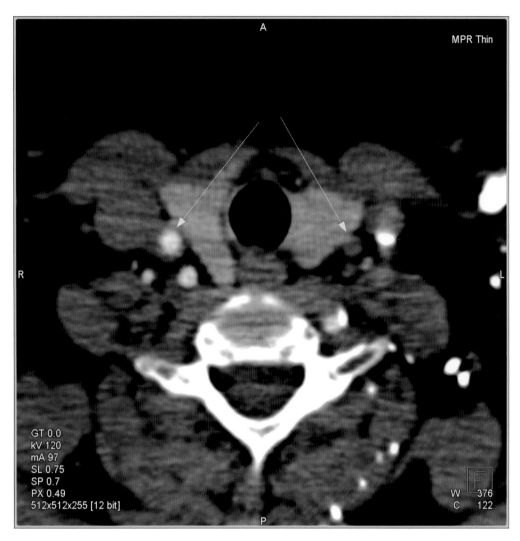

Figure 29.4 Carotid artery occlusion. The arrows indicate the common carotid arteries. No contrast enhancement is seen in the left common carotid artery, compatible with a complete occlusion. This image was acquired on a 64-slice scanner and the rapid scan acquisition combined with automated bolus tracking technique allow for a nearly exclusive arterial phase. Only reflux from the power injection is seen in the venous system. There is no antegrade venous opacification.

stroke.[80] Prospective confirmation of this finding has not been published to date.

While DSA and MRA are relatively insensitive with respect to assessing arterial calcification, plaque calcification can be detected and quantitatively estimated by CTA. MDCT-derived calcium measurement has been shown to represent a precise, reproducible equivalent of histological mineral content of vascular calcifications in ex vivo CEA specimens.[81,82] Preliminary work has shown that carotid bifurcation calcium volume, as measured by CT in vivo, may correlate strongly with the degree of carotid stenosis.[83,84] In addition, the presence of plaque calcification,[85] as well as higher absolute amount of[86] or higher relative proportion of[87] calcium in a plaque in patients with carotid stenosis as assessed by CTA, appear to be associated with plaque stability, based on decreased rates of ischemic symptoms.

NASCET data showed that in patients with severe stenosis treated medically, plaque ulceration was associated with an increased risk of stroke.[88] Although earlier studies, including one using NASCET data,[89] have documented the relative inability of DSA to detect ulceration, at least in part due to the limited number of views available, a more recent study suggests strong associations between plaque histology and angiographic plaque surface morphology.[90] While some earlier reports suggested the superiority of DSA, more recent studies indicate CTA (and MRA) may be more sensitive for plaque ulceration.[91] MRA may be more reliable than CTA in this regard.[73,74,92] Ideally, CTA and/or MRA will eventually routinely provide clinically useful information about plaque vulnerability, although other modalities, such as molecular imaging, are also likely to play a role.[93]

3.7 Additional applications

CTA capabilities in carotid atherosclerotic disease are not limited to assessing stenoses. Preliminary work has shown the ability of CTA to evaluate the intrastent luminal diameter in patients with carotid artery stents.[94,95] Stent assessment can be limited on US by overlying bone, postoperative hematoma and soft tissue emphysema, and on MRI by susceptibility artifact of the stent. Postoperative assessment for complications or residual disease is also possible.[96–98]

4 CAROTID AND VERTEBRAL ARTERY DISSECTIONS

Although relatively rare, extracranial arterial dissections are an established and important cause of ischemic stroke, particularly in young adults. These can be traumatic and nontraumatic in etiology. DSA is considered the gold standard for imaging of both carotid and vertebral artery dissections. However, DSA is not only associated with inherent risks, as described above, but it may also provide false negative results when there is lack of contrast opacification of the false lumen. DSA can be nonspecific and does not directly visualize intramural hematoma. Therefore, some authors recommend DSA only for an adjunct to endovascular therapy or for the uncommon cases in which noninvasive imaging techniques are equivocal.[99]

MRI/MRA has demonstrated high sensitivity and specificity for diagnosing cervical arterial dissections in prospective comparisons with DSA, particularly for the carotid arteries.[100] It is regarded as the method of choice for excluding this condition by many authors. This is largely because of its ability to see a positive finding, intramural hematoma, which is diagnostic of dissection. DSA and CTA rely more on vessel morphology and as such small dissections may be indistinguishable from vasospasm. Yet MRI/MRA is contraindicated in some patients and is not always available. Meanwhile, CTA has also demonstrated good results (see Figures 29.5 and 29.6), although the studies performed to date have all been relatively small. It is suspected that CTA is less sensitive in seeing dissection, as one relies less on identification of intramural hematoma and more on indirect signs of dissection, such as luminal narrowing and irregularity. In addition, CT is superior to MR in terms of visualizing the relationship of the dissection to bone and/or foreign bodies.

Initial reports of the CT appearance of carotid artery dissections were published in the 1980s.[101,102] Subsequent studies demonstrated sensitivities and specificities of up to 100%.[103,104] In a recent retrospective review of 7 patients with cervical internal carotid artery dissections, MDCTA identified the dissection in all 7 patients, while the combination of MRI and MRA identified dissection in 5 of the 7 patients, although the CT examination in one of these patients was performed 72 hours after the MR.[105] A recent retrospective review comparing MDCTA with DSA in 17 patients with vertebral artery dissections and 17 control patients demonstrated a sensitivity and specificity of MDCTA of 100% and 98%, respectively.[106] Like MRI/MRA, CTA has also been shown to be useful in the follow-up of patients with cervical carotid artery dissections.[107]

Based on a study of 18 angiographically confirmed extracranial carotid artery dissections, the most sensitive and specific finding of acute carotid artery dissections using single-detector row helical CTA is a narrowed eccentric lumen in association with an enlarged overall vessel diameter.[103] Increased external diameter has also been shown to be an accurate finding in vertebral artery dissections.[106] Additional less accurate findings of dissection include intimal flap, stenosis, mural thickening, occlusion, pseudoaneurysm formation, and thin annular contrast enhancement.

5 CAROTID AND VERTEBRAL ARTERY TRAUMA

Vascular injuries in the neck are associated with high morbidity and mortality. In fact, they are the leading cause of death in penetrating neck trauma. DSA is considered the imaging gold standard. However, its inherent risks, relatively high cost and the fact that the majority of angiographic evaluations in neck trauma are negative have led to the increased use of noninvasive imaging modalities for this indication. CTA is more readily available, faster and more conducive to the trauma setting than MRI/MRA. Meanwhile, US is operator dependent, relatively limited in accuracy for vessels near the skull base, and posttraumatic hematomas and soft tissue emphysema also decrease its sensitivity. In some centers CTA is used as the initial test for screening of suspected cervical arterial injury.[108–112] CTA has been shown to be able to detect a variety of cervical vascular injuries, including occlusion, pseudoaneurysm, extravasation, intimal flap, dissection and arteriovenous fistula. An additional advantage of CTA is that it can simultaneously provide information on the vertebral column, spinal canal, airway, other soft tissues, and location/trajectory of missiles or bone fragments.[113]

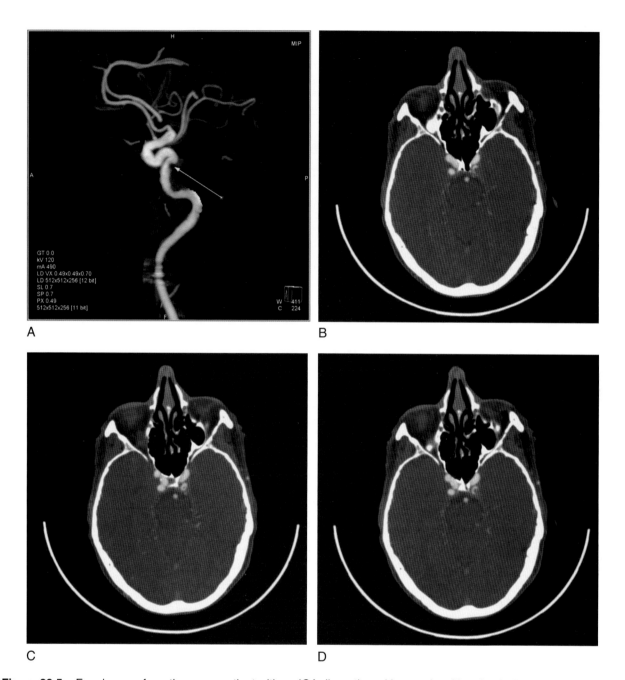

Figure 29.5 Four images from the same patient with an ICA dissection with associated intraluminal thrombus. (A) A MIP image from a matched-masked subtraction CTA demonstrates apparent stenosis of the proximal left cavernous ICA (arrow). (B–D) Three contiguous axial thin MPR images at this level demonstrate that the apparent stenosis actually represents a dissection with more distal intraluminal thrombus.

Initial reports of the accuracy of CTA for blunt cervical vascular injuries were disappointing.[114,115] However, in several prospective series comparing helical CTA and DSA for diagnosing blunt[110,116–119] or penetrating[120,121] arterial injuries to the neck, the sensitivity and specificity of CTA have been reported to be as high as 90% to 100%. Recent studies performed using MDCTA have shown particularly promising results.[109–111,116–119,122] For instance, Eastman et al. prospectively compared 16-channel MDCTA to DSA in 146

patients at risk for blunt cervical vascular injury. In the 43 patients with confirmed blunt cervical vascular injury, the sensitivity and specificity of MDCTA were 97.7% and 100%, respectively.[116] Several groups have also recently reported that the use of CTA as a guide to clinical decision-making for patients with penetrating neck trauma led to a significant decrease in the number of neck explorations, and essentially eliminated negative neck explorations at their institutions.[123,124]

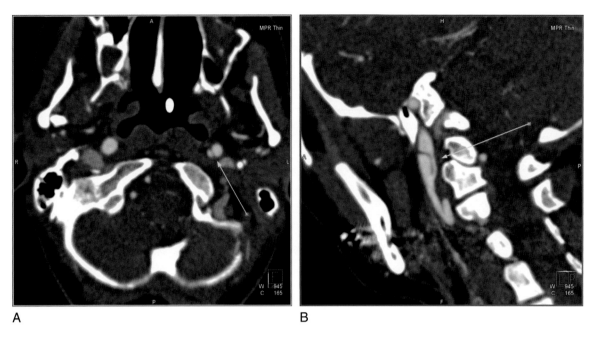

A   B

Figure 29.6   Two reformatted images from the same patient with ICA dissection. (A) An axial thin MPR demonstrates a dissection flap in the left ICA (arrow). (B) The same flap is seen in an oblique sagittal plane (arrow), with an additional flap seen more inferiorly.

REFERENCES

1. Willinsky RA, Taylor SM, terBrugge K et al. Neurologic Complications of Cerebral Angiography: Prospective Analysis of 2,899 Procedures and Review of the Literature. Radiology 2003; 227(2): 522–8.
2. Lell MM, Anders K, Uder M et al. New Techniques in CT Angiography. Radiographics 2006; 26(suppl 1): S45–62.
3. Takhtani D. CT neuroangiography: a glance at the common pitfalls and their prevention. AJR Am J Roentgenol 2005; 185(3): 772–83.
4. Fishman EK, Ney DR, Heath DG et al. Volume Rendering versus Maximum Intensity Projection in CT Angiography: What Works Best, When, and Why. Radiographics 2006; 26(3): 905–22.
5. Tomandl BF, Kostner NC, Schempershofe M et al. CT angiography of intracranial aneurysms: a focus on postprocessing. Radiographics 2004; 24(3): 637–55.
6. Beneficial effect of carotid endarterectomy in symptomatic patients with high-grade carotid stenosis. North American Symptomatic Carotid Endarterectomy Trial Collaborators. N Engl J Med 1991; 325(7): 445–53.
7. Rothwell PM, Eliasziw M, Gutnikov SA et al. Analysis of pooled data from the randomised controlled trials of endarterectomy for symptomatic carotid stenosis. Lancet 2003; 361(9352): 107–16.
8. Mayberg MR, Wilson SE, Yatsu F et al. Carotid endarterectomy and prevention of cerebral ischemia in symptomatic carotid stenosis. Veterans Affairs Cooperative Studies Program 309 Trialist Group. Jama 1991; 266(23): 3289–94.
9. Randomised trial of endarterectomy for recently symptomatic carotid stenosis: final results of the MRC European Carotid Surgery Trial (ECST). Lancet 1998; 351(9113): 1379–87.

10. MRC European Carotid Surgery Trial: interim results for symptomatic patients with severe (70–99%) or with mild (0–29%) carotid stenosis. European Carotid Surgery Trialists, Collaborative Group. Lancet 1991; 337(8752): 1235–43.
11. Barnett HJ, Taylor DW, Eliasziw M et al. Benefit of carotid endarterectomy in patients with symptomatic moderate or severe stenosis. North American Symptomatic Carotid Endarterectomy Trial Collaborators. N Engl J Med 1998; 339(20): 1415–25.
12. Rothwell PM, Gutnikov SA, Warlow CP. Reanalysis of the final results of the European Carotid Surgery Trial. Stroke 2003; 34(2): 514–23.
13. Endarterectomy for asymptomatic carotid artery stenosis. Executive Committee for the Asymptomatic Carotid Atherosclerosis Study. Jama 1995; 273(18): 1421–8.
14. Sabeti S, Schillinger M, Mlekusch W et al. Quantification of Internal Carotid Artery Stenosis with Duplex US: Comparative Analysis of Different Flow Velocity Criteria. Radiology 2004; 232(2): 431–9.
15. Powers WJ. Carotid arteriography: Still golden after all these years? Neurology 2004; 62(8): 1246–7.
16. Derdeyn CP. Catheter Angiography Is Still Necessary for the Measurement of Carotid Stenosis. AJNR Am J Neuroradiol 2003; 24(9): 1737–8.
17. Heinz E, Fuchs J, Osborne D et al. Examination of the extracranial carotid bifurcation by thin-section dynamic CT: direct visualization of intimal atheroma in man (Part 2). AJNR Am J Neuroradiol 1984; 5(4): 361–6.
18. Heinz E, Pizer S, Fuchs H et al. Examination of the extracranial carotid bifurcation by thin-section dynamic CT: direct visualization of intimal atheroma in man (Part 1). AJNR Am J Neuroradiol 1984; 5(4): 355–9.

19. Riles TS, Posner MP, Cohen WS et al. The totally occluded internal carotid artery. Preliminary observations using rapid sequential computerized tomographic scanning. Arch Surg 1982; 117(9): 1185–8.

20. Wardlaw JM, Chappell FM, Best JJ, Wartolowska K, Berry E. Non-invasive imaging compared with intra-arterial angiography in the diagnosis of symptomatic carotid stenosis: a meta-analysis. Lancet 2006; 367(9521): 1503–12.

21. Koelemay MJ, Nederkoorn PJ, Reitsma JB, Majoie CB. Systematic review of computed tomographic angiography for assessment of carotid artery disease. Stroke 2004; 35(10): 2306–12.

22. Hollingworth W, Nathens AB, Kanne JP et al. The diagnostic accuracy of computed tomography angiography for traumatic or atherosclerotic lesions of the carotid and vertebral arteries: a systematic review. Eur J Radiol 2003; 48(1): 88–102.

23. Kallmes DF, Omary RA, Dix JE, Evans AJ, Hillman BJ. Specificity of MR angiography as a confirmatory test of carotid artery stenosis. AJNR Am J Neuroradiol 1996; 17(8): 1501–6.

24. Layton KF, Huston J 3rd, Cloft HJ et al. Specificity of MR Angiography as a Confirmatory Test for Carotid Artery Stenosis: Is It Valid? Am J Roentgenol 2007; 188(4): 1114–16.

25. Berg M, Zhang Z, Ikonen A et al. Multi-Detector Row CT Angiography in the Assessment of Carotid Artery Disease in Symptomatic Patients: Comparison with Rotational Angiography and Digital Subtraction Angiography. AJNR Am J Neuroradiol 2005; 26(5): 1022–34.

26. Silvennoinen HM, Ikonen S, Soinne L, Railo M, Valanne L. CT angiographic analysis of carotid artery stenosis: comparison of manual assessment, semiautomatic vessel analysis, and digital subtraction angiography. AJNR Am J Neuroradiol 2007; 28(1): 97–103.

27. Jenkins RH, Mahal R, MacEneaney PM. Noninvasive imaging of carotid artery disease: critically appraised topic. Can Assoc Radiol J 2003; 54(2): 121–3.

28. Dillon E, van Leeuwen M, Fernandez M, Eikelboom B, Mali W. CT angiography: application to the evaluation of carotid artery stenosis. Radiology 1993; 189(1): 211–19.

29. Nonent M, Serfaty JM, Nighoghossian N et al. Concordance rate differences of 3 noninvasive imaging techniques to measure carotid stenosis in clinical routine practice: results of the CARMEDAS multicenter study. Stroke 2004; 35(3): 682–6.

30. Lell M, Fellner C, Baum U et al. Evaluation of carotid artery stenosis with multisection CT and MR imaging: influence of imaging modality and postprocessing. AJNR Am J Neuroradiol 2007; 28(1): 104–10.

31. Magarelli N, Scarabino T, Simeone AL et al. Carotid stenosis: a comparison between MR and spiral CT angiography. Neuroradiology 1998; V40(6): 367–73.

32. Patel SG, Collie DA, Wardlaw JM et al. Outcome, observer reliability, and patient preferences if CTA, MRA, or Doppler ultrasound were used, individually or together, instead of digital subtraction angiography before carotid endarterectomy. J Neurol Neurosurg Psychiatry 2002; 73(1): 21–8.

33. Cumming M, Morrow I. Carotid artery stenosis: a prospective comparison of CT angiography and conventional angiography. Am J Roentgenol 1994; 163(3): 517–23.

34. Hacklander T, Wegner H, Hoppe S et al. Agreement of multislice CT angiography and MR angiography in assessing the degree of carotid artery stenosis in consideration of different methods of postprocessing. J Comput Assist Tomogr 2006; 30(3): 433–42.

35. Josephson SA, Bryant SO, Mak HK et al. Evaluation of carotid stenosis using CT angiography in the initial evaluation of stroke and TIA. Neurology 2004; 63(3): 457–60.

36. Elgersma OEH, Wust AFJ, Buijs PC et al. Multidirectional Depiction of Internal Carotid Arterial Stenosis: Three-dimensional Time-of-Flight MR Angiography versus Rotational and Conventional Digital Subtraction Angiography. Radiology 2000; 216(2): 511–16.

37. Nederkoorn PJ, Elgersma OE, Mali WP et al. Overestimation of carotid artery stenosis with magnetic resonance angiography compared with digital subtraction angiography. J Vasc Surg 2002; 36(4): 806–13.

38. Nederkoorn PJ, Mali WPTM, Eikelboom BC et al. Preoperative Diagnosis of Carotid Artery Stenosis: Accuracy of Noninvasive Testing. Stroke 2002; 33(8): 2003–8.

39. Johnston DC, Eastwood JD, Nguyen T, Goldstein LB. Contrast-enhanced magnetic resonance angiography of carotid arteries: utility in routine clinical practice. Stroke 2002; 33(12): 2834–8.

40. Sameshima T, Futami S, Morita Y et al. Clinical usefulness of and problems with three-dimensional CT angiography for the evaluation of arteriosclerotic stenosis of the carotid artery: comparison with conventional angiography, MRA, and ultrasound sonography. Surg Neurol 1999; 51(3): 301–8; discussion 8–9.

41. U-King-Im JM, Trivedi RA, Graves MJ et al. Contrast-enhanced MR angiography for carotid disease: Diagnostic and potential clinical impact. Neurology 2004; 62(8): 1282–90.

42. Steger W, Vogl TJ, Rausch M et al. CT angiography in carotid stenosis. Diagnostic value compared to color-coded duplex ultrasonography and MR angiography. Rofo 1995; 162(5): 373–80.

43. Hoogeveen RM, Bakker CJ, Viergever MA. Limits to the accuracy of vessel diameter measurement in MR angiography. J Magn Reson Imaging 1998; 8(6): 1228–35.

44. Townsend TC, Saloner D, Pan XM, Rapp JH. Contrast material-enhanced MRA overestimates severity of carotid stenosis, compared with 3D time-of-flight MRA. Journal of Vascular Surgery 2003; 38(1): 36–40.

45. Borisch I, Horn M, Butz B et al. Preoperative Evaluation of Carotid Artery Stenosis: Comparison of Contrast-Enhanced MR Angiography and Duplex Sonography with Digital Subtraction Angiography. AJNR Am J Neuroradiol 2003; 24(6): 1117–22.

46. Cosottini M, Calabrese R, Puglioli M et al. Contrast-enhanced three-dimensional MR angiography of neck vessels: does dephasing effect alter diagnostic accuracy? European Radiology 2003; 13(3): 571–81.

47. Cosottini M, Pingitore A, Puglioli M et al. Contrast-Enhanced Three-Dimensional Magnetic Resonance Angiography of Atherosclerotic Internal Carotid Stenosis as the Noninvasive Imaging Modality in Revascularization Decision Making. Stroke 2003; 34(3): 660–4.

48. Berg MH, Manninen HI, Rasanen HT, Vanninen RL, Jaakkola PA. CT angiography in the assessment of carotid artery atherosclerosis. Acta Radiol 2002; 43(2): 116–24.

49. Heiserman JE. Measurement Error of Percent Diameter Carotid Stenosis Determined by Conventional Angiography: Implications for Noninvasive Evaluation. AJNR Am J Neuroradiol 2005; 26(8): 2102–7.

50. Eliasziw M, Fox A, Sharpe B, Barnett H. Carotid artery stenosis: external validity of the North American Symptomatic Carotid Endarterectomy Trial measurement method. Radiology 1997; 204(1): 229–33.

51. Anzalone N, Scomazzoni F, Castellano R et al. Carotid Artery Stenosis: Intraindividual Correlations of 3D Time-of-Flight MR Angiography, Contrast-enhanced MR Angiography, Conventional DSA, and Rotational Angiography for Detection and Grading. Radiology 2005; 236(1): 204–13.

52. Elgersma OEH, Buijs PC, Wust AFJ et al. Maximum Internal Carotid Arterial Stenosis: Assessment with Rotational Angiography versus Conventional Intraarterial Digital Subtraction Angiography. Radiology 1999; 213(3): 777–83.

53. Bosanac Z, Miller RJ, Jain M. Rotational digital subtraction carotid angiography: technique and comparison with static digital subtraction angiography. Clin Radiol 1998; 53(9): 682–7.

54. Netuka D, Benes V, Mandys V et al. Accuracy of angiography and Doppler ultrasonography in the detection of carotid stenosis: a histopathological study of 123 cases. Acta Neurochirurgica 2006; 148(5): 511–20.

55. Benes V, Netuka D, Mandys V et al. Comparison between degree of carotid stenosis observed at angiography and in histological examination. Acta Neurochirurgica 2004; 146(7): 671–7.

56. Bartlett ES, Walters TD, Symons SP, Fox AJ. Quantification of carotid stenosis on CT angiography. AJNR Am J Neuroradiol 2006; 27(1): 13–19.

57. Leclerc X, Godefroy O, Pruvo JP, Leys D. Computed Tomographic Angiography for the Evaluation of Carotid Artery Stenosis. Stroke 1995; 26(9): 1577–81.

58. Dix JE, Evans AJ, Kallmes DF, Sobel AH, Phillips CD. Accuracy and precision of CT angiography in a model of carotid artery bifurcation stenosis. AJNR Am J Neuroradiol 1997; 18(3): 409–15.

59. Papp Z, Patel M, Ashtari M et al. Carotid artery stenosis: optimization of CT angiography with a combination of shaded surface display and source images. AJNR Am J Neuroradiol 1997; 18(4): 759–63.

60. Ertl-Wagner BB, Bruening R, Blume J et al. Relative Value of Sliding-Thin-Slab Multiplanar Reformations and Sliding-Thin-Slab Maximum Intensity Projections as Reformatting Techniques in Multisection CT Angiography of the Cervicocranial Vessels. AJNR Am J Neuroradiol 2006; 27(1): 107–13.

61. Sparacia G, Bencivinni F, Banco A et al. Imaging processing for CT angiography of the cervicocranial arteries: evaluation of reformatting technique. La Radiologia Medica 2007; 112(2): 224–38.

62. Addis KA, Hopper KD, Iyriboz TA et al. CT Angiography: In Vitro Comparison of Five Reconstruction Methods. Am J Roentgenol 2001; 177(5): 1171–6.

63. Liu Y, Hopper KD, Mauger DT, Addis KA. CT Angiographic Measurement of the Carotid Artery: Optimizing Visualization by Manipulating Window and Level Settings and Contrast Material Attenuation. Radiology 2000; 217(2): 494–500.

64. Kaufmann TJ, Kallmes DF. Utility of MRA and CTA in the evaluation of carotid occlusive disease. Semin Vasc Surg 2005; 18(2): 75–82.

65. Zhang Z, Berg M, Ikonen AJ, Vanninen R, Manninen H. Carotid artery stenosis: reproducibility of automated 3D CT angiography analysis method. European Radiology 2004; V14(4): 665–72.

66. Fox AJ, Eliasziw M, Rothwell PM et al. Identification, Prognosis, and Management of Patients with Carotid Artery Near Occlusion. AJNR Am J Neuroradiol 2005; 26(8): 2086–94.

67. Bartlett ES, Walters TD, Symons SP, Fox AJ. Diagnosing carotid stenosis near-occlusion by using CT angiography. AJNR Am J Neuroradiol 2006; 27(3): 632–7.

68. Chen C-J, Lee T-H, Hsu H-L et al. Multi-Slice CT Angiography in Diagnosing Total Versus Near Occlusions of the Internal Carotid Artery: Comparison With Catheter Angiography. Stroke 2004; 35(1): 83–5.

69. Lev MH, Romero JM, Goodman DNF et al. Total Occlusion versus Hairline Residual Lumen of the Internal Carotid Arteries: Accuracy of Single Section Helical CT Angiography. AJNR Am J Neuroradiol 2003; 24(6): 1123–9.

70. Leclerc X, Godefroy O, Lucas C et al. Internal Carotid Arterial Stenosis: CT Angiography with Volume Rendering. Radiology 1999; 210(3): 673–82.

71. Rothwell PM, Warlow CP. Low Risk of Ischemic Stroke in Patients With Reduced Internal Carotid Artery Lumen Diameter Distal to Severe Symptomatic Carotid Stenosis: Cerebral Protection Due to Low Poststenotic Flow? Stroke 2000; 31(3): 622–30.

72. Morgenstern L, Fox A, Sharpe B et al. The risks and benefits of carotid endarterectomy in patients with near occlusion of the carotid artery. North American Symptomatic Carotid Endarterectomy Trial (NASCET) Group. Neurology 1997; 48(4): 911–15.

73. Walker LJ, Ismail A, McMeekin W et al. Computed Tomography Angiography for the Evaluation of Carotid Atherosclerotic Plaque: Correlation With Histopathology of Endarterectomy Specimens. Stroke 2002; 33(4): 977–81.

74. Oliver TB, Lammie GA, Wright AR et al. Atherosclerotic plaque at the carotid bifurcation: CT angiographic appearance with histopathologic correlation. AJNR Am J Neuroradiol 1999; 20(5): 897–901.

75. Toussaint J-F, LaMuraglia GM, Southern JF, Fuster V, Kantor HL. Magnetic Resonance Images Lipid, Fibrous, Calcified, Hemorrhagic, and Thrombotic Components of Human Atherosclerosis In Vivo. Circulation 1996; 94(5): 932–8.

76. von Ingersleben G, Schmiedl U, Hatsukami T et al. Characterization of atherosclerotic plaques at the carotid bifurcation: correlation of high-resolution MR imaging with histologic analysis – preliminary study. Radiographics 1997; 17(6): 1417–23.

77. Shinnar M, Fallon JT, Wehrli S et al. The diagnostic accuracy of ex vivo MRI for human atherosclerotic plaque characterization. Arterioscler Thromb Vasc Biol 1999; 19(11): 2756–61.

78. Estes JM, Quist WC, Lo Gerfo FW, Costello P. Noninvasive characterization of plaque morphology using helical computed tomography. J Cardiovasc Surg (Torino) 1998; 39(5): 527–34.

79. Gronholdt ML, Wagner A, Wiebe BM et al. Spiral computed tomographic imaging related to computerized ultrasonographic images of carotid plaque morphology and histology. J Ultrasound Med 2001; 20(5): 451–8.

80. Serfaty JM, Nonent M, Nighoghossian N et al. Plaque density on CT, a potential marker of ischemic stroke. Neurology 2006; 66(1): 118–20.

81. Hoffmann U, Kwait DC, Handwerker J et al. Vascular Calcification in ex Vivo Carotid Specimens: Precision and Accuracy of Measurements with Multi-Detector Row CT. Radiology 2003; 229(2): 375–81.

82. Denzel C, Lell M, Maak M et al. Carotid Artery Calcium: Accuracy of a Calcium Score by Computed Tomography – An In vitro Study with Comparison to Sonography and Histology. European Journal of Vascular and Endovascular Surgery 2004; 28(2): 214–20.

83. McKinney AM, Casey SO, Teksam M et al. Carotid bifurcation calcium and correlation with percent stenosis of the internal carotid artery on CT angiography. Neuroradiology 2005; 47(1): 1–9.

84. Nandalur KR, Baskurt E, Hagspiel KD et al. Carotid Artery Calcification on CT May Independently Predict Stroke Risk. Am J Roentgenol 2006; 186(2): 547–52.

85. Nandalur KR, Baskurt E, Hagspiel KD, Phillips CD, Kramer CM. Calcified Carotid Atherosclerotic Plaque Is Associated Less with Ischemic Symptoms Than Is Noncalcified Plaque on MDCT. Am J Roentgenol 2005; 184(1): 295–8.

86. Miralles M, Merino J, Busto M et al. Quantification and Characterization of Carotid Calcium with Multi-detector CT-angiography. European Journal of Vascular and Endovascular Surgery 2006; 32(5): 561–7.

87. Nandalur KR, Hardie AD, Raghavan P et al. Composition of the Stable Carotid Plaque: Insights From a Multidetector Computed Tomography Study of Plaque Volume. Stroke 2007; 38(3): 935–40.

88. Eliasziw M, Streifler J, Fox A et al. Significance of plaque ulceration in symptomatic patients with high-grade carotid stenosis. North American Symptomatic Carotid Endarterectomy Trial. Stroke 1994; 25(2): 304–8.

89. Streifler J, Eliasziw M, Fox A et al. Angiographic detection of carotid plaque ulceration. Comparison with surgical observations in a multicenter study. North American Symptomatic Carotid Endarterectomy Trial. Stroke 1994; 25(6): 1130–2.

90. Lovett JK, Gallagher PJ, Hands LJ, Walton J, Rothwell PM. Histological Correlates of Carotid Plaque Surface Morphology on Lumen Contrast Imaging. Circulation 2004; 110(15): 2190–7.

91. Randoux B, Marro B, Koskas F et al. Carotid Artery Stenosis: Prospective Comparison of CT, Three-dimensional Gadolinium-enhanced MR, and Conventional Angiography. Radiology 2001; 220(1): 179–85.

92. Alvarez-Linera J, Benito-Leon J, Escribano J, Campollo J, Gesto R. Prospective Evaluation of Carotid Artery Stenosis: Elliptic Centric Contrast-Enhanced MR Angiography and Spiral CT Angiography Compared with Digital Subtraction Angiography. AJNR Am J Neuroradiol 2003; 24(5): 1012–19.

93. Nighoghossian N, Derex L, Douek P. The Vulnerable Carotid Artery Plaque: Current Imaging Methods and New Perspectives. Stroke 2005; 36(12): 2764–72.

94. Orbach DB, Pramanik BK, Lee J et al. Carotid Artery Stent Implantation: Evaluation with Multi-Detector Row CT Angiography and Virtual Angioscopy – Initial Experience. Radiology 2006; 238(1): 309–20.

95. Leclerc X, Gauvrit JY, Pruvo JP. Usefulness of CT Angiography with Volume Rendering After Carotid Angioplasty and Stenting. Am J Roentgenol 2000; 174(3): 820–2.

96. Goddard AJP, Mendelow AD, Birchall D. Computed Tomography Angiography in the Investigation of Carotid Stenosis. Clinical Radiology 2001; 56(7): 523–34.

97. Moll R, Dinkel HP. Value of the CT angiography in the diagnosis of common carotid artery bifurcation disease: CT angiography versus digital subtraction angiography and color flow Doppler. Eur J Radiol 2001; 39(3): 155–62.

98. Marro B, Zouaoui A, Koskas F et al. Computerized tomographic angiography scan following carotid endarterectomy. Ann Vasc Surg 1998; 12(5): 451–6.

99. Flis CM, Jäger HR, Sidhu PS. Carotid and vertebral artery dissections: clinical aspects, imaging features and endovascular treatment. European Radiology 2007; 17(3): 820–34.

100. Levy C, Laissy J, Raveau V et al. Carotid and vertebral artery dissections: three-dimensional time-of-flight MR angiography and MR imaging versus conventional angiography. Radiology 1994; 190(1): 97–103.

101. Petro G, Witwer G, Cacayorin E et al. Spontaneous dissection of the cervical internal carotid artery: correlation of arteriography, CT, and pathology. Am J Roentgenol 1987; 148(2): 393–8.

102. Dal Pozzo G, Mascalchi M, Fonda C et al. Lower cranial nerve palsy due to dissection of the internal carotid artery: CT and MR imaging. J Comput Assist Tomogr 1989; 13(6): 989–95.

103. Leclerc X, Godefroy O, Salhi A et al. Helical CT for the Diagnosis of Extracranial Internal Carotid Artery Dissection. Stroke 1996; 27(3): 461–6.

104. Zuber M, Meary E, Meder J, Mas J. Magnetic resonance imaging and dynamic CT scan in cervical artery dissections. Stroke 1994; 25(3): 576–81.

105. Elijovich L, Kazmi K, Gauvrit JY, Law M. The emerging role of multidetector row CT angiography in the diagnosis of cervical arterial dissection: preliminary study. Neuroradiology 2006; 48(9): 606–12.

106. Chen C-J, Tseng Y-C, Lee T-H, Hsu H-L, See L-C. Multisection CT Angiography Compared with Catheter Angiography in Diagnosing Vertebral Artery Dissection. AJNR Am J Neuroradiol 2004; 25(5): 769–74.

107. Leclerc X, Lucas C, Godefroy O et al. Helical CT for the follow-up of cervical internal carotid artery dissections. AJNR Am J Neuroradiol 1998; 19(5): 831–7.

108. Rogers FB, Baker EF, Osler TM et al. Computed tomographic angiography as a screening modality for blunt cervical arterial injuries: preliminary results. J Trauma 1999; 46(3): 380–5.

109. Utter GH, Hollingworth W, Hallam DK, Jarvik JG, Jurkovich GJ. Sixteen-slice CT angiography in patients with suspected blunt carotid and vertebral artery injuries. J Am Coll Surg 2006; 203(6): 838–48.

110. Berne JD, Reuland KS, Villarreal DH et al. Sixteen-slice multi-detector computed tomographic angiography improves the accuracy of screening for blunt cerebrovascular injury. J Trauma 2006; 60(6): 1204–9; discussion 9–10.

111. Stuhlfaut JW, Barest G, Sakai O, Lucey B, Soto JA. Impact of MDCT Angiography on the Use of Catheter Angiography for the Assessment of Cervical Arterial Injury After Blunt or Penetrating Trauma. Am J Roentgenol 2005; 185(4): 1063–8.

112. Múnera F, Soto JA, Palacio DM et al. Penetrating Neck Injuries: Helical CT Angiography for Initial Evaluation. Radiology 2002; 224(2): 366–72.

113. Nuñez DB, Jr, Torres-León M, Múnera F. Vascular Injuries of the Neck and Thoracic Inlet: Helical CT-Angiographic Correlation. Radiographics 2004; 24(4): 1087–98.

114. Miller PR, Fabian TC, Croce MA et al. Prospective screening for blunt cerebrovascular injuries: analysis of diagnostic modalities and outcomes. Ann Surg 2002; 236(3): 386–93; discussion 93–5.

115. Biffl WL, Ray CE Jr., Moore EE et al. Noninvasive diagnosis of blunt cerebrovascular injuries: a preliminary report. J Trauma 2002; 53(5): 850–6.

116. Eastman AL, Chason DP, Perez CL, McAnulty AL, Minei JP. Computed tomographic angiography for the diagnosis of blunt cervical vascular injury: is it ready for primetime? J Trauma 2006; 60(5): 925–9; discussion 9.

117. Schneidereit NP, Simons R, Nicolaou S et al. Utility of screening for blunt vascular neck injuries with computed tomographic angiography. J Trauma 2006; 60(1): 209–15; discussion 15–16.

118. Biffl WL, Egglin T, Benedetto B, Gibbs F, Cioffi WG. Sixteen-slice computed tomographic angiography is a reliable noninvasive screening test for clinically significant blunt cerebrovascular injuries. J Trauma 2006; 60(4): 745–51; discussion 51–2.

119. Berne JD, Norwood SH, McAuley CE, Villareal DH. Helical computed tomographic angiography: an excellent screening test for blunt cerebrovascular injury. J Trauma 2004; 57(1): 11–7; discussion 7–9.

120. Múnera F, Soto JA, Palacio D, Velez SM, Medina E. Diagnosis of Arterial Injuries Caused by Penetrating Trauma to the Neck: Comparison of Helical CT Angiography and Conventional Angiography. Radiology 2000; 216(2): 356–62.

121. LeBlang SD, Nuñez DB, Rivas LA, Falcone S, Pogson SE. Helical computed tomographic angiography in penetrating neck trauma. Emergency Radiology 1997; 4(4): 200–6.

122. Bub LD, Hollingworth W, Jarvik JG, Hallam DK. Screening for blunt cerebrovascular injury: evaluating the accuracy of multidetector computed tomographic angiography. J Trauma 2005; 59(3): 691–7.

123. Bell RB, Osborn T, Dierks EJ, Potter BE, Long WB. Management of Penetrating Neck Injuries: A New Paradigm for Civilian Trauma. Journal of Oral and Maxillofacial Surgery 2007; 65(4): 691–705.

124. Woo K, Magner DP, Wilson MT, Margulies DR. CT angiography in penetrating neck trauma reduces the need for operative neck exploration. Am Surg 2005; 71(9): 754–8.

125. Kaufmann TJ, Huston J 3rd, Mandrekar JN, Schleck CD, Thielen KR, Kallmes DF. Complications of diagnostic cerebral angiography: evaluation of 19,826 consecutive patients. Radiology 2007 Jun; 243(3): 812–19.

30

Cardiovascular Computed Tomography: A Research Perspective

Yue Dong and Erik L. Ritman

1 INTRODUCTION

Continued developments in CT imaging are in part driven by the quest for increased accuracy, sensitivity and specificity of the measurements made from those CT images.

These can be achieved by 'brute force' improvement of the current CT scanner capabilities by technological advances applied to the systems. This approach is usually limited by the cost and technological possibilities. However, some plausible capabilities (which often cannot be fully evaluated as to their value until a system is made available), which are suggested from new insights obtained from research or clinical experience may only be achievable by use of aspects of x-ray interaction with matter different from the current use of attenuation of x-rays. All these potential developments must keep in mind the radiation exposure associated with a CT scan that has to be balanced against the possible harm done to a subject if the CT scan is not performed. Thus, for a person aged 65, repeated CT scans for monitoring of progression of coronary artery disease may be more readily justified than CT-based screening of 20-years-old.

A dilemma is that engineers and physicists may know what is technically possible, but have no reason to think of implementing those methods unless there is a clinical need for it. However, as clinicians may not know what is technically possible they have no reason to encourage the implementation of such new capabilities because they may not realize what new insights might be gained with them. The engineers and physicists also may not be aware as to which extensions of current technology would be useful. Consequently, this exploration of possible future developments in the CT imaging field and clinical needs (that might be susceptible to imaging advances) is broken down into possible expansion of existing CT technology and into technological implications of cardiological questions that can perhaps be better addressed with novel CT imaging methods.

2 EXTENSION OF CURRENT APPLICATIONS

With the introduction of helical scanning multi-slice CT we have seen, and continue to see, increased spatial and temporal resolution as well as increase in the cephalo-caudal extent of the body imaged. This evolution may possibly be further extended by the introduction of large flat panel detector arrays. These methods share certain challenges such as the need to suppress x-ray scatter contamination of the transmission measurements, the need for overcoming the cone-beam reconstruction problem and reducing the radiation consequences. Current knowledge can put some bounds on the upper limits of image resolution that may be needed, and tolerated to take full advantage of CT imaging in cardiovascular applications.

2.1 The upper limit of spatial resolution

Spatial resolution is determined by a number of technological factors and biomedical requirements. Generally speaking, the higher the resolution, the smaller the CT image voxel volume, and the higher the radiation exposure needed to maintain an adequate signal-to-noise ratio. Factors to be considered include:

2.1.1 Partial volume effect, reconstruction algorithm characteristics, etc.

Several technological and mathematical factors determine CT image resolution. The voxel size is a critical determinant of image resolution in that resolution can be no better than double the size of the voxel. However, voxel size does not guarantee that resolution because the scanner detector size, the reconstruction geometry, and reconstruction algorithm also impact on the information content of the voxel. Even if we assume that these technological factors provide a meaningful relationship between the voxel size and spatial resolution, the voxel can still affect spatial resolution via the partial volume effect. This effect is due to the 'misalignment' between the voxel and the anatomic structure such that a voxel that straddles an anisotropic region of roentgen opacity. This effect is reduced by having smaller detector pixels and CT image voxels, but even so there will always be a partial volume effect at interfaces where there is rapid change of radiopacity, such as occurs at the endothelial surface of a blood vessel during passage of a bolus of contrast agent through its lumen. This results in uncertainty in the measured location of the endothelial surface and in the CT value in the subendothelial tissues of the arterial wall. Removal of those voxels at the interface will reduce the contrast artifact but will impact on the dimensional measurement.[1]

2.1.2 Microvessel diameter

Intramyocardial microvessels greater than approximately 200 μm in diameter have different patho-physiological implications than vessels less than that diameter. It is unrealistic to expect to resolve these small vessels with

clinical CT, so models have to be developed to provide at least an index of the population characteristics of these two vessel types.

2.1.3 Basic Functional Unit diameter

The terminal arteriole (approximately 10 μm in lumen diameter) branches into a number of capillaries. These capillaries perfuse a number of myocytes (on average one capillary per cell). This ensemble is the myocardial basic functional unit and is approximately 200 μm in diameter.[2,3] Current multislice CT scanners almost achieve voxel sized of this magnitude, but it is unlikely that these units can be truly resolved in a routine clinical CT scanner. However, CT image analysis techniques may be able to extract information about the population behavior of these units from the CT images. Such perfusion territories are expected to not be perfused in certain condition such as microembolization resulting from intravascular interventions[4] or from pathological causes.[5]

2.1.4 Arterial wall thickness

The arterial wall of proximal coronary arteries is of great interest because any thickening (before encroachment into the lumen) is an early sign of atherosclerosis[6] and any change in CT number within the arterial wall can be an early sign of plaque development.[7] As the average normal wall thickness of a 4 mm diameter coronary artery is approximately 1 mm, this requires a spatial resolution of at least 0.25 mm, i.e., voxels less than 0.125 mm.

2.2 The upper limit of contrast resolution

2.2.1 Due to partial volume effect

As indicated above, there will always be voxels that straddle a region of changing radiopacity. Consequently, the measured CT number is open to question in regions such as the arterial wall where luminal contents 'mixes' with the subendothelial wall, and similarly opacities within the wall (e.g., calcium) may be smaller (but more opaque) than conveyed by the CT image. This effect can be partially overcome and the true volume of the contrasting materials estimated, if the true CT contrast value of the contrast accumulation is known (e.g., calcium plaque material or iodine concentration in lumen).[8]

2.2.2 Atherosclerotic plaque's fatty and fibrous components

Atherosclerotic plaque can consist of increased soft tissue (e.g., smooth muscle and/or collagen) which do not greatly affect local CT number, fatty infiltrates which have lower CT number or calcification which has a much increased CT number. Accurate measurement of the CT number is therefore critically important. The competing technological consequences of partial volume effect and adequate signal-to-noise ratio of the CT number here is a difficulty. Because of the inevitably limited contrast resolution at these high spatial resolutions needed, it is often impossible to separately delineate the calcium deposit from the contrast-enhanced lumen using combined CT imaging.

2.2.3 Iron accumulation following an intramural hemorrhage

Hemorrhage into an atherosclerotic plaque can have fatal consequences if it ruptures through the endothelium. If the hemorrhage remains constrained to the wall it could be a harbinger of a subsequent plaque rupture. Hence, detection of iron (from the hemoglobin) within the wall could be important clinical information. However, it is unlikely that it could be distinguished from calcification (which has much more benign implications at that site in the artery) by virtue of the CT number or any differences in their local spatial distribution pattern within the wall.

2.2.4 Transient opacification of myocardium and arterial wall following an IV contrast injection

The degree of transient opacification at these sites reflects local microvascular blood volume and blood flow. In the myocardium, reduction in these values can be expected when there is local ischemia due to narrowing of the epicardial or microvascular arteries or due to microembolism. In the arterial wall these values can change due to reduction or increase in the density of vasa vasorum in response to atherosclerosis or hypertension. Unlike the thick-walled myocardium (in which 10–15% of the normal myocardium is intravascular blood volume) where relatively large voxels (indeed ROIs) can provide useful information, the relatively thin arterial wall demands high contrast resolution at high spatial resolution because the vasa vasorum blood volume is normally only 2% of the wall (Figure 30.1).[9]

2.3 The upper limit of temporal resolution

Temporal resolution depends on a number of factors. The ultimate limit is set by the x-ray flux generated by the x-ray

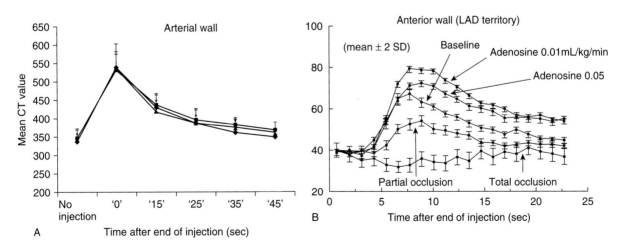

Figure 30.1 (A) Transient opacification of porcine coronary vessel wall measured with a cryostatic micro-CT shows that the maximal opacification occurs immediately after complete injection of contrast medium (0 s). All layers of the coronary vessel wall show a progressive decrease in opacification. (Reproduced with permission from Gössl, M et. al., Am J Physiol Heart Circ Physiol 2004; 287: H2346-H2351). (B) Transient opacification of porcine myocardium (measured with EBCT) shows impact of hyperemia and impaired perfusion on the myocardial dilution curve. Both the dilution curve in the arterial and ventricular walls allow quantitative of microvascular perfusion and blood volume in the tissues.

source as this governs the duration needed to obtain an adequate signal-to-noise ratio for any one angle-of-view. This limit can be ameliorated by having multiple x-ray sources which reduces the scan time roughly in inverse proportional to the number of sources. Dual-sources at 90° can reduce scan time by almost half for a 180° plus half fan-angle scan, but three sources at 120° can generate a 360° scan in 1/3 of the scanner rotation time. The 360° scan is preferable to the 180° plus half-angle scan because this eliminates the inevitable rotating scan artifact resulting from angle-dependent beam hardening.

2.3.1 Scan 'aperture time'

Scan 'aperture time' is the time required to obtain CT scan data over at least 180° plus the x-ray fan beam half-angle, although ideally 360° is scanned in that time. This duration is determined by the rate of movement of the structure of interest. Thus, as the normal heart wall thickens maximally during systole at about 50 mm/second (i.e., 1 mm in 20 msec),[10] an aperture time of 10 msec would be required if a spatial resolution of 1 mm is desired. However, in the slow filling phase of diastole this rate is more like 5 mm/second, so that an aperture time of 100 msec is adequate. This latter aperture time is now available in the latest 'fast' helical scanning multi-slice CT scanners.[11] While ECG-gated scanning can be used to obtain an effective aperture time less than the 'single shot' scan aperture time, this works only when the heart rate is steady and the level of blood opacification is sufficiently constant during the entire scan acquisition time (generally a single breath-hold). Thus, any events that are transient, such as the passage of a bolus of contrast agent through the myocardium or arterial wall, ECG-gated

scanning cannot be used. A 'single shot' scan is needed for such application.

2.3.2 Scan "frame rate"

If the information of interest is a time series (e.g., to show the maximum rate of ventricular wall thickening or thinning during the cardiac cycle), then the number of scans per second needed to adequately convey that dynamic process is governed by the maximal rate of motion during that process. Thus, even though the heart rate may be 60 beats per minute, the number of images needed to adequately capture the systolic phase is at least 15 frames per second.[12] At higher heart rates this will need to be more frequent.

2.3.3 Reproducibility of CT gray-scale values – role of calibration, beam hardening, partial volume effects

In current CT scanners the use of a contrast calibration to convert the CT number to mg/cm^3 of the desired material (e.g., calcium or iodine) increases the reproducibility of contrast values considerably. This has to be performed for each individual because the differences in beam hardening and scatter depends on body size and composition (as well as machine-related variations). Although algorithmic 'correction' of beam hardening is somewhat effective, the only way to overcome its pervasive effect is to use monochromatic radiation (Figure 30.2).[13] This has been achieved with a radioactive source (e.g., Am) but the x-ray flux is suitable only for small regions-of-interest such as the forearm, wrist or ankle regions.[14,15]

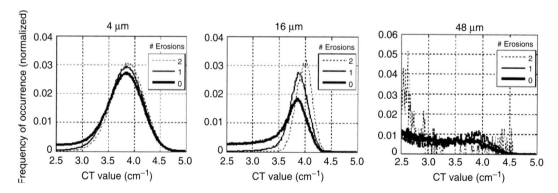

Figure 30.2 Frequency of CT image voxel gray-scale values for 3D images of the same specimen performed after increasing voxel size and following one or two erosions of voxels at the surfaces of the bone. The frequency data are normalized per voxel size in that a single value for a 16 μm cubic voxel would be (16/4)^3 of the value for the 4 μm cubic voxel images. Each data point represents all voxels with gray-scale spacing so as to span ten contiguous gray-scale values. (Modified with permission from Jorgensen SM et al., Proc SPIE 2006; 6143: 61433H-1–61433H-9).

2.4 'Tricks' for obtaining increased value from a scan

2.4.1 Use of a priori information

This is already done when prospective ECG-gated scanning is performed. Similarly, because the progression of an intravenous injected bolus of contrast agent through the vascular tree is well understood, the use of a monitoring image to determine the arrival of the bolus can be used to reduce the duration of the scan and hence radiation exposure. The frame rate of a sequence of scans can also be modulated on the basis of the known temporal 'shape' of an intravascular bolus of contrast agent. Thus, the initial frame rate might be every heart cycle whereas the latter half of the curve would require only once every second over third heart cycle.

2.4.2 Use of subject-specific scan characteristics – angle-dependent mA, local and PI-line reconstruction, etc.

Because the tissue pathlength differs in the lateral and the anteroposterior directions, the x-ray current can be adjusted so that the transmitted x-ray is always about the same intensity regardless of the angle-of-view. This has been implemented in a research setting.[16] Another approach that can be used involves restricting the x-ray exposure to the region-of-interest (in this case the heart). This can result in gross image artifacts, although some 'tricks' such as profile extension[17] (need information about the transverse extent of the not-imaged regions) can be used to mitigate these artifacts. Another approach is to use either local reconstruction[18] or PI-line reconstructions,[19] etc.

3 NEW QUESTIONS THAT REQUIRE NEW DEVELOPMENTS IN CT ALGORITHMS AND IMAGING APPROACH

3.1 Potential medical needs

3.1.1 Image conducting tissue within the heart wall

If the conducting tissue bundles of the heart could be imaged, then local damage might be detectable. Unfortunately, the conducting tissue has essentially the same CT number as the surrounding myocardium so that it is not feasible with current scanners.

3.1.2 Image the onset of a local myocardial contraction

Arrhythmias initiate in abnormal locations within the heart wall. If an image sequence could capture the initial local movement of the heart wall that would accompany the aberrant activation, then the localization could direct an intervention aimed at local destruction of the arrhythmia site. This would require a frame rate of at least 15 per second if the localization is to be accurate to within 1 mm.

3.1.3 Image hemorrhage within an arterial wall

Total hemoglobin in blood contains approximately 5 ng Fe/mm^3. Hence, a 1 mm^3 hemorrhage into an arterial wall should increase its radiopacity by 10 Hounsfield units. Histological information suggests that the volume of an hemorrhage into a non ruptured plaque can be up to 100 mm^3.[3,20] Hence, the contrast resolution at that spatial resolution has to be better than 10 HU (Figure 30.3).

3.1.4 Quantitate the surface area of infarcted region(s) within myocardium

The usual myocardial infarct consists of a relatively large continuous region of myocardium. The impact of those infarcts on LV function is reasonably proportional to the fraction of ventricular myocardium that has infarcted.[21] However, the impact of multiple discrete micro-infarcts (of the same total volume as a 'conventional' infarct) is much greater than that of a regular infarct.[22] This is because the surface area of the infarct becomes a dominant factor. Hence, the CT image should ideally resolve those micro-infarcts, but that is probably unrealistic in most instances as the micro-infarcts can be less than 1 mm^3.

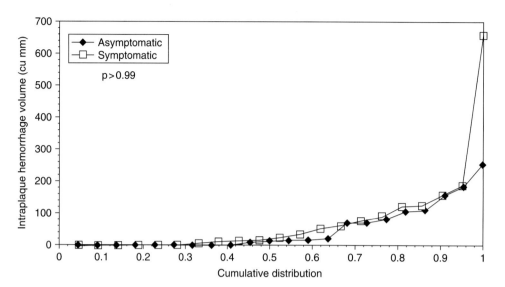

Figure 30.3   Cumulative distribution plot of the estimated volume of intraplaque hemorrhage in plaques harvested from asymptomatic and symptomatic individuals. There was no difference between asymptomatic and symptomatic plaques with regard to the volume of intraplaque hemorrhage (Reproduced with permission from Hatsukam TS et al., Stroke 1997; 28: 95–100).

3.2 Candidate x-ray imaging approaches to achieve the above proposed applications

3.2.1 Monochromatic x-ray, energy-selective photon detection and counting

Use of monochromatic x-ray provides a basis for discriminating most x-ray scatter from the transmitted x-ray by virtue of the generally reduced photon energy of the scattered photons. This capability could considerably increase the efficiency of photon detection because it could eliminate the use of a mechanical collimation. Counting of individual photons could help reduce noise by eliminating the noise introduced by the usual analog output before that is digitized.[23] If very short duration x-ray pulses are used, such as can be generated by field emission x-ray sources, use of a sub-nanosecond time-gate in the x-ray detector, such as is used in time-of-flight PET,[24,25] can discriminate the transmitted (ballistic) from the scattered photons. This could also be a means to improve the sensitivity of x-ray detection.

3.2.2 'Fractal' analysis

Nested multi-ROI image analysis (Figure 30.4) of CT images of the myocardium obtained during the passage of contrast agent through the coronary circulation can be used

to provide information about the size of sub-resolution perfusion defects (e.g., micro-infarcts).[26]

3.2.3 Iterative voxel sizing

If small voxels are reconstructed, even though the signal-to-noise ratio of those voxels is inadequate for clinical analysis, larger voxels can be generated retrospectively from those small voxels, thereby increasing the signal-to-noise ratio of each new, large voxel. The important aspect of this approach is that the location of each of those large voxels can be positioned with the precision of the small voxels. Thus, the large voxel can be positioned more appropriately near contrast edges in the image – e.g., across the wall of an artery – thereby reducing the partial volume effect.[18]

3.2.4 Dual-energy subtraction

This is a technique that has been explored in considerable depth for clinical CT scanners which use bremsstrahlung radiation[27] as well as K-edge absorption subtraction with, generally synchrotron-based, monochromatic radiation.[28–29] Although subtraction of images causes the noise to be additive, the contrast remaining in the images can be enhanced fivefold or more depending on the material of interest (Figure 30.5). Moreover, because the subtraction image is less complex, tomographic reconstruction of vascular trees

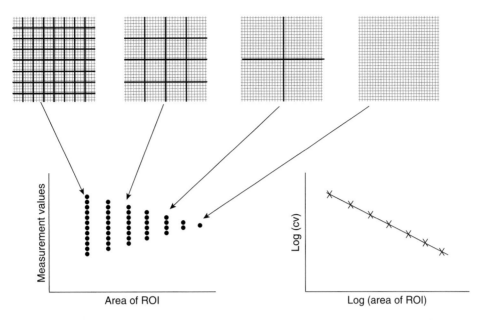

Figure 30.4   The imaged myocardial wall of the left ventricle can be subdivided into increasingly small nested regions-of-interest (ROI). The myocardial blood volume values estimated for each ROI show increasingly greater ranges of values with decreasing volume of ROI. The Log (SD/Mean) plotted against the Log (volume of nested ROI) results in a linear relationship if the heterogeneity follows a fractal pattern (Reproduced with permission of Springer Science and Business Media – Ritman, EL, Ann Biomed Eng 1998; 26: 519–525).

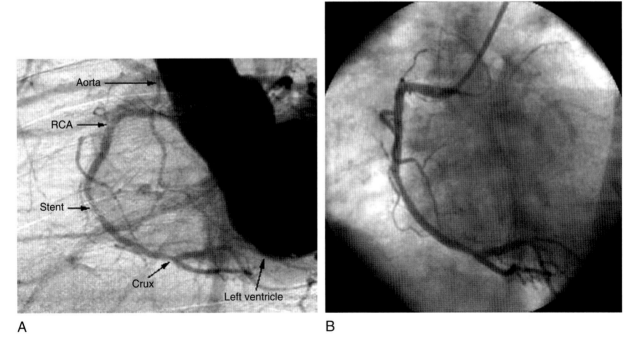

A   B

Figure 30.5   (A) Intravenous synchrotron angiogram of the first patient at the ESRF taken in a left anterior oblique (LAO) projection. Right coronary artery (RCA). The transit time between the injection of the contrast agent and the arrival of the bolus in the heart is then measured using a series of five synchrotron images at low x-ray dose (5 mGy) and with a small amount of contrast agent (10 ml). Forty-five minutes later, once the contrast agent used for the transit time estimation has disappeared totally from the venous circulation, the imaging sequence takes place. 30–45 ml of iodine (Iomeron® 350 mg ml^{-1}, Bracco, Italy) are injected into the superior vena cava using an auto-injector under remote control (15 ml s^{-1}). (B) Conventional selective coronary angiography of the same patient, in the LAO orientation, performed the same day at the cardiological unit of the hospital after arterial catheterization (Reproduced with permission from Elleaume, H, Phys Med Biol 2000; 45: L39-L43).[35]

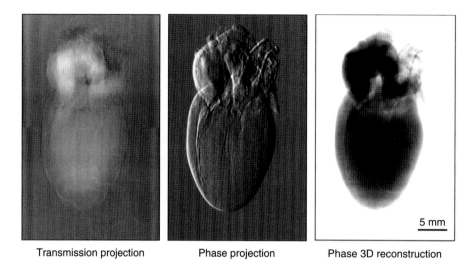

Transmission projection   Phase projection   Phase 3D reconstruction

Figure 30.6   X-ray phase contrast imaging of rat heart in saline – no contrast agent. Note outlines of lumens of the large vessel and ventricular chambers. (Image courtesy of F Pfeiffer in Stampanoni M, et al., Proc SPIE 2006; 6318: 63180M-1–63180M-14).

(subtraction aimed at highlighting iodine in contrast agent) may require fewer angles-of-view to provide a good reconstruction. A key element of this approach is that the two images are spatially registered and temporarily with great precision. Ideally, therefore, they are recorded simultaneously (e.g., by energy-selective detection of the two energies exposing the subject simultaneously) or in very close temporal relationship if the two separate images are recorded, such as is the case in the new dual-source Siemens CT scanner.[11,30] This method also can be used to reduce the dose of contrast agent needed. The use of europium or gadolinium-based contrast agents (instead of iodine) would better match the clinical x-ray photon energies used.[31–34]

3.2.5 X-ray scatter imaging

X-ray scatters from material in an angle-dependent manner that may be quite characteristic of the material.[30] Hence, different materials, with attenuation coefficients that are sufficiently close to prevent discrimination in the usual CT images, may be distinguishable when their x-ray scatter 'signatures' are used. This is now being done in some airport security scanners, which are basically converted multi-slice CT scanners.[36,37] Whether the spatial resolution for this mode of imaging can be made sufficiently high for clinical application remains to be demonstrated.

3.2.6 X-ray refractive index imaging

The x-ray refraction index of material consists of a real part and an imaginary part. The latter is the usual attenuation

coefficient whereas the former is related to the velocity of x-ray through the material. The contrast due to difference of refractive index can be orders of magnitude higher than achievable with attenuation imaging and it, therefore, requires fewer photons to generate a suitable signal. This is because the detected photon is the signal whereas with conventional imaging it is the absence of a photon that is the signal (Figure 30.6).[38–41]

Methods that have a chance of being clinically applicable include the use of the slight refraction of x-ray when these pass through material with very high contrast gradient but which are sub-resolution as far as the imaging device is concerned.[42] Another method is the use of interference grids positioned just after the patient and one in front of the detector.[43] The changing interference patterns generated by moving these grids slightly in sequential exposures can be used to determine the cumulative refractive index of the tissue.

4 CONCLUSION

(a) Current technologies need to be advanced to address the need to decrease radiation dose, to increase spatial and temporal resolution, and to address clinical problems not available to conventional, attenuation-based CT.

(b) The practical and resolution characteristics of new x-ray methods need to be replaced for possible clinical application.

REFERENCES

1. Jorgensen SM, Eaker DR, Vercnocke AJ, Ritman EL. Reproducibility of 3D micro-CT gray-scale and structural

dimension data in longitudinal studies. Proc SPIE 2006; 6143: 61433H-1–61433H-9.

2. Krogh A. The number and distribution of capillaries in muscles with calculations of the oxygen pressure head necessary for supplying the tissue. J Physiol 1919; 52: 409–15.

3. Jorgensen SM, Demirkaya O, Ritman EL. Three-dimensional imaging of vasculature and parenchyma in intact rodent organs with x-ray micro-CT. Am J Physiol Heart Circ Physiol 1998; 275: H1103–H1114.

4. Malyar NM, Lerman LO, Gössl M, Beighley PE, Ritman EL. Relation of nonperfused myocardial volume and surface area to left ventricular performance in coronary microembolization. Circulation 2004; 110: 1946–52.

5. Erbel R, Heusch G. Coronary microembolization. J Am Coll Cardiol 2000; 36: 22–4.

6. Zeiher A, Schachlinger V, Hohnloser S, Saurbier B, Just H. Coronary atherosclerotic wall thickening and vascular reactivity in humans. Elevated high-density lipoprotein levels ameliorate abnormal vasoconstriction in early atherosclerosis. Circulation 1994; 89: 2525–32.

7. Rumberger JA, Simons DB, Fitzpatrick LA, Sheedy PF, Schwartz RS. Coronary artery calcium area by electron-beam computed tomography and coronary atherosclerotic plaque area: A histopathologic correlative study. Circulation 1995; 92: 2157–62.

8. Scanlan JG, Gustafson DE, Chevalier PA, Robb RA, Ritman EL. Evaluation of ischemic heart disease with a prototype volume imaging computed tomographic (CT) scanner: preliminary experiments. Am J Cardiol 1980; 46: 1263–68.

9. Heistad DD, Marcus ML, Larsen GE, Armstrong ML. Role of vasa vasorum in nourishment of the aortic wall. Am J Physiol Heart Circ Physiol 1981; 240: H781–H787.

10. Dumesnil JG, Ritman EL, Frye RL et al. Quantitative determination of regional left ventricular wall dynamics by roentgen videometry. Circulation 1974; 50: 700–8.

11. Flohr TG, Bruder H, Petersilka M et al. First performance evaluation of a dual-source CT (DSCT) system. Eur Radiol 2006; 16: 256–68.

12. Bove AA, Block M, Smith HC, Ritman EL. Evaluation of coronary anatomy using high-speed volumetric computed tomographic scanning. Am J Cardiol 1985; 55: 582–4.

13. Carroll FE. Perspective. Tunable monochromatic x rays: A new paradigm in medicine. Am J Roentgenol 2002; 179: 583–90.

14. Ruegsegger P, Koller B, Muller R. A microtomographic system for the nondestructive evaluation of bone architecture. Calcif Tissue Int 1996; 58: 24–9.

15. Laib A, Hauselmann HJ, Ruegsegger P. In vivo high resolution 3D-QCT of the human forearm. Technol Health Care 1998; 6: 329–37.

16. Kalender WA, Wolf H, Suess C et al. Dose reduction in CT by on-line tube current control: Principles and validation on phantoms and cadavers. Eur Radiol 1999; 9: 323–8.

17. Lewitt RM. Processing of incomplete measurement data in computed tomography. Med Phys 1979; 6: 412–17.

18. Faridani A, Ritman EL. High-resolution computed tomography from efficient sampling. Inverse Problems 2000; 16: 635–50.

19. Zou Y, Pan X, Xia D, Wang G. PI-line-based image reconstruction in helical cone-beam computed tomography with a variable pitch. Med Phys 2005; 32: 2639–48.

20. Hatsukami TS, Ferguson MS, Beach KW et al. Carotid plaque morphology and clinical events. Stroke 1997; 28: 95–100.

21. Burns RJ, Gibbons RJ, Yi Q et al. The relationships of left ventricular ejection fraction, end-systolic volume index and infarct size to six-month mortality after hospital discharge following myocardial infarction treated by thrombolysis. J Am Coll Cardiol 2002; 39: 30–6.

22. Malyar NM, Lerman LO, Gossl M, Beighley PE, Ritman EL. Relation of nonperfused myocardial volume and surface area to left ventricular performance in coronary microembolization. Circulation 2004; 110: 1946–52.

23. Ignatiev KI, Lee W-K, Fezzaa K, Stock SR. Phase contrast stereometry: Fatigue crack mapping in three dimensions. Philos Mag 2005; 85: 3273–300.

24. Cobble JA, Kyrala GA, Hauer AA et al. Kilovolt x-ray spectroscopy of a subpicosecond-laser-excited source. Phys Rev A 1989; 39: 454–7.

25. Spinelli A, Davis L, Dautet H. Actively quenched single-photon avalanche diode for high repetition rate time-gated photon counting. Rev Sci Instrum 1996; 67: 55–61.

26. Dong Y, Beighley PE, Ritman EL, Malyar NM. Characterization of sub-resolution microcirculatory status using whole-body CT imaging. Proc SPIE 2005; 5746: 175–83.

27. Goldberg HI, Cann CE, Moss AA et al. Noninvasive quantitation of liver iron in dogs with hemochromatosis using dual-energy CT scanning. Invest Radiol 1982; 17: 375–80.

28. Thompson AC, Llacer J, Campbell Finman L et al. Computed tomography using synchrotron radiation. Nucl Instrum Methods Phys Res Sect A: Accelerators, Spectrometers, Detectors and Associated Equipment 1983; 222: 319–23.

29. Dilmanian FA, Wu XY, Parsons EC et al. Single- and dual-energy CT with monochromatic synchrotron x-rays. Phys Med Biol 1997; 42: 371–87.

30. Jaffray D, Battista J, Fenster A, Munro P. X-ray scatter in megavoltage transmission radiography: Physical characteristics and influence on image quality. Med Phys 1994; 21: 45–60.

31. Nakano Y, Gido T, Honda S et al. Improved computed radiography image quality from a BaFl: Eu photostimulable phosphor plate. Med Phys 2002; 29: 592–7.

32. Miyamoto A, Okimoto H, Shinohara H, Shibamoto Y. Development of water-soluble metallofullerenes as x-ray contrast media. Eur Radiol 2006; 16: 1050–53.

33. Spinosa DJ, Matsumoto AH, Hagspiel KD, Angle JF, Hartwell GD. Gadolinium-based contrast agents in angiography and interventional radiology. Am J Roentgenol 1999; 173: 1403–9.

34. Brasch RC. Introduction to the gadolinium class. J Comput Assist Tomogr 1993; 17: S14–S18.

35. Elleaume H, Fiedler S, Esteve F et al. First human transvenous coronary angiography at the European Synchrotron Radiation Facility. Phys Med Biol 2000; 45: L39–L43.

36. Harding G, Schreiber B. Coherent x-ray scatter imaging and its applications in biomedical science and industry. Radiat Phys and Chem 1999; 56: 229–45.

37. Speller R. Radiation-based security. Radiat Phys and Chem 2001; 61: 293–300.

38. Chapman D, Thomlinson W, Johnston RE et al. Diffraction enhanced x-ray imaging. Phys Med Biol 1997; 42: 2015–25.

39. Takeda T, Momose A, Wu J et al. Vessel imaging by interferometric phase-contrast x-ray technique. Circulation 2002; 105: 1708–12.

40. Takeda T, Momose A, Hirano K et al. Human carcinoma: early experience with phase-contrast x-ray CT with synchrotron

radiation-comparative specimen study with optical microscopy. Radiology 2000; 214: 298–301.

41. Stampanoni M, Groso A, Isenegger A et al. Trends in synchrotron-based tomographic imaging: the SLS experience. Proc SPIE 2006; 6318: 63180M-1–63180M-14.

42. Wernick MN, Wirjadi O, Chapman D et al. Multiple-image radiography. Phys Med Biol 2003; 48: 3875–95.

43. Weitkamp T, Diaz A, Nohammer B et al. Hard x-ray phase imaging and tomography with a grating interferometer. Proc SPIE 2004; 5535: 137–42.

31

Computed Tomographic Coronary Angiography for Subclinical Coronary Artery Disease, Coronary Artery Remodeling, and Plaque Imaging

Paul Schoenhagen

The introduction of coronary imaging with *conventional* x-ray angiography in the late 1950s has revolutionized the care of patients with advanced coronary artery disease (CAD).[1-3] In modern practice, the identification of high-grade stenoses in symptomatic patients has become the basis to determine the need for percutaneous and surgical intervention. However, despite the success of revascularization therapies, CAD remains the leading cause of death in the United States and Europe. It is increasingly obvious that only interventions at earlier stages of disease development can significantly reduce morbidity and mortality of atherosclerotic disease.

Almost 50 years after the introduction of coronary catheterization, recent advances in computerized tomography (CT) technology have allowed routine, non-invasive imaging of coronary arteries. A major focus of the scientific evaluation of this technology has been the identification of significant luminal stenosis in comparison to conventional angiography. Based on early results, many proponents have argued that CT angiography (CTA) has the potential to replace angiography. However, a comparison of the strengths and limitations of invasive angiography and MDCT demonstrates that this perception may be misguided.

As a non-invasive imaging modality with significantly lower spatial and temporal resolution than conventional angiography, the clinical value of CT for the assessment of advanced high-grade lesions will remain limited. Furthermore, the non-invasive identification of a high-grade stenosis would only confirm the need for subsequent invasive diagnostic and therapeutic approaches. On the other hand, evolving data suggest that CTA provides unique information in the evaluation of intermediate risk populations. The high negative predictive value allows the exclusion of stenotic disease. At the same time, as a tomographic imaging modality, MDCT shows the vessel wall and atherosclerotic plaque burden, which may provide important prognostic information.

It is therefore important to examine aspects of coronary CTA, which are beyond coronary luminology. Based on results from other atherosclerosis imaging modalities including intravascular ultrasound (IVUS), carotid ultrasound (CIMT), and CT calcium scoring, important imaging endpoints are plaque burden, plaque morphology, and arterial remodeling. The non-invasive identification of subclinical coronary artery disease could have a profound impact on disease prevention. However, the value of CTA for plaque imaging is still unclear and there is no evidence-based data to support its clinical use. This chapter will describe the current status of imaging early stages of coronary artery disease by CTA.

1 LIMITATIONS OF LUMINOGRAPHY

Based on the success of coronary revascularization, cardiologists have increasingly relied on the angiographic identification and quantification of luminal stenosis to guide both clinical practice and research. However, it is well known that angiographic lumen imaging is a limited standard on which to base therapeutic decisions. Comparative studies demonstrate major anatomic discrepancies between the apparent angiographic severity of lesions and postmortem histology.[4–6]

Beside others, diffuse disease and arterial remodeling are major reasons for these discrepancies. Diffuse disease involving the reference site leads to angiographic underestimation of the extent of atherosclerosis, because estimation or measurement of angiographic lesion severity relies on comparison of the luminal dimensions between the narrowed segment and an adjacent 'normal' reference segment.[7] The phenomenon of coronary 'remodeling,' first described in 1987 by Glagov et al., refers to the outward expansion of the external vessel wall overlying the atheroma.[8] The adventitial enlargement opposes luminal encroachment, concealing the presence of atheroma. Although remodeled lesions do not restrict blood flow, clinical studies have demonstrated that plaque rupture in these low-grade lesions represents the most important cause of acute coronary syndromes.[9–11]

In addition to these anatomic discrepancies, there is discordance between angiographic lesion severity and the physiological effects of the stenosis.[12,13] In chronic ischemic coronary disease, symptoms occur because coronary stenoses blunt the increase in coronary blood flow that is usually induced by increased metabolic demands of the myocardium. This increase in blood flow is called coronary flow reserve (CFR) and was originally described by Gould et al. in the 1970s.[14] Animal and human studies have documented that a normal CFR, in the absence of epicardial stenoses, should exceed 5:1 (ratio of hyperemic to basal flow) and that flow reserve remains normal until the stenosis severity approaches 75% of the luminal reference diameter. As stenosis severity increases from 75% to 95%, CFR falls progressively to reach values approaching a 1:1 ratio. Accordingly, the angiographic difference between a 'moderate' and a 'severe' coronary stenosis may be only a few tenths of a millimeter. Such differences are difficult to discern, given

the limitations in spatial and temporal resolution of coronary imaging modalities. Modern angiographic equipment can resolve about four or five line pairs per millimeter, which corresponds to a spatial resolution of about 0.2 mm. Adequate image quality typically requires cineangiographic pulse durations, and hence temporal resolution, of 4 to 10 ms.

These limitations are even more pronounced in non-invasive coronary imaging with CT angiography, because CTA has lower spatial and temporal resolution. Current 64-slice MDCT scanners have a spatial resolution of 0.45×0.45 mm in the axial plane with almost isotropic voxels (equal in-plane and through-plane resolution). The time required for the acquisition of individual axial CT images with multidetector scanners is limited by the rotation time of the x-ray tube/ detector system (currently $\geq$330 ms/rotation). The resulting temporal resolution of 165 ms is relatively long for coronary imaging. Recently introduced dual source CT scanners will have better temporal resolution,[15,16] but will still be limited in comparison to invasive angiography. In addition to the impact of spatial and temporal resolution, CTA is limited by vascular calcification, which is frequently present in advanced lesions. Small amounts of calcium in a given voxel increase the overall Hounsfield Unit (gray scale) of the entire voxel, giving the appearance of a larger calcification. This 'calcium blooming' leads to overestimation of lesion severity and often precludes assessment of calcified segments altogether.

These limitations of CT are reflected in the results of comparative studies demonstrating inferiority of CTA (similar to MRI) for the assessment of luminal stenosis in comparison to invasive angiography.[17,18] Advances in scanner technology (>64 slice systems, faster gantry rotation, dual source systems) will improve the sensitivity and specificity of CT for the evaluation of coronary artery stenosis, but the clinical value of CT for the assessment of advanced high grade lesions will likely remain limited. As stated previously, it should also be recognized that, even if advances in scanner technology will significantly narrow the gap to invasive angiography, non-invasive identification of advanced lesions would only confirm the need for subsequent invasive diagnostic and therapeutic approaches.

Therefore, a non-invasive test such as coronary CTA is not optimally suited for the evaluation of patients with high pretest probability of significant luminal disease.[19] (Figure 31.1) Similar to stress-testing, non-invasive angiography may be more appropriate in patients with lower pretest probability of highly stenotic disease. In these patients, the diagnostic goal is the exclusion of significant disease and the assessment of risk of future events. It is important to

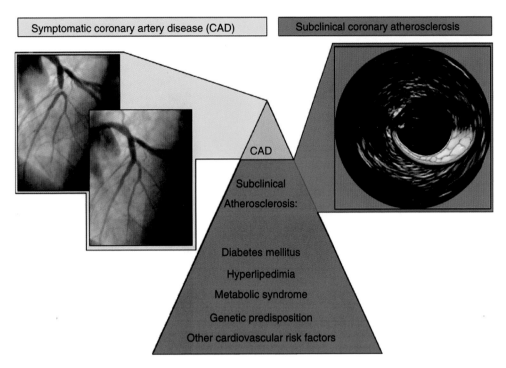

Figure 31.1 This figure demonstrates differences between imaging of patients with symptomatic coronary artery disease and subclinical coronary atherosclerosis. While the assessment of high-grade symptomatic luminal stenosis is well established with invasive coronary angiography, the assessment of early disease developing in the vessel wall requires a tomographic imaging modality.

address the role of atherosclerosis imaging in general and of CTA in particular for this purpose.

2 BEYOND LUMINOGRAPHY: THE ROLE OF NON-INVASIVE VESSEL WALL IMAGING

Coronary atherosclerosis is a systemic disease of the vessel wall, characterized by subclinical plaque build-up over long periods of time.[20] Secondary prevention trials have demonstrated that aggressive risk factor modification reduces the risk for cardiovascular events, likely by affecting subclinical atherosclerosis. It has therefore been hypothesized that visualization of subclinical disease burden in vivo, many years before onset of clinical symptoms, would allow reduction of cardiovascular events by targeted, early risk intervention.[21] Confirming the findings of pathological studies, studies using invasive intravascular ultrasound (IVUS) imaging have shown a high prevalence of subclinical atherosclerosis in patients without established CAD (Figure 31.2).[22–25] Subsequent studies have demonstrated the value of serial imaging of plaque burden as a surrogate endpoint in pharmacological intervention trials.[26–32] The validity of this approach is best documented for coronary intravascular

ultrasound (IVUS) and carotid ultrasound (CIMT). For these two imaging modalities, changes of plaque burden during clinical studies of lipid-lowering therapy have been documented[27,32] which parallel the reduction of the hard clinical endpoint of mortality.[33]

Non-invasive coronary atherosclerosis imaging has become possible with MDCT. Cardiac CT imaging without contrast enhancement allows the quantification of coronary calcification, which is a pathognomonic sign of chronic atherosclerosis,[34,35] and is very sensitive in detecting and quantitating coronary arterial calcification[36,37] (Figure 31.3). The use of coronary artery calcium scanning by CT is discussed exhaustively in other chapters of this book. In short, total calcium load in the coronary tree can be quantified using one of several calcium scoring algorithms, including Agatston scoring,[36] volume scoring[38] and mass scoring.[39] EBCT is the most established imaging modality for coronary calcium scoring, but MDCT has recently emerged as an alternative.[40,41] Coronary calcium scores have been shown to correlate with the total atherosclerotic plaque burden (calcified and non-calcified plaque), but the absolute burden is significantly underestimated.[42,43] The predictive value of the overall calcium score for future coronary events has been demonstrated.[34,44] An incremental value of calcium scores over 'traditional' multi-variate risk-assessment models in

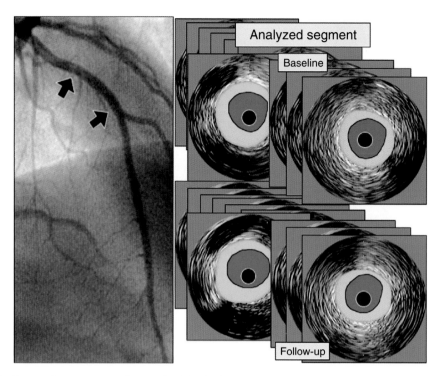

Figure 31.2 This figure demonstrates the methodological approach in serial IVUS studies. A vessel segment with minimal angiographic disease is identified and plaque burden assessed in multiple cross-sections. Plaque burden is the primary endpoint and is compared before and after several months of pharmacologic intervention.

selected patient groups with intermediate risk has been shown in recently published studies.[45,46] However, the site of calcification does not necessarily localize the plaque prone to rupture. High-grade stenotic lesions causing chronic, stable angina pectoris often demonstrate dense calcifications. In contrast, high-risk culprit lesions causing acute coronary events are frequently not calcified and may not be reflected by calcium scoring.[47,48] It is not well understood how plaque stabilization affects individual lesion calcification. It is therefore not surprising that the results of CT studies examining dynamic changes in the calcium volume score during pharmacological therapy have been inconclusive.[49–52] It has been suggested that discordant changes in calcified and overall plaque burden are responsible for these discrepancies. In particular, a reduction in overall plaque burden during disease stabilizing therapy may be associated with increased calcification in some lesions.

This is the rationale to image overall plaque burden and differentiate plaque components. Several recent studies using contrast-enhanced CT imaging have established the ability of MDCT to identify calcified and non-calcified atherosclerotic plaque and therefore overall plaque burden and remodeling[53–56] (Figure 31.4). The following paragraphs will describe the preclinical and clinical experience with MDCT imaging of coronary artery plaque.

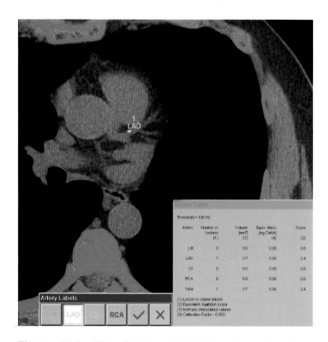

Figure 31.3 This figure demonstrates the concept of CT calcium-scoring. In a non-contrast enhanced scan, calcified plaque is identified by its high Hounsfield unit. The overall score for the entire coronary tree is calculated and has a relationship to future cardiovascular risk.

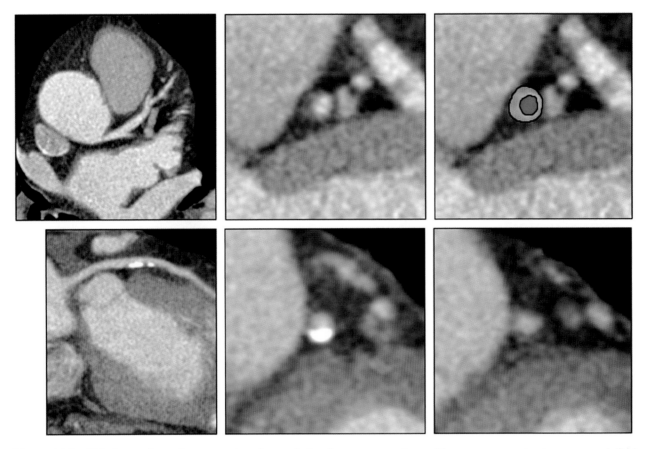

Figure 31.4   This figure shows two examples of non-obstructive coronary plaque. The upper example shows non-calcified plaque in the proximal LAD. In the right-hand cross-section, the plaque is highlighted in yellow. The lower example shows partially calcified plaque. The middle panel shows calcified plaque, the right hand panel adjacent non-calcified plaque.

2.1 Ex-vivo and animal models

Ex-vivo MDCT imaging of explanted arteries has been compared to the findings of histologic examination.[57–60] A study by Nikolaou[57] tested the ability of multidetector-row computed tomography (MDCT) and magnetic resonance imaging (MRI) to identify and characterize atherosclerotic lesions in human coronary arteries ex vivo. For both modalities, the sensitivity for the detection of any atherosclerotic lesion was evaluated, and a retrospective analysis of plaque morphology according to criteria defined by the American Heart Association (AHA) was performed. At histopathology, 28 atherosclerotic lesions were found. 21 and 23 of these lesions were identified by MDCT and MRI, respectively. Both modalities detected a small number of lesions that were not present on histology. After retrospective matching with histopathology, MDCT and MRI were able to differentiate typical morphological features for fatty, fibrous or calcified plaque components.

However, clinical imaging is more complicated than ex-vivo imaging due to phasic contrast flow and the constant cardiac motion. A more physiologic model than static filling of the vessels with a contrast/gel mix is the use of perfusion systems.[61,62] Studies using such systems describe vessel wall enhancement during contrast injection and the effect on plaque characterization. Our group investigated the effect of contrast injection on atherosclerotic coronary plaque attenuation.[62] Using a pressurized perfusion system, 10 human coronary arteries were examined postmortem with multidetector-row computed tomography and histology. Pre-enhanced, peak-enhanced, and delayed enhanced multidetector-row computed tomography images were acquired during continuous perfusion of the vessel. A total of 37 focal atherosclerotic plaques were identified. Vessel wall attenuation was measured from multidetector-row computed tomography images during all three enhancement phases. On the basis of the histology, plaques were categorized as noncalcified (predominantly fibrous or predominantly fibrofatty), mixed calcified (calcified fibrous or calcified necrotic core), or densely calcified. The mean Hounsfield unit was compared among contrast phases for all plaques and in plaque subgroups. We observed contrast enhancement of atherosclerotic plaques within the vessel wall. For noncalcified plaques, including both fibrous and fibrofatty plaques, the mean Hounsfield unit of the vessel wall during and after contrast injection exceeded the mean value before injection (t-test, P<0.002). This empirical evidence of contrast-enhancement of the vessel wall does not reveal the origin of this enhancement. One hypothesis is that vessel wall enhancement results from perfusion of contrast agent through the vasa vasorum serving the arterial wall. These microscopic vessels in the coronary wall are increasingly seen as important contributors in the pathogenesis of plaque development and rupture.[63–65] Recent studies showing a correlation between plaque inflammation and density of the vasa vasorum suggest that plaques with intense inflammation could demonstrate increased contrast enhancement.[66,67]

Similarly, arterial imaging of animal models with subsequent histologic examination provides a controlled experiment closer to clinical studies.[68,69] A study by Viles[68] compared the ability of MDCT and MRI to assess noncalcified, atherosclerotic plaques in the aorta. Six atherosclerotic rabbits underwent in vivo imaging by MDCT and 1.5-T MRI. Blinded analysis of 3-mm axial reconstructions from MDCT and the carefully matched MRI images (182 sections) showed good agreement between both modalities. MDCT yielded a slightly larger lumen area, with no significant differences in total vessel area. The sensitivity and specificity to detect noncalcified, atherosclerotic plaques were 89% and 77% for MDCT and 97% and 94% for MRI. Fibrous-rich and lipid-rich plaque could not be differentiated visually although they showed different attenuation properties on CT imaging (116 ± 27 vs. 51 ± 25 Hounsfield units, P<0.01).

2.2 Clinical studies

In clinical studies, contrast-enhanced protocols have demonstrated the ability of CTA to differentiate calcified and noncalcified plaque in comparison to IVUS.[53–55,70] Our group analyzed with IVUS and contrast-enhanced MDCT mildly stenotic segments of the left coronary artery identified by coronary angiography.[54] Independent reviewers evaluated the accuracy of MDCT for determining presence, composition and distribution of atherosclerotic plaque and the remodeling response in comparison to IVUS using receiver operating characteristic (ROC) data analysis. Of 46 segments in 14 patients, diagnostic characterization by MDCT was possible in 37 (80.4%) segments. In these segments, the accuracy of MDCT for identifying presence of plaque, calcification, distribution and positive remodeling

was consistently greater than 0.87. In 19.6% of segment analysis was not possible secondary to motion artifact (n = 3) or due to small vessel caliber (n = 6). Mean lumen diameter of the segments not analyzed due to small caliber was 3.0±0.5 mm.

Other studies demonstrate the potential value of plaque characterization based on the Hounsfield unit value. Schroeder et al. analyzed 34 plaques with IVUS and MDCT.[53] Plaque echodensity was classified by IVUS as soft (n = 12), intermediate (n = 5) and calcified (n = 17). On MDCT imaging, soft plaques had a density of 14±26 HU (range −42 to +47 HU), intermediate plaques of 91±21 HU (61 to 112 HU) and calcified plaques of 419±194 HU (126 to 736 HU). The differences between plaque densities among the three groups were significant (p<0.0001). A similar study by Leber et al. included 46 consecutive patients with cardiovascular risk factors.[71] Nine of these 46 consecutive patients could not be studied by MDCT because of high heart rate (n = 7) or renal insufficiency (n = 2). In the 37 patients, 68 vessels were investigated by IVUS. Of those, 58 were visualized by MDCT with image quality sufficient for analysis. The vessels were divided into 3-mm segments. MDCT correctly classified 62 of 80 (78%) sections containing hypoechoic plaque areas, 87 of 112 (78%) sections containing hyperechoic plaque areas, and 150 of 158 (95%) sections containing calcified plaque tissue. In 484 of 525 (92%) sections, atherosclerotic lesions were correctly excluded. The MDCT-derived density measurements within coronary lesions revealed significantly different values for hypoechoic (49 HU [Hounsfield Units] ±22), hyperechoic (91 HU±22), and calcified plaques (391 HU±156, p < 0.02).

However, there is a large overlap of attenuation values between the different plaque types, which can make differentiating between soft and fibrous plaque components difficult. In addition, recent CT studies suggest that the attenuation of plaques may be altered by vessel wall enhancement with contrast medium, demonstrating the need for standard image acquisition and contrast administration protocols and advanced analysis systems.[61,62] In contrast, clinical studies have demonstrated excellent plaque characterization in carotid arteries with MRI.[72]

Based on the observed correlation between CT Hounsfield Units and plaque echogenicity by IVUS, Leber et al. examined whether MDCT can show differences of plaque composition in patients with different acuity of coronary artery disease.[73] The authors examined 21 patients with recent acute myocardial infarction (AMI) and 19 stable angina pectoris (SAP). MDCT was performed with a Somatom VZ scanner (4-slice scanner). Total calcium scores were significantly higher in patients with SAP (631.4±676.3, 36–2374) compared with patients with AMI (322±366.2, 0–1345) (p<0.04). In the SAP group, all patients showed detectable coronary calcium. Three of 19 patients showed only mild calcium scores (Agatston score <100). In the AMI group, 2 of 21 patients had no coronary calcium, and in 7 of 21 patients we found low Agatston scores of <100. In the SAP group the authors found 230 coronary plaques in 19 patients. In this group, 132 segments (57%) showed heavy calcification, 51 (22%) showed spotty calcium, 30 (13%) of plaques were mixed, and 17 (7%) were non-calcified. In the AMI group (21 patients), of 217 plaques, 71 (32%) were heavy calcified, 54 (24%) were spotty calcified, 39 (18%) were mixed, and 53 (24%) were noncalcified. The mean CT density of non-calcified plaques was 63±46 HU, of mixed plaques, 278±83 HU, of spotty calcified plaque, 315±86 HU, and heavily calcified plaques, 472±93 HU (p<0.05). This and other studies[74,75] demonstrated that differences in coronary plaque composition between patients with myocardial infarction and SAP can determined noninvasively by contrast-enhanced multidetector CT.

However, to date there are no prospective data demonstrating that presence of plaque or differences in plaque characteristics determined by CT can predict plaque rupture or future events. In fact, similar to the experience with IVUS, recent MDCT studies demonstrated the frequent presence of atherosclerotic plaque in angiographically normal coronary artery segments.[76] (Figure 31.5)

In this study, Hausleiter et al. investigated the prevalence and characteristics of noncalcified coronary plaques in 161 consecutive patients with an intermediate risk for having CAD with 64-slice computed tomography (0.6-mm collimation, 330-ms gantry rotation time). The CT images were evaluated for presence of coronary calcifications, noncalcified plaques, and lumen narrowing. Noncalcified coronary plaques were detected in 48 patients (29.8%). Noncalcified plaques together with coronary calcifications were present in 38 of 161 (23.6%) patients. The prevalence of noncalcified plaques as the only manifestation of CAD was 6.2% (10 of 161 patients). Patients with noncalcified plaques were characterized by significantly higher total cholesterol, low-density lipoprotein, and C-reactive protein levels, as well as a trend for more diabetes mellitus than those who had no evidence of non-calcified plaque. The majority of noncalcified plaques resulted in lumen narrowing of <50%. CAD and coronary calcifications were absent in 53 of 161 (32.9%) patients, and 60 of 161 (37.3%) patients had coronary calcifications but no noncalcified plaque.

In order to establish the relationship between plaque burden and coronary events, quantitative assessment of plaque burden and remodeling will be necessary (Figure 31.6). Achenbach et al. investigated the feasibility of quantitating coronary plaque burden in 83 coronary segments in 22 patients without significant luminal coronary stenoses with contrast-enhanced MDCT (0.75-mm collimation, 420-ms rotation) in comparison to IVUS as a reference standard.[55]

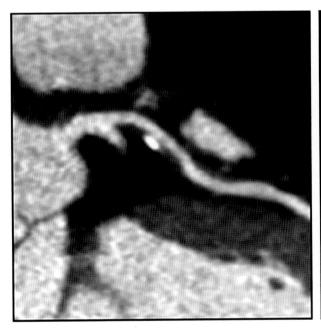
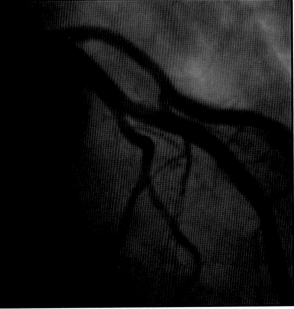

Figure 31.5 This figure shows partially calcified plaque in a CT image and the corresponding coronary angiogram. Because of expansive remodeling, the significant plaque burden causes only mild luminal stenosis.

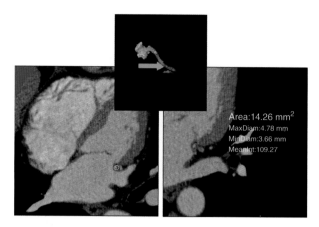

Figure 31.6 Eventually, quantitative assessment of plaque burden will be necessary. Current system can identify a vessel segment and allow area measurement. However, the lower spatial resolution is still a limiting factor in comparison to e.g. IVUS.

MDCT data sets were evaluated for the presence and volume of plaque in the coronary artery segments. Results were compared with IVUS in a blinded fashion. For the detection of segments with any plaque, MDCT had a sensitivity of 82% and specificity of 88%. For the detection of calcified plaque, sensitivity was 94% and specificity 94%. Coronary segments containing only noncalcified plaque were detected with a sensitivity of 78% and specificity of 87%, but presence of exclusively noncalcified plaque was detected with only 53% sensitivity. In quantitative analysis, MDCT substantially underestimated plaque volume per segment compared with IVUS (24±35 mm^3 versus 43±60 mm^3, p<0.001). Building on previous qualitative studies,[54,74,77] quantitative assessment of arterial remodeling has been examined[78,79] Achenbach et al.[78] examined 44 patients who had atherosclerotic plaque in a proximal coronary artery segment detected by MDCT coronary angiography. In multiplanar reconstructions orthogonal to the course of the coronary artery, the cross-sectional vessel area was measured for the segment with plaque and for a proximal reference segment. The 'Remodeling Index' was calculated by dividing the vessel area at the lesion site and the reference segment. Results were correlated to the presence of 'significant' luminal stenosis (>50% diameter reduction) assessed with invasive angiography. In a subset of 13 patients, quantitative MDCT measurements were verified by IVUS. The authors found that reference vessel area was not significantly different between vessels with nonstenotic and with stenotic plaques (20±8 mm^2, n = 23 vs. 22±8 mm^2, n = 21). However, the mean Remodeling Index was significantly

higher in vessels without than those with 'significant' stenoses (1.3±0.2 vs. 1.0±0.2, p<0.001). In vessels with 'significant' stenoses, 'negative remodeling' (Remodeling Index = 0.95) was observed. Cross-sectional vessel areas and Remodeling Indices measured by MDCT correlated closely with IVUS (r^2 = 0.77 and r^2 = 0.82, respectively). However, a study by Leber et al., evaluating the accuracy of 64-slice computed tomography (CT), compared with intravascular ultrasound, found different results.[80] In 20 patients, MDCT and intravascular ultrasound of vessels without stenosis >50% was performed. Diagnostic image quality with CT was obtained in 36 vessels in 19 patients. In these vessels, which were divided in 3-mm sections, CT enabled correct detection of plaque in 54 of 65 (83%) sections containing noncalcified plaques, 50 of 53 (94%) sections containing mixed plaques, and 41 of 43 (95%) sections containing calcified plaques. In 192 of 204 (94%) sections, atherosclerotic lesions were excluded correctly. In addition, CT enabled the visualization of 7 of 10 (70%) sections revealing a lipid pool and could identify a spotty calcification pattern in 27 of 30 (90%) sections. The correlation coefficient to determine plaque volumes per vessel was r^2 = 0.69 (p<0.001) with an underestimation of mixed and noncalcified plaque volumes (p<0.03) and a trend to overestimate calcified plaque volumes by CT. Interobserver agreement to identify atherosclerotic sections was good (Cohen's kappa coefficient = 0.75). However, the interobserver variability to determine plaque volumes was 37%. The authors conclude that the ability of 64-slice CT to determine plaque burden currently is still hampered by mainly an insufficient reproducibility.

Quantification of remodeling and plaque burden will eventually allow serial non-invasive examination of coronary anatomy and plaque burden in pharmacological studies, similar to previous noninvasive serial studies in femoral arteries, carotid arteries, and the aorta using B-mode ultrasound or magnetic resonance imaging (MRI).[81–85] Using MRI, Corti et al. compared the effects of aggressive and conventional lipid lowering by two different dosages of the same cholesterol-lowering drug on early human atherosclerotic lesions using serial noninvasive magnetic resonance imaging (MRI).[85] Using a double-blind design, newly diagnosed hypercholesterolemic patients (n = 51) with asymptomatic aortic and/or carotid atherosclerotic plaques were randomized to 20 mg/day (n = 29) or 80 mg/day (n = 22) of simvastatin. Mean follow-up was 18.1 months. A total of 93 aortic and 57 carotid plaques were detected and sequentially followed by MRI every six months after initiation of lipid-lowering pharmacologic therapy. The primary

MRI end point was change in vessel wall area (VWA) as a surrogate for atherosclerotic burden. Both statin doses significantly (p<0.001) reduced total cholesterol (TC) and low-density lipoprotein cholesterol (LDL-C) compared to baseline values. Total cholesterol decreased by 26% versus 33% and LDL-C by 36% versus 46% in the conventional (20 mg) versus aggressive (80 mg) simvastatin groups, respectively. Although the patient group receiving 80 mg of simvastatin had significantly higher baseline TC and LDL-C levels, both groups reached similar absolute values after treatment. A significant reduction in VWA was observed beginning at 12 months after the initiation of therapy. There was no difference in the magnitude of the effect on VWA reduction between the two dosages of simvastatin. However, post-hoc analysis showed that patients attained a mean on-treatment LDL-C < or = 100 mg/dl had larger decreases in plaque size.

To date, no studies have reported the results of serial measurements of plaque burden by CT but such measurements are the subject of ongoing studies. Such studies will also examine the relationship between imaging markers of cardiovascular atherosclerotic burden and other makers of cardiovascular risk, including systemic serum markers of inflammation. This important relationship has been examined previously in invasive fashion with IVUS.[86–88]

3 CONCLUSION

Early identification and quantification of subclinical plaque burden, combined with traditional clinical risk factor assessment and biochemical markers of cardiovascular risk, could identify those patient subgroups that would benefit the most from aggressive primary prevention.[89] Targeted early intervention including exercise, diet and weight control, and systemic pharmacological treatment of risk factors could potentially prevent a large number of adverse cardiovascular events. In addition, atherosclerosis imaging with MDCT has the potential to define new standards for the development and evaluation of drug therapies that are designed to reduce the progression of atherosclerosis.

However, the use of CT in patients with low pretest probability or low risk of cardiovascular events must be justified against the (potentially repeated) exposure to ionizing radiation. Further validation studies are needed to address the accuracy and reproducibility of lesion characterization and quantification of plaque burden by MDCTA before this modality can be applied to research and clinical settings similar to how CIMT and IVUS are used now.

REFERENCES

1. Sones FM, Shirey EK. Cine coronary arteriography. Mod Concepts Cardiovasc Dis 1962; 31: 735–8.
2. Judkins MP. Selective coronary arteriography: a percutaneous transfemoral technique. Radiology 1967; 89: 815–17.
3. Proudfit WL, Shirey EK, Sones FM Jr. Selective cine coronary arteriography. Correlation with clinical findings in 1,000 patients. Circulation 1966; 33: 901–10.
4. Arnett EN, Isner JM et al. Coronary artery narrowing in coronary heart disease: comparison of cineangiographic and necropsy findings. Ann Intern Med 1979; 91: 350–6.
5. Grodin CM, Dyrda I, Pasternac A, Campeu L, Bourassa MG. Discrepancies between cineangiographic and post-mortem findings in patients with coronary artery disease and recent myocardial revascularization. Circulation 1974; 49: 703–9.
6. Galbraith JE, Murphy ML, Desoyza N. Coronary angiogram interpretation: interobserver variability. JAMA 1981; 240: 2053–9.
7. Mintz GS, Painter JA, Pichard AD et al. Atherosclerosis in angiographically "normal" coronary artery reference segments: an intravascular ultrasound study with clinical correlations. J Am Coll Cardiol 1995; 25: 1479–85.
8. Glagov S, Weisenberg E, Zarins CK, Stankunavicius R, Kolettis GJ. Compensatory enlargement of human coronary arteries. N Engl J Med 1987; 316: 1371–5.
9. Little WC, Constantinescu M, Applegate RJ et al. Can arteriography predict the site of a subsequent myocardial infarction in patients with mild-to-moderate coronary artery disease? Circulation 1988; 78: 1157–66.
10. Pasterkamp G, Schoneveld AH, van der Wal AC et al. Relation of arterial geometry to luminal narrowing and histologic markers for plaque vulnerability: the remodeling paradox. J Am Coll Cardiol 1998; 32: 655–62.
11. Schoenhagen P, Ziada KM, Kapadia SR et al. Extent and direction of arterial remodeling in stable versus unstable coronary syndromes. Circulation 2000; 101: 598–603.
12. White CW, Wright CB, Doty DB et al. Does visual interpretation of the coronary arteriogram predict the physiologic importance of a coronary stenosis? N Engl J Med 1984; 310: 819–24.
13. Kern MJ, Donohue TJ, Aguirre FV et al. Assessment of angiographically intermediate coronary artery stenoses using the Doppler flow wire. Am J Cardiol 1993; 71: 26D–33D.
14. Gould KL, Lipscomb K, Hamilton GW. Physiologic basis for assessing critical coronary stenosis: instantaneous flow response and regional distribution during coronary hyperemia as measures of coronary flow reserve. Am J Cardiol 1974; 33: 87–93.
15. Flohr TG, McCollough CH, Bruder H et al. First performance evaluation of a dual-source CT (DSCT) system. Eur Radiol 2006; 16: 256–68.
16. Achenbach S, Ropers D, Kuettner A et al. Contrast-enhanced coronary artery visualization by dual-source computed tomography – initial experience. Eur J Radiol 2006; 57: 331–5.
17. Garcia MJ, Lessick J, Hoffmann MH, CATSCAN Study Investigators. Accuracy of 16-row multidetector computed tomography for the assessment of coronary artery stenosis. JAMA 2006; 296: 403–11.
18. Kim WY, Danias PG, Stuber M et al. Coronary magnetic resonance angiography for the detection of coronary stenoses. N Engl J Med 2001; 345: 1863–9.

19. Schoenhagen P, Stillman AE, Garcia MJ et al. Coronary artery imaging with multidetector computed tomography: a call for an evidence-based, multidisciplinary approach. Am Heart. 2006; 151: 945–8.

20. Strong JP, Malcom GT, McMahan CA et al. Prevalence and extent of atherosclerosis in adolescents and young adults: implications for prevention from the Pathobiological Determinants of Atherosclerosis in Youth Study. JAMA 1999; 281: 727–35.

21. Sankatsing RR, de Groot E, Jukema JW et al. Surrogate markers for atherosclerotic disease. Curr Opin Lipidol 2005; 16: 434–41.

22. Tuzcu EM, Hobbs RE, Rincon G et al. Occult and frequent transmission of atherosclerotic coronary disease with cardiac transplantation. Insights from intravascular ultrasound. Circulation 1995; 91: 1706–13.

23. Tuzcu EM, Kapadia SR, Tutar E et al. High prevalence of coronary atherosclerosis in asymptomatic teenagers and young adults: evidence from intravascular ultrasound. Circulation 2001; 103: 2705–10.

24. St Goar FG, Pinto FJ, Alderman EL et al. Detection of coronary atherosclerosis in young adult hearts using intravascular ultrasound. Circulation 1992; 86: 756–63.

25. Larsen J, Brekke M, Sandvik L et al. Silent coronary atheromatosis in type 1 diabetic patients and its relation to long-term glycemic control. Diabetes 2002; 51: 2637–41.

26. Schartl M, Bocksch W, Koschyk DH et al. Use of intravascular ultrasound to compare effects of different strategies of lipid-lowering therapy on plaque volume and composition in patients with coronary artery disease. Circulation 2001; 104: 387–92.

27. Nissen SE, Tuzcu EM, Schoenhagen P et al. REVERSAL Investigators. Effect of intensive compared with moderate lipid-lowering therapy on progression of coronary atherosclerosis: a randomized controlled trial. JAMA 2004; 291: 1071–80.

28. Nissen SE, Tsunoda T, Tuzcu EM et al. Effect of recombinant ApoA-I Milano on coronary atherosclerosis in patients with acute coronary syndromes: a randomized controlled trial. JAMA 2003; 290: 2292–300.

29. Nissen SE, Tuzcu EM, Libby P et al. CAMELOT Investigators. Effect of antihypertensive agents on cardiovascular events in patients with coronary disease and normal blood pressure: the CAMELOT study: a randomized controlled trial. JAMA 2004; 292: 2217–25.

30. Okazaki S, Yokoyama T, Miyauchi K et al. Early statin treatment in patients with acute coronary syndrome: demonstration of the beneficial effect on atherosclerotic lesions by serial volumetric intravascular ultrasound analysis during half a year after coronary event: the ESTABLISH Study. Circulation 2004; 110: 1061–8.

31. Nicholls SJ, Sipahi I, Schoenhagen P et al. Application of intravascular ultrasound in anti-atherosclerotic drug development. Nat Rev Drug Discov 2006; 5: 485–92.

32. Taylor AJ, Kent SM, Flaherty PJ et al. ARBITER: Arterial Biology for the Investigation of the Treatment Effects of Reducing Cholesterol: a randomized trial comparing the effects of atorvastatin and pravastatin on carotid intima medial thickness. Circulation 2002; 106: 2055–60.

33. Cannon CP, Braunwald E, McCabe CH et al. Pravastatin or Atorvastatin Evaluation and Infection Therapy-Thrombolysis in Myocardial Infarction 22 Investigators. Intensive versus moderate lipid lowering with statins after acute coronary syndromes. N Engl J Med 2004; 350: 1495–504.

34. O'Rourke RA, Brundage BH, Froelicher VF et al. American College of Cardiology/ American Heart Association expert consensus document on electron-beam computed tomography for the diagnosis and prognosis of coronary artery disease. Circulation 2000; 102: 126–40.

35. Hoff JA, Daviglus ML, Chomka EV et al. Conventional coronary artery disease risk factors and coronary artery calcium detected by electron beam tomography in 30.908 healthy individuals. Ann Epidemiol 2003; 13: 163–9.

36. Agatston AS, Janowitz WR, Hildner FJ et al. Quantification of coronary artery calcium using ultrafast computed tomography. J Am Coll Cardiol 1990; 15: 827–32.

37. Shemesh J, Apter S, Rozenman J et al. Calcification of coronary arteries. Radiology 1995; 197: 779–83.

38. Callister TQ, Cooil B, Raya SP et al. Coronary artery disease: improved reproducibility of calcium scoring with and electron-beam CT volumetric method. Radiology 1998; 208: 807–14.

39. Detrano R, Tang W, Kang X et al. Accurate coronary calcium phosphate mass measurements from electron beam computed tomograms. Am J Card Imaging 1995; 3: 167–73.

40. Becker CR, Kleffel T, Crispin A et al. Coronary artery calcium measurement: agreement of multirow detector and electron beam CT. Am J Roentgenol 2001; 176: 1295–8.

41. Nasir K, Budoff MJ, Post WS et al. Electron beam CT versus helical CT scans for assessing coronary calcification: current utility and future directions. Am Heart J 2003; 146: 969–77.

42. Rumberger JA, Simons DB, Fitzpatrick LA, Sheedy PF, Schwartz RS. Coronary artery calcium area by electron-beam computed tomography and coronary atherosclerotic plaque area. Circulation 1995; 92: 2157–62.

43. Sangiorgi G, Rumberger JA, Severson A et al. Arterial calcification and not lumen stenosis is highly correlated with atherosclerotic plaque burden in humans. J Am Coll Cardiol 1998; 31: 126–33.

44. Secci A, Wong N, Tang W et al. Electron beam computed tomographic coronary calcium as a predictor of coronary events. Circulation 1997; 96: 1122–9.

45. Shaw LJ, Raggi P, Schisterman E, Berman DS, Callister TQ. Prognostic value of cardiac risk factors and coronary artery calcium screening for all-cause mortality. Radiology 2003; 228: 826–33.

46. Greenland P, LaBree L, Azen SP, Doherty TM, Detrano RC. Coronary artery calcium score combined with Framingham score for risk prediction in asymptomatic individuals. JAMA 2004; 291: 210–15.

47. Schmermund A, Erbel R. Unstable coronary plaque and its relation to coronary calcium. Circulation 2001; 104: 1682–7.

48. Schoenhagen P, Tuzcu EM. Coronary artery calcification and end-stage renal disease: vascular biology and clinical implications. Cleve Clin J Med. 2002; 69 Suppl 3: S12–20.

49. Budoff MJ, Raggi P. Coronary artery disease progression assessed by electron-beam computed tomography. Am J Cardiol 2001; 88: 46E–50E.

50. Callister TQ, Raggi P, Cooil B, Lippolis NJ, Russo DJ. Effect of HMG-CoA reductase inhibitors on coronary artery disease by electron-beam computed tomography. N Engl J Med 1998; 339: 1972–8.

51. Achenbach S, Ropers D, Pohle K et al. Influence of Lipid-Lowering Therapy on the Progression of Coronary Artery Calcification. A Prospective Evaluation. Circulation 2002; 106: 1077–82.

52. Schmermund A, Achenbach S, Budde T et al. Effect of Intensive Versus Standard Lipid-Lowering Treatment With Atorvastatin on the Progression of Calcified Coronary Atherosclerosis Over 12 Months: A Multicenter, Randomized, Double-Blind Trial. Circulation 2006; 113: 427–37.

53. Schroeder S, Kopp AF, Baumbach A et al. Noninvasive detection and evaluation of atherosclerotic coronary plaques with multislice computed tomography. J Am Coll Cardiol 2001; 37: 1430–5.

54. Schoenhagen P, Tuzcu EM, Stillman AE et al. Non-invasive assessment of plaque morphology and remodeling in mildly stenotic coronary segments: comparison of 16-slice computed tomography and intravascular ultrasound. Coron Artery Dis 2003; 14: 459–62.

55. Achenbach S, Moselewski F, Ropers D et al. Detection of calcified and noncalcified coronary atherosclerotic plaque by contrast-enhanced, submillimeter multidetector spiral computed tomography: a segment-based comparison with intravascular ultrasound. Circulation 2004; 109: 14–17.

56. Fayad ZA, Fuster V, Nikolaou K, Becker C. Computed tomography and magnetic resonance imaging for noninvasive coronary angiography and plaque imaging: Current and potential future concepts. Circulation 2002; 106: 2026–34.

57. Nikolaou K, Becker CR, Muders M et al. Multidetector-row computed tomography and magnetic resonance imaging of atherosclerotic lesions in human ex vivo coronary arteries. Atherosclerosis 2004; 174: 243–52.

58. Nikolaou K, Becker CR, Flohr T et al. Optimization of ex vivo CT- and MR-imaging of atherosclerotic vessel wall changes. Int J of Cardiovasc Imaging 2004; 20: 275–82.

59. Schroeder S, Kuettner A, Leitritz M et al. Reliability of differentiating human coronary plaque morphology using contrast-enhanced multislice spiral computed tomography: a comparison with histology. J Comput Assist Tomogr 2004; 28: 449–54.

60. Schroeder S, Kuettner A, Wojak T et al. Non-invasive evaluation of atherosclerosis with contrast enhanced 16 slice spiral computed tomography: results of ex vivo investigations. Heart 2004; 90: 1471–5.

61. Mollet NR, Cademartiri F, Runza G et al. In vivo assessment of attenuation of different plaque tissue components using multislice CT coronary angiography. Circulation 2004; 110: III-523, abst. 2451.

62. Halliburton SS, Schoenhagen P, Nair A et al. Contrast enhancement of coronary atherosclerotic plaque: a high-resolution, multidetector-row computed tomography study of pressure-perfused, human ex-vivo coronary arteries. Coron Artery Dis 2006; 17: 553–60.

63. Williams JK, Armstrong ML, Heistad DD. Vasa vasorum in atherosclerotic coronary arteries: responses to vasoactive stimuli and regression of atherosclerosis. Circ Res 1988; 62: 515–23.

64. Gossl M, Malyar NM, Rosol M, Beighley PE, Ritman EL. Impact of coronary vasa vasorum functional structure on coronary vessel wall perfusion distribution. Am J Physiol Heart Circ Physiol 2003; 285: H2019–26.

65. Wilson SH, Herrmann J, Lerman LO et al. Simvastatin preserves the structure of coronary adventitial vasa vasorum in experimental hypercholesterolemia independent of lipid lowering. Circulation 2002; 105: 415–18.

66. Fleiner M, Kummer M, Mirlacher M et al. Arterial neovascularization and inflammation in vulnerable patients: early and late signs of symptomatic atherosclerosis. Circulation 2004; 110: 2843–50.

67. Moreno PR, Purushothaman KR, Fuster V et al. Plaque neovascularization is increased in ruptured atherosclerotic lesions of human aorta: implications for plaque vulnerability. Circulation 2004; 110: 2032–8.

68. Viles-Gonzalez JF, Poon M, Sanz J et al. In vivo 16-slice, multidetector-row computed tomography for the assessment of experimental atherosclerosis: comparison with magnetic resonance imaging and histopathology. Circulation 2004; 110: 1467–72.

69. Schneider JE, McAteer MA, Tyler DJ et al. High-resolution, multicontrast three-dimensional-MRI characterizes atherosclerotic plaque composition in ApoE-/-mice ex vivo. J Magn Reson Imaging 2004; 20: 981–9.

70. Becker CR, Knez A, Ohnesorge B, Schoepf UJ, Reiser MF. Imaging of noncalcified coronary plaques using helical CT with retrospective ECG gating. Am J Roentgnol 2000; 175: 423–4.

71. Leber AW, Knez A, Becker A et al. Accuracy of multidetector spiral computed tomography in identifying and differentiating the composition of coronary atherosclerotic plaques; A comparative study with intracoronary ultrasound. J Am Coll Cardiol. 2004; 43: 1241–7.

72. Yuan C, Mitsumori LM, Ferguson MS et al. In vivo accuracy of multispectral magnetic resonance imaging for identifying lipid-rich necrotic cores and intraplaque hemorrhage in advanced human carotid plaques. Circulation 2001; 104: 2051–6.

73. Leber AW, Knez A, White CW et al. Composition of coronary atherosclerotic plaques in patients with acute myocardial infarction and stable angina pectoris determined by contrast-enhanced multislice computed tomography. Am J Cardiol. 2003; 91: 714–18.

74. Imazeki T, Sato Y, Inoue F et al. Evaluation of coronary artery remodeling in patients with acute coronary syndrome and stable angina by multislice computed tomography. Circ J 2004; 68: 1045–50.

75. Caussin C, Ohanessian A, Ghostine S et al. Characterization of vulnerable nonstenotic plaque with 16-slice computed tomography compared with intravascular ultrasound. Am J Cardiol 2004; 94: 99–104.

76. Hausleiter J, Meyer T, Hadamitzky M et al. Prevalence of noncalcified coronary plaques by 64-slice computed tomography in patients with an intermediate risk for significant coronary artery disease. J Am Coll Cardiol 2006; 48: 312–18.

77. Kim WY, Stuber M, Börnert P et al. Three-Dimensional Black-Blood Cardiac Magnetic Resonance Coronary Vessel Wall Imaging Detects Positive Arterial Remodeling in Patients With Nonsignificant Coronary Artery Disease. Circulation 2002; 106: 296–9.

78. Achenbach S, Ropers D, Hoffmann U et al. Assessment of coronary remodeling in stenotic and nonstenotic coronary atherosclerotic lesions by multidetector spiral computed tomography. J Am Coll Cardiol 2004; 43: 842–7.

79. Moselewski F, Ropers D, Pohle K et al. Comparison of measurement of cross-sectional coronary atherosclerotic plaque and vessel areas by 16-slice multidetector computed tomography versus intravascular ultrasound. Am J Cardiol 2004; 94: 1294–7.

80. Leber AW, Becker A, Knez A et al. Accuracy of 64-slice computed tomography to classify and quantify plaque volumes in the proximal coronary system: a comparative study using intravascular ultrasound. J Am Coll Cardiol. 2006; 47: 672–7.

81. Trogan E, Fayad ZA, Itskovich VV et al. Serial studies of mouse atherosclerosis by in vivo magnetic resonance imaging detect lesion regression after correction of dyslipidemia. Arterioscler Thromb Vasc Biol 2004; 24: 1714–19.

82. de Groot E, Jukema JW, Montauben van Swijndregt AD et al. B-mode ultrasound assessment of pravastatin treatment effect on carotid and femoral artery walls and its correlation with coronary arteriogarphic findings: a report of the Regression Growth Evaluation Statin Study (REGRESS). J Am Coll Cardiol 1998; 31: 1561–7.

83. Taylor AJ, Kent SM, Flaherty PJ et al. ARBITER: Arterial Biology for the Investigation of the Treatment Effects of Reducing Cholesterol. A Randomized Trial Comparing the Effects of Atorvastatin and Pravastatin on Carotid Intima Medial Thickness. Circulation 2002; 106: 2055–60.

84. Corti R, Fayad ZA, Fuster V et al. Effects of lipid-lowering by simvastatin on human atherosclerotic lesions: a longitudinal study by high-resolution, noninvasive magnetic resonance imaging. Circulation 2001; 104: 249–52.

85. Corti R, Fuster V, Fayad ZA et al. Effects of aggressive versus conventional lipid-lowering therapy by simvastatin on human atherosclerotic lesions: a prospective, randomized, double-blind trial with high-resolution magnetic resonance imaging. J Am Coll Cardiol 2005; 46: 106–12.

86. Nissen SE, Tuzcu EM, Schoenhagen P et al. Statin therapy, LDL cholesterol, C-reactive protein, and coronary artery disease. N Engl J Med 2005; 352: 29–38.

87. Ridker PM, Cannon CP, Morrow D et al. C-reactive protein levels and outcomes after statin therapy. N Engl J Med 2005; 352: 20–8.

88. Schoenhagen P, Tuzcu EM, Apperson-Hansen C et al. Determinants of arterial wall remodeling during lipid-lowering therapy: serial intravascular ultrasound observations from the Reversal of Atherosclerosis with Aggressive Lipid Lowering Therapy (REVERSAL) trial. Circulation 2006; 113: 2826–34.

89. Naghavi M, Falk E, Hecht HS et al.; for the SHAPE Task Force. From Vulnerable Plaque to Vulnerable Patient-Part III: Executive Summary of the Screening for Heart Attack Prevention and Education (SHAPE) Task Force Report. Am J Cardiol 2006; 98(2 Suppl 1): 2–15.

32

Imaging of Myocardial Viability and Infarction

Andreas H. Mahnken and Arno Buecker

I INTRODUCTION

Imaging of myocardial infarction (MI) and myocardial viability is one of the fastest-developing fields in medical imaging. Visualization of myocardial viability is an important concept because dysfunctional, but viable, myocardium has the potential for functional recovery after revascularization. In contrast, non-viable myocardium is unlikely to recover function.[1] It is estimated that 23%–40% of patients with chronic ischaemic ventricular dysfunction have potential for improvement of left ventricular (LV) function after revascularization.[2] This is of great importance for the clinical practice of cardiology, because non-invasive assessment of myocardial viability allows selection of patients who will benefit from coronary revascularization. With more than 865,000 MIs in 2003 in the USA, and estimated costs of US$83,919 per surgical revascularization and US$38,203 per percutaneous coronary intervention targeting patients appropriate for these resource-consuming interventions is of enormous socio-economic relevance.[3] Moreover, percutaneous coronary angioplasty or coronary artery bypass grafting both are associated with relevant risks in terms of morbidity and mortality that must be justified by expected benefits in terms of quality of life or survival.

MI size is a direct predictor for the development of LV dysfunction and maladaption of LV geometry in patients with acute MI.[4] Moreover, spatial extent and degree of myocardial injury determine the individual patient's long

term outcome and survival.[5] In patients with viable myocardium, the annual death rate after revascularization is only half as high as in patients without viable myocardium.[6] The transmural extent of infarction is also a relevant determinant of functional recovery and long term outcome. In MI with a transmural extent of less than 25% myocardium normally shows a globally improved LV function after revascularization. Even in cases of up to 50% irreversibly damaged myocardium an improvement of regional function can be achieved by revascularization therapy.[7] In the presence of MI with an extent of 75% or more of LV wall thickness, improvement of LV function is extremely rare[8] and areas of entirely transmural infarction will not recover function (Figure 32.1). Consequently assessment of myocardial viability is essential not only for risk assessment but also treatment planning.

Several techniques for myocardial viability imaging have been established. These techniques include low-dose dobutamine stress echocardiography, single photon emission computed tomography (SPECT) and ^{18}F-fluorodeoxyglucose positron emission tomography (PET) and magnetic resonance (MR) imaging. Among these techniques, MR imaging has evolved as a clinically accepted gold standard for the assessment of myocardial viability.[9] One of its most important advantages when compared with SPECT or PET is the potential to differentiate between transmural and non-transmural infarction. In addition, MR imaging provides detailed information on contractile function and myocardial perfusion if needed.

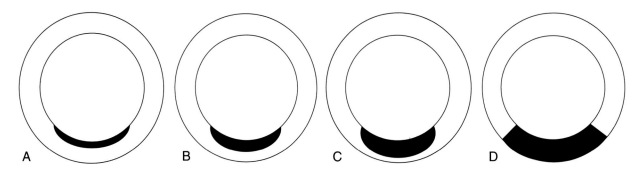

Figure 32.1 Dysfunctional but viable myocardium may experience functional improvement after revascularization therapy. Functional recovery depends on the transmural extent of MI. If less than 25% of the left ventricular wall thickness is necrotic global improvement of left ventricular function can be expected (A). If hyperenhancement comprises less than 50% of the transmural extent regional wall motion improvement can be expected (B). Segments with more than 75% (C) delayed contrast enhancement have very little chance for functional improvement. In transmural hyperenhancement (D) there will be no functional recovery after revascularization.

Over the last decade, great strides have been made in non-invasive cardiac imaging. Multislice-spiral computed tomography (MSCT) has become a widely used cardiac imaging modality. MSCT not only allows visualization of the coronary arteries and global LV function, but also of myocardial viability. Similar to MR imaging, MSCT is also capable of differentiating transmural from non-transmural infarction.[10] Initial CT approaches to the assessment of myocardial infarction and viability were developed in the late 1970s.[11] Electron beam computed tomography (EBCT)[12] or, at the Mayo Clinic, the dynamic spatial reconstructor[13] were successfully evaluated for their ability to visualize MI. However, for a number of reasons these techniques never became part of the clinical routine. With introduction of cardiac MR imaging in clinical routine, CT techniques for MI imaging disappeared from the radiologists' and cardiologists' sight. Although MR imaging is a reliable standard of reference for imaging myocardial viability, alternative techniques are needed, e.g. for the large patient population with cardiac pacemakers or deep brain stimulators. Moreover, there is a need for comprehensive and cost-effective imaging strategies that can assess both myocardial viability and coronary arteries, a combination that can be achieved with the current CT technique.

2 PATHOPHYSIOLOGICAL BASICS

Although classification of ischemic injury of the myocardium into specific categories may be artificial, it is important to differentiate between irrevocably necrotic myocardium on the one hand, and the various types of viable myocardium on the other. In order to understand CT imaging of myocardial viability and infarction, an understanding of the different categories of myocardial injury and their etiology is essential. In general, ischemic injury of the myocardium can be differentiated in reversible and irreversible conditions in the acute and chronic state.

2.1 Reversible – acute (stunning)

Exercise induced ischemia, heart transplantation, acute myocardial ischemia and peri-infarction dysfunction are associated with single or repeated short periods of myocardial ischemia. The latter may induce myocardial stunning,[14] a postischemic myocardial dysfunction that persists even if the coronary flow is restored.[15]

2.2 Reversible – chronic (hibernation)

Chronic impairment of the regional blood flow may result in hibernation, which is characterized by viable but non-functional myocardium.[16] The most common reason for myocardial hibernation is hemodynamically relevant multivessel disease. In hibernating myocardium, contractile function is diminished due to reduced myocyte metabolism in reaction to prolonged impairment of perfusion. Revascularization therapy may restore myocardial function to some degree.[17] When compared with myocardial stunning, functional recovery takes longer in hibernating myocardium.[18]

Moreover, after a certain time, chronically hypoperfused myocardium may become irreversibly damaged.[19]

2.3 Irreversible – acute (acute MI)

Irreversible myocardial damage is marked by the loss of the cell membrane integrity. In acute MI the intracellular space of the necrotic myocytes becomes accessible to extracellular contrast media. Interstitial edema further increases the distribution volume for contrast material. Compared to the intravascular space, wash-in and wash-out of contrast material is delayed in these regions. These altered kinetics provide the pathophysiological basis for delayed myocardial contrast enhancement.

In acute MI, not all myocytes within the infarct zone die simultaneously.[20] Most of the myocardial thickening during cardiac contraction, and therefore the highest local energy demand, occurs within the endocardial half of the myocardium.[21] Hence, myocyte necrosis in acute MI starts in the subendocardial layer and spreads like a wave front towards the subepicardial myocardium. As a result, location, spatial extent, and lateral boundaries of myocyte necrosis are a function of which coronary artery segment is occluded, but the transmural extent of MI is determined by the duration of ischemia. Early coronary artery revascularization prior to the development of transmural MI may salvage the myocardium at risk in the mid-myocardial and subepicardial layer.[8]

If myocardial ischemia persists for more than two hours, restoration of blood flow in the epicardial coronary arteries does not necessarily result in restoration of microvascular flow. As a consequence, so-called microvascular obstruction (no-reflow) occurs, which is characterized clinically by increased cardiac mortality during the acute period, and a reduced long-term prognosis.[22]

2.4 Irreversible – chronic (chronic MI)

At the chronic stage of MI, starting approximately 72 h after the acute event, thinning of the necrotic myocardium may be observed. Within 6 weeks, the necrotic myocardium is replaced by scar tissue that is markedly thinner than normal myocardium. The severity of the underlying coronary artery disease and the occurrence of secondary events, such as recurrent MI, define the exact time course of this myocardial remodeling process.[23]

3 CT IMAGING OF MYOCARDIAL ISCHEMIC INJURY

Several years before spiral CT and sub-second gantry rotation became available, several promising reports on the application of CT for imaging MI were published.[24] A straight-forward approach for the detection of MI is the visualization of hypoenhancing myocardium during the arterial phase of contrast enhanced CT. While this is the most obvious and basic CT approach for evaluating the myocardium, several other techniques for imaging MI were developed. Some of these techniques, including the assessment of left ventricular wall motion, thickness, and thickening, or of myocardial perfusion, were previously validated for cardiac MR imaging. Imaging of delayed myocardial contrast enhancement by CT goes one step beyond these approaches by directly visualizing myocardial viability.

3.1 First-pass CT perfusion imaging

The myocardial microvasculature plays a key role in regulating myocardial perfusion and flow reserve. Intramyocardial microvascular dysfunction occurs in early stages of coronary artery disease and precedes MI. Quantification of microvascular function allows assessing the physiological relevance and therefore significance of coronary artery lesions before irreversible damage to the myocardium occurs. Microvascular function can be quantified by first-pass myocardial perfusion imaging, and decreased myocardial perfusion represents the first consequence of obstructive coronary artery disease.[25] EBCT has been used to non-invasively quantify intramyocardial microcirculatory function in the animal model, including the quantification of the microvascular blood volume distribution.[26]

For a first-pass perfusion study, sequential ECG-gated images are obtained without table advance during at least every second heart beat. Starting with baseline images of the myocardium without contrast-enhancement, the passage of a bolus of contrast medium is followed from the right heart to the LV and through the myocardium. From carefully placed regions of interest, time-attenuation curves for different myocardial segments can be computed. For inter- and intraindividual comparisons, the data must be corrected for variations in the hemodynamic status by normalizing the myocardial attenuation values to the attenuation values measured in the LV cavity. These time-attenuation curves can then be analyzed quantitatively and semi-quantitatively.

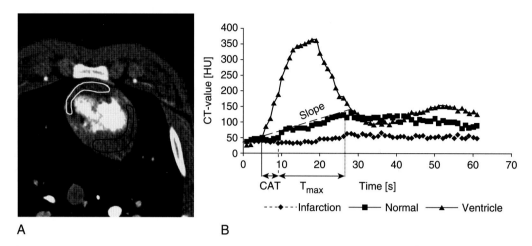

A   B

Figure 32.2   For first-pass perfusion analysis time-attenuation curves (B) are computed from regions of interest that are placed in the area of MI (A; white) and healthy remote myocardium (A; black). Results are normalized to the enhancement in the left ventricular cavity. Several semi-quantitative parameters like slope, contrast-arrival time (CAT) or time-to-maximum (T_{max}) may be computed from time-attenuation curves.

For more than a decade this technique could reliably be performed only with EBCT. Quantitative perfusion analysis, including computation of transit time, myocardial blood volume or myocardial perfusion has been reported for EBCT.[26] More recently, the temporal resolution of MSCT has become sufficient for myocardial perfusion studies. In animal and human studies, the potential of contrast enhanced MSCT to provide information about myocardial perfusion has been demonstrated.[27,28] In the MSCT perfusion studies to date, mostly semi-quantitative parameters previously validated for MR imaging including maximum signal intensity, wash-in time and slope have been examined.[29] In the animal model, the combination of CT rest and stress perfusion imaging can allow the assessment of regional differences of myocardial perfusion.[30] Theoretically, assessment coronary perfusion reserve and even myocardial blood flow quantification[27] from MSCT data should be possible. The concepts of, and available data on, first-pass CT perfusion imaging are discussed in more detail in chapter X.X. To date, MSCT perfusion techniques are not used in the clinical setting and optimized scan protocols have not yet been developed.

Compared to MR imaging, the linear relationship between iodine concentration and contrast enhancement in CT imaging offers the great advantage of permitting direct quantification of myocardial blood flow without the complex mathematical modeling required for quantitative MR myocardial perfusion studies. However, first-pass CT perfusion imaging has the disadvantage of requiring exposure to ionizing radiation. Another relevant limitation of first-pass CT perfusion imaging is the limited myocardial

volume that can be examined and that is determined by the detector width. With introduction of new CT detectors that can acquire 256 or more slices per rotation simultaneously, whole organ perfusion imaging will become feasible albeit most likely at the price of increased radiation exposure.[31]

3.2 Arterial phase CT imaging

Arterial phase imaging of the myocardium is a routine part of CT coronary angiography, and does not require extra exposure of the patient to ionizing radiation or contrast material. These images are obtained during the first pass of contrast material. Consequently, contrast enhancement is directly related to myocardial perfusion. For many organ regions, lack of contrast enhancement is an accepted surrogate marker of infarction. This concept also holds true for the myocardium, where hypoattenuation during arterial phase CT imaging reflects diminished or delayed contrast delivery due to reduced blood flow.[32] The direct relationship between absent perfusion, hypoenhancement on CT and MI has been demonstrated in several animal models of acute MI.[33,34] Thus, it is justified to consider reduced contrast enhancement during arterial phase CT as a marker of MI or myocardial perfusion deficit. Interestingly, even in CT scans without contrast enhancement, hypoattenuation of infarcted myocardium may be seen in some patients.[35,36]

In the early 1980s, single slice CT[24-38] and EBCT were successfully used to detect MI in patients.[39] At that time, CT imaging of the heart with mechanical scanners was limited by difficulty visualizing the inferior wall of the LV on ungated axial images. With introduction of MSCT scanners with subsecond gantry rotation time and submillimeter spatial resolution, cardiac CT imaging, including the assessment of MI, has become eminently feasible and widely available.

Several recent studies reported sensitivities and specificities ranging from 79–91% for the detection of MI from ECG-gated MSCT data (Table 32.1). With current CT scanners, even non-gated chest CT permits reliable detection of MI.[40] Although the attenuation values of normal myocardium are typically more than twice as high as those of infarcted myocardium, a threshold of 20 HU is typically used to differentiate normal from infarcted myocardium. Advanced visualization strategies are likely to further improve the detection of MI from arterial phase CT (Figure 32.3).[41] Analysis of regional myocardial function that is possible from MSCT examinations performed for coronary angiography can corroborate the classification of hypoattenuating myocardium as infarcted.[42,43] Because both acute and chronic MI present as hypoattenuating areas during arterial phase, additional imaging characteristics are needed to separate acute from chronic MI. Wall thickness is a good marker for this purpose. Chronic MI typically presents with wall thinning due to scar formation.[44,45] Thus, the presence of hypoattenuating myocardium in combination with regional wall thinning is likely to represent chronic MI.

There are several limitations to arterial phase CT for assessing MI. Although the sensitivity for the detection of MI is in the clinically acceptable range, MI size is typically underestimated by CT when compared to MR imaging.[10] Microvascular obstruction, as known from MR imaging of acute and subacute MI, likely contributes to this finding. During the healing phase of MI, capillary infiltration from the periphery may not extend to the central portion of the infarct, resulting in a central area of hypoattenuation on contrast-enhanced CT.[35] The gradual ingrowth of capillaries

from the periphery may lead to the appearance on CT imaging of progressively decreasing MI size as the organization of infarcted myocardium progresses. The main limitation of arterial phase CT for imaging of myocardial infarction, however, is that hypoattenuating myocardium does not necessarily represent MI, but may simply be the result of reduced perfusion resulting from high-grade coronary luminal obstruction. As a consequence, myocardial segments with reduced contrast enhancement may be viable or not (Table 32.2).

Arterial phase CT of the myocardium does not provide dynamic information such flow reserve, because it is performed under resting conditions from data obtained for coronary CT angiography. In one small patient series, arterial phase adenosine stress CT imaging for the detection of myocardial ischemia was performed.[46] The agreement with stress thallium-201 myocardial perfusion scintigraphy was 83%. This approach may allow differentiating between acute MI and reversible perfusion deficits. However, at the current stage of technical development, the need for repeated exposure to ionizing radiation and contrast material limit the clinical usefulness of CT for myocardial stress imaging, especially since less invasive techniques such as stress MR imaging and stress echocardiography are available.

3.3 Late phase CT imaging

The limitations of arterial phase CT imaging of MI fueled the quest for CT techniques that are more specific for myocardial viability or lack thereof. In 1978, Higgins et al. demonstrated that extracellular contrast material accumulates in areas of acute MI on CT imaging,[47] presenting as delayed myocardial contrast enhancement 5 to 20 minutes after contrast material injection. During the 1980s, several

Table 32.1 Studies on the detection of MI from arterial phase CT

Author		Patients MI /total	Reference	Sensitivity (%)	Specificity (%)	Attenuation MI [HU]	Attenuation healthy [HU]
Gosalia[40]	2004	18 / 69*	clinical	83	95	8-87	66-147
Nikolaou[44]	2004	27 / 106	clinical	85	91	54±19	117±28
Nikolaou[61]	2005	11 / 30	MR imaging	91	79	54±34	122±26
Mahnken[10]	2005	110 / 448[2]	MR imaging	83	91	59±17	101±14
Francone[45]	2006	29 / 187	clinical	83	91	39±14	104±16
Sanz[35]	2006	21 / 42	MR imaging	91	81	42±39	119±20

*ungated CT; [2]segment based analysis; HU, Hounsfield Units.

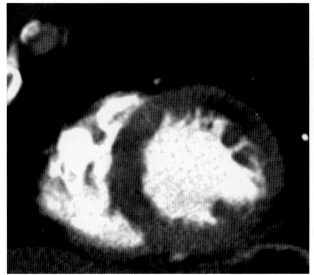

A

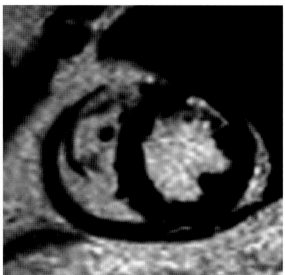

B

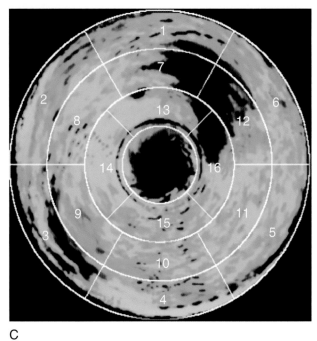

C

Figure 32.3   On arterial phase CT MI is depicted as an area of reduced contrast enhancement (A). MI size is typically underestimated, when compared with MR imaging (B). By application of advanced visualization techniques like perfusion weighted color maps sensitivity for the detection of MI can be improved (C; blue areas).

Table 32.2   Classification ischemic injury and the typical CT imaging features

	Acute		Chronic	
	Reversible stunning	Irreversible acute MI	Reversible hibernation	Irreversible chronic MI
arterial phase	hypodense or normal	hypodense	hypodense or normal	hypodense, wall thinning
late phase	hypodense	occlusive = hypodense; reperfused = hyperdense	hypodense	occlusive = hypodense; reperfused = hyperdense

Table 32.3 Animal studies proving delayed contrast enhanced CT feasible for the detection of MI

Author	Animal	MI age	delay [min]	MI size MSCT [%]	MI size MR imaging [%]	MI size TTC [%]	Attenuation MI [HU]	Attenuation healthy [HU]
Buecker 2005[50]	14 pigs	acute	5-60	22.8±9.2	20.8±11	20.6±12	-	-
Baks 2006[59]	10 pigs	acute	15	21±15	22±16	20±15	126±20	66±6
Lardo 2006[57]	10 dogs	acute	5-40	21.4	-	20.8	261±57	134±11
	7 pigs	chronic		4.2±1.9		4.9±2.1	181±39	97±15

min, minutes.

studies on the use of delayed contrast enhancement in EBCT for the assessment of MI were published.[48,49] At that time, however, CT imaging of MI was not valued as clinical tool.

With the rapid spread of cardiac MSCT, the role of CT imaging in MI is being re-examined. Within the last few years, several studies in animals (Table 32.3) and in patients (Table 32.4) have compared delayed contrast enhancement on retrospectively ECG-gated MSCT for the detection of MI with single photon emission computed tomography (SPECT), MR imaging, and 2,3,5-triphenyl tetrazolium chloride (TTC) staining. The imaging characteristics of acute, subacute and chronic as well as of reperfused and occlusive MIs have been investigated.

Reperfused MI typically presents with delayed contrast enhancement in areas of infarction. The delayed enhancement is much less pronounced than in delayed-enhanced MR imaging. Depending on the amount of iodine injected and the timing of imaging relative to contrast injection, the attenuation values in infarcted myocardium are typically approximately double those in normal myocardium.

In contrast, MI with an occluded infarct-related artery presents as an area of diminished attenuation that persists up to one hour after injection of contrast material. The lack of contrast enhancement in occlusive MI is attributed to a lack of inflow of contrast material into the area of infarction resulting from a lack of collaterals. These simple imaging features reliably allow differentiating occlusive from reperfused MI.[50]

While arterial phase CT typically underestimates the size of MI, several studies suggest that delayed contrast enhancement on CT slightly overestimates the size of acute MI. This is thought to be due to an increased distribution volume in the periinfarction zone.[51] In chronic MI, not only regional wall thinning, but also a decrease in infarct size may be observed, as discussed above. An animal study on chronic MI with sequential CT examinations over a period of three months suggested shrinkage of the damaged myocardium with subsequent fibrosis.[52] Overall, the size of reperfused MI on delayed myocardial enhancement by CT correlates well with that on delayed myocardial enhancement MRI at all stages of infaction.[52A]

Given the submillimeter spatial resolution of MSCT, subendocardial infarctions can be differentiated from transmural MIs based on the transmural extent of delayed enhancement (Figure 32.4). Detection of prognostically important microvascular obstruction is feasible, as well. These so called 'no-reflow' areas present on delayed CT imaging as hypodense regions surrounded by hyperenhanced myocardium.[53] Although imaging of delayed myocardial contrast enhancement has been developed to image myocardial viability, it is not specific for MI and also may be found in other conditions that are associated with

Table 32.4 Patient studies show a good agreement between late enhanced CT and the standard of reference indicating the reliability of CT for assessing myocardial viability

Author	Patient / segment	Reference	MI age	delay [min]	Sensitivity [%]	Specificity [%]	Attenuation MI [HU]	Attenuation healthy [HU]
Paul 2005[62]	34 / 578	SPECT	acute	5	78	91	-	-
Mahnken 2005[10]	28 / 448	MR imaging	acute	15	97	98	108±16	75±11
Gerber 2006[58]	16 / 256	MR imaging	acute	10	85	90	97±11	131±16
	21 / 336	MR imaging	chronic	10	59	92		

min, minutes; HU, Hounsfield Units.

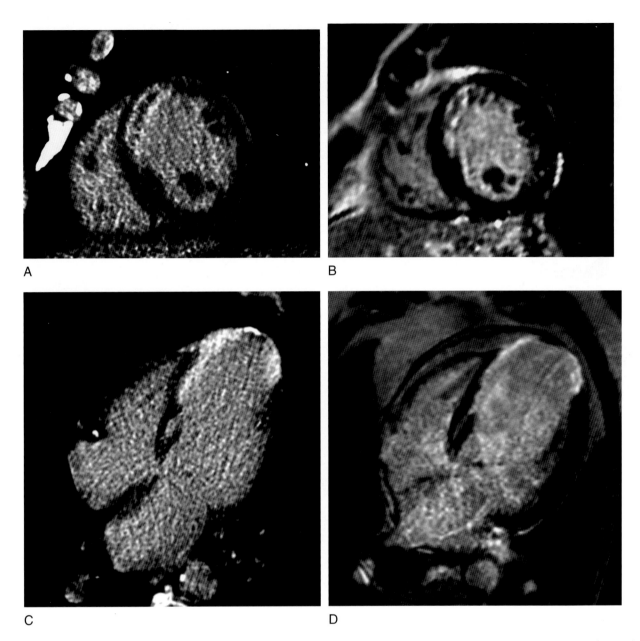

A   B

C   D

Figure 32.4   CT allows differentiation of subendocardial (A) from transmural (C) infarction. Extent and location of actual infarction on delayed enhanced CT (A,C) correlate well with MR imaging (B,D).

myocardial scarring such as cardiomyopathies, myocarditis or cardiac sarcoidosis.[54,55]

When arterial and late phase MSCT imaging are combined, various contrast enhancement patterns can be observed that may allow conclusion regarding the completeness of reperfusion. Some patients with myocardial contrast enhancement on late phase CT have hypoattenuating areas during arterial phase, while others do not. After reperfusion therapy, the absence of a hypoattenuating area during arterial phase CT may indicate successful reperfusion at both the epicardial and the microvascular level. Koyama et al. described three different enhancement patterns and evaluated their relation to the recovery of global and regional LV

function (Figure 32.5). Wall thickening and ejection fraction recovered best in patients who did not have perfusion defects during the arterial phase. In contrast, LV function recovered least in patients who had non-enhancing areas during both arterial and late phase CT.[53] Based on animal data, the different lesion sizes in arterial and late phase CT are thought to reflect reperfusion in the area at risk.[56] Because the combination of arterial and late phase CT appears to provide prognostic information on the likelihood of LV function recovery, a CT examination protocol for the assessment of MI should include an arterial phase scan that can also be used for the assessment of the coronary arteries, and a late phase scan (Figure 32.6).

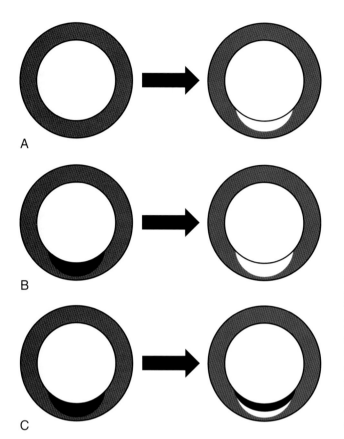

Figure 32.5 When comparing arterial phase (left) and late-phase (right) CT of the heart, myocardial infarction presents with different contrast enhancement patterns. These patterns are related to functional recovery after myocardial infarction. Best results with respect to wall thickening and left ventricular ejection fraction have to be expected if no early perfusion deficit but delayed contrast enhancement (white regions) is seen (A). Prognosis decreases if hypoattenuating areas (black regions) are also present during arterial phase (B). In patients with hypoattenuating areas during arterial and late phase CT, so called no-reflow areas, poorest results have to be expected (C).

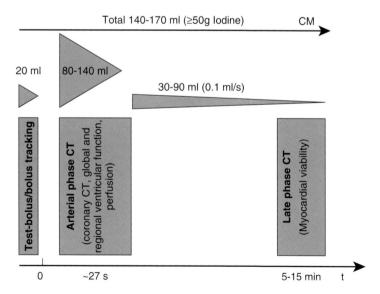

Figure 32.6 There are no recommendations for a uniform scan and contrast injection protocol for imaging myocardial viability with CT. For a comprehensive analysis of the coronary arteries, cardiac function and myocardial viability a contrast-enhanced dual phase scan protocol can be recommended. Most groups use a single contrast material injection. Others, however, maintain a low flow contrast injection after the arterial phase scan.

To date, there is no universal agreement on how to best tailor scan protocols to the sensitive detection of delayed contrast enhancement in CT. Key issues are the mode of contrast administration and the optimal delay for late phase image acquisition. Contrast delivery to non-viable tissue will take several minutes. Consequently, a relatively long delay after contrast injection is needed. Delays ranging from 5 to 60 minutes have been evaluated.[50,57,58] Some studies reported excellent results with a delay of 15 minutes,[59] but others showed the best contrast between infarcted and normal myocardium at a delay of 5 minutes between contrast injection and CT imaging.[58]

The low contrast between the area of infarction and the blood pool is an important challenge for delayed contrast enhanced MSCT imaging of MI. The delay of several minutes that is needed to allow contrast material to accumulate in infarcted myocardium leads to near-absence of contrast enhancement in the LV cavity. Dedicated contrast injection protocols to optimize contrast between infarcted myocardium and normal myocardium or the LV blood pool must be developed. To ensure sufficient contrast on late phase CT images, the total amount of iodine administered should exceed 50g. Some authors advocate lowering the tube voltage to improve contrast in late phase CT. This approach will result in better iodine contrast and lower radiation exposure at the expense of an increased image noise.[60] With dual source CT (see chapter x.x), enough power scanning of the heart at 80kVp with acceptable image noise will be available. An attractive clinical approach in patients with acute myocardial infarction has been reported that avoids excessive exposure to contrast medium by utilizing the contrast material injected for invasive, selective coronary angiography for delayed enhancement CT imaging, and reduces additional radiation exposure by setting the tube voltage to 80 kVp.[59A] At an average delay of up to 51 minutes after the end of invasive coronary angiography, delayed enhancement CT, compared to low-dose dobutamine echocardiography, had 98% sensitivity, 94% specificity, 97% accuracy, and 99% positive and 79% negative predictive values for detecting viable myocardial segments in this setting.

The combination of myocardial viability imaging of non-invasive coronary MSCT angiography and analysis of global and regional LV function offers a comprehensive examination strategy for evaluation of patients with known or suspected heart disease.

REFERENCES

1. Rahimtoola SH. A perspective on the three large multicenter randomised clinical trials of coronary bypass surgery for chronic stable angina. Circulation 1985; 72: V123–V135.

2. Bonow RO. Identification of viable myocardium. Circulation 1996; 94: 2674–80.

3. American Heart Association. Heart Disease and Stroke Statistics – 2006 Update. Dallas, Texas: American Heart Association, 2006.

4. Baks T, van Geuns RJ, Biagini E et al. Recovery of left ventricular function after primary angioplasty for acute myocardial infarction. Eur Heart J 2005; 26: 1070–7.

5. Gersh BJ, Anderson JL. Thrombolysis and myocardial salvage. Results of clinical trials and the animal paradigm - paradoxic or predictable? Circulation 1993; 88: 296–306.

6. Allman KC, Shaw LJ, Hachamovitch R, Udelson JE. Myocardial viability testing and impact of revascularization on prognosis in patients with coronary artery disease and left ventricular dysfunction: a meta-analysis. J Am Coll Cardiol 2002; 39: 1151–8.

7. Choi KM, Kim RJ, Gubernikoff G et al. Transmural extent of acute myocardial infarction predicts long-term improvement in contractile function. Circulation 2001; 104: 1101–7.

8. Kim RJ, Wu E, Rafael A et al. The use of contrast-enhanced magnetic resonance imaging to identify reversible myocardial dysfunction. N Engl J Med 2000; 343: 1445–53.

9. Wagner A, Mahrholdt H, Holly TA et al. Contrast-enhanced MRI and routine single photon emission computed tomography (SPECT) perfusion imaging for detection of subendocardial myocardial infarcts: an imaging study. Lancet 2003; 361: 374–9.

10. Mahnken AH, Koos R, Katoh M et al. Assessment of myocardial viability in reperfused acute myocardial infarction using 16-slice computed tomography in comparison to magnetic resonance imaging. J Am Coll Cardiol 2005; 45: 2042–7.

11. Adams DF, Hessel SJ, Judy PF, Stein JA, Abrams HL. Computed tomography of the normal and infarcted myocardium. AJR Am J Roentgenol 1976; 126: 786–91.

12. Hamada S, Naito H, Takamiya M. Evaluation of myocardium in ischemic heart disease by ultrafast computed tomography. Jpn Circ J 1992; 56: 627–31.

13. Scanlan JG, Gustafson DE, Chevalier PA, Robb RA, Ritman EL. Evaluation of ischemic heart disease with a prototype volume imaging computed tomographic (CT) scanner: preliminary experiments. Am J Cardiol 1980; 46: 1263–8.

14. Braunwald E, Kloner RA. The stunned myocardium: prolonged, postischemic ventricular dysfunction. Circulation 1982; 66: 1146–9.

15. Bolli R, Marban E. Molecular and cellular mechanisms of myocardial stunning. Physiol Rev 1999; 79: 609–34.

16. Shen YT, Vatner SF. Mechanism of impaired myocardial function during progressive coronary stenosis in conscious pigs. Hibernation versus stunning? Circ Res 1995; 76: 479–88.

17. Tillisch J, Brunken R, Marshall R et al. Reversibility of cardiac wall motion abnormalities predicted by positron emission tomography. N Engl J Med 1986; 314: 884–8.

18. Bax JJ, Visser FC, Poldermans D et al. Time course of functional recovery of stunned and hibernating segments after surgical revascularization. Circulation 2001; 104(12 Suppl 1): I314–I318.

19. Kloner RA, Bolli R, Marban E, Reinlib L, Braunwald E. Medical and cellular implications of stunning, hibernation, and preconditioning: an NHLBI workshop. Circulation 1998; 97: 1848–67.

20. Reimer KA, Lowe JE, Rasmussen MM, Jennings RB. The wavefront phenomenon of ischemic cell death.

1. Myocardial infarct size vs duration of coronary occlusion in dogs. Circulation 1977; 56: 786–94.

21. Myers JH, Stirling MC, Choy M, Buda AJ, Gallagher KP. Direct measurement of inner and outer wall thickening dynamics with epicardial echocardiography. Circulation 1986; 74: 164–72.

22. Wu KC, Zerhouni EA, Judd RM et al. Prognostic significance of microvascular obstruction by magnetic resonance imaging in patients with acute myocardial infarction. Circulation 1998; 97: 765–72.

23. Cohn JN, Ferrari R, Sharpe N. Cardiac remodeling-concepts and clinical implications: a consensus paper from an international forum on cardiac remodeling. Behalf of an International Forum on Cardiac Remodeling. J Am Coll Cardiol 2000; 35: 569–82.

24. Huber DJ, Lapray JF, Hessel SJ. In vivo evaluation of experimental myocardial infarcts by ungated computed tomography. AJR Am J Roentgenol 1981; 136: 469–73.

25. Nesto RW, Kowalchuk GJ. The ischemic cascade: temporal sequence of hemodynamic, electrocardiographic and symptomatic expressions of ischemia. Am J Cardiol 1987; 59: 23C–30C.

26. Mohlenkamp S, Lerman LO, Lerman A et al. Minimally invasive evaluation of coronary microvascular function by electron beam computed tomography. Circulation 2000; 102: 2411–16.

27. Wintersperger BJ, Ruff J, Becker CR et al. Assessment of regional myocardial perfusion using multirow-detector computed tomography (MDCT). Eur Radiol 2002; 12 (Suppl 1): S294.

28. Mahnken AH, Bruners P, Katoh M et al. Dynamic multi-section CT imaging in acute myocardial infarction: preliminary animal experience. Eur Radiol 2006; 16: 746–52.

29. al-Saadi N, Gross M, Bornstedt A et al. Comparison of various parameters for determining an index of myocardial perfusion reserve in detecting coronary stenosis with cardiovascular magnetic resonance tomography. Z Kardiol 2001; 90: 824–34 [German].

30. Stantz KM, Liang Y, Meyer CA, Teague SD, March K. In vivo myocardial perfusion measurements by ECG-gated multi-slice computed tomography. Radiology 2002; S225: 308.

31. Funabashi N, Yoshida K, Tadokoro H et al. Cardiovascular circulation and hepatic perfusion of pigs in 4-dimensional films evaluated by 256-slice cone-beam computed tomography. Circ J 2005; 69: 585–9.

32. Doherty PW, Lipton MJ, Berninger WH et al. Detection and quantitation of myocardial infarction in vivo using transmission computed tomography. Circulation 1981; 63: 597–606.

33. Slutsky RA, Mattrey RF, Long SA, Higgins CB. In vivo estimation of myocardial infarct size and left ventricular function by prospectively gated computerized transmission tomography. Circulation 1983; 67: 759–65.

34. Hoffmann U, Millea R, Enzweiler C et al. Acute myocardial infarction: contrast-enhanced multi-detector row CT in a porcine model. Radiology 2004; 231: 697–701.

35. Sanz J, Weeks D, Nikolaou K et al. Detection of healed myocardial infarction with multidetector-row computed tomography and comparison with cardiac magnetic resonance delayed hyperenhancement. Am J Cardiol 2006; 98: 149–55.

36. Winer-Muram HT, Tann M, Aisen AM et al. Computed tomography demonstration of lipomatous metaplasia of the left ventricle following myocardial infarction. J Comput Assist Tomogr 2004; 28: 455–8.

37. Kramer PH, Goldstein JA, Herkens RJ, Lipton MJ, Brundage BH. Imaging of acute myocardial infarction in man with contrast-enhanced computed transmission tomography. Am Heart J 1984; 108: 1514–23.

38. See reference 24.

39. Schmermund A, Gerber T, Behrenbeck T et al. Measurement of myocardial infarct size by electron beam computed tomography: a comparison with 99 mTc sestamibi. Invest Radiol 1998; 33: 313–21.

40. Gosalia A, Haramati LB, Sheth MP, Spindola-Franco H. CT detection of acute myocardial infarction. Am J Roentgenol 2004; 182: 1563–6.

41. Mahnken AH, Klotz E, Lautenschläger S et al. Assessment of myocardial infarction with cardiac MSCT using model based heart segmentation and perfusion weighted color maps. Eur Radiol 2005; 14 (Suppl 2): S250.

42. Mahnken AH, Katoh M, Bruners P et al. Acute myocardial infarction: assessment of left ventricular function with 16-detector row spiral CT versus MR imaging-study in pigs. Radiology 2005; 236: 112–17.

43. Mahnken AH, Koos R, Katoh M et al. Sixteen-slice spiral CT versus MR imaging for the assessment of left ventricular function in acute myocardial infarction. Eur Radiol 2005; 15: 714–20.

44. Nikolaou K, Knez A, Sagmeister S et al. Assessment of myocardial infarctions using multirow-detector computed tomography. J Comput Assist Tomogr 2004; 28: 286–92.

45. Francone M, Carbone I, Danti M et al. ECG-gated multidetector row spiral CT in the assessment of myocardial infarction: correlation with non-invasive angiographic findings. Eur Radiol 2006; 16: 15–24.

46. Kurata A, Mochizuki T, Koyama Y et al. Myocardial perfusion imaging using adenosine triphosphate stress multi-slice spiral computed tomography alternative to stress myocardial perfusion scintigraphy. Circ J 2005; 69: 550–7.

47. Higgins CB, Sovak M, Schmidt W, Siemers PT. Uptake of contrast materials by experimental acute myocardial infarctions: a preliminary report. Invest Radiol 1978; 13: 337–9.

48. Naito H, Saito H, Ohta M, Takamiya M. Significance of ultrafast computed tomography in cardiac imaging: usefulness in assessment of myocardial characteristics and cardiac function. Jpn Circ J 1990; 54: 322–7.

49. Masuda Y, Yoshida H, Morooka N, Watanabe S, Inagaki Y. The usefulness of x-ray computed tomography for the diagnosis of myocardial infarction. Circulation 1984; 70: 217–25.

50. Buecker A, Katoh M, Krombach GA et al. A feasibility study of contrast enhancement of acute myocardial infarction in multislice computed tomography: comparison with magnetic resonance imaging and gross morphology in pigs. Invest Radiol 2005; 40: 700–4.

51. Saeed M, Lund G, Wendland MF et al. Magnetic resonance characterization of the peri-infarction zone of reperfused myocardial infarction with necrosis-specific and extracellular nonspecific contrast media. Circulation 2001; 103: 871–6.

52. Mahnken AH, Wildberger JE. Multislice spiral computed tomography for assessment of myocardial viability in myocardial infarction. Eur Radiol 2006; 16 (Suppl 1): S493.

52A. Mahnken AH, Bruners P, Kinzel S et al. Late-phase MSCT in the different stages of myocardial infarction: animal experiments. Eur Radiol 2007; 17: 2310–17.

53. Koyama Y, Matsuoka H, Mochizuki T et al. Assessment of reperfused acute myocardial infarction with two-phase contrast-enhanced helical CT: prediction of left ventricular function and wall thickness. Radiology 2005; 235: 804–11.

54. Smedema JP, Truter R, de Klerk PA et al. Cardiac sarcoidosis evaluated with gadolinium-enhanced magnetic resonance and contrast-enhanced 64-slice computed tomography. Int J Cardiol 2005; 112: 261–3.

55. Kaminaga T, Naito H, Takamiya M, Hamada S, Nishimura T. Myocardial damage in patients with dilated cardiomyopathy: CT evaluation. J Comput Assist Tomogr 1994; 18: 393–7.

55A. Dambrin G, Laissy JP, Serfaty JM, Caussin C, Lancelin B, Paul JF. Diagnostic value of ECG-gated multidetector computed tomography in the early phase of suspected acute myocarditis. A preliminary comparative study with cardiac MRI. Eur Radiol 2007; 17: 331–8.

56. Park JM, Choe YH, Chang S et al. Usefulness of multidetector-row CT in the evaluation of reperfused myocardial infarction in a rabbit model. Korean J Radiol 2004; 5: 19–24.

57. Lardo AC, Cordeiro MA, Silva C et al. Contrast-enhanced multidetector computed tomography viability imaging after myocardial infarction: characterization of myocyte death, microvascular obstruction, and chronic scar. Circulation 2006; 113: 394–404.

58. Gerber BL, Belge B, Legros GJ et al. Characterization of acute and chronic myocardial infarcts by multidetector computed tomography: comparison with contrast-enhanced magnetic resonance. Circulation 2006; 113: 823–33.

59. Baks T, Cademartiri F, Moelker AD et al. Multislice computed tomography and magnetic resonance imaging for the assessment of reperfused acute myocardial infarction. J Am Coll Cardiol 2006; 48: 144–52.

59A. Habis M, Capderou A, Ghostine S et al. Acute Myocardial Infarction Early Viability Assessment by 64-Slice Computed Tomography Immediately After Coronary Angiography: Comparison With Low-Dose Dobutamine Echocardiography. J Am Coll Cardiol 2007; 49: 1178–85.

60. Sigal-Cinqualbre AB, Hennequin R, Abada HT, Chen X, Paul JF. Low-kilovoltage multi-detector row chest CT in adults: feasibility and effect on image quality and iodine dose. Radiology 2004; 231: 169–74.

61. Nikolaou K, Sanz J, Poon M et al. Assessment of myocardial perfusion and viability from routine contrast-enhanced 16-detector-row computed tomography of the heart: preliminary results. Eur Radiol 2005; 15: 864–71.

62. Paul JF, Wartski M, Caussin C et al. Late defect on delayed contrast-enhanced multi-detector row CT scans in the prediction of SPECT infarct size after reperfused acute myocardial infarction: initial experience. Radiology 2005; 236: 485–9.

33

Computed Tomography for the Assessment of Myocardial Perfusion

Richard T. George, Albert C. Lardo, and Joao A.C. Lima

1 INTRODUCTION

Recent advances in multidetector computed tomography (MDCT) technology have extended its use to the comprehensive evaluation of cardiovascular disease. Improvements in temporal and spatial resolution along with wider detector coverage have made practicable the non-invasive imaging of the coronary artery lumen and surrounding atherosclerotic plaque. Single center studies of the current generation of 64 slice MDCT scanners have demonstrated that MDCT non-invasive angiography has good sensitivity and specificity for identifying stenoses ≥50 % severity when compared to invasive angiography.[1-4] Moreover, it appears that its greatest power is in its negative predictive value, meaning its ability to exclude coronary artery disease in those patients without disease.[5] However, it is in those patients with coronary artery disease that the MDCT angiogram becomes more limited in its diagnostic accuracy due to the presence of coronary calcification and intracoronary stents.[6-8]

Although multidetector computed tomography provides unsurpassed non-invasive imaging of coronary atherosclerosis, we need to be cautious not to go back to the days of 'lumenography' when the physiological significance of stenoses was largely ignored. The invasive coronary angiography literature has made clear that percent diameter stenosis is poorly correlated with vasodilatory reserve and myocardial blood flow (MBF) measurements.[9,10] Furthermore, the radionuclide myocardial perfusion

imaging (MPI) literature has demonstrated that perfusion imaging adds valuable prognostic value above and beyond the invasive coronary angiogram and the identification and quantification of ischemia can risk stratify patients into groups who will or will not benefit from invasive over medical therapies.[11,12]

Recent evidence reveals that MDCT angiography alone has a poor positive predictive value for identifying atherosclerosis contributing to ischemia.[13-14] This has lead to the development of hybrid imaging systems that combine MDCT scanning systems with single photon emission computed tomography (SPECT) or positron emission tomography (PET) systems capable of acquiring the non-invasive coronary angiogram and radionuclide MPI. However, adding radionuclide perfusion imaging to the MDCT angiogram can more than double the effective radiation dose to patients.[15] Alternatively, there is great interest in evaluating myocardial perfusion with MDCT alone. MDCT perfusion imaging, combined with the MDCT angiogram, has the potential to not only detect the presence of coronary atherosclerosis, but also its physiologic impact on MBF. This chapter aims to review those aspects of X-ray computed tomography that make it a candidate for MPI. In doing so, we will review cardiac CT perfusion imaging over the last 20 years and how today's multidetector CT systems can be used in conjunction with the non-invasive angiogram to detect atherosclerosis and its physiologic significance.

2 THEORETICAL CONSIDERATIONS

The measurement of MBF by non-invasive means has required using the principles of indicator-dilution theory first developed by Stewart and Hamilton in the late 19th and early 20th centuries, respectively.[16,17] In the case of computed tomography, iodinated contrast is typically used as the indicator (or tracer) and serial imaging of regions of interest within the heart is performed to record the transit of iodinated contrast through the vasculature. These images are used to construct a time-attenuation curve in the aorta (or LV blood pool) and myocardium from which MBF and myocardial blood volume (MBV) measurements can be derived (Figure 33.1). There are certain assumptions that are made when applying indicator-dilution theory to the measurement of MBF with CT. Adopting the assumptions described by Rumberger and colleagues,[18,19] they are as follows:

1. Complete mixing of the indicator proximal to arrival to the heart.
2. Volume of indicator is negligible to the volume of the vasculature.
3. The indicator does not cause hemodynamic or physiologic changes as it traverses the cardiac vasculature.
4. The recorded CT attenuation number accurately reflects the concentration of the indicator.
5. Recirculation of the indicator can be ignored or accounted for.
6. There is no extravascular diffusion of the indicator during its first pass circulation through the vasculature.

Assumptions 1, 2, 3, and 5 can be justified using an intravenous injection of today's non-ionic contrast agents. However, assumptions 4 and 6 require further discussion.

Several characteristics of X-ray computed tomography and iodinated contrast make it an ideal candidate for MPI. In regards to the assumption 4, iodinated contrast is used in CT due to its ability to attenuate X-rays. In fact, the attenuation of X-rays, measured in Houndsfield units, is directly proportional to the concentration of iodine in tissue (Figure 33.2). Therefore, if you know the volume of tissue sampled and its CT number, you can calculate the concentration of iodine in the tissue. This is, of course, dependent on the accuracy of recording the actual attenuation number in the tissue which can be hindered by beam hardening (Compton scatter) and motion artifacts (Figure 33.3). These artifacts can increase or decrease the CT attenuation number that is measured and cause error in the calculation of flow measurements. Thus care needs to be taken not to violate assumption 4 by identifying these artifacts visually or correcting for them using beam hardening correction algorithms during image reconstruction.

In regards to assumption 6, iodinated contrast agents are mostly intravascular during early first pass circulation through the vasculature. However, their diffusion over time to the extravascular space increases over time and, after about 1 minute, the concentration of iodinated contrast in the extravascular space becomes higher than the intravascular space.[20,21] Furthermore, extravascular diffusion may be more pronounced in myocardial beds supplied by stenosed versus non-stenosed arteries.[22] Therefore, in order to accurately measure perfusion, imaging during the early portion

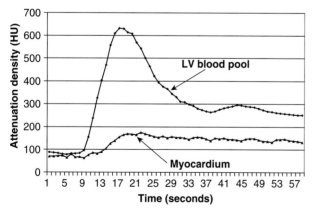

Figure 33.1 Time-attenuation curves for the left ventricular (LV) blood pool and myocardium. Dynamic imaging of the LV was performed during an intravenous injection of iodinated contrast at time zero. The attenuation density was measured in a region of interest in the LV blood pool and myocardium and plotted over time.

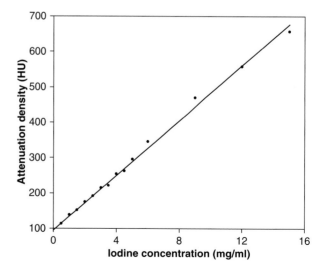

Figure 33.2 Multidetector computed tomography imaging of increasing concentrations of iodine. The attenuation of X-rays measured in Houndsfield units (y-axis) is directly proportional to the concentration of iodine (x-axis).

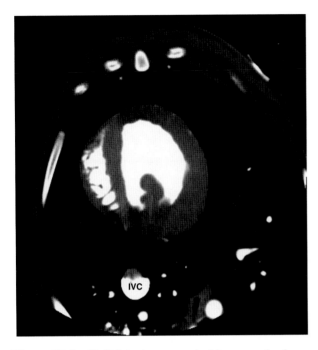

Figure 33.3 Multidetector computed tomography imaging of a canine heart at the mid left ventricle level after the administration of iodinated contrast through femoral venous access. Note iodinated contrast pooled in the inferior vena cava (IVC) is causing a beam hardening artifact (arrows) in the inferior myocardial wall.

of first pass circulation is critical. Alternatively, mathematical models can be applied that account for the diffusion of contrast agents to the extravascular space.[23]

3 MYOCARDIAL PERFUSION IMAGING USING FAST COMPUTED TOMOGRAPHY

The measurement of perfusion is not new to X-ray computed tomography. Leon Axel first described the Fermi function deconvolution method for the analysis of CT derived cerebral perfusion measurements in 1983, a method commonly used to calculate perfusion using magnetic resonance.[24] Beginning in the late 1980s, myocardial perfusion studies were first reported using electron beam tomography (EBT). Rumberger and colleagues used two different methods to derive MBF measurements from axial tomographic data: (1) the ratio of peak myocardial opacification from baseline to the area under the left ventricular cavity curve and (2) the ratio of the left ventricular to posterior papillary muscle curve areas divided by the full width/half maximal contrast transit time in the region of the posterior papillary muscle. Using these two methods they demonstrated good correlations with microsphere derived MBF with correlation coefficients of 0.7 and 0.82 respectively.

However, this study and others demonstrated an underestimation of MBF at rates above 2.5 to 3.5 ml/g/min.[25,26]

Around this same time, a multislice fast CT scanner known as the dynamic spatial reconstructor (DSR) was used to derive MBF and MBV measurements. The DSR was a one of a kind device with a gantry weighing in at nearly 17 US tons. Wang et al. used the DSR to image the heart over time and record indicator-dilution curves in the aorta and myocardium. Using an aortic root contrast injection they demonstrated an excellent correlation between DSR derived and microsphere derived MBF.[27] They also postulated that underestimations of MBF derived by fast CT were secondary to increases in regional MBV during vasodilation and, by applying a volume correction, you could extend the linear range of fast CTs capability to measure MBF up to 4.5 ml/g/min.

Bell et al. validated the use of indicator curves or time attenuation curves (TAC) in an animal study that was then applied to the measurement of myocardial perfusion in normal volunteers during maximal vasodilation and baseline conditions.[28] The exact details of the mathematical algorithms to derive MBV and MBF are beyond the scope of this chapter. But, to summarize, MBV was derived from the ratio of the area under the myocardial TAC and the area under the left ventricular blood pool TAC. MBF was calculated by multiplying MBV by the mean transit time and then applying a volume correction. Using this volume correction, they showed a good correlation between EBT derived and microsphere derived MBF measurements up to 3.5–4.0 ml/g/min (r = 0.82). Applying this method to healthy volunteers, they confirmed they could measure MBF in the range of normal coronary flow reserve of 2.8.

EBT studies demonstrated the feasibility of performing MPI using X-ray computed tomography. EBT scanning systems were designed with cardiac imaging in mind and, without the physical limitations of a rotating gantry, were capable of providing cardiac images with excellent temporal resolution (33–100 msec). However, the cost of these systems, limited spatial resolution in the z-axis, and recent improvements in MDCT scanner technology, have shifted cardiac CT imaging to MDCT scanning systems.

4 MULTIDETECTOR COMPUTED TOMOGRAPHY MYOCARDIAL PERFUSION IMAGING

The current generation of MDCT scanners can image the entire heart in as little as 5–10 seconds with spatial resolution as low as 350 μm³. These technologic improvements have made MDCT coronary angiography for the non-invasive evaluation of coronary stenoses and atherosclerotic plaque possible. However, as previously noted, the technology falls short of determining the functional significance of coronary stenoses. It is important to point out that MDCT scanners differ from EBT. While MDCT scanners have improved spatial resolution, temporal resolution is slower due the physical limits of a rotating gantry that contains the X-ray source and a set of detectors. Depending on scanner manufacturer and the reconstruction algorithm used (e.g. half-scan vs. segmental reconstruction), images of the heart can be acquired with an effective temporal resolution of approximately 80–200 msec. These scanners can be programmed in either helical mode, commonly used for coronary angiography, or dynamic mode and we will discuss the prospects for CT perfusion imaging using each image acquisition mode.

4.1 Dynamic MDCT perfusion imaging

Similar to EBT, 64 slice CT systems can be programmed to image in dynamic mode. In this mode, the subject lies on a stationary table and the detectors are aligned over a portion of the heart in the axial plane. It is important to note that not all 64 slice CT scanners actually have 64 detectors and, depending on the manufacturer, detector widths vary from 0.5 mm to 0.625 mm. Therefore 64 detector scanners with 0.5 mm or 0.625 mm detectors have 32 mm and 40 mm coverage in the z-axis, respectively. Even more complicated are 64 slice scanners that contain 32 detectors with a 0.6 mm detector width flanked on each side by 4 detectors with a 1.2 mm width for a total coverage of 28.8 mm coverage in the z-axis. What this means is that dynamic imaging with today's generation of scanners can only cover approximately 2 to 4 cm of the heart, thus limiting this method of perfusion imaging. This will change as manufacturers push for whole heart coverage, for example with 256 detector CT.[29,30]

Dynamic MDCT has been used in the preclinical setting of acute non-reperfused MI. Mahnken et al. studied several parameters of time-attenuation curves obtained with 16 slice MDCT in a porcine model of MI. When comparing infarcted and normal myocardium, they found significant differences in the maximum attenuation density, time to maximal attenuation density and upslopes of the myocardial time attenuation curves. When comparing the size of the hypoperfused area noted on MR and MDCT dynamic imaging to TTC, the mean difference was −1.4% and 0.7% respectively.[31]

Recently, a comparison between dynamic MDCT and EBT was published by Daghini et al.[32] Time-attenuation curves was obtained in 12 pigs at rest and during adenosine infusion using the two scanning systems, EBT and MDCT. They measured two indices of endothelial function and microvascular perfusion: microvascular permeability-surface area (MPSP) and fractional vascular volume (FVV) using both indicator-dilution and Patlak models. They showed that dynamic MDCT could accurately assess MPSP and FVV using the Patlak method, compared with EBT. However, using the indicator dilution method, which requires a gamma variate function be fitted to the time-attenuation curve, measurements of MPSP and FVV were not well correlated between EBT and MDCT. The authors concluded that the lower temporal resolution of MDCT contributes more noise to the TACs, making gamma variate curve fitting error prone. We have had the same experience in our laboratory trying to apply gamma variate fit functions to dynamic MDCT time-attenuation data (unpublished data). Patlak plot analyses, however, do not require curve fitting and instead use fewer points during the upslope of the TACs and then applies a linear fit to the data that may cancel out some of the noise found in the MDCT data.

Studies from our laboratory have studied dynamic MDCT in a canine model of moderate to severe coronary stenosis. Similar to the previous described study, we performed dynamic imaging of a portion of the LV and constructed TACs for the LV blood pool and the myocardium (Figure 33.1 and Figure 33.4).[33] We applied several semi-quantitative and quantitative analysis methods, including upslope and model-based deconvolution methods. We showed a strong correlation between the ratio of the myocardial upslope and LV upslope and MBF ($R^2 = 0.92$). Absolute quantification of MBF derived from the model-based deconvolution analysis also strongly correlated with microspheres ($R^2 = 0.90$). Furthermore, the model-based deconvolution approach provided measurements of MPSP and MBV.

Dynamic MDCT perfusion imaging is currently limited due to restricted cardiac coverage in the z axis. This will change with the introduction of scanners with full cardiac coverage. Additionally, the radiation dose required for serial imaging of only a portion of left ventricle is relatively high. This will be overcome by protocols capable of prospective ECG-gating that will limit the exposure to just the phase of the R-R interval that is of interest. Dynamic MDCT, like EBT, has the potential for the evaluation of myocardial perfusion and microvascular function and could be used to determine the early microvascular changes in

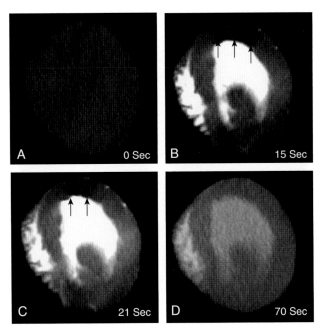

Figure 33.4 Adenosine stress dynamic multidetector computed tomography (d-MDCT) imaging of the mid left ventricle in a canine model of left anterior descending artery stenosis. Panels A–D demonstrate d-MDCT at 0, 15, 21, and 70 seconds. Note the area of hypoenhancement (arrows) in the anterior myocardial wall as contrast first arrives in the left ventricle (panel B and panel C). No visually significant differences are noted at the end of imaging (Panel D). (George RT et al. Invest Radiol; In Press)

patients with atherosclerosis, diabetes, hypercholesterolemia, hypertension, etc.[34]

4.2 Helical MDCT perfusion imaging

Currently, non-invasive coronary angiography is achieved with an MDCT scanner imaging in helical mode. Helical CT is performed with the scanner table moving the patient through a rotating gantry at a set rate. Image data is acquired as the X-ray source and detectors move around the patients in spiral fashion (Figure 33.5). In this mode, the entire heart is imaged over 5 to 10 heartbeats. This is fundamentally different from dynamic CT imaging since, in helical mode, different parts of the heart are imaged at different times during the relative peak of coronary arterial contrast enhancement. Therefore, the traditional time-attenuation curves imaged from dynamic CT are not acquired and the absolute quantification of MBF would pose great difficulty. However, there is evidence that important semi-quantitative metrics of myocardial perfusion can be extracted from helical MDCT imaging protocols.

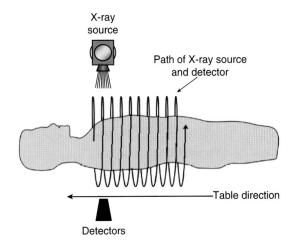

Figure 33.5 Schematic demonstrating helical multidetector computed tomography imaging. The patient lies on a table between an X-ray source and a set of detectors. The table moves the patient in the direction shown while the gantry rotates the X-ray source and detectors about the patient. The X-ray source and detectors image the patient in spiral fashion as shown.

Myocardial viability imaging will be extensively covered elsewhere (Chapter 32). There is evidence that decreased MBF and microvascular obstruction associated with myocardial infarction can be detected with helical MDCT. Using 16 slice MDCT, Hoffman et al. demonstrated in a porcine model of acute non-reperfused myocardial infarction (MI) that hypoenhanced regions of myocardium represent areas of decreased perfusion secondary to an occluded coronary artery during the first pass circulation of contrast.[35] Lardo et al. studied MDCT perfusion imaging in a canine model of acute occlusion and reperfusion MI.[36] They also noted that hypoenhanced areas representing decreased perfusion following MI could be detected within the infarcted territory. During delayed enhanced imaging, persisting areas of hypoenhancement were shown to represent areas of microvascular obstruction by thioflavin S staining and they confirmed the absence of blood flow in these areas using microsphere injections. Similar findings of hypoenhancement have been confirmed in patients with a history of recent MI and chronic myocardial scar (Figure 33.6).[37–39]

As noted above, there is great interest in combining MDCT angiography with MPI. Since, percent diameter stenosis determined from MDCT angiography has a poor positive predictive value for predicting ischemia when compared to SPECT MPI.[13–15] Preclinical evidence from our laboratory has demonstrated that myocardial perfusion information can be extracted from MDCT coronary angiography protocols when performed during maximal vasodilation.[40] Using a canine model of left anterior

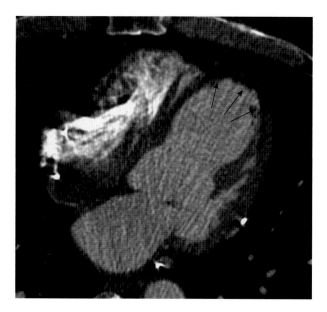

Figure 33.6 First-pass MDCT imaging in a patient with a chronically occluded left anterior descending artery. Note the hypoenhancement in the anterior/apical wall as a result of reduced perfusion in this territory (George RT et al. J Invasive Cardiology, 2005;17C:15–17).

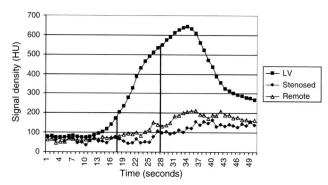

Figure 33.7 Time-attenuation curves in a canine model of left anterior descending artery stenosis imaged by dynamic MDCT during the infusion of adenosine and intravenous iodinated contrast (2.5 ml/sec). Myocardial curves were measured from the anterior myocardial wall (stenosed) and the inferior myocardial wall (remote). Vertical lines illustrate the period that helical MDCT scanning took place during this study. Helical scanning was triggered when bolus tracking detected a signal density of 180 HU in the ascending aorta (HU = Hounsfield units, George RT et al. J Am Coll Cardiol 2006; 48(1): 153–60).

descending artery stenosis, we performed MDCT imaging towards the end of a 5 minute infusion of adenosine (0.14 mg/kg/min). The imaging protocol was modeled after our clinical CT angiography protocol. This study aimed to capture myocardial perfusion data using a helical acquisition during early first-pass circulation of contrast (Figure 33.7). When comparing the attenuation density from stenosed and non-stenosed territories, there were significant differences seen in each experiment both visually and quantitatively (Figure 33.8). Furthermore, when normalizing the myocardial attenuation densities to the LV blood pool attenuation density, there was a semiquantitative relationship between the signal density ratio and MBF. This relationship was curvilinear and MDCT measurements underestimated blood flow at higher flows above 6 ml/g/min. This study, for the first time, showed that relative differences in myocardial perfusion could be measured using protocols designed for MDCT angiography when performed during adenosine infusion.

Based on the results of this study, we have translated this method into an ongoing clinical study of patients at high risk for coronary artery disease. Patients with a history of an abnormal SPECT myocardial perfusion study undergo MDCT angiography during adenosine infusion prior to invasive angiography. Pre-scan beta-blockers are used to blunt the tachycardia caused by adenosine. Preliminary results have documented that CT perfusion imaging is more

sensitive and specific compared with SPECT for identifying abnormal perfusion in territories supplied by a significantly stenosed artery.[41] Furthermore, the high spatial resolution of MDCT allows for the identification transmural differences in myocardial perfusion. Specifically, subendocardial perfusion deficits are visually evident and can be quantified in territories with stenoses >50% on invasive coronary angiography. Advances in CT perfusion software allow for the quantification of perfusion differences and their display on 17-segment polar maps (Figure 33.9).[42] The measurement

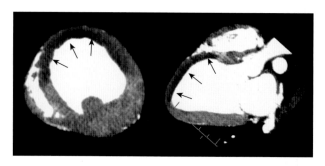

Figure 33.8 Results from helical MDCT perfusion imaging in a canine model of left anterior descending artery coronary stenosis. Shown on the left is a mid ventricular slice in the axial plane showing a perfusion deficit (arrows) in the anteroseptal, anterior, and anterolateral myocardial territories. To the right is a multi-planar reconstruction showing the extent of the perfusion deficit (arrows) extending from the anteroseptal and anterior walls to the apex (George RT et al. J Am Coll Cardiol 2006; 48(1):153–60).

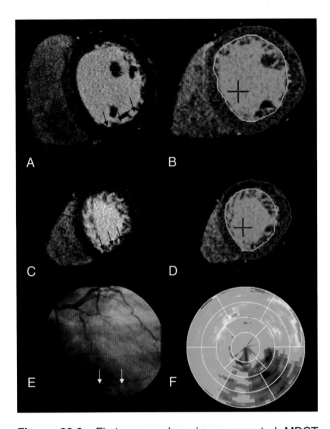

Figure 33.9 First-pass, adenosine augmented MDCT myocardial perfusion imaging in a patient referred for invasive angiography after single photon emission computed tomography showed a fixed perfusion deficit in the inferior and inferolateral territories. Panels A and C demonstrate an inferior and inferolateral subendocardial perfusion deficit in the mid and distal left ventricle, respectively (arrows). Using semi-automated function/perfusion software, myocardium meeting the perfusion deficit signal density threshold of one standard deviation below the remote myocardial signal density is designated blue in panels B and D. Invasive angiography shows a chronically occluded distal right coronary artery with left to right collaterals filling the posterior descending (arrows) and posterolateral branches, panel E. Panel F, seventeen-segment polar plot of MDCT derived myocardial signal densities. Note the hypoperfused inferior and inferolateral regions displayed in blue. (J Am Coll Cardiol. 2006; 48(1): 153–60.)

of myocardial perfusion, when added to MDCT angiography protocols, could change the way we diagnose and manage coronary artery disease. In the setting of coronary calcifications, where blooming artifacts can cause the coronary arterial lumen to appear stenosed, CT perfusion imaging could act as a second lens to determine if perfusion to the myocardium is impacted. This would also assist in the assessment of coronary segments containing stents and determine if in-stent restenosis is impacting MBF. Ultimately, it would provide valuable functional information to determine if a stenosis of physiologic significance is

present and whether medical versus invasive therapies are indicated.

There are limitations of helical MDCT perfusion imaging that need to be overcome. Beam hardening artifacts can increase or decrease the externally recorded attenuation number in the myocardium. Care needs to be taken to identify these artifacts and take them into consideration. One concern is the beam hardening that occurs due to iodinated contrast in the LV cavity itself. This can lower the attenuation number of the subendocardial layer of myocardium immediately adjacent to the LV cavity. Adenosine mediated tachycardia is also of concern; however, with the use of beta-blockers, most patients can be imaged at an acceptable heart rate. The use of beta-blockers during vasodilatory stress testing has raised the concern that their use could mask the identification of ischemia in radionuclide myocardial perfusion studies.[43,44] In our experience, this does not seem to be an issue with helical MDCT perfusion imaging.[40]

5 FUTURE DIRECTIONS

The evaluation of myocardial perfusion by X-ray computed tomography shows great promise. There are technological improvements in scanner systems and software that are on the horizon that could bring MDCT perfusion imaging closer to reality.

One strategy that looks promising is 256 detector computed tomography. With 256 detectors covering 12.8 cm of the chest in the z-axis, whole heart imaging can be acquired in as little as one heart beat. Lower radiation and contrast doses make the acquisition of rest and stress imaging feasible. Additionally, scanners that cover the entire heart with one rotation of the gantry will have the potential for dynamic CT perfusion imaging of the entire LV myocardium. This will allow for the quantification of MBF for the entire heart.

Another strategy using current 64 slice MDCT scanners that may show promise is shuttle imaging of the heart. This approach could perform dynamic imaging on portions of the heart every 2 heart beats by moving the scanner table back and forth to image the basal and distal LV multiple times during first-pass contrast enhancement. And yet another approach aimed at improved temporal resolution with dual source CT may allow helical MDCT perfusion imaging to be performed at the higher heart rates sometimes encountered in patients receiving coronary vasodilators such as adenosine.

6 CONCLUSIONS

Based on previous CT perfusion work with EBT and the DSR, it has been established that MPI can be performed using iodinated contrast as an indicator and X-ray computed tomography as a detection system. The newer generation of 64 slice MDCT scanners with unsurpassed spatial resolution is revolutionizing the non-invasive diagnosis of CAD. In the future, the combination of non-invasive coronary angiography and MDCT perfusion imaging could solidify X-ray computed tomography as the test of choice for the non-invasive diagnosis of atherosclerosis and its physiologic impact on myocardial perfusion.

REFERENCES

1. Leber AW, Knez A, von Ziegler F et al. Quantification of obstructive and nonobstructive coronary lesions by 64-slice computed tomography: a comparative study with quantitative coronary angiography and intravascular ultrasound. J Am Coll Cardiol 2005; 46(1): 147–54.
2. Leschka S, Alkadhi H, Plass A et al. Accuracy of MSCT coronary angiography with 64-slice technology: first experience. Eur Heart J 2005; 26(15): 1482–7.
3. Mollet NR, Cademartiri F, Nieman K et al. Multislice spiral computed tomography coronary angiography in patients with stable angina pectoris. J Am Coll Cardiol 2004; 43(12): 2265–70.
4. Raff GL, Gallagher MJ, O'Neill WW, Goldstein JA. Diagnostic accuracy of noninvasive coronary angiography using 64-slice spiral computed tomography. J Am Coll Cardiol 2005; 46(3): 552–7.
5. Ropers D, Pohle FK, Kuettner A et al. Diagnostic accuracy of noninvasive coronary angiography in patients after bypass surgery using 64-slice spiral computed tomography with 330-ms gantry rotation. Circulation 2006; 114(22): 2334–41; quiz.
6. Cordeiro MA, Miller JM, Schmidt A et al. Non-invasive half millimetre 32 detector row computed tomography angiography accurately excludes significant stenoses in patients with advanced coronary artery disease and high calcium scores. Heart 2006; 92(5): 589–97.
7. Gaspar T, Halon DA, Lewis BS et al. Diagnosis of coronary in-stent restenosis with multidetector row spiral computed tomography. J Am Coll Cardiol 2005; 46(8): 1573–9.
8. Ehara M, Kawai M, Surmely JF et al. Diagnostic accuracy of coronary in-stent restenosis using 64-slice computed tomography: comparison with invasive coronary angiography. J Am Coll Cardiol 2007; 49(9): 951–9.
9. Uren NG, Melin JA, De Bruyne B et al. Relation between myocardial blood flow and the severity of coronary-artery stenosis. N Engl J Med 1994; 330(25): 1782–8.
10. White CW, Wright CB, Doty DB et al. Does visual interpretation of the coronary arteriogram predict the physiologic importance of a coronary stenosis? N Engl J Med 1984; 310(13): 819–24.
11. Hachamovitch R, Hayes SW, Friedman JD, Cohen I, Berman DS. Comparison of the short-term survival benefit associated with revascularization compared with medical therapy in patients with no prior coronary artery disease undergoing stress myocardial perfusion single photon emission computed tomography. Circulation 2003; 107(23): 2900–7.
12. Iskandrian AS, Chae SC, Heo J et al. Independent and incremental prognostic value of exercise single-photon emission computed tomographic (SPECT) thallium imaging in coronary artery disease. J Am Coll Cardiol 1993; 22(3): 665–70.
13. Schuijf JD, Wijns W, Jukema JW et al. Relationship between noninvasive coronary angiography with multi-slice computed tomography and myocardial perfusion imaging. J Am Coll Cardiol 2006; 48(12): 2508–14.
14. Hacker M, Jakobs T, Matthiesen F et al. Comparison of spiral multidetector CT angiography and myocardial perfusion imaging in the noninvasive detection of functionally relevant coronary artery lesions: first clinical experiences. J Nucl Med 2005; 46(8): 1294–300.
15. Rispler S, Keidar Z, Ghersin E et al. Integrated single-photon emission computed tomography and computed tomography coronary angiography for the assessment of hemodynamically significant coronary artery lesions. J Am Coll Cardiol 2007; 49(10): 1059–67.
16. Bateman TM, Maddahi J, Gray RJ et al. Diffuse slow washout of myocardial thallium-201: a new scintigraphic indicator of extensive coronary artery disease. J Am Coll Cardiol 1984; 4(1): 55–64.
17. Hamilton WF, Moore JW, Kinsman JM, Spurling RG. Studies on the circulation. IV. Further analysis of the injection method and of changes in hemodynamics under physiological and pathological conditions. Am J Physiol 1932; 99: 534.
18. Rumberger JA, Bell MR. Measurement of myocardial perfusion and cardiac output using intravenous injection methods by ultrafast (cine) computed tomography. Invest Radiol 1992; 27 Suppl 2: S40–6.
19. Rumberger JA, Feiring AJ, Lipton MJ et al. Use of ultrafast computed tomography to quantitate regional myocardial perfusion: a preliminary report. J Am Coll Cardiol 1987; 9(1): 59–69.
20. Newhouse JH, Murphy RX Jr. Tissue distribution of soluble contrast: effect of dose variation and changes with time. AJR Am J Roentgenol 1981; 136(3): 463–7.
21. Newhouse JH. Fluid compartment distribution of intravenous iothalamate in the dog. Invest Radiol 1977; 12(4): 364–7.
22. Canty JM Jr., Judd RM, Brody AS, Klocke FJ. First-pass entry of nonionic contrast agent into the myocardial extravascular space. Effects on radiographic estimates of transit time and blood volume. Circulation 1991; 84(5): 2071–8.
23. George RT, Jerosch-Herold M, Silva C, Lima JAC, Lardo AC. Absolute Quantification of Myocardial Blood Flow Using Dynamic Multidetector (64 Slice) Computed Tomography. Circulation 2006; 114: Supplement II.
24. Axel L. Tissue mean transit time from dynamic computed tomography by a simple deconvolution technique. Invest Radiol 1983; 18(1): 94–9.
25. Gould RG, Lipton MJ, McNamara MT et al. Measurement of regional myocardial blood flow in dogs by ultrafast CT. Invest Radiol 1988; 23(5): 348–53.

26. Wolfkiel CJ, Ferguson JL, Chomka EV et al. Measurement of myocardial blood flow by ultrafast computed tomography. Circulation 1987; 76(6): 1262–73.

27. Wang TWX, Chung N et al. Myocardial Blood Flow Estimated by Synchronous Multislice, High-Speed Computed Tomography. IEEE Trans Med Imaging 1989; 8: 70–7.

28. Bell MR, Lerman LO, Rumberger JA. Validation of minimally invasive measurement of myocardial perfusion using electron beam computed tomography and application in human volunteers. Heart 1999; 81(6): 628–35.

29. Mori S, Kondo C, Suzuki N et al. Volumetric coronary angiography using the 256-detector row computed tomography scanner: comparison in vivo and in vitro with porcine models. Acta Radiol 2006; 47(2): 186–91.

30. Kondo C, Mori S, Endo M et al. Real-time volumetric imaging of human heart without electrocardiographic gating by 256-detector row computed tomography: initial experience. J Comput Assist Tomogr 2005; 29(5): 694–8.

31. Mahnken AH, Bruners P, Katoh M et al. Dynamic multi-section CT imaging in acute myocardial infarction: preliminary animal experience. Eur Radiol 2006; 16(3): 746–52.

32. Daghini E, Primak AN, Chade AR et al. Evaluation of Porcine Myocardial Microvascular Permeability and Fractional Vascular Volume Using 64-Slice Helical Computed Tomography (CT). Invest Radiol 2007; 42(5): 274–82.

33. George RT, Jerosch-Herold M, Silva C et al. Quantification of myocardial perfusion using dynamic 64 detector computed tomography. Invest Radiol 2007; In Press.

34. Mohlenkamp S, Lerman LO, Lerman A et al. Minimally invasive evaluation of coronary microvascular function by electron beam computed tomography. Circulation 2000; 102(19): 2411–6.

35. Hoffmann U, Millea R, Enzweiler C et al. Acute myocardial infarction: contrast-enhanced multi-detector row CT in a porcine model. Radiology 2004; 231(3): 697–701.

36. Lardo AC, Cordeiro MA, Silva C et al. Contrast-enhanced multidetector computed tomography viability imaging after myocardial infarction: characterization of myocyte death, microvascular obstruction, and chronic scar. Circulation 2006; 113(3): 394–404.

37. Gerber BL, Belge B, Legros GJ et al. Characterization of acute and chronic myocardial infarcts by multidetector computed tomography: comparison with contrast-enhanced magnetic resonance. Circulation 2006; 113(6): 823–33.

38. Mahnken AH, Koos R, Katoh M et al. Assessment of myocardial viability in reperfused acute myocardial infarction using 16-slice computed tomography in comparison to magnetic resonance imaging. J Am Coll Cardiol 2005; 45(12): 2042–7.

39. George RT, Lardo AC, Lima JA. Multidetector computed tomography for viability and perfusion imaging. The J Invasive Cardiol 2005; Volume 17, Supplement C: 15–7.

40. George RT, Silva C, Cordeiro MA et al. Multidetector computed tomography myocardial perfusion imaging during adenosine stress. J Am Coll Cardiol 2006; 48(1): 153–60.

41. George RT, Resar J, Silva C et al. Combined Computed Tomography Coronary Angiography and Perfusion Imaging Accurately Detects the Physiological Significance of Coronary Stenoses in Patients with Chest Pain. Circulation 2006: 114: (Supplement) II–691.

42. George RT, Lardo AC, Silva C et al. Subendocardial perfusion deficits predict the functional significance of coronary stenoses during adenosine stress multidetector computed tomography in patients with chest pain. J Am Coll Cardiol 2007; 49: (Supplement A) 161A.

43. Bottcher M, Czernin J, Sun K, Phelps ME, Schelbert HR. Effect of beta 1 adrenergic receptor blockade on myocardial blood flow and vasodilatory capacity. J Nucl Med 1997; 38(3): 442–6.

44. Koepfli P, Wyss CA, Namdar M et al. Beta-adrenergic blockade and myocardial perfusion in coronary artery disease: differential effects in stenotic versus remote myocardial segments. J Nucl Med 2004; 45(10): 1626–31.

34

Dual-Energy Computed Tomography

Bernhard Schmidt and Cynthia McCollough

I BASIC PRINCIPLES OF DUAL ENERGY IMAGING

In 1895, Wilhelm Conrad Röntgen discovered X-rays when performing measurements with a cathode ray tube. Accidentally, he noticed that these rays – till then unknown – were able to pass though matter. Immediately, the benefit for medical care was clear – the ability to look into the human body without a dangerous surgery.

One of the earliest X-ray images is shown in Figure 34.1. The anatomy of the bones is clearly visible. In addition to that, one observes that bones cause a higher attenuation than the surrounding tissue. However, when ignoring the anatomical information and only looking at gray scale values, one also sees that it is difficult – only from the gray scale values – to differentiate between the ring around the finger and the bones.

Over the years, X-ray tubes, radiographic films and other components of X-ray equipment for radiography were improved so that better images at a lower dose were possible. Nevertheless, two limitations were not overcome: the superposition of anatomical structures and the inability to differentiate materials with the same attenuation but different chemical compositions.

Godfrey Newbold Hounsfield performed the first measurements with a computed tomographic (CT) system in 1968. This revolutionary acquisition method solved the problem of superposition of structures. For the first time, images of the brain were possible without the interference of overlaying

bony structures. However, even for CT images, the second limitation remained: tissues of different chemical composition appeared the same in CT images, having the same or similar Hounsfield-value (CT number). This makes the differentiation and classification of tissue types challenging. Classical examples are the differentiation between calcified plaques and iodinated blood or hyper-dense and contrast enhanced lesions.

The reason for this ambiguity is that the measured and displayed CT numbers are related to the **linear** attenuation coefficient $\mu(E)$ of the respective volume element (voxel). However, $\mu(E)$ is not specific for any given material; it is determined by the effective atomic number Z and mass density ρ of the material. The **mass** attenuation coefficient μ / ρ, however, is a function only of the X-ray energy E and the material atomic number Z. Hence, the mass attenuation coefficient μ / ρ is determined only by the elemental composition of a tissue (i.e., the effective atomic number Z of the tissue) irregardless of the mass density ρ.[6] The relationship between these two attenuation coefficients is given in Equation 1.

$$\mu(E) = \left(\frac{\mu}{\rho}\right)(E, Z) \cdot \rho \qquad (1)$$

Thus, for different values of μ / ρ, and therefore different materials, the same $\mu(E)$ can be measured, depending on the value of the mass density ρ (Figure 34.2).

Besides the issue of differentiation and classification, the ambiguity of CT numbers hampers the reliability of

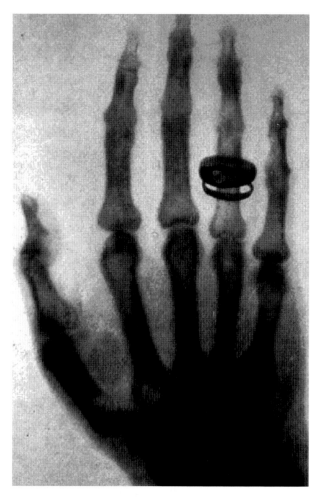

Figure 34.1   X-ray picture (radiograph) taken by Wilhelm Röntgen.

quantitative measurements. For example, in the case of the assessment of vertebral bone mineral density, the accuracy is limited mainly by unknown marrow and fat concentrations in trabecular bone.[1,2] Since both vary in individuals and with age and health, generic corrections can reduce the error only on population averages[1,3,4] as they do not increase accuracy on an individual basis. Even for the more seemingly straight-forward task of quantitating iodine concentration, the accuracy of the measured values is limited by the presence of other tissue types. For example, when determining the amount of iodine enhancement of a soft tissue lesion within some region of interest (ROI) in that lesion, the measured mean CT number will reflect not only the enhancement due to iodine, but also the underlying tissue.

To overcome this limitation, additional information is required. Referring to the schematic illustration in Figure 34.2, one can see that additional information can be obtained by a second measurement at another energy. Assuming that mono-energetic X-ray photons are used, for example at about 100 keV, the same linear attenuation coefficients are obtained for bone and iodine. However, data acquired at an energy around 40 keV allows the differentiation of the two materials. Hence, by looking at the attenuation of a material at two different energies, materials such as bone and iodine can be differentiated.

Although medical X-ray tubes generate a polychromatic spectra of x-ray quanta (that is, many energies of photons are produced), the general principle remains valid. Attenuation values are acquired with different energy spectra and the changes in attenuation between the two spectra provide the needed information to differentiate and classify tissue type.

In conventional projection X-ray imaging, the principles of dual energy imaging are well known and in routine clinical use. The most widespread application is for bone densitometry. Here Dual Energy X-ray Absorptiometry (DEXA) is used for improved diagnosis and monitoring of osteoporosis by determining the bone mineral density from the projection images acquired at different energies.

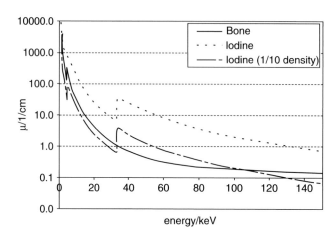

Figure 34.2   Linear attenuation coefficients for bone (assuming ρ = 1g/cm³), iodine (assuming ρ = 1g/cm³) and iodine with lower density (assuming ρ = 0.1g/cm³). Since the linear attenuation coefficient is determined by the mass attenuation coefficient and the density, the same values for $\mu(E)$ can be obtained although the materials are different.

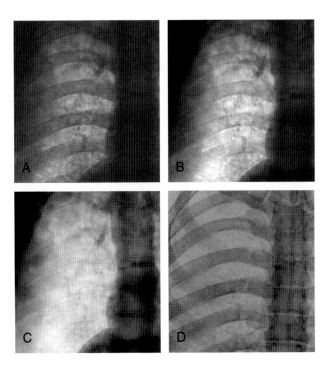

Figure 34.3 Chest radiograph acquired using a low (a) and high (b) energy spectrum (tube potential). With dual energy techniques, post processed 'soft tissue' (c) and 'bone' (d) images can be calculated.

In a similar but not quantitative manner, chest radiographs can be acquired with dual energy methods (Figure 34.3 a–d). Utilizing the information from the high and the low energy image, a bone image can be calculated which allows the assessment of bony structures and calcifications. Alternatively, the bone image can be suppressed, so that a soft tissue image is generated which improves the visualization of structures previously hidden by bony anatomy.

2 PROJECTION-BASED TWO-MATERIAL DECOMPOSITION FOR CT

2.1 Previous work

The first investigations of dual energy methods for CT were made by Alvarez and Macovski in 1976.[5,6] They demonstrated that, using a conventional X-ray source having a broad energy spectrum, one can still separate the attenuation coefficient into the contributions from the photoelectric effect and Compton scattering. Thereafter, several applications were reported utilizing dual energy CT, focusing primarily on lung, liver and tissue characterization.[7–12] However, all of the approaches were limited in some manner and not able to be used routinely in clinical practice. The primary limitation was that data for

the different tube voltages were acquired at two different times. Patient motion that occurred between the two acquisitions severely degraded the quality of the resultant images.

In the 1980s, it was possible to acquire dual energy data nearly simultaneously using a modified commercial CT system (Siemens DR scanner).[13] During the rotation of the tube-detector pair, the tube voltage was switched quickly for each detector reading between the high and low settings so that two sets of raw data (projections) were acquired nearly simultaneously at two different tube voltages. After phantom and initial clinical studies, Siemens Medical Solutions was the first company to offer a dual energy application as a commercial CT product. Specifically, bone densitometry measurements were made using the above mentioned voltage switching technique.

2.2 Principle and applications

The basic assumption of two material decomposition, or basis material decomposition, is that the mass attenuation coefficient μ/ρ of all materials can be expressed with sufficient accuracy as a linear combination of the photoelectric and Compton attenuation coefficients. As a consequence, μ/ρ of any material can be expressed as a linear combination of μ/ρ of two basis materials, where both materials differ in their photoelectric and Compton characteristics. In CT, the line integrals P of the attenuation of the object are measured. Hence, for each ray from the X-ray source to the respective detector elements, P can be expressed as

$$P(E) = \left(\frac{\mu}{\rho}\right)_1 (E) \cdot \rho_1 \cdot d_1 + \left(\frac{\mu}{\rho}\right)_2 (E) \cdot \rho_2 \cdot d_2 \qquad (2)$$

whereas $\rho_i \cdot d_i$ represents the area density in g/cm^2 of base material i. Measuring P at two different tube voltages and solving Equation 2 for the area densities allows for the characterization of the two materials.[5,6]

A practical implementation is illustrated in Figure 34.4. Using simulated data for the two different spectra, line integrals P for different pairs of thicknesses d of soft tissue and bone are calculated. After inverting the data, thicknesses for water and bone can be obtained from the line integral measurements at the two different spectra. Those data can now be used, for example, to generate pseudo monochromatic raw data. Depending on the values selected for the attenuation coefficients μ_W and μ_B, either pseudo monochromatic images (i.e., reduced beam hardening) or material selective images can be reconstructed (Figures 34.5–34.6).

Simulation for two different spectra:

low: $(d_W, d_B) \rightarrow P_1(d_W, d_B)$
low: $(d_W, d_B) \rightarrow P_1(d_W, d_B)$

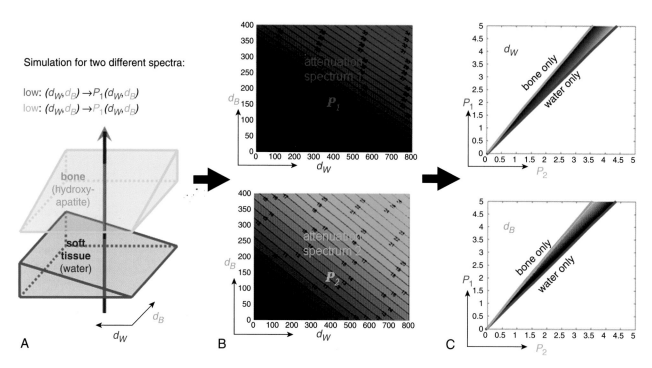

A   B   C

Figure 34.4   Basic principle of raw data-based two material decompositions: (a) Simulation of the polychromatic line integral P for low and high energy spectra. Values for P are simulated for multiple combinations of different thicknesses of water d_W and bone d_B. (b) 2D-matrixes for the two different spectra. (c) By inverting the results shown in (b), measured P_1 and P_2 values can be translated into thickness of water d_W and bone d_B. For practical purpose data should be available as pairwise lookup table.[18]

2.3 Limitations

The biggest challenge of projection data based methods is data consistency between the low and high energy data. Any kind of motion, change in contrast agent concentration, or internal pulsation will lead to severe artifacts in the reconstructed dual energy data. Rapid voltage switching between the different readings addresses this limitation. However,

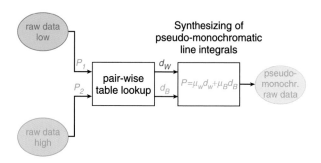

Figure 34.5   Using a pair-wise lookup table, measured raw (projection) data are converted into thicknesses of water and bone. By selecting μ_W and μ_B at a certain energy, pseudo monochromatic raw data are calculated and a pseudo monochromatic image can be generated.

the tube current can not be adapted in the same rapid manner to deliver comparable photon flux in both datasets. Hence, there is increased noise in the low voltage dataset. For applications like bone densitometry, which do not demand a low noise level, voltage switching is an option. However, for most other applications, the difference in noise between the two data sets remains a limiting factor.

Apart from switching the tube voltage, dual energy acquisitions are conceivable with appropriate alternate detector designs. So-called 'sandwich' detectors have two layers of detector elements. These detectors are able to provide dual energy data by detecting photons with lower energies in the upper detector layer and photons with higher energies in the lower detector layer. However, the technique suffers from the same limitation as the voltage switching. The low energy data are noisier than the high energy data.

A robust solution to this limitation is the use of energy sensitive detectors. These detectors are able to amplify the signal contribution of the lower part of the X-ray spectrum, resulting in a similar noise level for the low and high energy data sets. Although energy sensitive detectors are currently available, they are not yet able to deal with the photon flux used in CT imaging.

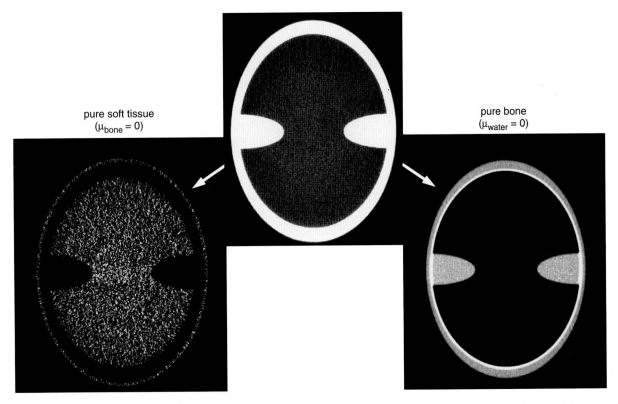

pure soft tissue
($\mu_{bone} = 0$)

pure bone
($\mu_{water} = 0$)

Figure 34.6 Application of raw data-based methods: From a dual-energy CT image dataset, a pure bone and pure soft tissue image can be calculated.

3 NEW APPROACHES FOR DUAL ENERGY WITH DUAL SOURCE CT SYSTEMS

The technical issues discussed above have limited the clinical use of dual energy methods in CT imaging. Up to 2006, the only clinically used dual energy application in CT was for bone densitometry measurements on the Siemens SOMATOM DR CT system in the 1980s, which was realized by tube voltage switching. However, this application alone did not justify the additionally technical requirements and cost, so dual energy capabilities were not implemented on subsequent CT scanners. With the introduction of dual source CT in 2006, a new approach for dual energy CT became clinically feasible.

3.1 Technical implementation of dual-source CT

The technical design of a dual source CT system is shown in Figure 34.7. In contrast to a single source system, dual source CT systems have two separate tube/detector pairs that are mounted orthogonally on the rotating slip ring. This design provides the flexibility to adjust not only the tube voltage but also the tube current for both tube/detector pairs and allows simultaneous data acquisition. Although the raw projection data do not match identically because of the 90 degree offset between the detectors, reconstructed images – although measured at different tube positions – are acquired at exactly the same time. This is true for spiral or sequential scans and also for the gated scans used in cardiac examinations.

To utilize the advantages of the simultaneous acquisition of similar noise low and high energy data sets, one has to work with reconstructed image data and not with raw projection data. Therefore, images from both tube/detector pairs are reconstructed separately into two different image stacks. Image-based post processing then is used to extract the dual energy information (Figure 34.8).

3.2 Alternative acquisition approaches and their limitations

Apart from the dual source approach, also other acquisition approaches for image-based dual energy CT using single source systems have been proposed.[14] Approaches with two subsequent spiral acquisitions or two subsequent sequential scans have been reported. The latter can be realized in a

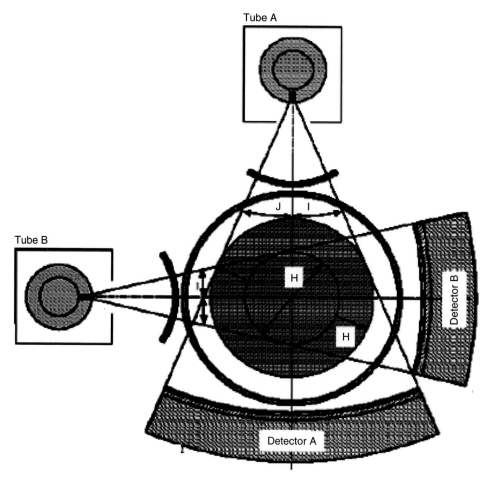

Figure 34.7   Schematic illustration of the geometry of a dual source CT system. In contrast to a single source system, dual source CT systems have two separate tube/detector pairs. This allows data at different tube voltages to be acquired at the same time. In cardiac dual energy mode, after half a rotation both systems have acquired enough data to reconstruct images at the different energies.

kind of 'step-and shoot' mode using partial (180° based) image reconstructions. During the first rotation, 180° of data are acquired with a high voltage setting. During the remaining portion of the rotation, the tube voltage is switched and then, during the next rotation, images are acquired with a low voltage setting. After incrementing the table, the procedure is repeated. For static anatomical structures without any contrast enhancement dynamics this acquisition technique appears feasible. However, for most patient scans, this prerequisite is not fulfilled. Motion, pulsation or changes in contrast agent concentration between both the acquisitions would lead to registration artifacts or false dual energy information. Acquisitions could be triggered to the cardiac cycle, but with the proposed rotation time of about one second, the scan time and temporal resolution would not be clinically acceptable.

3.3 Image based methods and three material decomposition

The simplest way to process dual energy data is by performing a weighted subtraction. The low voltage images (typically 80 kVp) are multiplied by a weighting factor and subtracted from the high voltage images (140 kVp) to obtain dual energy information. Similar to what is shown in Figure 34.3, bone can be suppressed or enhanced. In addition to this, weighted subtraction may allow discrimination between iron and calcium. In a feasibility study, McCollough et al.[15,16] have shown that using the dual energy subtraction method, iron (Fe) and calcium (Ca) can be differentiated. This indicates the possibility for differentiation between hemorrhagic and calcified plaques, which both appear bright in single energy CT images.

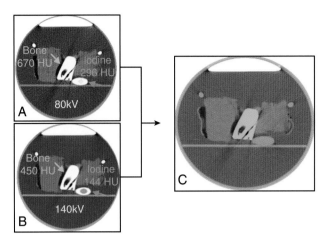

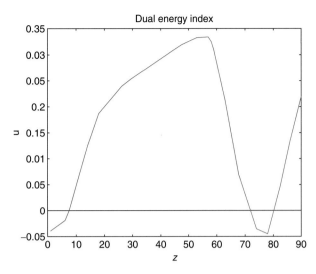

Figure 34.9 Dual energy index u for different atomic numbers Z. Up to $Z = 55$ or an equivalent effective atomic number of 55, u is monotonically increasing and unique.

Figure 34.8 Illustration of a dual energy image-based approach: Vessels filled with a mixture of saline and iodinated contrast media, soft tissue and bone were placed in a water tank. Using CT numbers alone, differentiation between the bones and the iodine-enhanced vessels is not possible. However, acquiring data at 80 kVp and 140 kVp provides the additional information necessary to differentiate the two materials. The CT numbers increase for iodine from 144 HU at 140 kV to 296 HU at 80 kV, which is nearly a factor of 2. However, the CT numbers for bone only increase from 450 HU at 140 kV to 670 HU at 80 kV. The differences in these enhancement ratios allows the discrimination between materials, which can be marked with color: Bone is colored green and iodine is colored orange. Alternative displays of the information might be a bone-only or iodine-only image.

Another, more sophisticated way to process dual energy information is by using the so-called dual energy index u.

$$u = \frac{CT_{low} - CT_{high}}{CT_{low} + CT_{high} + 2000\,HU} \qquad (3)$$

Processing data in this way allows the estimation of effective atomic mass and therefore chemical composition. By definition, u is independent of the density of the material and its value for water is zero. As shown in Figure 34.9, up to an atomic number of 55, the dual energy index allows the unique identifications of pure materials.

A third, more sophisticated and clinically oriented method to post-process images acquired at two different tube voltages uses a so-called three material decomposition approach.[17] The principle is illustrated in Figure 34.10. First, three adequate base-materials have to be selected, e.g. fat, tissue and iodine. Ideally, the three base-materials span a triangle in a plot of the CT number at one tube potential versus the CT number at the other tube potential. The typical CT numbers of the three materials are plotted on this low/high voltage diagram. Thereafter, corresponding CT

number pairs from the low/high voltage images are mapped onto the calibration diagram. Depending on their position in the diagram, the material or percent composition of a certain material is determined. By processing all the pixels of the low/high voltage image stacks, a material map is generated. For example, pure soft tissue images can be calculated by only displaying the contribution of fat and tissue, suppressing the iodine signal and creating a virtual non-contrast image set (Figure 34.11). Alternatively, bone can be suppressed and the iodine containing vascular structures displayed. This automatic bone removal allows CT angiographic applications in regions where complex bone anatomic previously interfered with the visualization of vascular anatomy.

3.4 Clinical examples and considerations for cardiovascular dual energy

With simultaneously acquired spiral dual-energy data sets and post-processing algorithms for bone and plaque removal, dual-energy CT can be expected to play a new and evolving role in routine clinical practice. The first clinical uses of dual-energy CT have already been reported,[17] and include both cardiovascular and soft tissue applications. One of the applications most likely to be widely adopted is that of direct CT angiography, whereby the dual energy algorithm identifies and removes bone in a 3-D CT angiographic data set, allowing direct visualization of iodinated vessels without the need for user intervention to remove overlying bony anatomy. In the case of dual-source CT, advanced bone

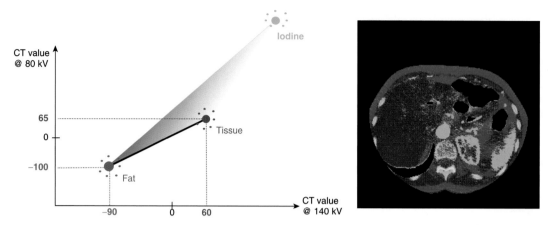

Figure 34.10 Principle of the three material decomposition: for each pixel, the CT numbers for the low and high voltage images are mapped into a low- vs. high-voltage CT number diagram. Predefined values for fat, tissue and iodine mark areas of known material types. The location of a certain pixel-pair in the resulting triangle determines the contribution of a certain material to a respective volume element. The parameters can be altered to differentiate between any three appropriately different materials, for example tissue, fat and calcium/bone or tissue, iodine and xenon.

removal algorithms are applied to the Tube A data to remove large bony anatomy in the periphery of the patient, beyond the 26-cm FOV of Tube B (see Figure 34.8).

The use of dual-energy information to perform automatic bone removal in the skull is shown in Figure 34.12. The bone removal algorithm identifies each voxel within

the data set as either bone, soft-tissue or iodine. This allows the user to toggle back and forth between the merged data set, containing all voxels, or the angiographic data set where bone voxels have been suppressed. This technique provides subtraction of bone, without operator intervention, in even complex anatomical regions such as the skull base.

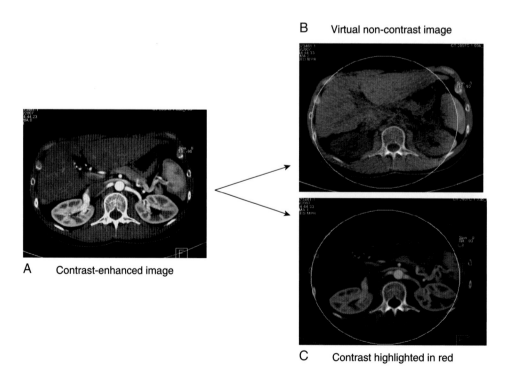

Figure 34.11 Three material decomposition: Although data are acquired after the iodinated contrast agent has been injected (a), the dual energy information can be used to produce images wherein the contrast agent is removed (b) or color coded and shown on top of the non-iodine image (c).

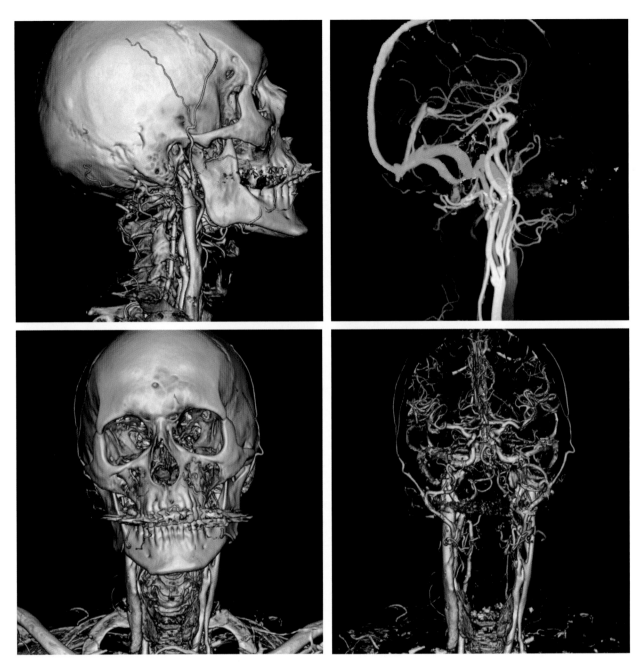

Figure 34.12   Dual-energy material decomposition allows for the classification of voxels in this 3-D cerebral angiogram as either bone or iodine. At left, both bone and vessles are shown, while at right, direct visualization of the cerebral vessels can be accomplished automatically by suppressing the bone voxels in the sagital MIP and volume rendered images. Courtesy of University Hospital of Munich, Grosshadern, Munich, Germany.

An extension of the bone removal algorithm is the removal of smaller hard plaques within the vessel lumen. Figures 34.13 and 34.14 provide examples of bone and plaque removal in the abdominal and peripheral vasculature, respectively. The removal of hard plaques may allow more rapid and clearer visualization of patent lumens in MIP projections.

In addition to removing bone to see iodine, the identification of iodine voxels allows the enhancement of iodinated areas. One potential application is for visualization of the perfused blood volume, also referred to as blood pool imaging. In Figure 34.15, this capability is used to identify areas with a deficit in the perfused blood volume of the lung. The pulmonary emboli in this patient result in a focal perfusion

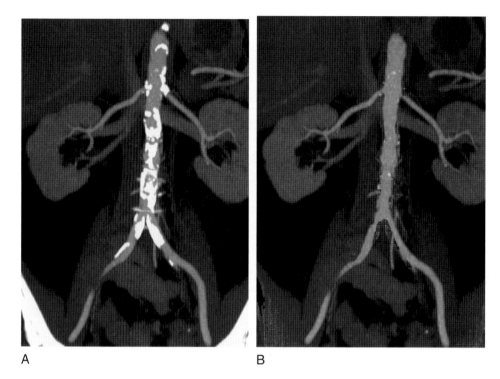

A   B

Figure 34.13   Coronal MIP images of a heavily calcified abdominal aorta. In (a), the calcified plaques make it difficult to appreciate the aortic lumen. In (b), after removal of aortic plaque, the lumen is much more clearly visualized.

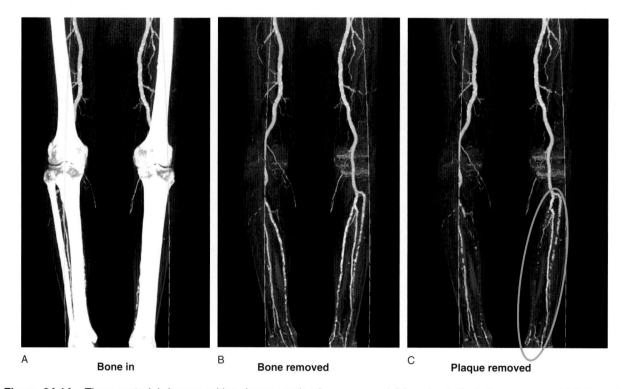

A   **Bone in**   B   **Bone removed**   C   **Plaque removed**

Figure 34.14   Three material decomposition demonstrating bone removal (b) and calcified plaque removal (c). Bone is detected and removed without manual editing. In (c), the detection of calcified plaques and the removal of corresponding voxels from the maximum intensity (MIP) image is shown. This allows for the quicker and easier assessment of lumen dimensions. After the plaque removal, one can better appreciate the total occlusion of the posterior tibial artery (circled).

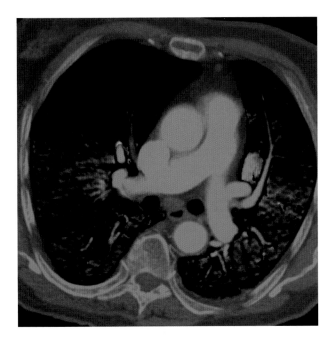

Figure 34.15 In the lung, dual energy processing is used to identify areas with a deficit in the perfused blood volume. In this example, a pulmonary emboli results in a focal perfusion deficit, shown as black. Only the lung tissue is color coded, allowing a hybrid display of morphological and perfused blood volume information. Courtesy of University Hospital of Munich, Grosshadern, Munich, Germany.

deficit, which is shown as black in the dual-energy image. This tool color-codes only the lung tissue, allowing a hybrid display where the morphological data of the vasculature is presented in the same image as the perfused blood volume information. Tissue outside of the 26 cm FOV of tube B can not be assessed with the perfused blood volume algorithm. It is important to note that this is not a time resolved perfusion image, requiring multiple scans over time, but rather a display of the iodine content of the lung at the time of the scan that reflects the amount of blood being supplied to the tissue. The radiation dose to the patient is the same as for a routine pulmonary emboli CT examination.

The presence of calcified plaque within a vessel creates artifactual elevation of the CT numbers in adjacent voxels, obscuring the dimension of the true lumen. Known as calcium blooming, this can result in an overestimation of the degree of stenosis, or so limits the reader's confidence in the luminal assessment that the exam is considered nondiagnostic in the region. The artificial increased brightness of CT values in adjacent voxels is often accompanied by an artificial decreased brightness in voxels somewhat further away from the plaque, often referred to as undershoot or ringing. These errors in CT numbers caused by calcified plaque are

relevant to all of vascular imaging, but are of particular significance in smaller vessels such as those of the neck, heart, and extremities.

The dual energy bone and plaque removal techniques discussed above can also be applied in retrospectively-gated cardiac imaging. In this case, Tube A and B are each used to acquire partial scan cardiac images at 165 ms temporal resolution at 140 and 80 kVp, respectively. Thus, temporal resolution is inferior to single-energy, dual-source CT (83 ms), but allows the acquisition of energy resolved information. Figure 34.16 shows a cardiac dual-energy CT angiogram acquired in a patient with a known proximal LAD calcification. In the volume rendered image, the calcified plaque is suppressed, providing visualization of the stenotic lumen. Because the dual-energy technique used here is based on reconstructed data at each tube potential, any calcium blooming present in the Tube A and B reconstructions will affect the bone-suppressed image. Investigations into methods to overcome significant calcium blooming effects are ongoing.

In summary, dual energy CT represents a new field of clinical and research CT imaging. The ability to differentiate material composition may allow an improved ability to visualize cardiovascular anatomy, as well as creating new clinical applications for the detection and diagnosis of cardiovascular disease.

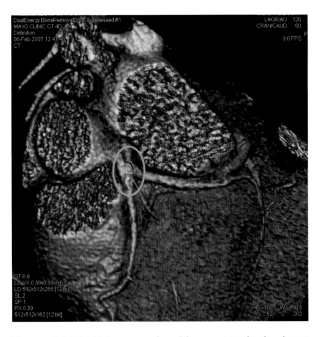

Figure 34.16 Volume rendered image acquired using a dual energy cardiac CT acquisition. The calcified plaque in the proximal left coronary artery (circled) is suppressed, allowing visualization of the highly stenotic lumen.

BIBLIOGRAPHY

1. Genant HK, Boyd D. Quantitative bone mineral analysis using dual energy computed tomography. Invest Radiol 1977; 12: 545–51.
2. Vetter JR, Perman WH, Kalender WA, Mazess RB, Holden JE. Evaluation of a prototype dual-energy computed tomographic apparatus. II. Determination of vertebral bone mineral content. Med Phys 1986; 13: 340–3.
3. Kalender WA. Computed Tomography. Publis MCD Verlag, Munich (2000).
4. Kalender WA, Perman WH, Vetter JR, Klotz E. Evaluation of a prototype dual-energy computed tomographic apparatus. I. Phantom studies. Med Phys 1986; 13: 334–9.
5. Macovski A, Alvarez RE, Chan JL, Stonestrom JP, Zatz LM. Energy dependent reconstruction in X-ray computerized tomography. Comput Biol Med 1976; 6: 325–36.
6. Alvarez RE, Macovski A. Energy-selective reconstructions in X-ray computerized tomography. Phys Med Biol 1976; 21: 733–44.
7. Johnson RJ, Zhu XP, Isherwood I et al. Computed tomography: qualitative and quantitative recognition of liver disease in haemophilia. J Comput Assist Tomogr 1983; 7: 1000–6.
8. Cann CE, Gamsu G, Birnberg FA, Webb WR. Quantification of calcium in solitary pulmonary nodules using single- and dual-energy CT. Radiology 1982; 145: 493–6.
9. Goldberg HI, Cann CE, Moss AA et al. Noninvasive quantitation of liver iron in dogs with hemochromatosis using dual-energy CT scanning. Investigative Radiology 1982; 17: 375–80.
10. Adams JE, Chen SZ, Adams PH, Isherwood I. Measurement of trabecular bone mineral by dual energy computed tomography. J Comput Assist Tomogr 1982; 6: 601–7.
11. Chiro GD, Brooks RA, Kessler RM et al. Tissue signatures with dual-energy computed tomography. Radiology 1979; 131: 521–3.
12. Wang B, Gao Z, Zou Q, Li L. Quantitative diagnosis of fatty liver with dual-energy CT. An experimental study in rabbits. Acta Radiol 2003; 44: 92–7.
13. Kalender WA, Klotz E, Suess C. Vertebral bone mineral analysis: an integrated approach with CT. Radiology 1987; 164: 419–23.
14. Ueno A. Evaluation and assessment of material decomposition between bone/calcification and iodine for CT angiography using 40 mm coverage volumetric CT with novel high-speed pulsed dual energy scanning, RSNA 2006 (abst).
15. McCollough CH, Kantor B, Primak AN et al. Fast, Dual-energy, Multi-slice CT Can Discriminate Fe and Ca, Circulation 2006; 114(18 Suppl) II: 724–5.
16. Langheinrich AC, Michniewicz A, Sedding DG et al. Quantitative x-ray imaging of intraplaque hemorrhage in aortas of apoE$^{-/-}$/LDL$^{-/-}$ double knockout mice by synchrotron-based micro-CT and x-ray fluorescence microscopy. Invest Radiol 2006; 41: 645–50.
17. Johnson TRC, Krauss B, Sedlmair M et al. Material differentiation by dual energy CT: initial experience. European Radiology 2007; In Press.
18. Raupach R, Bruder H, Krauss B et al. Raw data based beam hardening correction for dual energy CT data. RSNA 2006 (abst).

35

Hybrid Imaging Combining Cardiovascular Computed Tomography with Positron Emission Tomography

Roman Fischbach, Klaus Schäfers, and Kai Uwe Juergens

1 INTRODUCTION

Imaging of cardiac structure and function, myocardial perfusion, and coronary artery lumen has become a routine component in the diagnosis and management of almost all patients with manifest or suspected heart disease. The recent technologic advances in cardiac computed tomography (CT), cardiac magnetic resonance (CMR) and positron emission tomography (PET) have delivered high-resolution and robust noninvasive imaging of coronary arteries, cardiac morphology and corresponding functional data regarding perfusion, metabolism, and myocardial viability. Each modality by itself has seen a remarkable development in the last decade, with the greatest excitement generated by the introduction and rapid advance of multislice cardiac computed tomography.

While noninvasive CT coronary artery imaging has become an accepted clinical application to detect or exclude coronary artery stenosis, a detailed characterization of coronary pathology requires information on global and regional myocardial function, which to some extent can be provided by CT,[1] and even more importantly relies on data on myocardial perfusion, metabolism, and viability.[2] PET provides unique physiologic information by specific tracers that track perfusion, metabolism, innervation, and receptor activity.[3–6] Fusion imaging with combined PET-CT systems in

a hybrid device with the potential to deliver both the exquisite anatomic detail of CT and the corresponding functional information of PET using a common bed thus is a logical consequence.[7–9]

Recently 16-slice and 64-slice CT scanners that are fast enough to permit cardiac gating have begun to be marketed with PET scanners. Experience with these hybrid systems in cardiac imaging is scarce and several open technical issues have to be resolved before hybrid scanners will find their way into routine clinical practice. Today, only ideas exist on how these systems might be best used for cardiac imaging. This chapter will therefore focus on technical considerations related to PET-CT in cardiac imaging and can only point out potential future indications.

2 SINGLE PHOTON EMISSION COMPUTED TOMOGRAPHY

The goal of all cardiac nuclear imaging is to trace the fate of radioactively labeled biochemical compounds (tracers) within the blood pool or myocardium.[2] Either a static image of the distribution of the tracer or dynamic information from a series of images of uptake and clearance of the tracer with time is acquired. Functional cardiovascular imaging by nuclear medicine techniques has been performed traditionally by single-photon emission tomography (SPECT), a well accepted low-cost and highly sensitive imaging technique. SPECT uses a rotating tomographic gamma camera to register gamma photons emitted by a radioactive tracer.[10,11] Special tomographic reconstruction algorithms are then applied to the projection images to calculate a 3D volume dataset of radionuclide distribution.

SPECT has been used for a long time in cardiac imaging and is used for assessment of the extent and severity of myocardial ischemia. The most frequent indication is to determine whether a patient should be referred to coronary angiography for further diagnosis or treatment.[12,13] Results from SPECT perfusion measurement provide useful prognostic information regarding future myocardial events.[14,15] Due to it's proven value in patient management myocardial perfusion SPECT has become an integral part of the evaluation of patients with suspected coronary artery disease. The principle of stress-rest myocardial perfusion imaging is that reduced myocardial blood flow results in decreased tracer uptake and thus reduced activity in the affected myocardium. Coronary lesions, which do not impair blood flow to the myocardium at rest will manifest as flow limiting lesions if coronary blood flow is increased above a certain threshold by either pharmaceutical or physical stress. Stress myocardial perfusion imaging by SPECT is performed with thallium-201 or technetium-99m based perfusion tracers.

As SPECT reflects the perfusion situation of the myocardium it depicts the effect of coronary atherosclerosis on coronary blood flow and thus provides information that can not be obtained by anatomic-morphologic imaging as with cardiac CT. Coronary CT angiography is a sensitive tool to visualize coronary atherosclerosis and has an excellent negative predictive value for detection of coronary artery stenosis.[16–18] Technological progress has improved on diagnostic limitations of coronary CT angiography but moderate specificity and positive predictive value for the diagnosis of hemodynamically significant coronary lesions, motion artifacts at high heart rate, and heavily calcified coronary arteries or metallic stents are major challenges.[19–22] A recent study comparing CT and SPECT showed that, despite an overall positive relationship between the severity of coronary artery disease on multislice CT and myocardial perfusion abnormalities on SPECT, only moderate agreement between coronary lesions and perfusion impairment existed on a segment level.[23] This observation indicates that SPECT and CT provide complementary rather than overlapping information with potential impact on patient management decisions,

especially in patients with equivocal findings on coronary CT angiography.

Despite the wide use of SPECT in cardiac imaging diagnostic limitations prevail. Conventional SPECT acquisition suffers from physical limitations related to photon detection sensitivity and a limited spatial resolution over 10 mm. Inaccurate measurements of left ventricular volumes and ejection fraction can be attributed to limited spatial resolution, which also causes difficulties when differentiating visceral and subdiaphragmatic activity from inferior left ventricular myocardium. Furthermore, soft tissue attenuation causes inhomogeneous attenuation artifacts in anterior or inferior walls that can mimic perfusion deficits. The use of CT attenuation information has been successfully applied to attenuation correction in SPECT, resulting in improved diagnostic accuracy for detection of coronary stenosis.[24] In patients with chest pain hybrid imaging with SPECT-CT resulted in an increase in sensitivity and positive predictive value for detection of coronary artery stenosis when using the combination of SPECT/CTA (specificity 95%, PPV 77%) compared to CT angiography alone (specificity 63%, PPV 31%).[25]

3 POSITRON EMISSION TOMOGRAPHY

Positron emission tomography functions in a manner very similar to SPECT but some significant differences have to be considered. PET tracers decay by emission of a positron (β^+-decay). Except for their opposite charge, both positron and electron have nearly the same properties. As positrons are the 'antimatter' of electrons close proximity of a positron and an electron will lead to their 'annihilation' and their masses will be converted into energy in the form of two gamma rays (annihilation photons) that both have a characteristic energy of 511 keV. The emission angle between these photons is 180°, making the two photons travel in nearly opposite directions.

3.1 Coincidence scanning

The positron usually annihilates with an electron while traveling through tissue within a millimeter of its emission from the tracer. PET scanners detect pairs of gamma rays resulting from annihilation in a ring of detectors (or multiple rings for simultaneous acquisition of several sections) that encircle the patient. Since the location of the β^+-decay is determined by measuring coincident pairs of gamma photons, each detector element has to be connected with all other elements. Whenever two detectors record a gamma photon of 511 keV within a certain coincidence time, it is assumed that a β^+-decay has occurred on a line between these two detectors. This line is known as the line of response (LOR, Figure 35.1). The number of coincidences seen by each detector pair during the scan time represents the amount of radioactivity in the volume between the detector pair. The reconstruction process to generate tomographic sections from multiple 2D projection images consists of several steps or mathematical operations, similar to image reconstruction in computed tomography.[26]

3.2 Attenuation correction

The measured raw data has to be processed during image reconstruction to correct for a wide range of possible artifacts and misregistrations. These corrections include decay correction for the specific radionuclide, normalization (correction of different detector sensitivities), correction for random and scattered coincidences and 'attenuation.' Since most photons that travel toward the detector pass through tissue, interaction (attenuation) occurs. This attenuation depends on the intensity of radiation I, the length of the path x and a tissue and radiation energy dependant constant μ, and is described by a simple mathematical rule: $I(x) = I_0 * \exp(-\mu x)$. This attenuation effect

has to be accounted for when measuring PET coincidences, since only a fraction of all gamma photon pairs leave the body and can be potentially detected.

Attenuation correction in a conventional PET scanner is usually performed by an accompanying transmission scan with a β^+-source (^{68}Ge) rod that is rotated around the patient. The 511 keV gamma radiation passes through the patient's body and is then detected by opposite detector elements. Comparing this scan with a blank scan without attenuation from a patient yields a direct multiplicative attenuation factor for each LOR in the projection data.

In contrast to the conventional method of attenuation correction, PET-CT scanners use CT images to compute the tissue depending PET absorption coefficients μ.[27] When using a CT scan for attenuation correction, the much slower ^{68}Ge rod source transmission scan (which is also a source of noise in the corrected images) is not necessary, thus improving image quality and decreasing examination time substantially. As CT uses radiation energies of typically ~70 keV, a transformation to 511 keV PET energy must be performed first.[27,28] The computed attenuation values for the scanned object can then be included in the reconstruction process to calculate attenuation corrected PET images.

3.3 Radiopharmaceuticals

Several β^+-active radionuclides are in use for PET. For assessment of myocardial viability, the fluorine-18 isotope (^{18}F, half-life $t_{1/2} = 110$ min) in the form of a modified glucose molecule (2-[^{18}F]-fluoro-2-deoxy-D-glucose, ^{18}FDG) has shown its value.[6,9,10] ^{18}FDG is the tracer of choice for a wide range of PET applications in oncology, since ^{18}FDG is accumulated in tissues with high glucose metabolism. For myocardial perfusion studies, nitrogen-13 (^{13}N, $t_{1/2} = 10$ min) in the radioactive form of ammonia ([^{13}N]-NH$_3$) and oxygen-15 (^{15}O, $t_{1/2} = 2$ min) in the form of radioactive water ([^{15}O]-H$_2$O) and Rubidium-82 (^{82}Rb, $t_{1/2} = 75$ sec), a potassium analog, can be used. Apart from ^{18}FDG with an almost 2 hour half-life and ^{82}Rb, which can be produced in a special generator, the other isotopes must be produced locally with an on-site cyclotron due to their short half-life.

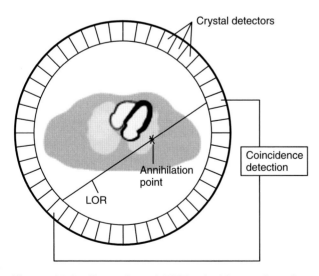

Figure 35.1 Illustration of PET coincidence detection. When two crystal elements detect a gamma photon within a small coincidence time window, a line of response (LOR) is defined by the two detector elements involved. The annihilation point, where the positron is 'converted' into two gamma photons ideally lies on the LOR.

4 CARDIAC PET-CT

4.1 Technical considerations

The gold standard in noninvasive PET cardiac imaging is conventional PET with transmission-based attenuation correction.[5,9,29] In this case both the transmission scan and the PET scan are performed in the order of minutes, so both data sets contain practically the same amount of motion, thus resulting in blurred, but artifact-free images. Using high resolution fast CT cardiac scanning for attenuation correction of cardiac PET poses special challenges, the most important is spatial misalignment of CT and emission data when performing attenuation correction for PET image reconstruction.[30,31] Relatively small misalignments can cause significant differences in the display of tracer uptake in PET, e.g. resulting in artificial uptake defects in healthy myocardium. One source of misalignment is inadvertent patient movement between the CT scan and the subsequent emission acquisition. Clear patient instructions and patient cooperation should control this potential source of error. Unavoidable misalignments due to patient respiration and cardiac motion are more difficult to deal with.[32]

The CT scan is usually performed during a short inspiratory breath hold and subsecond CT cardiac image reconstruction represents only a specific phase of the cardiac cycle with the highest possible temporal resolution to avoid coronary motion artifacts. PET emission data, on the other hand, is acquired over many minutes and thus averages information over many respiration and cardiac cycles. The two data sets therefore do not perfectly match, which causes artifacts at boundaries of high and low attenuation regions. This may result in wrong tracer uptake quantification due to false attenuation correction results, e.g. if the CT scan was acquired in a state of deep inspiration, while the average respiration phase in a PET scan corresponds to normal expiration.[33] For oncology chest scans a major source of uptake miscalculation is the air–tissue interface at the dome of the diaphragm.[34,35] In cardiac PET-CT the lung-myocardium interface, especially of the free left ventricular wall, represents a similar problem area.[36]

To reduce the effects of respiratory motion and/or heart contraction, different possibilities have been proposed.[37] One way to overcome the problem of respiratory motion artifacts includes a very slow low dose CT scan for attenuation correction that captures several respiration cycles and therefore corresponds to a PET transmission scan.[31] Another solution would be to use respiratory and cardiac gating, which adds considerably to the complexity of the acquisition (Figure 35.2). This approach divides the heart cycle into a certain number of gates for both the CT and the PET scan. Every PET image is then reconstructed using the corresponding CT image from the same cardiac phase as basis for attenuation correction. If PET raw data are continuously saved during the scan (list mode PET) raw data can be reconstructed even with an

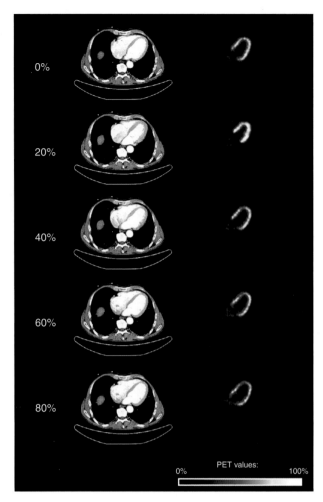

Figure 35.2 ECG-gated [18]FDG PET-CT scan of the heart, 45 minutes after intravenous injection of 575 MBq [18]FDG an ECG-gated CT scan of the heart was performed. The CT data was reconstructed in 10% steps throughout the heart cycle. Five gates are shown on the left side. A subsequent retrospectively ECG-gated PET list mode scan was performed and reconstructed corresponding to the CT images, which were then used to correct the PET gates for attenuation. The resulting PET images are shown on the right. The contraction and relaxation of the myocardium are clearly visible. Maximum systolic contraction is reached in the 20% gate.

additional respiratory gating technique (Figure 35.3). The aim of this method is to use only those coincidences that fall in a respiratory gate that corresponds to the inspiration CT scan to avoid spatial misalignment between CT and PET. Some techniques that were developed for this purpose include the use of pressure sensors that are attached to the patient to monitor respiratory motion, temperature sensors that measure the temperature of the breath, thus marking the start of inspiration, and small radioactive sources placed inside the PET field of view.[30] Another promising development is the use of a camera system that films a marker placed on the patient's abdomen.

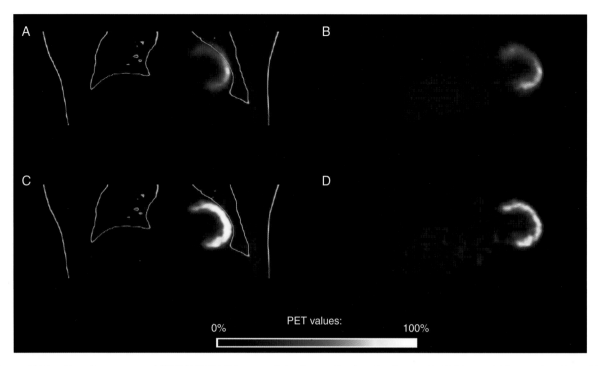

Figure 35.3   Respiratory-gated ^{18}FDG PET-CT scan of the heart. During the list mode PET acquisition patient breathing was monitored by video recording markers attached to patient. Eight respiration gates were retrospectively produced. (A) Comparison of the non-attenuation-corrected, full list mode PET image with the CT (contour plot) reveals a spatial mismatch due to strong inspiration during the CT scan. (B) The attenuation-corrected full list mode PET image shows seemingly reduced tracer uptake in the left ventricular wall in close proximity to the lung. (C) Non-attenuation-corrected PET image of the CT-fitting respiration gate. No mismatch is visible. (D) Attenuation-corrected PET image of the CT-fitting respiration gate. The misquantification of tracer uptake in the left ventricular wall has vanished. Additionally, the image is less blurred than figure (B).

This method not only shows the beginning of the respiration cycle, it also accounts for different respiration amplitudes that can be evaluated in the gating scheme.[30]

Another type of artifact may arise if a contrast-enhanced CT scan is used for attenuation correction (Figure 35.4). The presence of intravenous contrast agent in the CT image is critical due to two facts: first, the contrast agent is washed out of the heart very quickly after the CT scan and will thus hardly affect the subsequent PET scan.[36] Second, iodine cannot be treated properly by the standard CT to PET attenuation transformation since iodine absorbs x-rays very well, whereas 511 keV gamma rays are attenuated only to a disproportionately low degree.[38] This leads to an overestimation of absorption values for PET attenuation correction and thereby to wrong quantification of radioactivity in the respective region by PET. Usage of such CT data therefore results in artificially high absorption coefficients in the PET μ-map and may lead to potential overestimation in tracer uptake in the reconstructed PET images. In the case of oncological PET-CT studies indicate that these contrast agent-induced artifacts are not of clinical importance.[39–41] However, the bolus passage of contrast agents in cardiac PET-CT causes high concentration of these agents in the great vessels and heart cavities, and pronounced artifacts and misquantification of tracer uptake have been observed.[36,42] A recent study reported an average mean signal increase in left ventricular myocardium of 23% when contrast enhanced cardiac CT scans were used for attenuation correction compared to unenhanced CT.[43] Using a simple threshold based segmentation of high attenuation areas to exclude contrast effects from CT images effectively corrected for contrast media induced artifacts (Figure 35.4d).

4.2 PET cardiac imaging

PET provides unique physiologic information by specific tracers that can show molecular processes in vivo.[9] Since almost every substance can be labeled with radioactive elements, potential tracers in PET imaging are unlimited. In clinical cardiology assessment of myocardial function and viability are of special importance as only ischemic but viable myocardium will benefit from a revascularization procedure. ^{18}FDG activity represent ongoing myocardial glucose

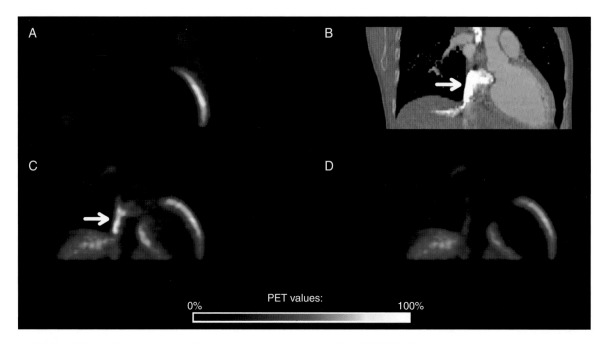

Figure 35.4 Effects of iodine-containing contrast agents on cardiac PET-CT. The outcome of a myocardial perfusion study using ^{13}N-ammonia is presented. (A) Non-attenuation-corrected PET image, oblique slice showing the left ventricle. (B) The same slice in the contrast-enhanced CT scan (bone window). High concentration of contrast agent is visible in the superior vena cava (arrow). (C) Attenuation-corrected PET image using the contrast-enhanced CT image shown in (B). A massive contrast agent-induced artifact is seen in the vena cava (arrow). (D) Reducing the attenuation values in the heart to a normal value of 50 HU results in a PET image where the artifact has vanished. Additionally, the overall uptake in the heart has been reduced to some extent.

metabolism and thus differentiates living myocardial tissue from scar tissue, the hallmark of viability imaging with PET. ^{18}FDG uptake indicates viable myocardium and a revascularization of ischemic myocardium will result in improvement of regional and global function. Scar tissue will not benefit from revascularization procedures. Viability imaging with ^{18}FDG can be combined with perfusion imaging for assessment of match/mismatch.

Myocardial perfusion and coronary flow reserve are assessed using ^{13}N ammonia, ^{15}O water or ^{82}Rb. By acquiring dynamic gated myocardial perfusion data PET provides an insight into impairment of regional coronary blood flow reserve due to epicardial coronary artery stenosis, microvascular disease and endothelial dysfunction.[44,45] Quantitative analysis with PET is based on dynamic acquisition protocols, which allow assessment of the retention fraction and the washout time of the radiotracer. Combining these parameters with net tracer uptake allows accurate quantitative evaluation of myocardial perfusion in mL/min/gram of tissue. Myocardial perfusion can be quantified after pharmaceutical stress (direct vasodilation) or cold pressor test (reactive endothelium dependent vasodilation) and is compared to myocardial perfusion data at rest.[5,10]

Assessment of blood flow reserve with PET allows early identification of coronary artery disease characterized by endothelial dysfunction, which is a relevant prognostic marker of future cardiac events.[46] Endothelial dysfunction causes impaired stress-induced coronary artery vasodilation, which leads to diminished myocardial blood flow reserve, long before hemodynamically significant coronary artery stenosis develops. Impaired myocardial blood flow has been shown in asymptomatic subjects with elevated cholesterol, smoking, hypertension and diabetes either during pharmaceutical stress or cold pressor test.[45,47–49]

With this, PET perfusion assessment will be of increasing interest when it comes to early detection of coronary artery disease and initiation of preventive therapy.[50] Since the majority of coronary events occur in coronary arteries without distinct angiographic stenosis, identification of preclinical atherosclerosis could prove clinically important. Medical therapy in 'preclinical patients' will have to be tailored to the individual person to avoid unnecessary healthcare costs and side effects. Therefore detailed information on clinical risk factors, morphological indicators of coronary atherosclerosis (plaque burden) and functional data reflecting the effect on myocardial blood flow and myocardial metabolism will all be necessary. Furthermore, monitoring the perfusion parameters in response to medical treatment may provide additional information on a particular individual.

4.3 Combined PET and CT cardiac imaging

PET perfusion and CT angiography depict complimentary aspects of coronary artery disease. While CT angiography reveals detailed information on the presence and extent of luminal narrowing of coronary arteries as well as coronary plaque burden, PET perfusion provides information on the down-stream functional consequence of such coronary lesions. The advantage of the combined scanner is that the images are spatially aligned and both data sets can be acquired at a single imaging session. Since PET-CT in cardiac imaging is a new and not widely available technology, clinical experience is limited and no guidelines exist on its use. From a theoretical point of view, the clinical advantage of combining PET perfusion and CT angiographic information will depend on the results of each scan. Several clinical scenarios can illustrate this:

(i) If PET shows an abnormal perfusion result, CT may provide detailed information on coronary artery anatomy and location of coronary artery narrowing. This information is then used to plan a revascularization procedure.

(ii) Equivocal results of PET perfusion imaging will probably benefit the most from additional CT information. In the case of a normal CT further invasive testing or medical treatment can be avoided. A significant stenosis depicted by CT will direct the patient to a revascularization attempt. An intermediate stenosis or a high coronary artery calcium score should trigger clinical risk factor modification and medical therapy and probably also follow up testing.

(iii) If PET results are normal, CT seems to have the least impact, as normal perfusion results preclude further therapeutic or invasive diagnostic measures, even if CT should depict a significant stenosis. Information on calcium score or total plaque burden could prove to be of interest when making decisions on preventive medical interventions. On the other hand, significance of coronary lesions, especially in patients with diffuse or pronounced calcification that impair coronary artery

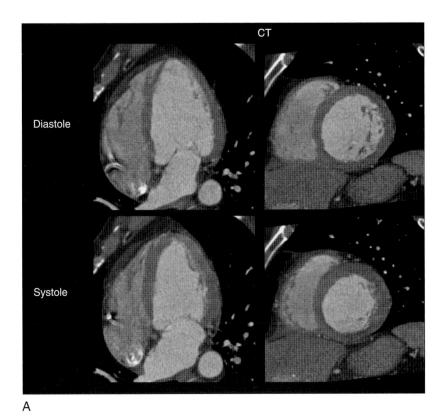

A

Figure 35.5 Fusion imaging of [18]FDG-PET and 16-slice cardiac CT in a patient with ischemic myocardial scar in the apical and midventricular inferior segments. (A) CT shows thinning of the myocardium in the diastolic reconstruction without systolic increase in wall thickness. Note the heavily calcified right coronary artery.

Continued

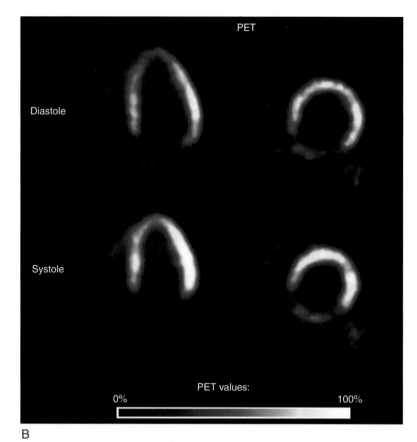

B

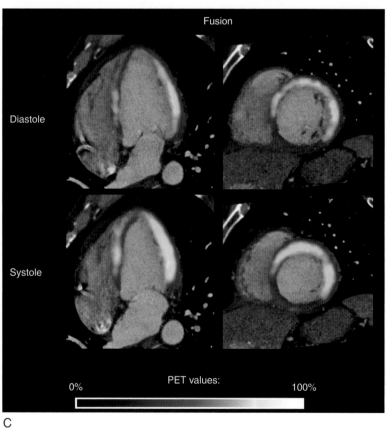

C

Figure 35.5, cont'd   (B) [18]FDG activity is significantly decreased. (C) Fusion image shows near perfect alignment of CT and PET in both cardiac phases and very good agreement of [18]FDG activity and myocardial wall contours from CT.

lumen assessment, will be much easier to assess in the light of supplementary perfusion information.

In PET perfusion and viability assessment CT will provide complementary information on myocardial wall thickness and dynamic changes of wall thickness within the cardiac cycle, both of which are of significant prognostic value.[1,51] Furthermore, retrospective cardiac gating for CT and PET will form the basis for perfect alignment of the two scans, which in turn will improve attenuation correction and as a result image quality and reliability of the quantification of perfusion data and metabolic activity (Figure 35.5). However, robust correction methods for respiration and cardiac motion as well as contrast-induced artifacts are not readily available. This is still an area of ongoing research.

5 CONCLUSIONS

Combining PET with CT in oncology imaging has almost replaced single modality conventional PET imaging. A similar development can be expected in cardiac PET imaging as soon as technical issues like motion correction and attenuation correction have been solved. The additional information associated with overlaying physiologic data with CT angiographic data, coupled with information about wall thickness and wall thickening, clearly will advance noninvasive cardiac imaging.

REFERENCES

1. Juergens KU, Fischbach R. Left ventricular function studied with MDCT. Eur Radiol 2006; 16(2): 342–57.
2. Machac J. Radionuclear assessment in ischemic heart disease. Curr Opin Cardiol 1990; 5(4): 397–402.
3. Rimoldi O, Schafers KP, Boellaard R et al. Quantification of subendocardial and subepicardial blood flow using 15O-labeled water and PET: experimental validation. J Nucl Med 2006; 47(1): 163–72.
4. Schafers M, Riemann B, Levkau B et al. Current status and future applications of cardiac receptor imaging with positron emission tomography. Nucl Med Commun 2002; 23(2): 113–15.
5. Schwaiger M. Myocardial perfusion imaging with PET. J Nucl Med 1994; 35(4): 693–8.
6. Travin MI, Bergmann SR. Assessment of myocardial viability. Semin Nucl Med 2005; 35(1): 2–16.
7. Townsend DW, Carney JP, Yap JT, Hall NC. PET/CT today and tomorrow. J Nucl Med 2004; 45 Suppl 1: 4S–14S.
8. Di Carli MF, Dorbala S. Integrated PET/CT for cardiac imaging. Q J Nucl Med Mol Imaging 2006; 50(1): 44–52.
9. Machac J. Cardiac positron emission tomography imaging. Semin Nucl Med 2005; 35(1): 17–36.
10. Slart RH, Bax JJ, van Veldhuisen DJ et al. Imaging techniques in nuclear cardiology for the assessment of myocardial viability. Int J Cardiovasc Imaging 2006; 22(1): 63–80.
11. Mowatt G, Brazzelli M, Gemmell H et al. Systematic review of the prognostic effectiveness of SPECT myocardial perfusion scintigraphy in patients with suspected or known coronary artery disease and following myocardial infarction. Nucl Med Commun 2005; 26(3): 217–29.
12. Berger BC, Watson DD, Taylor GJ et al. Quantitative thallium-201 exercise scintigraphy for detection of coronary artery disease. J Nucl Med 1981; 22(7): 585–93.
13. Mahmarian JJ, Boyce TM, Goldberg RK et al. Quantitative exercise thallium-201 single photon emission computed tomography for the enhanced diagnosis of ischemic heart disease. J Am Coll Cardiol 1990; 15(2): 318–29.
14. Berman DS, Hachamovitch R, Kiat H et al. Incremental value of prognostic testing in patients with known or suspected ischemic heart disease: a basis for optimal utilization of exercise technetium-99m sestamibi myocardial perfusion single-photon emission computed tomography. J Am Coll Cardiol 1995; 26(3): 639–47.
15. Klocke FJ, Baird MG, Lorell BH et al. ACC/AHA/ASNC guidelines for the clinical use of cardiac radionuclide imaging–executive summary: a report of the American College of Cardiology/American Heart Association Task Force on Practice Guidelines (ACC/AHA/ASNC Committee to Revise the 1995 Guidelines for the Clinical Use of Cardiac Radionuclide Imaging). Circulation 2003; 108(11): 1404–18.
16. Leschka S, Alkadhi H, Plass A et al. Accuracy of MSCT coronary angiography with 64-slice technology: first experience. Eur Heart J 2005; 26(15): 1482–7.
17. Hoffmann MH, Shi H, Schmitz BL et al. Noninvasive coronary angiography with multislice computed tomography. Jama 2005; 293(20): 2471–8.
18. Ropers D, Rixe J, Anders K et al. Usefulness of multidetector row spiral computed tomography with 64- × 0.6-mm collimation and 330-ms rotation for the noninvasive detection of significant coronary artery stenoses. Am J Cardiol 2006; 97(3): 343–8.
19. Kuettner A, Beck T, Drosch T et al. Image quality and diagnostic accuracy of non-invasive coronary imaging with 16 detector slice spiral computed tomography with 188 ms temporal resolution. Heart 2005; 91(7): 938–41.
20. Gilard M, Cornily JC, Pennec PY et al. Accuracy of multislice computed tomography in the preoperative assessment of coronary disease in patients with aortic valve stenosis. J Am Coll Cardiol 2006; 47(10): 2020–4.
21. Rixe J, Achenbach S, Ropers D et al. Assessment of coronary artery stent restenosis by 64-slice multi-detector computed tomography. Eur Heart J 2006; 27(21): 2567–72.
22. Hacker M, Jakobs T, Hack N et al. Sixty-four slice spiral CT angiography does not predict the functional relevance of coronary artery stenoses in patients with stable angina. Eur J Nucl Med Mol Imaging 2007; 34(1): 4–10.
23. Schuijf JD, Wijns W, Jukema JW et al. A comparative regional analysis of coronary atherosclerosis and calcium score on multislice CT versus myocardial perfusion on SPECT. J Nucl Med 2006; 47(11): 1749–55.

24. Utsunomiya D, Tomiguchi S, Shiraishi S et al. Initial experience with X-ray CT based attenuation correction in myocardial perfusion SPECT imaging using a combined SPECT/CT system. Ann Nucl Med 2005; 19(6): 485–9.

25. Rispler S, Keidar Z, Ghersin E et al. Integrated single-photon emission computed tomography and computed tomography coronary angiography for the assessment of hemodynamically significant coronary artery lesions. J Am Coll Cardiol 2007; 49(10): 1059–67.

26. Parker J. Image reconstruction in radiology. Boca Raton: CRC Press, 1990.

27. Burger C, Goerres G, Schoenes S et al. PET attenuation coefficients from CT images: experimental evaluation of the transformation of CT into PET 511-keV attenuation coefficients. Eur J Nucl Med Mol Imaging 2002; 29(7): 922–7.

28. Koepfli P, Hany TF, Wyss CA et al. CT attenuation correction for myocardial perfusion quantification using a PET/CT hybrid scanner. J Nucl Med 2004; 45(4): 537–42.

29. Berman DS, Hachamovitch R, Shaw LJ et al. Roles of nuclear cardiology, cardiac computed tomography, and cardiac magnetic resonance: assessment of patients with suspected coronary artery disease. J Nucl Med 2006; 47(1): 74–82.

30. Schafers KP, Dawood M, Lang N et al. Motion correction in PET/CT. Nuklearmedizin 2005; 44 Suppl 1: S46–50.

31. Martinez-Moller A, Souvatzoglou M, Navab N, Schwaiger M, Nekolla SG. Artifacts from Misaligned CT in Cardiac Perfusion PET/CT Studies: Frequency, Effects, and Potential Solutions. J Nucl Med 2007; 48(2): 188–93.

32. Lang N, Dawood M, Buther F et al. Organ movement reduction in PET/CT using dual-gated list-mode acquisition. Z Med Phys 2006; 16(1): 93–100.

33. Osman MM, Cohade C, Nakamoto Y, Wahl RL. Respiratory motion artifacts on PET emission images obtained using CT attenuation correction on PET-CT. Eur J Nucl Med Mol Imaging 2003; 30(4): 603–6.

34. Goerres GW, Kamel E, Heidelberg TN et al. PET-CT image co-registration in the thorax: influence of respiration. Eur J Nucl Med Mol Imaging 2002; 29(3): 351–60.

35. Weckesser M, Stegger L, Juergens KU et al. Correlation between respiration-induced thoracic expansion and a shift of central structures. Eur Radiol 2006; 16(7): 1614–20.

36. Buther F, Schafers KP, Stegger L et al. Artifacts caused by contrast agents and patient movement in cardiac PET-CT. Nuklearmedizin 2006; 45(5): N53–4.

37. Dawood M, Lang N, Jiang X, Schafers KP. Lung motion correction on respiratory gated 3-D PET/CT images. IEEE Trans Med Imaging 2006; 25(4): 476–85.

38. Kinahan PE, Hasegawa BH, Beyer T. X-ray-based attenuation correction for positron emission tomography/computed tomography scanners. Semin Nucl Med 2003; 33(3): 166–79.

39. Mawlawi O, Erasmus JJ, Munden RF et al. Quantifying the effect of IV contrast media on integrated PET/CT: clinical evaluation. AJR Am J Roentgenol 2006; 186(2): 308–19.

40. Yau YY, Chan WS, Tam YM et al. Application of intravenous contrast in PET/CT: does it really introduce significant attenuation correction error? J Nucl Med 2005; 46(2): 283–91.

41. Dizendorf E, Hany TF, Buck A, von Schulthess GK, Burger C. Cause and magnitude of the error induced by oral CT contrast agent in CT-based attenuation correction of PET emission studies. J Nucl Med 2003; 44(5): 732–8.

42. Nakamoto Y, Chin BB, Kraitchman DL et al. Effects of nonionic intravenous contrast agents at PET/CT imaging: phantom and canine studies. Radiology 2003; 227(3): 817–24.

43. Buther F, Dawood M, Stegger L et al. Effective methods to correct contrast agent-induced errors of PET quantification in cardiac PET-CT. J Nucl Med 2007; in press.

44. Cecchi F, Olivotto I, Gistri R et al. Coronary microvascular dysfunction and prognosis in hypertrophic cardiomyopathy. N Engl J Med 2003; 349(11): 1027–35.

45. Prior JO, Quinones MJ, Hernandez-Pampaloni M et al. Coronary circulatory dysfunction in insulin resistance, impaired glucose tolerance, and type 2 diabetes mellitus. Circulation 2005; 111(18): 2291–8.

46. Cohn JN, Quyyumi AA, Hollenberg NK, Jamerson KA. Surrogate markers for cardiovascular disease: functional markers. Circulation 2004; 109(25 Suppl 1): IV31–46.

47. Czernin J, Sun K, Brunken R et al. Effect of acute and long-term smoking on myocardial blood flow and flow reserve. Circulation 1995; 91(12): 2891–7.

48. Guethlin M, Kasel AM, Coppenrath K et al. Delayed response of myocardial flow reserve to lipid-lowering therapy with fluvastatin. Circulation 1999; 99(4): 475–81.

49. Masuda D, Nohara R, Tamaki N et al. Evaluation of coronary blood flow reserve by 13N-NH3 positron emission computed tomography (PET) with dipyridamole in the treatment of hypertension with the ACE inhibitor (Cilazapril). Ann Nucl Med 2000; 14(5): 353–60.

50. Berman DS, Hachamovitch R, Shaw LJ et al. Roles of nuclear cardiology, cardiac computed tomography, and cardiac magnetic resonance: Noninvasive risk stratification and a conceptual framework for the selection of noninvasive imaging tests in patients with known or suspected coronary artery disease. J Nucl Med 2006; 47(7): 1107–18.

51. Fischbach R, Juergens KU, Ozgun M et al. Assessment of regional left ventricular function with multidetector-row computed tomography versus magnetic resonance imaging. Eur Radiol 2007; 17(4): 1009–17.

36

Full-Field Cardiac Imaging using Ultra-High Resolution Flat-Panel Volume-Computed Tomography

Rajiv Gupta, Soenke H. Bartling, Mannudeep K. Kalra, and Thomas J. Brady

1 INTRODUCTION

Coronary artery disease (CAD) is the leading cause of death in the United States, accounting for approximately 540,000 myocardial infarctions, ~515,000 total deaths, and ~250,000 sudden deaths per year, most of which result from ruptured vulnerable plaques.[1] Initial diagnostic evaluation of symptomatic patients with suspected CAD includes risk assessment and stress testing.[2,3] Coronary angiography with diagnostic catheterization remains the cornerstone for detecting flow-limiting lesions (>75% stenosis) and is paramount for percutaneous coronary interventions (PCI). While there is concern regarding the expense and potential complications of diagnostic catheterization, the major limitation of coronary angiography is its inability to visualize atherosclerotic plaque within the vessel wall. This is of critical importance since the majority of patients with acute coronary syndromes (unstable angina, myocardial infarction, sudden death) have plaques that did not have a hemodynamically significant stenosis prior to rupture and thrombosis. Indeed, more than 60% of myocardial infarctions are caused by lesions, which are previously associated with a less than 50% luminal narrowing of coronary arteries.[4]

Currently, Intravascular Ultrasound (IVUS) is the only established modality for imaging the coronary artery wall with atherosclerotic plaques, but it requires cardiac catheterization, which is an invasive procedure. Non-invasive imaging techniques such as multidetector-row CT

(MDCT) and Magnetic Resonance Imaging (MRI) are often limited because of their temporal and spatial resolution.

Recent advances in flat panel volume CT enable acquisition of image data with an isotropic spatial resolution of about 150 µm and electrocardiographically gated volumetric acquisition with the use of digital detector arrays. In this article, the basic concepts and fundamental principles underlying a high-resolution flat-panel Volume-CT are briefly described by means of a prototype scanner. The primary focus will be describing and illustrating potential applications of this technology in the field of cardiac imaging.

2 FUNDAMENTALS OF FLAT-PANEL VOLUME CT DESIGN

2.1 System gantry

A flat-panel detector may be integrated with a variety of different types of mechanical gantries, depending on the functional requirements of the system. In one design, a CT gantry integrated with a modified X-ray tube and a 2-D digital flat-panel detector system forms the basis of a Volumetric-CT or cone-beam CT scanner (Figures 36.1 and 36.2; other variations on this basic design will be presented later in this chapter). As the CT gantry rotates, projection images of the anatomy are acquired. These 2-D projections

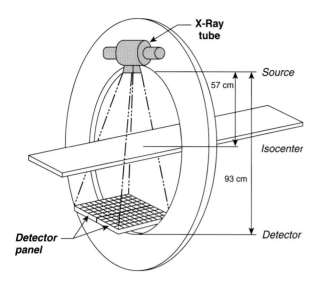

Figure 36.1   Schematic of a flat-panel volume-CT system.

are reconstructed into a volumetric stack of slices using a 3-D reconstruction algorithm.

A flat panel detector produces large amounts of data. For example, a flat-panel detector with a 2k × 2k matrix of pixels, operating at 100 frames per second (fps), will produce 800 mega-bytes of data every second (assuming 2 bytes/pixel). Given the amount of data generated, a less apparent but equally important aspect of the CT gantry based design is the need for fast connection between the rotating flat-panel detector and the stationary control computer. This connection has to be provided by a large bandwidth slip-ring, or by

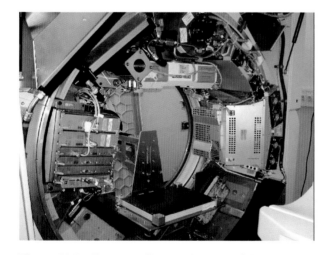

Figure 36.2   Prototype flat-panel volume-CT based on a Sensation-64 CT gantry. The flat-panel detector is at the bottom of the bore of the gantry, while the X-ray tube is on the top. The size of the field-of-view, and the area that it occupies in the bore of the gantry, can be appreciated from this picture by imagining a cone-beam emanating from the X-ray tube and illuminating the detector (courtesy of Siemens Medical Solutions, Germany).

an optical coupling between the rotor and the stator. Another consideration with the fpVCT gantry is that a closed CT gantry somewhat restricts free access to the patient for interventional procedures. On the other hand, a CT gantry provides fast rotation time on a stable platform that is free of significant vibrations.

In order to provide open access to the patient, one can mount a flat-panel detector on a C-arm system. All major vendors have C-arm based flat-panel systems that are capable of limited tomographic reconstructions. The emphasis in these systems, however, is on traditional radiography and fluoroscopy, with rotational tomography as an additional feature. The gantries are very slow compared to CT rotation times, and cannot turn freely and continuously around an axis. Since the detector is always connected to the control computer, there is no need for a high-bandwidth slip ring.

2.2 X-ray tube

The X-ray tube used in the fpVCT system needs to be modified to incorporate the following changes.

- **Cone angle:** Wide anode angle (~16) is needed to enable a true cone-beam geometry in the primary X-ray beam.
- **Pulsed operation:** This mode ensures that the tube is 'on' only during the acquisition of a projection. A duty cycle of 50% was used.
- **Focal spot size:** A small focal spot size of approximately 0.57 mm is typically used to minimize the penumbra effect in high-resolution imaging.
- **Filter:** An aluminum filter is used to remove low energy photons that will be completely absorbed by the patient and will not contribute to the projection image. The thickness of the filter can be configured according to the application. Additional filters such as a wedge filter or a bow-tie filter can be used to further shape the photon flux in the incident X-ray beam. Typically, a source-side collimator is used to eliminate extraneous radiation beyond the field of view.

2.3 Flat-panel detector

A digital flat-panel detector is constructed by growing a thin-film of scintillator crystals on a matrix of photo-cells. The photo-cells are fabricated directly on an amorphous silicon (a-Si) wafer using photolithographic techniques. These manufacturing techniques, which are commonly used in silicon foundries for manufacturing integrated circuits (ICs), ensure very small detector element size and direct digital read-out. The scintillator converts incident X-ray energy to light. The generated light is sensed by a photo-cell, which generates and stores signal as a charge. A thin-film field effect transistor transfers the collected charge to external circuit.

Cesium Iodide (CsI) is typically used as the scintillating material. Needle-shaped crystals of CsI act as fibre optic channels and guide the light generated by the scintillation process down to the photodiodes. Because the scintillator is deposited directly on the a-Si photocell, there is an intimate optical contact between the two. This construction, when combined with the novel columnar structure of the CsI, serves to significantly enhance the efficiency with which X-rays are converted into an electronic image.

The flat-panel detectors were originally developed as a substitute for film in conventional X-ray radiography and mammography. Both of these applications demand ultra-high spatial resolution (~150 μm) in 2-D images. A flat-panel detector based Volume CT (fpVCT) scanner combines the advances in CT with digital flat-panel detector technology.[31,32]

Flat-panel Volume CT represents a fundamental shift in the design of CT scanners: it employs a digital flat panel detector instead of a small number of 1-D detector rows used in-state-of-the-art MDCT scanners. Modern semiconductor fabrication technology allows a flat-panel detector to be built with much smaller X-ray detection elements as compared with the discrete detectors used in MDCT. The high resolution available in individual projection images is transferred to the reconstructed volumetric CT images. By virtue of the large area of the flat-panel detector, unlike micro-CT,[33] fpVCT is suitable for in vivo imaging of large animals and humans.[34]

In current clinical practice, three different radiologic modalities – radiography and fluoroscopy (R&F), X-ray angiography, and computed tomography (CT) – play a central role. Even though these modalities are all based on X-ray imaging, they provide different and often complementary information about a disease process. Due to detector technology, these three X-ray modalities have remained separated, even though at a block-diagram level they seem to utilize similar components. The R&F and C-arm based systems require a detector that can provide 2-D projections at the video frame rate. Consequently, these systems use image intensifiers for image capture at the video frame rate of 25–30 frames/sec. This allows for fast, real-time image capture, but the dynamic range of the data is limited to 8–10 bits/pixel. Consequently, only high-contrast structures such as opacified vessels and bones can be visualized.

On the other side of the spectrum, the detectors used for MDCT have very high dynamic range. This enables contrast resolution of almost 256,000 shades of gray (i.e., a dynamic range of 18 bits) at the detector level. Also, the detector panel can be read-out at an incredibly fast frame rate: in one rotation lasting about 330–440 milliseconds, approximately 1,000 projections are acquired and read out. However, the MDCT detector elements are bigger, measuring approximately 1 mm in their smallest dimension. In addition, these detectors are not available in large area arrays, and they are made long in the axial dimension to provide better sensitivity, which leads to anisotropic volumetric data.

FpVCT scanners that employ the recent advent flat-panel detectors could potentially satisfy the demands of these three different X-ray modalities, which would be a significant leap forward.

In the prototype system reported here, a 30 cm × 40 cm a-Si flat-panel detector was used in the prototype fpVCT (Varian 4030CB). This detector provides a matrix of 2048 × 1536 detector elements, each with a dimension of $194 \times 194\ \mu m^2$.

2.4 Reconstruction algorithm

The reconstruction algorithm converts the set of projections into a set of tomographic slices. A simple and robust reconstruction algorithm, an adaptation of direct 3-D Feldkamp algorithm, was used in the current prototype system. Using approximately 600 projections, the geometric parameters for each projection, and a de-convolution kernel that describes what to emphasize in the tomographic image (i.e., bone, soft tissue, etc.), this reconstruction algorithms produces a stack of slices. The 3-D nature of this algorithm ensures that each voxel, at least at the isocenter, has isotropic dimensions.

3 PERFORMANCE CHARACTERIZATION OF FPVCT

3.1 Spatial resolution

The fpVCT can be operated in a mode where all detector elements are used individually. This so called 1 × 1 binning

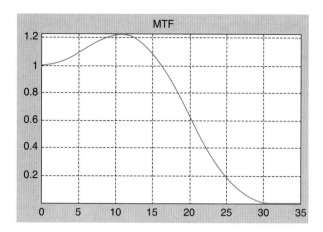

Figure 36.3 The modulation transfer function (MTF) curve from fpVCT image of a 100 μm tungsten wire phantom and 1 × 1 binning mode (courtesy of Siemens Medical Solutions, Germany).

mode gives highest possible spatial resolution. However, the image noise is high because of low photon flux. The signal-to-noise ratio can be improved by averaging neighboring pixels. Pixels can be averaged in groups of 2 × 2 (i.e., four neighboring pixels) leading to a 2 × 2 binning mode. This results in increased SNR at the expense of resolution. Figure 36.3 depicts the MTF curve obtained from a fpVCT scan of a 100 μm tungsten wire phantom at 120 kV reconstructed with a sharp kernel and 1 × 1 binning mode. As can be seen from the MTF curve, at 10% modulation cut-off, the spatial frequency is approximately 28 line-pairs/cm in 1 × 1 binning mode. Figure 36.4 shows the image of a high-resolution line-pair phantom. Once again, 28 line-pairs/cm can be distinguished.

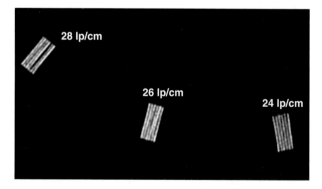

Figure 36.4 A portion of a fpVCT image of a high resolution CATPHAN phantom scanned using 1 × 1 binning mode. Notice that the 24 line-pair/cm inserts (right and middle) are well seen as individual lines. The 28 lp/cm insert (left) is at the limit of resolution (courtesy of Siemens Medical Solutions, Germany).

3.2 Contrast resolution

Contrast resolution refers to the ability to visualize small density differences over the background. FpVCT image of a low-contrast phantom (a 16 cm PMMA phantom) is illustrated in Figure 36.5. The image shown has a slice width of 10 mm and was acquired on fpVCT using 500 mAs and 120 kV. The dose from such an exposure ($CTDI_{100, center}$) is 64.2 mGy and is quite comparable to that from a standard head scan from a multidetector CT (MDCT).

As can be seen, fpVCT has the ability differentiate structures with a difference of 5 HU over the background. This is slightly inferior to MDCT that can differentiate structures to within approximately 3 HU. The difference is largely due to lower dynamic range of the CsI based flat-panel detector. Although such difference in the contrast resolution may have bearing on characterization of some plaques, it is inconsequential for calcium scoring and for most coronary CT angiographies.

3.3 X-ray dose

Initial studies had suggested that scattered radiation dose associated with fpVCT might result in incremental increase in dose to the patients as compared to the MDCT scanners.

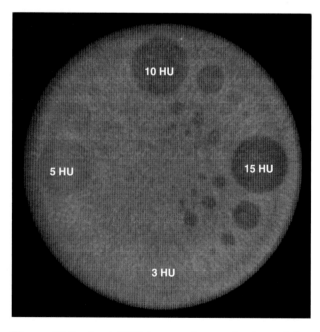

Figure 36.5 An fpVCT image of a contrast resolution phantom showing low contrast inserts that are 15, 10, 5, and 3 HU away from the background in density. The 5HU insert is clearly visible, while the 3HU insert can be faintly discerned (courtesy of Siemens Medical Solutions, Germany).

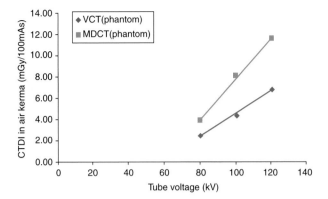

Figure 36.6 CTDI in air kerma of fpVCT and MDCT scans as a function of tube voltage (courtesy of Siemens Medical Solutions, Germany).

In order to assess the X-ray dose, CT dose index ($CTDI_{100}$) was measured with a 10 cm ionization chamber and oval water-equivalent phantom (27×18 cm) (QRM, Möhrendorf, Germany) for fpVCT and Sensation-16. Air kerma (in units of mGy/100 mAs) and effective dose (mSv) were calculated to obtain normalized values that represent X-ray dose under identical conditions (Figure 36.6). X-ray dose expressed in air kerma is the measured dose normalized to 100 mAs. Effective dose takes into account the dose length product, DLP = (CTDI in air kerma) × (Irradiated scan length), and a normalization factor according to the body part being irradiated. The normalization factor for various body regions incorporates the damage a certain amount of absorbed dose may inflict.

As can be seen from the above comparison, the radiation exposure from fpVCT, normalized to 100 mAs, is less than that from MDCT. Normalization to 100 mAs is essential to keep the two scans comparable. The lower dose of fpVCT essentially reflects reduced filtration and lack of scatter rejection, with associated decrease in the effective signal-to-noise ratio.

4 VARIATIONS OF THE FLAT-PANEL VOLUME-CT CONCEPT

The system described in detail above uses a single flat-panel detector mounted on a CT-grantry. Other ways of integrating a gantry, X-ray tube, and one or more plat-panel detectors are possible, depending of the ultimate application being conceived. In this section, we briefly describe some of these variations.

4.1 Systems with multiple flat-panel detectors

With a single flat-panel detector measuring 40 cm in the plane of the gantry, the size of the scan field of view (sFOV) is limited to about 25 cm. The sFOV is a function of the geometry of a scanner and the width of the flat-panel detector. The scanned object needs to fit within the sFOV during the whole rotation. If structures protrude out of the sFOV, the protruding portions (which will not be imaged in all projections) will cause artifacts. For high contrast structures that are relatively near the iso-center, these artifacts can often be tolerated. In fact in some flat-panel scanner designs – e.g., those dedicated maxillo-facial imaging or orthopedic applications – these artifacts are accepted as an unavoidable part of the image in order to keep the price and complexity low.[48]

For other applications, such as thoracic or abdominal imaging, a bigger sFOV without artifacts is essential. Multiple flat-panel detectors can be placed next to each other on a gantry in order to increase sFOV while keeping the same magnification factor and resolution. This is schematically shown in Figure 36.7.

Several engineering challenges need to be addressed to make this concept practical. First, there is the engineering challenge of fitting all this hardware in the confined space of a closed gantry. The task of bringing all the data generated by multiple flat-panel detectors from the rotating gantry into the stationary reconstruction computer also poses a challenge. Very high bandwidth slip-rings are typically employed for this task. Then there is the problem of fast, artifact-free reconstruction. If the data from the flat-panels is used as is, it is incomplete because of missing projection data at the seams between two adjacent flat-panels. This 'seam correction' problem is solved by appropriately positioning the seams in the X-ray cone beam. If the seams are off-center, then the data sets acquired from 180° away can be used to fill in the missing data at the seams. A multiprocessor system that takes advantage of the inherent parallelism in a cone-beam reconstruction problem is employed for fast hardware based reconstruction.[49]

4.2 C-arm based fpVCT systems

A wide angle cone-beam X-ray tube and a flat-panel detector can be integrated with C-arm gantry. If the C-arm allows simultaneous image acquisition and rotation around an iso-center, as most of them do, 3-D reconstruction can be

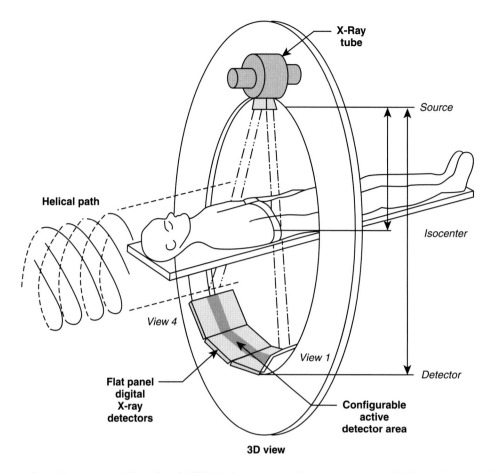

Figure 36.7 A schematic representation of an fpVCT design using multiple detector panels. The missing projections at the seams can be obtained by using projections that are 180 degrees away from the current position. Such a design is discussed by Ross et al.[49]

performed using the resulting projection data-set. Most modern flat-panel based angiography systems offer such spin angiography and tomographic scanning capability.

The difference between CT-gantry based and C-arm based systems lies in their basic engineering. The CT-gantry based systems are more stable and have less geometric inaccuracies as compared to the C-arm based systems. The iso-center of any CT-gantry, by virtue of its mechanical design, is much more narrowly defined than the best C-arm gantries. Because of these reasons, the CT-gantry based designs offer better spatial resolution. The high-resolution offered by the detector panel is typically not fully utilized by the mechanical gantry.

In a C-arm, the detector and the X-ray tube are connected to the control hardware by a spool of cables. Therefore, the C-arm cannot continuously spin around its iso-center as it lacks the slip-rings for getting the data off from a rotating component. Lack of continuous rotation forbids dynamic imaging of temporally evolving processes. Also, there are safety concerns with a fast moving C-arm.

Elaborate collision avoidance schemes have been implemented to ensure operator safety.

C-arm systems have the advantage of being more flexible in terms of orienting the imager around a patient. They also provide better access to a patient than a closed CT gantry. This is especially important if fpVCT is to be used for interventional or intra-operative applications.

Another variation of C-arm based flat-panel systems are the so called 'seat-scanners': The patient sits on a chair while a small C-arm with a small flat-panel detector revolves around his or her head. These scanners are dedicated to maxillo-facial and temporal bone applications because of their relatively small sFOV.[48] There is no fundamental reason why their sFOV cannot be increased. They are currently limited to these niche applications primarily because of cost and marketing reasons.

Because of their more favorable imaging characteristics flat-panel detectors are slowly replacing the image-intensifiers in angiography and fluoroscopy systems. Most of these C-arm based systems offer rotational tomography modes.

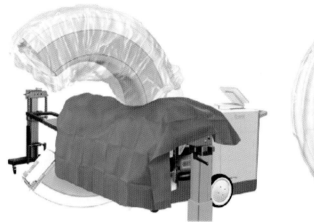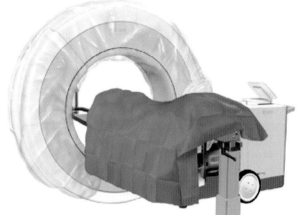

Figure 36.8   A flat-panel detector based O-arm system with the arm in the C-configuration (left), and in the O-configuration (right). The O-configuration, that is achieved using a telescoping mechanism in the C-arm, provides a closed gantry that allows continuous rotation of the imaging chain (courtesy of Breakaway Technologies, LLC).

It is to be expected that, in future, flat-panel volume tomography scanning capability will be much widely available.

4.3 O-arm flat-panel detector system

An O-arm system provides a system that tries to combine the advantages of a CT-gantry based design and a C-arm based design. It provides a mobile imaging platform that is optimized for intra-operative imaging. An O-arm system (Breakaway Imaging, LLC) is shown in Figure 36.8. It is essentially a C-arm system with a telescoping gantry. The gantry can function as standard C-arm, or one can complete the O-ring, and turn the system into a CT-like gantry where the flat-panel detector and the X-ray tube freely rotate. The system allows both fluoroscopy and 3-D imaging. Given the bulk of the gantry, a robotic positioning system is provided for ease of use. Such a compact design is a direct outcome of the lightweight and compactness of a digital flat panel detector.

5 PRACTICAL CONSIDERATIONS WITH CARDIAC CT EXAMINATIONS

5.1 EKG gating

Complex motion of the heart during the cardiac cycle makes it necessary to acquire image data in a short period of time to avoid motion related artifacts in the image. As a single gantry rotation is typically longer than 300 milliseconds,

substantial cardiac motion occurs during one complete rotation. If no special technique is employed to sort the projections or reduce the image reconstruction time, there will be motion blurring. In addition, since diastole accounts for about 70% of the acquired projection data, the images reconstructed from the entire projection set will look like a blurred version of a heart in diastole.

EKG tagging of projection data is essential for multi-phase reconstruction of the cardiac cycle. The EKG is used either prospectively or retrospectively to gather enough projections for a given phase of cardiac cycle so that a volumetric reconstruction can be performed. Gating, therefore, works as a trick to freeze the motion of the heart so that enough projections of a moving heart can be acquired.

In prospective gating different angular projections are acquired each time the cardiac cycle is at a defined phase. Using this method, motion-compensated still images as well as 4D time series can be reconstructed. The principal disadvantages of prospective methods are long scan times and complex setups.

In retrospective gating, the scanning is performed continuously over multiple rotations. Each projection is tagged with an EKG time-stamp during data acquisition. This dataset is then retrospectively sorted in order to reconstruct various phases of the cardiac cycle. Traditionally, two types of reconstruction techniques have been used: half-sector reconstruction and multi-sector reconstruction.

5.2 Half-sector reconstruction for MDCT

In order to reconstruct a volumetric stack, projection data from (180° + the cone angle) are required. Assuming a cone angle of approximately 60°, we need projections from 240° around the heart. In half-sector reconstruction, the entire projection set needed for reconstructing a volume is acquired during diastole of one heart beat. At a heat rate of 60 beats per minute or 1 beat/second, the diastole is about 0.7 second long. Thus the gantry must rotate at about 240°/0.7 second. Clearly, this scheme requires a sub-second rotation and a high rate for acquisition of projections. MDCT, because of a fast scintillator, are able to employ this scheme. To date, all fpVCT systems that employ a CsI scintillator cannot use a half sector recon because of slow gantry rotation time and slow acquisition of projection data.

5.3 Multi-sector reconstruction for MDCT

In multi-sector recon, the required set of projections is collected over multiple cardiac cycles. Therefore, this reconstruction scheme assumes repeatability of the cardiac cycle and heart position from beat to beat.

If gantry rotation cycle is not in phase with the cardiac motion cycle, a geometric phase difference exists between gantry rotation cycle and heart motion cycle. In other words, for a given phase of cardiac cycle, the angular position of the detector is different from one cycle to the next. This makes it possible to combine different angular positions from multiple cardiac cycles to make up the dataset necessary for image reconstruction. The improvement in the temporal resolution improvement can be multiple folds using this scheme. Typically, 4 to 5 cardiac cycles, each contributing approximately 50 to 60 degrees worth of projection data for a given phase of the cardiac cycle, are needed. The scheme of projection collection for angles between 0 and 240 degrees

is depicted in Figures 36.9 and 36.10. A 3-D reconstruction with this data set will result in rendering of the heart morphology right before the P wave of the EKG.

5.4 Gated cardiac reconstructions for fpVCT

Recently, fpVCT scanners have also started allowing EKG gating and gated reconstructions. Since these systems are not FDA approved, all imaging to date has been performed on animals or using ex vivo specimens from cadaver parts. While the images obtained are not from living humans, they leave no doubt about potential clinical utility of this technology.

For the purpose of illustrating the technique and the practical considerations that need to be employed, we now briefly describe EKG gated fpVCT scanning technique for evaluation of heart in mice (C3H/HeN wild type mice each weighing ~30 g). For the contrast-enhanced scan, 0.5 ml blood-pool contrast media (Fenestra VC, 50 mg Iodine/ml; ART Advanced Research Technologies, Saint-Laurent, CA)[16] was injected into a tail vein. The animals were anesthetized by continuous inhalation of 3% (by volume) Sevoflurane (Sevorane, Abbot, Maidenhead, UK) in oxygen during preparation, injection of contrast media and scanning. ECG electrodes and the pneumatic cushion from a commercially available small animal monitoring unit (1025L and Signal Breakout Module, SA Instruments, Stony Brook, NY, USA) were attached to the animal to record the physiological data.

The physiological data recorded by ECG electrodes and pneumatic cushion for respiratory gating were time-stamped on each X-ray projection. The ECG electrodes provided

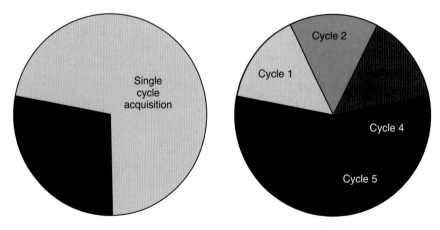

Figure 36.9   Schematic representation of data acquisition for half-sector reconstruction (left) and multi-sector reconstruction using 5 cycles (right).

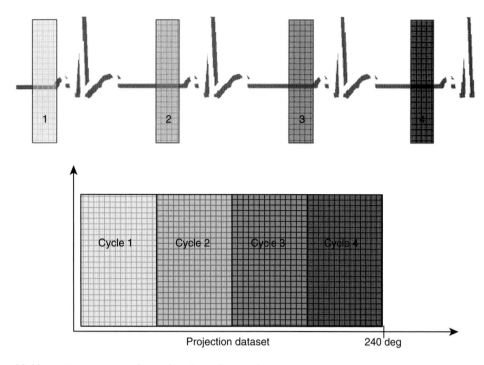

Figure 36.10 Multi-sector reconstruction using 4 cardiac cycles.

information about the cardiac cycle while the pneumatic cushion recorded the information about the respiratory cycle. An example of the recorded ECG as well as respiratory curves is shown in Figure 36.11.

The animals were free breathing during the scan. Total scan duration was 80s with a rotation time of 5s resulting in 16 full rotations per scan. A tube voltage of 80 kV and a tube current of 50 mA were selected.

For motion-gated reconstruction from the projection data, a multi-sector reconstruction technique was used. Several rotations were retrospectively sorted to compose new 'multi-phase' dataset as follows. For each phase, projections that were acquired within certain time frames of the

cardiac and respiratory cycle were selected for image reconstruction. Each phase was defined by its start and end points expressed as percentage of the cardiac or respiratory cycle.

The cardiac cycle in an RR interval was divided into 10 distinct phases. From all acquired projections, those corresponding to a given phase of cardiac and respiratory cycle were assembled into a new 360 data set consisting of 600 evenly distributed projections. Angularly weighted interpolation was used to fit the actual projection positions to the new projection positions within this dataset.

The reconstruction field-of-view was 4.5 cm transaxially with a reconstruction matrix of 512 × 512 pixels and an axial slice spacing 0.2 mm resulting in a voxel size of 0.08 ×

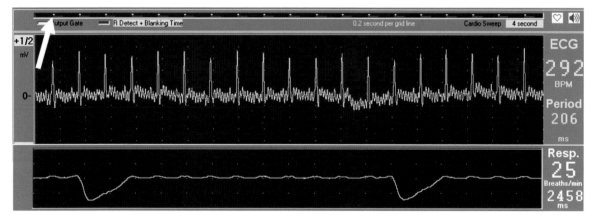

Figure 36.11 ECG signal (top curve) and respiratory gating signal (bottom curve) showing the fast heart rate and respiratory cycles. The white arrow shows the trigger pulse that was used for gating.

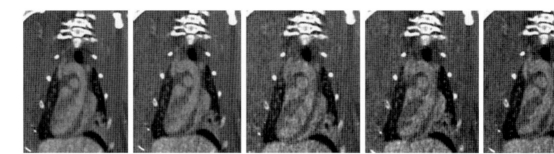

Figure 36.12   A multi-phasic reconstruction of the cardiac cycle of a mouse from a 4-D time series of the heart with respiratory and cardiac gating. Various 10% wide segments (10%, 30%, 50%, 60%, and 70%) of the cardiac cycle in oblique coronal plane are shown. The heart rate was approximately 300 beats/minute.

0.08×0.2 mm^3. A high spatial resolution kernel (H80s) was used for image reconstruction. Figure 36.12 shows a sample multi-phase reconstruction. Despite the small size of the anatomy being studied, and the fast cardiac rate approaching 300 beats/minute, the widening of the ventricle from an end-systole to end-diastole can be easily appreciated.

6 POTENTIAL ADVANTAGES AND APPLICATIONS OF CARDIAC fpVCT IMAGING

There are four main advantages of fpVCT as compared with MDCT:

1. High resolution,
2. Volumetric coverage,
3. Dynamic imaging, and
4. Omni-scanning (combined fluoroscopy and tomography).

In the following subsections, we discuss the potential applications of each of these four key attributes of fpVCT in the domain of cardiac imaging.

6.1 High resolution imaging

FpVCT provides a spatial resolution of 150 microns, which is a factor of 3 better than MDCT. However, the contrast resolution of fpVCT is about 5 HU, which is slightly inferior to that available on MDCT. Therefore, applications that require imaging of high contrast objects in exquisite detail will benefit most from fpVCT. Imaging of calcified coronary atherosclerotic plaque, contrast enhanced coronary arteries, and imaging of cardiac stents fall in this category.

Pathological examinations of human lesions have found that plaque rupture of unstable plaques is the most common

cause of acute coronary events. It is widely accepted that the severity of a coronary stenosis is not an accurate predictor of the site responsible for future plaque rupture. Imaging approaches that produce luminograms are necessary for the accurate identification of flow-limiting stenoses which are typically caused by stable plaques. One major limitation of luminograms is that the main artery lumen can appear normal, albeit advanced atherosclerotic disease may exit within the vessel wall.

Currently, IVUS (80–150 μm in plane resolution) is the only established modality for imaging coronary plaques within the artery wall, but it requires cardiac catheterization. IVUS can measure vessel wall structures including luminal area, plaque area, positive remodeling and can provide an estimate of total plaque burden.[13,14] Based on ultrasound reflection, IVUS can differentiate calcified from soft plaques, however, differentiation of fibrous and lipid tissue is difficult.

While intravascular approaches may be of value for patients already scheduled for coronary catheterization, a non-invasive measure to detect and characterize plaques is needed to manage the majority of patients with asymptomatic CAD and for the large cohort of patients at very high risk for cardiac events. Recent developments in MDCT and dual-source CT allow ECG-gated acquisition of up to 256 images in 83–165 seconds, enabling evaluation of cardiac vessels, structure and function during a single breath hold.[24] Several investigators have demonstrated high sensitivity and specificity of the 64-slice MDCT to identify coronary stenoses in patients in artifact free segments (i.e., those segments that have not been rendered non-evaluable by calcium, motion artifact, or scanner resolution).[25–27]

While conventional 64-slice MDCT imaging, and more recently dual source CT scanning, can identify lesions within the coronary wall, the spatial, temporal, and contrast resolution are still limited for assessment of plaque vulnerability, in-stent luminal evaluation, and coronary arteries with heavy calcification. Due to relatively large voxel size of MDCT, there is accentuation of partial volume effect in MDCT images. When imaging sharply delimited high-contrast objects such as calcified atherosclerotic plaques in coronary arteries, this partial volume artefact manifests itself as broadening of the edge of the calcium, resulting in the so-called 'calcium blooming' artefact.

The calcium blooming artefact not only obscures important structures in the surroundings (e.g., the lipid core of an atheromatous calcified plaque), it makes the lumen of the coronary artery appear artificially narrower than it

actually is. The resulting overcall can easily lead to up-staging the state of the atherosclerotic disease. For example, such an artefact may turn a *moderate* stenosis into *severe* stenosis. This may result in up-staging the disease burden, with potentially serious consequences. Such a false-positive result may convert a patient who potentially could have been managed using conservative medical treatment into a candidate for surgical coronary-artery bypass graft.

Our initial experiments with ex-vivo coronary arteries suggest that fpVCT is associated with substantially less calcium blooming as compared to MDCT (Figure 36.13). Higher resolution of fpVCT also results in better metal

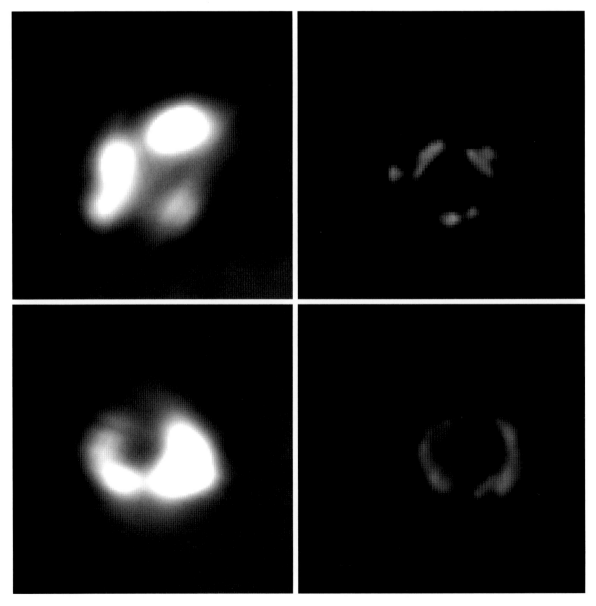

Figure 36.13 Comparison of cross-sections through calcified plaques using MDCT (left) and fpVCT (right) on coronary specimens (top – LAD, bottom – RCA). Notice that the calcium blooming artifacts are substantially reduced by the small voxel size offered by fpVCT.

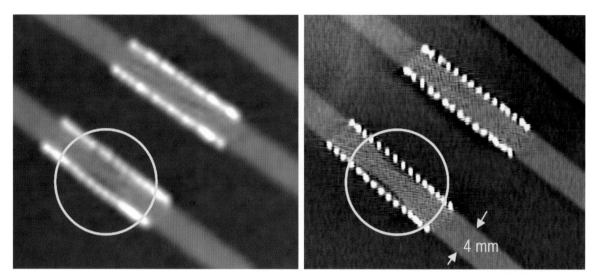

Figure 36.14 Multiplanar reformatted image of coronary stents. Note the fidelity in fpVCT images (right) for visualization of the stent struts and in-stent lumen as compared with MDCT images (left). (Image courtesy of Jennifer Lisauskas, Fabian Moselewski and Ray Chan.)

artifact profile for coronary stent evaluation. Thus metallic stents can be visualized, and their lumen can be interrogated (Figure 36.14).

6.2 Volumetric coverage

The size of the flat-panel along the axial dimension (i.e., along Z) is 30 cm. This translates into a field of view of about 18 cm along Z. For comparison, the traditional 16 or 64 row CT scanners have a FOV of about 2 to 4 cm. Thus both projection and tomographic views of an entire organ or a large tissue volume are possible using fpVCT.

An example of larger volumetric coverage with fpVCT is illustrated in Figure 36.15. A New Zealand rabbit was anesthetized and a peripheral IV line was started via the left femoral vein. Post-contrast (I+) scans were performed by continuously rotating the gantry for 40 seconds with a rotation time of 5 seconds. For the I+ scan, 15cc of non-ionic, hypo-osmolar contrast (Omnipaque, Amersham Health) was injected 5 seconds after the start of the scan. This ensured that the first scan was a pre-contrast scan, while the subsequent scans showed the evolution of the contrast bolus through the heart. The 3-D images, and the generated movies (not shown) from the resulting datasets demonstrated excellent image quality and wide coverage

available from a single rotation of the scanner. Even with non-optimized injection time, fpVCT was able to show fine cardiac and vascular details (Figure 36.15).

6.3 Dynamic imaging

The ability of fpVCT to cover a large volume during one rotation, together with relatively short rotation times and ability to rotate continuously, allow dynamic imaging studies of tissue or vessels. If the temporal resolution is short enough – and the imaging is conducted for an appropriate length of time depending on the tissue type being studied – the evolution of a contrast bolus can be followed through the arteries, soft-tissue, veins, viscera, and bone. Using such a dataset, a perfusion study of these tissues can be performed, making it possible to combine fpVCT-angiography and fpVCT-perfusion in one dynamic imaging process.

Once projection data is acquired through multiple, continuous rotations, a continuous sequence of projections that captures the dynamics of the scene in evolution is available. In order to reconstruct a volumetric dataset at any time T, one can simply use the projections from 360° centered on time T. A 4-D sequence of a dynamic process, using overlapping or non-overlapping 3-D datasets, can thus be acquired. The temporal resolution of this dataset will be

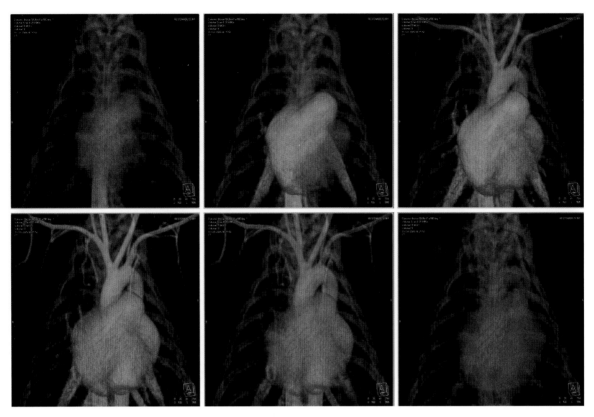

Figure 36.15 Multiple volume rendered images from a dynamic 4-D acquisition of a rabbit heart and large thoracic vessels acquired using fpVCT.

equal to the rotation time of the gantry. The time increment between successive 3D volumes can be arbitrarily chosen.

Figure 36.15 shows the dynamic evolution of the injected bolus as it travels from the IVC, to the right atrium, right ventricle, pulmonary artery, pulmonary veins, the left side of the heart, the systemic circulation, and then into the venous return phase.

Dynamic fpVCT can be adapted to the requirements of various imaging problems. For example, the temporal resolution can be increased by acquiring less projections allowing for a faster rotation. Partial read out of the flat-panel detector can further increase the temporal resolution at the expense of volumetric coverage.

6.4 Omni-scanning

The fpVCT technology can be used as an 'omni-scanner,' that is, a CT scanner that combines X-ray fluoroscopy and computed tomography (CT) in one highly flexible system. The scanner can be parked in one position to obtain fluoroscopic imaging from any arbitrary angle in space, or can be rotated continuously to visualize temporal evolution of a dynamic process. These features form the basis of omni-scanner capability.

These features are independent of what type of gantry the flat-panel detector is mounted in. In fact, one can already find these features in the newer angiographic C-arm gantries that utilize the digital flat-panel detector technology. Figure 36.16 shows one such gantry (Axiom Artis dTC, Siemens Medical Solutions, Germany). Besides all the traditional capabilities of a C-arm system, these systems allow 3-D spin angiography and tomographic capabilities. For spin angiography, one can obtain pre- and post-contrast image sets and do a 3-D reconstruction using the subtracted images. This facility is quite useful in visualization of aneurysms and other vascular pathologies. One can also acquire a set of projection images and reconstruct them in 3-D. If these images are gated, it is possible to perform gated cardiac reconstructions of different

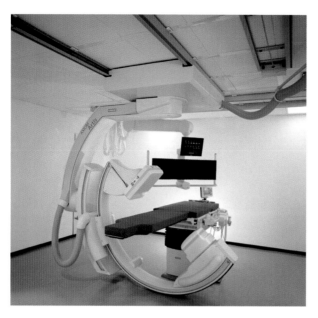

Figure 36.16 A C-arm system with a digital flat-panel detector (Axiom Artis, Siemens Medical Solutions, Germany).

phases of the cardiac cycle. On such example is shown in Figure 36.17 (courtesy of Drs. Rebecca Fahrig and Amin Alahmad, Stanford University). To generate this figure, a set of EKG-gated projections were acquired and sorted into different bins representing the phase of the cardiac cycle. Each bin was then independently reconstructed. As can be seen in

Figure 36.17, the expansion of the LV between systole and diastole can be appreciated. Such data can be used, among other things, to estimate the ejection fraction. The fact that this data is truly a set of 3-D volumes evolving over time is illustrated in Figure 36.18. In this figure short axis views of the heart at different phases of cardiac cycle, and in different cardiac planes are shown. The image quality and spatial resolution are good enough to show the cross-section of coronary arteries.

Other potential applications of such ultra-high resolution imaging include 3-D cardiac angiography, intra-operative CT-imaging, and dynamic studies of time evolving processes such as myocardial function, first-pass of contrast bolus through the heart, and myocardial perfusion.

7 SUMMARY

In summary, flat panel volume CT technology has made tremendous advances in terms of superior spatial resolution, scan volume coverage, and omni-scanning. Initial animal and ex-vivo human specimen experiments suggest that fpVCT may have important application in human cardiac scanning. However, higher radiation dose, and relatively poor temporal resolution compared to MDCT of the heart, are potential limitations of fpVCT for cardiac imaging.

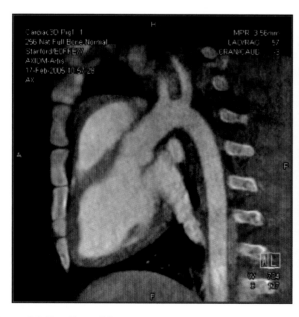
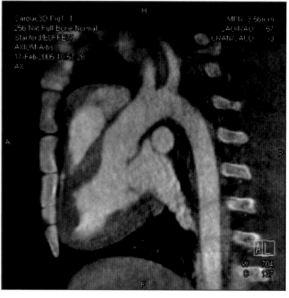

Figure 36.17 Two oblique sagittal views through a pig thorax showing the heart in diastole (left) and systole (right). (Images courtesy of Drs. Rebecca Fahrig and Amin Al-Ahmad, Stanford University).

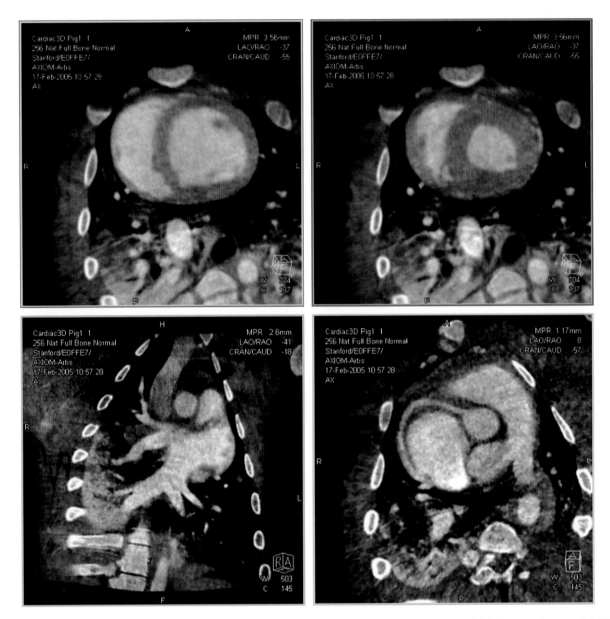

Figure 36.18   Short axis views through the LV in diastole (upper left) and systole (upper right) in a porcine model. The ejection fraction can be accurately estimated using such views. A view of the pulmonary veins from an oblique sagittal perspective (lower left). An oblique axial image showing the origin of the RCA in the sinus of Valsalva. (Images courtesy of Drs. Rebecca Fahrig and Amin Al-Ahmad, Stanford University).

REFERENCES

1. American Heart Association. Heart Disease and Stroke Statistics – 2003 Update. Dallas, TX: American Heart Association, 2003.

2. Chandrasekar B, Doucet S, Bilodeau L et al. Complications of cardiac catheterization in the current era: a single-center experience. Catheter Cardiovasc Interv 2001; 52: 289–95.

3. Kaandorp TA, Lamb HJ, Bax JJ, van der Wall EE, de Roos A. Magnetic resonance imaging of coronary arteries, the ischemic cascade, and myocardial infarction. Am Heart J 2005; 149: 200–8.

4. Yeh EN, McKenzie CA, Ohliger MA, Sodickson DK. Parallel magnetic resonance imaging with adaptive radius in k-space (PARS): Constrained image reconstruction using k-space locality in radiofrequency coil encoded data. Magn Reson Med 2005; 53: 1383–92.

5. Hoffmann U, Dunn E, d'Othee BJ. Is CT angiography ready for prime time? A meta-analysis. J Am Coll Cardiol 2004; 43 (Suppl A): 312A.

6. Nieman K, Cademartiri F, Lemos PA et al. Reliable noninvasive coronary angiography with fast submillimeter multislice spiral computed tomography. Circulation 2002; 106: 2051–4.

7. Ropers D, Baum U, Pohle K et al. Detection of coronary artery stenoses with thin-slice multi-detector row spiral computed tomography and multiplanar reconstruction. Circulation 2003; 107: 664–6.

8. Hoffmann U, Moselewski F, Cury RC et al. Predictive value of 16-slice multidetector spiral computed tomography to detect significant obstructive coronary artery disease in patients at high risk for coronary artery disease: patient-versus segment-based analysis. Circulation 2004; 110: 2638–43.

9. Mollet NR, Cademartiri F, Nieman K et al. Multislice spiral computed tomography coronary angiography in patients with stable angina pectoris. J Am Coll Cardiol 2004; 43: 2265–70.

10. Mollet NR, Cademartiri F, Krestin GP et al. Improved diagnostic accuracy with 16-row multi-slice computed tomography coronary angiography. J Am Coll Cardiol 2005; 45: 128–32.

11. Kuettner A, Trabold T, Schroeder S et al. Noninvasive detection of coronary lesions using 16-detector multislice spiral computed tomography technology: initial clinical results. J Am Coll Cardiol 2004; 44: 1230–7.

12. Kuettner A, Beck T, Drosch T et al. Diagnostic accuracy of noninvasive coronary imaging using 16-detector slice spiral computed tomography with 188 ms temporal resolution. J Am Coll Cardiol 2005; 45: 123–7.

13. Dewey M, Laule M, Krug L et al. Multisegment and halfscan reconstruction of 16-slice computed tomography for detection of coronary artery stenoses. Invest Radiol 2004; 39: 223–9.

14. Achenbach S, Giesler T, Ropers D et al. Comparison of image quality in contrast-enhanced coronary-artery visualization by electron beam tomography and retrospectively electrocardiogram-gated multislice spiral computed tomography. Invest Radiol 2003; 38: 119–28.

15. Achenbach S, Ulzheimer S, Baum U et al. Noninvasive coronary angiography by retrospectively ECG-gated multislice spiral CT. Circulation 2000; 102: 2823–8.

16. Nieman K, Oudkerk M, Rensing BJ et al. Coronary angiography with multi-slice computed tomography. Lancet 2001; 357: 599–603.

17. Achenbach S, Giesler T, Ropers D et al. Detection of coronary artery stenoses by contrast-enhanced, retrospectively electrocardiographically-gated, multislice spiral computed tomography. Circulation 2001; 103: 2535–8.

18. Gerber TC, Kuzo RS, Lane GE et al. Image quality in a standardized algorithm for minimally invasive coronary angiography with multislice spiral computed tomography. J Comput Assist Tomogr 2003; 27: 62–9.

19. Giesler T, Baum U, Ropers D et al. Noninvasive visualization of coronary arteries using contrast-enhanced multidetector CT: influence of heart rate on image quality and stenosis detection. AJR Am J Roentgenol 2002; 179: 911–6.

20. Morgan-Hughes GJ, Marshall AJ, Roobottom CA. Multislice computed tomographic coronary angiography: experience in a UK centre. Clin Radiol 2003; 58: 378–83.

21. Leber AW, Knez A, Becker C et al. Non-invasive intravenous coronary angiography using electron beam tomography and multislice computed tomography. Heart 2003; 89: 633–9.

22. Ferencik M, Moselewski F, Ropers D et al. Quantitative parameters of image quality in multidetector spiral computed tomographic coronary imaging with submillimeter collimation. Am J Cardiol 2003; 92: 1257–62.

23. Martuscelli E, Romagnoli A, D'Eliseo A et al. Accuracy of thin-slice computed tomography in the detection of coronary stenoses. Eur Heart J 2004; 25: 1043–8.

24. Schuijf JD, Bax JJ, Salm LP et al. Noninvasive coronary imaging and assessment of left ventricular function using 16-slice computed tomography. Am J Cardiol 2005; 95: 571–4.

25. Morgan-Hughes GJ, Roobottom CA, Owens PE, Marshall AJ. Highly accurate coronary angiography with submillimetre, 16 slice computed tomography. Heart 2005; 91: 308–13.

26. Kitagawa T, Fujii T, Tomohiro Y et al. Ability for visualization, reasons for nonassessable image, and diagnostic accuracy of 16-slice multidetector row helical computed tomography for the assessment of the entire coronary arteries. The American Journal of Cardiology 2005; 95: 1079.

27. Thompson BH, Stanford W. Imaging of coronary calcification by computed tomography. J Magn Reson Imaging 2004; 19: 720–33.

28. Barrett JF, Keat N. Artifacts in CT: recognition and avoidance. Radiographics 2004; 24: 1679–91.

29. Hsieh J. Image artifacts, causes, and correction. In: Goldman L, Fowlkes J, eds. Medical CT and Ultrasound, current technology and applications. Madison: Advanced Medical Publishing, 1995: 487–518.

30. DeMan B, Nuyts J, Dupont P, Marchal G, Suetens P. Metal Streak Artifacts in X-Ray Computed Tomography: A simulation study. IEEE Trans Nuclear Sci 1999; 46: 691–6.

31. Nikolaou K, Flohr T, Stierstorfer K, Becker CR, Reiser MF. Flat panel computed tomography of human ex vivo heart and bone specimens: initial experience. Eur Radiol 2005; 15(2): 329–33.

32. Kalender WA, The use of flat-panel detectors for CT imaging. Radiology 2003; 43: 379–87.

33. Engelke K, Karolczak M, Lutz A et al. [Micro-CT. Technology and application for assessing bone structure]. Radiology 1999; 39(3): 203–12.

34. Kalender WA. [The use of flat-panel detectors for CT imaging]. Radiology 2003; 43(5): 379–87.

35. Grasruck M, Suess C, Stierstorfer K, Popescu S, Flohr T. Evaluation of Image Quality and Dose on a Flat-Panel CT-Scanner 2005.

36. Bartling S, Gupta R, Torkos A et al. Flat-panel Volume-CT (fpVCT) for cochlear implant electrode array examination in isolated temporal bone specimens. Otology & Neurootology 2005.

37. Gupta R, Bartling SH, Basu SK et al. Experimental flat-panel high-spatial-resolution volume CT of the temporal bone. AJNR Am J Neuroradiol. 2004; 25(8): 1417–24.

38. Baba R, Ueda K, Okabe M. Using a flat-panel detector in high resolution cone beam CT for dental imaging. Dentomaxillofac Radiol 2004; 33(5): 285–90.

39. Groh BA, Siewerdsen JH, Drake DG, Wong JW, Jaffray DA. A performance comparison of flat-panel image-based MV and kV cone-beam CT. Med Phys 2002; 29(6): 967–75.

40. Marten K, Funke M, Engelke C. Flat panel detector-based volumetric CT: prototype evaluation with volumetry of small artificial nodules in a pulmonary phantom. J Thorac Imaging 2004; 19(3): 156–63.

41. Marten K, Engelke C, Grabbe E, Rummeny EJ. [Flat-panel detector-based computed tomography: accuracy of experimental growth rate assessment in pulmonary nodules]. Rofo 2004; 176(5): 752–7.

42. Mahnken AH, Seyfarth T, Flohr T et al. Flat-panel detector computed tomography for the assessment of coronary artery stents: phantom study in comparison with 16-slice spiral computed tomography. Invest Radiol 2005; 40(1): 8–13.

43. Lee SC, Kim HK, Chun IK et al. A flat-panel detector based micro-CT system: performance evaluation for small-animal imaging. Phys Med Biol 2003; 48(24): 4173–85.

44. Kiessling F, Greschus S, Lichy MP et al. Volumetric computed tomography (VCT): a new technology for noninvasive, high-resolution monitoring of tumor angiogenesis. Nat Med 2004; 10(10): 1133–8.

45. Greschus S, Kiessling F, Lichy MP et al. Potential applications of flat-panel volumetric CT in morphologic and functional small animal imaging. Neoplasia 2005; 7(8): 730–40.

46. Siewerdsen JH, Moseley DJ, Burch S et al. Volume CT with a flat-panel detector on a mobile, isocentric C-arm: pre-clinical investigation in guidance of minimally invasive surgery. Med Phys 2005; 32(1): 241–54.

47. Rafferty MA, Siewerdsen JH, Chan Y et al. Investigation of C-Arm Cone-Beam CT-Guided Surgery of the Frontal Recess. Laryngoscope 2005; 115(12): 2138–2143.

48. Dalchow CV, Weber AL, Bien S, Yanagihara N, Werner JA. Value of digital volume tomography in patients with conductive hearing loss. Eur Arch Otorhinolaryngol 2005.

49. Ross W, Cody DD, Hazle JD. Design and performance characteristics of a digital flat panel computed tomography system. Med Phys 2006 Jun; 33(6): 1888–901.

37

Micro Computed Tomography

Marc Kachelrieß

I INTRODUCTION

Tomographic imaging started with clinical x-ray computed tomography (CT) in 1972.[1] Since then, CT technology has advanced significantly and clinical CT became radiology's powerhouse. In addition to clinical CT imaging there is an increasing need for pre-clinical examinations such as scans of tissue samples, organs or whole animals (in-vitro or in-vivo) that are used as models to evaluate human diseases and therapies.[2] For example non-invasive imaging of mice gains in importance due to recent advances in mouse genomics and the production of transgenic mouse models. Longitudinal studies that use a single animal population can provide internally consistent long-term data and help to reduce the number of sacrificed animals and to cut down the costs.

Since many of the objects of interest are far smaller than a human body, and since one is interested in imaging vessels, bone structures or other details of microscopic size, clinical CT scanners are not suitable for many pre-clinical imaging tasks. For example laboratory mice or rats have a diameter of less than 5 cm. Compared to the 50 cm diameter of a clinical CT scanner's field of measurement (FOM) this is 10% or less. Only one tenth of the detector elements would be used when scanning such a specimen in a clinical CT scanner and, evidently, the small animal anatomy cannot be imaged in a clinical CT scanner with an image quality equivalent to the human anatomy. This low efficiency calls for dedicated scanners that are specialized for small objects and high spatial resolution, which is the reason why all clinical imaging modalities have been scaled down during the last years.

Higher spatial resolution requires dedicated micro-CT scanners which are usually defined to achieve a spatial resolution of 100 µm or better.[3] Micro-CT scanners have a smaller FOM compared with clinical CT scanners and their design ranges from micro-CTs as large as clinical CT scanners to small desktop scanners that easily integrate into the laboratory (Figure 37.1).

The basic principles of micro-CT are the same as in clinical CT: attenuation is measured for a large number of line integrals and image reconstruction is typically based on the filtered backprojection (FBP) algorithm. For cone-beam geometries, such as the flat panel detector-based micro-CT geometries, the Feldkamp image reconstruction algorithm is used[4] which is of filtered backprojection type. In contrast to clinical CT where spiral scans are dominant one uses circle scans in micro-CT. The reason is the large coverage that can be achieved by a simple circular scan due to the large size of the area detector.

2 GEOMETRY

Modern micro-CT scanners are equipped with an x-ray tube and a flat panel area detector consisting of at least 1,000 by 1,000 detector pixels. (The older designs where only a single slice is measured will not be discussed in this chapter.) Either the object rotates relative to the source-detector-arrangement or the source and detector rotate around the object (Figure 37.2). Collimators are used to avoid radiation

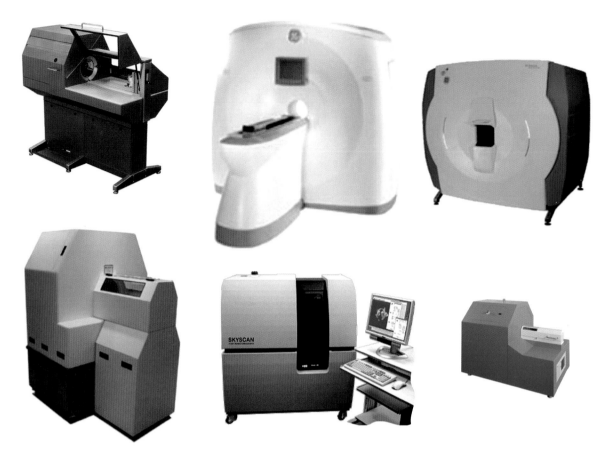

Figure 37.1   Typical micro-CT scanners as they can be used for preclinical imaging. From top left to bottom right: Gamma Medica, GE, Scanco, Siemens, Skyscan, and VAMP.

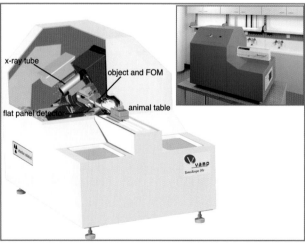

Figure 37.2   Rotating object type micro-CTs are typically used for non-destructive material testing or for in-vitro studies. Dedicated in-vivo small animal micro-CT scanners have a stationary object and a rotating source-detector-system.

in those regions that are not covered by the detector. They can also be used to limit the longitudinal exposure range (z-range) if only a few slices shall be reconstructed. For today's rectangular flat-panel detectors the shape of the x-ray ensemble is a pyramid; due to mathematical and historical reasons it is loosely called a cone-beam.

The rotation axis of the scanner defines the z-axis (longitudinal axis), the x- and y-axes are perpendicular thereto and define the lateral plane. The lateral opening angle of the cone is called fan angle and the longitudinal angle is called cone angle, respectively (Figure 37.3). For square detectors that are perfectly aligned the fan angle equals the cone angle. The distance of the focal spot to the isocenter (rotation center) R_F and the distance focus detector R_{FD} are important parameters in micro-CT imaging. Together with the radial size U and the longitudinal size V of the detector they define the size of the cylinder that is measured in each projection during a 360° scan. This cylinder is called the field of measurement (FOM) and the object of interest must not exceed this volume laterally unless special techniques are used to enlarge the FOM (e.g. shifted detector, multiple scans or detruncation algorithms). For square detectors that are aligned parallel to the z-axis the cylinder's diameter always exceeds the cylinder's length.

Objects that exceed the FOM longitudinally are typically assessed by combining several circle scans.

3 MEASUREMENT, RECONSTRUCTION, DISPLAY

During a full rotation about 1,000 readouts of the detector are performed. Flat panel detectors with 1024^2 to 4096^2 detector pixels are in use. Altogether in the order of 10^9 intensity measurements are taken per rotation. Physically, micro-CT is the measurement of the object's x-ray absorption along straight lines, just as it is the case in clinical CT.

Image reconstruction is one of the key components of a micro-CT scanner. The Feldkamp algorithm that is typically used is of filtered backprojection type and similar to the image reconstruction implemented in clinical CT scanners for step-and-shoot scans. Reconstruction times can range from some minutes up to one hour or even more, depending on the number of voxels used and the number of projections acquired. Image reconstruction is an $O(N)^4$ process when N projections are backprojected into a volume of size N^3. The constant of proportionality lies in the range of 2 ns to 10 ns for today's micro-CT reconstruction engines, which means

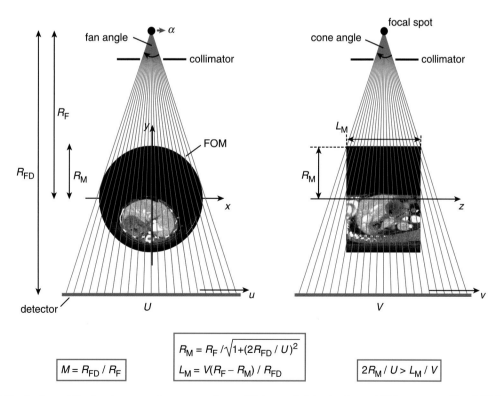

$$M = R_{FD} / R_F$$

$$R_M = R_F / \sqrt{1+(2R_{FD} / U)^2}$$
$$L_M = V(R_F - R_M) / R_{FD}$$

$$2R_M / U > L_M / V$$

Figure 37.3 Illustration of the basic geometry parameters of flat panel detector-based CT scanners. The FOM shown here is of 40 mm diameter and filled with an anesthetized mouse. The magnification M depends on the ratio of the distance focal spot to detector to the distance focal spot to isocenter.

that a 512^3 reconstruction from 512 projections should be definitely finished in less than five minutes.

Alike in clinical CT the reconstructed voxel values are often converted into CT values prior to storage: the gray values are approximately proportional to the mass density, air has a CT value of –1000 HU (Hounsfield units) and water has a CT value of 0 HU.

Micro-CT images are either stored in a proprietary image format or in DICOM format. In the first case the micro-CT manufacturer's viewing workstation must be used for image display and analysis. In case of DICOM images the user is free to select any other state-of-the-art viewing workstation.

4 MICRO-CT DESIGN

As previously indicated two basic design concepts are realized in micro-CT: the stationary tube-detector system with rotating object and the rotating gantry with stationary object. Many of the commercial products are self-shielded and need no further radiation shielding.

For in-vitro imaging the design using a rotating object with fixed focal spot detector is the method of choice (Figure 37.2, left). The design is robust and cost-efficient since the number of components moving during the scan – these must be of highest precision to allow for high spatial resolution – is minimized to the rotation stage only. Further on, this design easily allows to change the magnification of the scanner by repositioning the rotation stage. Hence variable spatial resolution values can be achieved with minimum technical effort.

A serious drawback of the rotating object scanners is the object placement since the rotation axis and thus the object are usually oriented vertically. Regardless of what the actual orientation of the rotation axis is, be it vertical or horizontal or something else, the object is subject to centrifugal or varying gravitational forces. This plays no role for rigid samples but motion artifacts may impair image quality when flexible objects or liquids are scanned, in particular animals or animal samples.

Scanners with a rotating source-detector system are more complicated with respect to the mechanical setup but they provide far more comfort regarding the object placement. The rotating gantry is usually mounted with a horizontal rotation axis to allow placing the object on a simple table (Figure 37.2, right). This resembles clinical CT scanners that also have a patient bed and a rotating gantry. The mechanical design of rotating source-detector scanners is far more demanding, since high precision rotation

components must be used and care must be taken that the varying gravitational forces do neither change the rotation speed nor change the mechanical alignment of the source and the detector relative to each other and relative to the rotation axis. Typically, in-vivo scanners use the rotating source-detector micro-CT but there are also industrial applications for non-destructive material testing where the use at conveyor belts dictates this design.

5 TYPICAL PARAMETERS, IMAGE QUALITY AND DOSE

At first sight, micro-CT appears very similar to clinical CT, except for the higher spatial resolution and the smaller field of measurement. However, tube technology and flat-panel detector technology are quite different. First of all, the high spatial resolution requires a small x-ray focal spot which in turn implies very low tube power. A rule of thumb is that the maximum power per focal spot area lies in the order of $1 \text{ W}/\mu\text{m}^2$. In some cases, scan speed may be limited by the low tube power; the need for dose accumulation that is required to obtain low-noise images requires to increase the scan time. The detector, however, is limiting scan speed more drastically since the read-out of millions of detector pixels is technically demanding. The frame rates achieved by modern flat-panel detectors are in the range of 1 to 50 frames per second. High frame rates often require a detector binning where 2 by 2 physical detector pixels are combined to yield one logical detector element. Needless to say that binning yields a reduced spatial resolution. If the achievable frame rate is too low a fast scan time can only be achieved by taking less projections per rotation than actual necessary. This angular undersampling yields an angular blurring and hence significantly reduced image quality in the peripheral regions of the images. Today, typical scan times in micro-CT range from 1 second to many minutes. Given the high heart rates of small animals and the low temporal resolution of today's micro-CT devices, and compared to clinical CT, there is currently little potential of in-vivo motion-resolved cardiovascular imaging with micro-CT.

Another drawback of current micro-CT detector technology is the low dynamic range of the flat panel detectors. In contrast to clinical CT detectors, which offer 20 or even 22 bits of dynamic range, flat panel detectors achieve a dynamic range of only 12 to 14 bits. Consequently, the low contrast resolution achieved with micro-CT is inferior to clinical CT where 5 to 10 HU contrast resolution can be easily observed.

Altogether these points, high image noise due to lower count rates and lower contrast resolution due to low detector dynamics, show that micro-CT image quality still is inferior to clinical CT image quality. Obviously, there is room for improvement and certainly the detector generations coming up will provide improved image quality with flat panel detector-based CT.

Further on, dose is an issue in in-vivo micro-CT imaging of animals where radiation damage to the object must be avoided. Even if there is no deterministic risk to be expected – this is the case whenever dose levels are far below, say, 1 Gy – the measurement may influence those parameters that shall be observed in pre-clinical imaging. Tumor growth, for example, may be modified by a micro-CT scan with high dose levels. Especially for longitudinal studies that require multiple scans of the very same animal dose levels may become critical.

There are two reasons why dose in micro-CT is increased compared to clinical CT. One is that the dose required to saturate the detector is determined by the absorption efficiency of the detector. A high absorption efficiency means a good dose usage and can reduce the total scan time. In clinical CT, where the detectors are structured and septa between the detectors avoid that light travels from one detector element to its neighbors, thick scintillator layers are used and an absorption efficiency of above 95% can be easily achieved. However, in flat panel detectors unstructured scintillators are used and a high absorption efficiency would require thick layers of scintillators, which in turn would significantly impair spatial resolution. Here the absorption efficiency lies in the order of 50% for typical detectors. Hence about 50% of the x-ray photons and thereby about 50% of the animal dose remain unused.

Another reason for higher dose levels in micro-CT is the spatial resolution itself. It can be shown that the dose required to achieve a given spatial resolution level in tomographic imaging is proportional to the fourth power of spatial resolution.[5,6] As an example assume one wants to switch from 100 μm to 50 μm spatial resolution. If one cannot accept an increase of image noise for the 50 μm scan compared with the 100 μm scan one would have to use the 16-fold mAs-value, and hence apply the 16-fold dose. Therefore one must always compromise between spatial resolution and image noise or dose – just as in clinical CT image noise decreases with the square-root of dose – and high resolution scans will have a low low-contrast detectability due to large image noise unless dose is significantly increased.

The tube voltage largely determines the x-ray spectrum that is used for CT scanning. Image quality is also a function of the x-ray spectrum, object size, shape and density.[7,8] This is the case for clinical CT as well as for micro-CT. The tube voltage should be decreased with decreasing object size and density. This dependence on object size is more significant for small objects than it is for large objects, since for low energies photon attenuation is dominated by the photo effect that is strongly energy-dependent. Tube voltages typical for micro-CT can be as low as 10 kV whereas a clinical CT scanner's lowest tube voltage is 80 kV. For example objects of a diameter of 3 to 4 cm, such as small rodents, are best scanned at voltages around 40 kV.

The table below lists important parameters as they are typically provided in today's clinical CT scanners and in flat-panel detector CT scanners (C-arm CT and micro-CT).

Although the previous discussion lists numerous disadvantages of micro-CT technology compared to clinical CT

	Clinical CT	C-arm CT	In-vivo micro-CT	In-vitro micro-CT
Dominant trajectory	Spiral	Circle	Circle	Circle
Spatial resolution	250–1000 μm	200–400 μm	50–200 μm	1–200 μm
FOM diameter	500–700 mm	100–250 mm	30–100 mm	1–200 mm
Tube voltage	80–140 kV	50–125 kV	10–160 kV	10–160 kV
Tube current	10–600 mA	10–800 mA	0.04–2 mA	0.04–2 mA
Tube power	20–100 kW	20–80 kW	1–30 W	1–30 W
Scan time	0.3–20 s	5–20 s	10 s–10 min	<1 h
mAs$_{eff}$	10–750 mAs	10–750 mAs	5–200 mAs	5–200 mAs
Detector	≈1000 × 64	1024^2–2048^2	1024^2–4096^2	1024^2–4096^2
Dose	1–70 mGy	1–70 mGy	50–500 mGy	≤1500 mGy
Acquisition rate	≤600 MB/s	≤60 MB/s	≤20 MB/s	≤20 MB/s

technology, one must emphasize that the increase in spatial resolution achieved with micro-CT is an enormous benefit or even a prerequisite for many applications, especially when thinking of preclinical imaging. Three prominent examples of the wide application spectrum are: (1) non-destructive material testing, such as the evaluation of stent implants, (2) the in-vivo bone densitometry and bone morphology assessment in small animals, and (3) in-vivo scans of complete animals with good soft tissue contrast resolution for longitudinal preclinical imaging studies. Typical micro-CT images are shown in Figure 37.4.

With respect to cardiovascular imaging micro-CT scans of specimen allow to detect atherosclerotic lesions in coronary vessels and to characterize lesion morphology (see chapter [Micro-CT-based plaque imaging, Langheinrich] of this book). Those examinations are done in vitro and not in vivo, however. Due to the limited temporal resolution, that is primarily dictated by the rotation time, one cannot apply similar techniques for phase-correlated imaging (4D imaging) as is the case in clinical CT, today (see chapter [Physics of and Approaches to Cardiovascular Computed Tomography, Kachelrieβ] of this book).

6 DISCUSSION AND OUTLOOK

Modern micro-CT scanners allow for micrometer spatial resolution and good contrast resolution. Image quality and dose usage have not approached clinical CT standards yet; compared to clinical CT micro-CT is still in its infancy. Further advances in micro-focus tube technology and flat-panel detector technology are expected to improve micro-CT dose usage, increase scan speed and to widen the dynamic range of the detectors until the physics of the underlying x-ray absorption mechanisms determine and thereby limit image quality.

Temporal resolution is probably the most critical issue, at least for in-vivo studies, and must still be improved to allow for dynamic studies or for phase-correlated imaging of the beating heart. Increased temporal resolution would

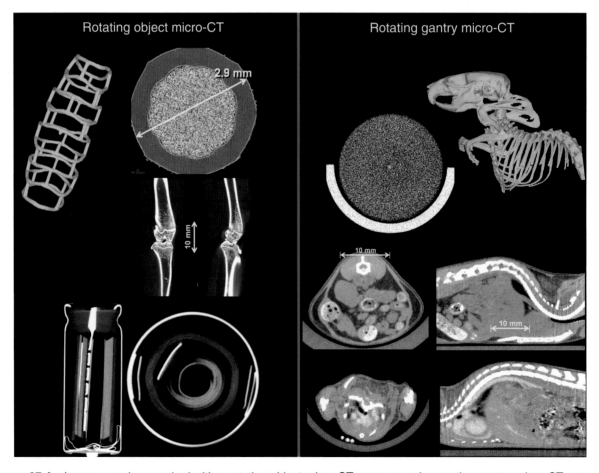

Figure 37.4 Image samples acquired with a rotating object micro-CT scanner and a rotating gantry micro-CT scanner. The objects shown are a tiny stent implanted in a pig's coronary artery, a butterfly catheter filled with glass particles, a rat knee, an electrolytic capacitor, a water phantom, a shaded surface display of an in-vivo mouse, and contrast-enhanced axial and sagittal displays of two in-vivo mice. The data were acquired with the scanners shown in Figure 37.2.

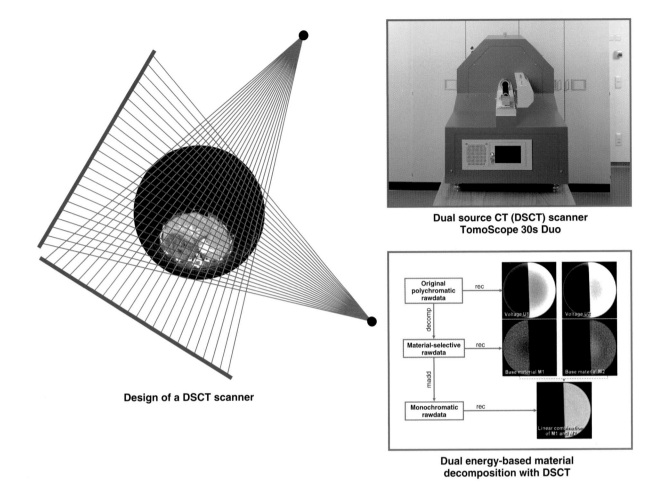

Design of a DSCT scanner

**Dual source CT (DSCT) scanner
TomoScope 30s Duo**

**Dual energy-based material
decomposition with DSCT**

Figure 37.5 Dual source CT scanners (DSCT), such as the TomoScope 30s Duo scanner (VAMP GmbH, Erlangen, Germany) allow for the simultaneous acquisition of the object with two spectra. These dual energy CT (DECT) scans allow to decompose the rawdata to show material-selective images.[10] These can be used to distinguish between tissue, plaques, calcification and contrast media, for example.

allow for the assessment of tissue kinematics and of cardiac motion and function. Higher detector frame-rates will certainly improve micro-CT temporal resolution in the near future. Combined with new scanner concepts that utilize two or three x-ray sources and detectors simultaneously the goal of high temporal resolution can be achieved more easily.[9]

These dual source CT (DSCT) scanners are in clinical use since 2005 and their micro-CT counterparts became available in early 2007. Besides aiming at increased temporal resolution – only a quarter gantry rotation is required with dual source CT – the simultaneous use of two different tube voltages opens the way to dual energy CT (DECT) and material-selective imaging. Here, new contrast mechanisms can be exploited that, for example, allow for an easy discrimination between plaque types or between contrast agent and calcifications (Figure 37.5). Dual source CT together with dual energy CT techniques have the potential to enter preclinical imaging routinely.[10]

Above all, there is a great need for specialized and dedicated micro-CT scan protocols with respect to animal handling, contrast agent and others. Certainly, micro-CT will grow up to finally keep up with clinical CT standards.

REFERENCES

1. Hounsfield GN. Computerized transverse axial scanning (tomography). Part I. Description of system. Br. J. Radiol. 1973; 46: 1016.
2. IEEE. Special issue on molecular imaging. IEEE Trans on Medical Imaging 2004; 24(7).
3. Kalender WA. Computed Tomography. Fundamentals, System Technology, Image Quality, Applications, 2005; 2nd ed. Publicis Erlangen.
4. Feldkamp LA, Davis LC, Kress JW. Practical cone-beam algorithm. J Optical Society America A 1984; 1(6): 612–19.
5. Brooks RA, Di Chiro G. Statistical limitations in X-ray reconstruction tomography. Med Phys 1976; 3: 237–40.
6. Ford NL, Thornton MM, Holdsworth DW et al. Fundamental image quality limits for microcomputed tomography in small animals. Med Phys 2003; 30(11): 2869–77.

7. Sekihara K, Kohno H, Yamamoto S. Theoretical prediction of X-ray CT image quality using contrast-detail diagrams. IEEE Trans Nucl Science NS-26 1982; (6): 2115–21.
8. Gkanatsios NA, Huda W. Computation of energy imparted in diagnostic radiology. Med Phys 1997; 24(4): 571–9.

9. Kachelrieβ M, Knaup M, Kalender WA. Multi-threaded cardiac CT. Med Phys 2006; 33(7): 2435–47.
10. Stenner P, Berkus T, Kachelrieβ M. Empirical dual energy calibration (EDEC) for cone-beam computed tomography. Med Phys 2007; 34(9): 3630–41.

38

Imaging of Plaques and Vasa Vasorum with Micro-computed Tomography: Towards an Understanding of Unstable Plaque

Alexander C. Langheinrich

There have been great advances in our knowledge of the cellular biology underlying atherosclerotic plaque formation and progression. A hot topic in vascular biology is the role of abnormal plaque vascularization in atherogenesis. In normal arteries, microvessels, vasa vasorum (VV), are observed only in the adventitia and in the outer media of artery walls that exceed a thickness of 250 μm. Neovascularization in atherosclerotic arteries occurs primarily by growth from the adventitia into the neointima of advanced plaques. New microvessels in plaques appear fragile and are susceptible to rupture which may contribute to intraplaque hemorrhage. Intraplaque hemorrhage is a hallmark of unstable plaques, which are at high risk for rupture. Plaque rupture is the dominant cause of myocardial infarction (MI). Repeated cycles of plaque rupture and healing may also explain the finding that there is layering in arterial plaques, which reflects an intermittent growth pattern of the developing plaque.

I MICROSCOPIC-COMPUTED TOMOGRAPHY (MICRO-CT) FOR THE ASSESSMENT OF ATHEROSCLEROTIC PLAQUES

Screening for atherosclerotic plaques using CT has evolved from coronary calcium CT scans[1,2] to luminal scanning by CT coronary angiography and to the assessment of coronary

arterial wall CT numbers as an index of fatty or fibrous material.[3] Developing imaging technologies capable of identifying vulnerable atheromatous plaques non-invasively and in vivo is a major focus of current research efforts. In the past decade, micro-CT has become a powerful research technique as technical advances of processing speed and memory have enabled micro-CT systems to generate high-resolution images of small specimens.[4–6] While the early implementation of 3D micro-CT focused on the technical and methodological aspects of these systems, more recent work has emphasized the study of physiological aspects.[7–11] The focus of this chapter is micro-CT applications to study VV in normal and atherosclerotic arteries.

The current understanding of the initiation and progression of human atherosclerotic coronary artery disease is mainly based on morphological data from autopsies[12] observations derived from clinical invasive[13,14] and non-invasive studies[15] and on experimental animal models.[16] These data, however, are not entirely consistent. In particular, a long-standing discordance between angiographic and pathological studies exists with respect to differentiating stable from vulnerable plaques, the lesion underlying the majority of acute coronary events. These discrepancies are probably the result of important limitations of the different approaches.

Micro-CT can render vessel-wall alterations in human coronary arteries[6] (Figure 38.1). Histology is the gold standard for the identification of cellular components of the

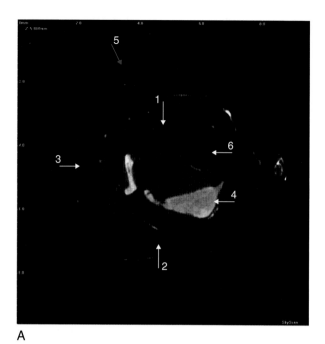

A

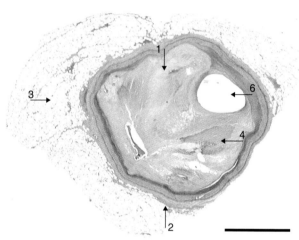

B

Figure 38.1 Example of an advanced fibrocalcific atherosclerotic lesion of a human coronary artery visualized by transverse micro-CT imaging (A) or conventional histomicroscopy (B, magnification × 10, bar = 500 μm). Samples were scanned by micro-CT and reconstructed at a resolution of 8 μm and displayed at 21 μm resolution. The corresponding cross-section of the same specimen was subsequently stained with hematoxylin and eosin with elastica counterstaining for histomicroscopical examination. Note eccentric neointimal thickening (1), boundary between media and adventitia (2), adventitia (3), calcification (4), and vessel lumen (6). Coronary artery was stored in paraffin (5) to prevent distorsions during the scan (with permission from Ref. 20).

plaque, but micro-CT imaging of atherosclerosis may offer several additional advantages:

(i) Micro-CT imaging is a research technology which is ideal for the rapid qualitative and quantitative evaluation of atherosclerotic lesions. With a general acquisition time

of ~10 cross-sections per minute, micro-CT clearly exceeded the mechanical process of conventional histology. This technical benefit might become more important considering a recent study in which morphological predictors of arterial remodeling in coronary atherosclerosis have been evaluated by processing 2885 coronary cross-sections for histological examination.[17] Up to now, detailed plaque classification is a major advantage of histopathology with additional immunhistochemistry, but remains a lab-intensive and time-consuming method which might be complemented with micro-CT imaging.

(ii) Micro-CT has emerged as a research technique to detect atherosclerotic lesions in coronary vessels in excised arteries. Micro-CT has been shown to detect even small, early lesions that can be missed by conventional histology. Histomorphometric results are reported by sections, and for volumetric determinations, the results are often estimated by interpolation. Micro-CT is particularly helpful for continuous visualization of the entire vessel compared to the rather time-consuming segmental examination of tissue specimen during histological cross-sectioning.

(iii) Micro-CT can accurately characterize lesion dimensions. Measurements of morphometric indices performed by micro-CT led to the same results obtained by conventional histological analysis. This finding indicates that micro-CT is an appropriate tool to quantitatively analyze atherosclerotic plaques size. Based on differences in gray-scale attenuations, micro-CT correctly identified atherosclerotic lesions histologically classified as fibrous plaques, calcified lesions, fibroatheroma (Figure 38.2), and lipid rich lesions. It is conceivable that, with future technical advances (increasing spatial resolution, antibody-labeling, dual-energy scanning), micro-CT imaging might enable radiographic visualization of distinct cellular plaque compositions.

(iv) Histology may be limited in that, once sliced, the intact volume is lost so that the study of three-dimensional structures such as VV or the tissue distribution of calcium are challenging. Micro-CT imaging does not prevent subsequent histomorphological analyses and does not interfere with standard paraffin-embedded immunohistological techniques performed on the same coronary vessel segments. Since further histological analysis can be done on the same specimens, the use of micro-CT may be of great advantage in clinical or experimental studies.

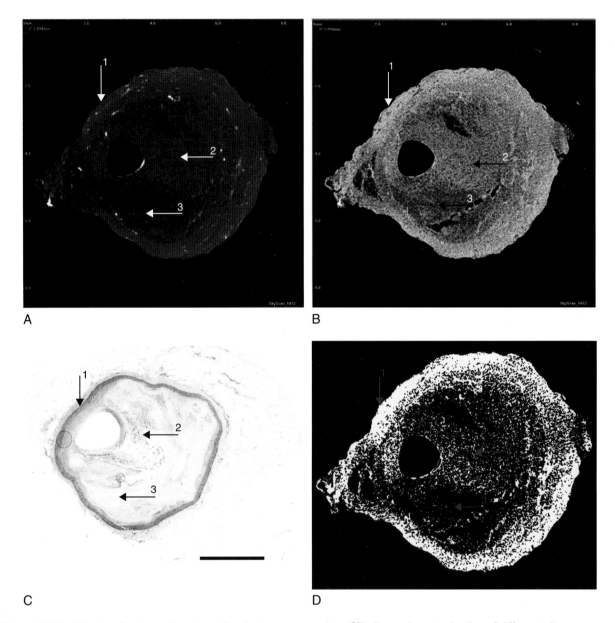

Figure 38.2 Display of gray-scale attenuation by transverse micro-CT allows characterization of different plaque compositions (A: raw data; B: colored; D: thresholding technique). Comparison to the corresponding immunohistological cross-section (C; stained for smooth muscle actin, bar = 500 μm) shows that micro-CT visualizes smooth muscle cell rich media (1), plaque areas predominantly composed of smooth muscle cells (2) and areas containing no or sparse smooth muscle cells (3) (with permission from Ref. 20).

Quantitative ex-vivo analysis of atherosclerotic lesions is typically done by microscopy on thin histological sections. Two problems with this approach are the difficulty in obtaining adjacent slices and the distorsions that occur during the sectioning process. Histologic microscopy may be limited in that it does not provide three-dimensional information and – as a destructive technique – it does not allow continuous measurements and in that it limits tissue quantification to a small number of two-dimensional sections. With micro-CT imaging, a complete digital data set of the vessel wall is now available. As a non-destructive approach, micro-CT allows three-dimensional analysis of the several plaque characteristics such as plaque area, lumen size, calcification, or lipid core over the entire length of the selected vessel segment. Using tomographic reconstruction algorithms, three-dimensional images of the vessel wall can be generated which allow total stereoscopic visualization of the plaques 3D micro-architecture. As tomography allows convenient extraction of appropriate slices from the 3 D-images, micro-CT can also be used to analyze distinct regions of interest more accurately (e.g. high-risk lesions with thin fibrous caps can be detected prior to dissection of the specimen) thus 'steering' the pathologist's knife to distinct local alterations within the tissue specimen.

1.1 Vasa vasorum

Experimental and clinical data strongly suggest that vasa vasorum play a role in proliferative vascular disorders. Multiple studies have shown a high correlation between number of VV and the degree of atherosclerotic stenoses.[18–20] Recent studies have emphasized the involvement of VV in the inflammatory aspect of atherosclerosis. Both number of VV and the degree of inflammation in the adventitia are significantly higher in advanced atherosclerotic plaques compared to early stages.[18] In apoE–/–/LDL–/– mice, this relationship varies in different vascular beds.[21] In this model, the spatial distribution of VV, their density, and the magnitude of adventitial inflammation were strongly correlated with advanced atherosclerotic lesion types.

Moreno and colleagues[22] demonstrated a similar association between presence of VV and inflammatory cells in human aortas. Microvessel density was low in lesions with mild plaque inflammation and increasingly higher in lesions with moderate or severe inflammation. In normal arteries, inflammation was absent, but once atheromas started to occur adventitial inflammation increased with plaque development.[23,24]

One study suggested that patients with symptomatic atherosclerosis had a denser network of VV than patients with asymptomatic disease. The increased number of VV was accompanied by a strong inflammatory reaction of the vascular wall.[25] These findings are supported by several other papers showing that the inflammatory response in the adventitia with increased expression of IL-6, TNF-alpha, MCP-1, VCAM-1 can alter atherogenesis.[26,27]

Further support comes from Judah Folkman's group. In apoE-deficient mice, VV density correlated better with the number of inflammatory cells within the plaque than with plaque size.[28] These findings, based on micro-CT imaging and histopathology, suggest a role of plaque neovascularization in initiating and promoting atherosclerotic lesions. One possible mechanism may be facilitation of the inflammatory milieu within the vessel wall.

1.2 Vasa vasorum and intraplaque hemorrhage

Intraplaque hemorrhage is a marker of instability in advanced atherosclerotic lesions.[29] Iron, a main component of red blood cells, can accumulate in the plaque after extravasation of erythrocytes, whether isolated or within macrophage-derived cells that have phagocytosed red blood cells.[30] Supporting this idea, Lee et al.[31] suggested that hemoglobin/heme released from the phagocytosed erythrocytes may contribute to at least part of the iron deposition seen in atherosclerotic lesions in apoE-deficient mice.

Recently, neoangiogenesis as a source of intraplaque hemorrhage has been reported in carotid arteries in apoE-deficient mice.[32] In this study, CD31, a marker of endothelial cells (Platelet Endothelial Cell Adhesion Molecle-1) staining revealed colocalization of plaque microvessels and sites of extravasated and degraded erythrocytes, consistent with intimal neo-angiogenesis as a feasible source for intraplaque hemorrhage.

Kolodgie et al.[33] showed that the degree of glycophorin A reactivity, a specific marker of erythrocyte membranes, and the magnitude of iron accumulation in plaques corresponded to the size of the necrotic core, indicating that iron deposits may be a sign of plaque hemorrhage and instability. Capillary-like microvessels have been shown in very early atherosclerotic lesions (type II) in human carotid artery samples, associated with accumulations of macrophages, mast cells, and T-cells.[34] Evidence of local microvascular damage with subsequent intraplaque hemorrhage within the shoulder regions of human carotid arteries are demonstrated by extravascular red blood cells, macrophages containing hemosiderin, and perivascular fibrin deposition.[35] Such findings indicate that plaque neovascularization is a prominent feature of plaque development, possibly providing an important source of intraplaque hemorrhage.[36]

In Pedro Moreno's study of human aortas,[37] lesions with intraplaque hemorrhage had increased numbers of intraplaque microvessels. High-resolution synchrotron-based micro-CT demonstrated iron deposits within plaques that showed evidence of prior intraplaque hemorrhage.[38] The strong spatial, punctate colocalization of the elements Fe and Ca indicated that iron within the lesion resulted from intraplaque hemorrhage. The schematic in Figure 38.5 summarizes the current paradigm of the role of vasa vasorum in advanced atherosclerotic lesions.

1.3 Dual-energy computed tomography of vulnerable plaques

Methological applications of dual-energy CT imaging have been described over the last 20 years[39,40] and have been used to quantify iron deposits in the liver in an animal model of hemochromatosis.[41] Advanced iron accumulations in the liver were visible using dual energy CT scanning at 80 and 120 kVp as a change of 24 HU/100mg% iron. Recently, first experiences with a new, commercially available, clinical dual-energy CT system have been reported.[42] The ability to use two different tube voltages simultaneously to differentiate two materials with different atomic number may open new possibilities for detailed tissue and plaque characterization.

A high temporal and spatial resolution is a basic requirement to image increased vascularization by virtue of enhanced lesion perfusion reflected by an increase of transient opacification of the artery wall during an intravascular contrast injection. Contrast-enhanced multi-detector computed tomography (MDCT) permits visualization of epicardial coronary arteries. Recent studies showed high sensitivity and specifity of 16- and 64-slice MDCT for the detection of hemodynamically significant coronary stenosis. It has bcome apparent that MDCT can also visualize atherosclerotic vessel walls in addition to luminal narrowings.[43]

The role of atherosclerotic calcifications has been investigated extensively during the past years, suggesting an association of overall calcium burden and cardiovascular event risk. But up to now, although clinically very important, non-invasive imaging of non-calcified 'vulnerable' plaque remains elusive.

As discussed above, neoangiogenesis may be a source of intraplaque hemorrhage. Using synchrotron-based micro-CT at 2 μm voxel resolution, we have recently scanned the aortic arch of old apoE-/-LDL-/-mice which develop severe atherosclerosis and proliferation of vasa vasorum. Advanced atherosclerotic plaques showed local accumulations of punctate bright spots (~8μm diameter) consistent with iron deposits resulting from individual extravascular erythrocytes[38] (Figures 38.3 and 38.4). Comparisons of micro-CT and

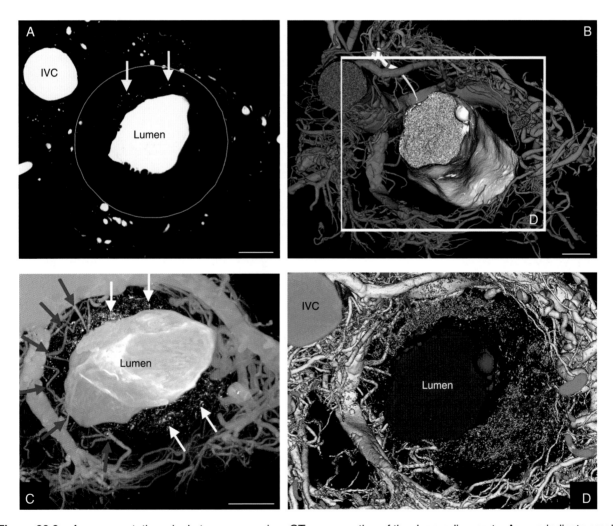

Figure 38.3 A, representative, single transverse micro-CT cross-section of the descending aorta. Arrows indicate small, unconnected, radiopaque spots within the lesion (superimposed gray circle demonstrates the border between media and adventitia). B, Volume-rendered 3D-micro-CT image in the same region viewed axially, demonstrating arterial (red) and venous (blue) vasa vasorum. The spots are not displayed in this image because they have no anatomic connection to the vessels. C, Maximum intensity projection confirms the interconnectivity of adventitial VV and plaque microvessels (red arrows). D, Volume-rendered micro-CT image show that small opacities are distributed (gold colored spots) between the aortic lumen (red) and the VV. Bar = 200 μm, voxels size 2 μm (with permission from Ref. 38).

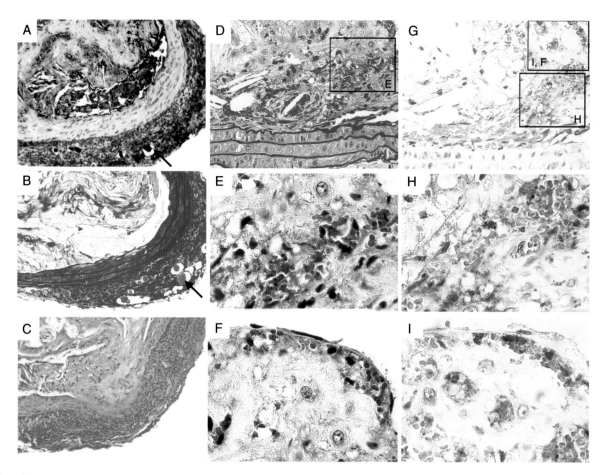

Figure 38.4   Intraplaque hemorrhage in aortas of apoE–/–/LDL–/– double knockout mice at the age of 80 weeks. A, erythrocyte membranes are demonstrated by using antibodies against glycophorin A (CD23 A, ×100). VV are present within the adventitia (black arrow). B, C, contrast-enhanced VV are present in the adventitia surrounded by clusters of inflammatory cells stained for Movat pentachrome (×100) and HE (×100). Recent intraplaque hemorrhage at low (D, G, × 20; E, H, × 40) and high-power field magnification (F, I ×100) stained for Movat pentachrome (D, E, F) and Iron (Perls' stain, G, H, I) demonstrated by extravasated erythrocytes and iron (hemosiderin) deposits in a lesion with a thin-fibrous cap in serial sections.

histology showed that calcium and iron are frequently co-localized in advanced plaques. Both appear bright white on single energy CT which makes them undistinguishable and computed tomography of iron deposits challenging. However, the discrimination of iron and calcium is necessary because the presence of calcium is not associated with vulnerability, unlike iron, which appears to be specifically located in vulnerable plaque.[44]

Based on the different attenuation coefficients of calcium and iron, dual energy micro-CT and dual-source CT seems to be a suitable technology to discriminate these two elements. Images obtained from the aortic arch of the ApoE–/–LDL–/– mice at 16 and 20 keV were subtracted after the high-energy images were biased such that bone had the same gray scale as the lower-energy images. Areas identified as calcified lesions cancelled out,

whereas bright spots identified as iron on histology remained in the subtracted image. Because the attenuation coefficient of calcium decreases more rapidly than iron at higher energies, we achieved a 'positive' signal in the descending aorta for iron using dual-energy 64-slice CT scanning.

1.4 Cinical implications and conclusion

While these micro-CT and 64-slice CT data on plaque neo-vascularization and intraplaque hemorrhage are encouraging, clinical studies have to assess the in vivo accuracy, sensitivity, and specifity in patients. Testing this hypothesis in vulnerable and ruptured plaques will depend on

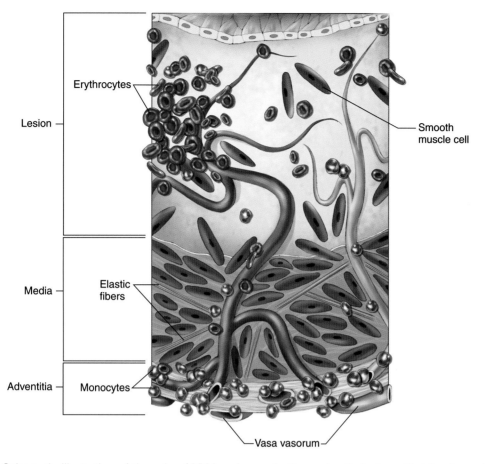

Figure 38.5 Schematic illustration of the role of VV in advanced atherosclerotic lesion with intraplaque hemorrhage. Remnants of red blood cells and hemosiderin-laden macrophages are detectable by iron deposits (with permission from Langheinrich AC et al. Atherosclerosis and VV: Quid Novi? Thrombosis and Haemostasis, 2007; 42: 263–273).

technologies that allow noninvasive serial imaging of advanced lesions in appropriate animal models and humans. If iron deposits can be identified and quantified noinvasively in hemorrhagic plaques it may be possible to selectively treat asymptomatic patients who are at high risk for rupture and myocardial infarction. Outcome studies need to prove that early imaging and subsequent therapeutic intervention improve long-term morbidity and survival.

One other imaging marker of vulnerable lesions could be the vasa vasorum themselves. It may be possible to detect and quantify enhanced plaque vascularization due to proliferation of vasa vasorum by virtue of increased lesion perfusion, reflected by the increase in transient opacification of the arterial wall during an intravascular contrast injection. Consequently, combined imaging of plaque perfusion as an index of vasa vasorum density and iron deposits as a marker of plaque hemorrhage in atherosclerotic plaques may form a basis for advanced CT imaging of vulnerable plaques.

REFERENCES

1. Cordeiro MA, Lima JA. Atherosclerotic plaque characterization by multidetector row computed tomography angiography. J Am Coll Cardiol 2006; 47(8 Suppl): C40–C47.
2. Leber AW, Knez A, von Ziegler F et al. Quantification of obstructive and nonobstructive coronary lesions by 64-slice computed tomography: a comparative study with quantitative coronary angiography and intravascular ultrasound. J Am Coll Cardiol 2005; 46(1): 147–54.
3. Leber AW, Becker A, Knez A et al. Accuracy of 64-slice computed tomography to classify and quantify plaque volumes in the proximal coronary system: a comparative study using intravascular ultrasound. J Am Coll Cardiol 2006; 47(3): 672–7.
4. Gossl M, Rosol M, Malyar NM et al. Functional anatomy and hemodynamic characteristics of vasa vasorum in the walls of porcine coronary arteries. Anat Rec A Discov Mol Cell Evol Biol 2003; 272(2): 526–37.
5. Langheinrich AC, Bohle RM, Breithecker A, Lommel D, Rau WS. [Micro-computed tomography of the vasculature in parenchymal organs and lung alveoli]. Rofo 2004; 176(9): 1219–25.
6. Langheinrich AC, Bohle RM, Greschus S et al. Atherosclerotic lesions at micro CT: feasibility for analysis of coronary

artery wall in autopsy specimens. Radiology 2004; 231(3): 675–81.

7. Galili O, Herrmann J, Woodrum J et al. Adventitial vasa vasorum heterogeneity among different vascular beds. J Vasc Surg 2004; 40(3): 529–35.

8. Gossl M, Zamir M, Ritman EL. Vasa vasorum growth in the coronary arteries of newborn pigs. Anat Embryol (Berl) 2004; 208(5): 351–7.

9. Gossl M, Beighley PE, Malyar NM, Ritman EL. Role of vasa vasorum in transendothelial solute transport in the coronary vessel wall: a study with cryostatic micro-CT. Am J Physiol Heart Circ Physiol 2004; 287(5): H2346–H2351.

10. Langheinrich AC, Leithauser B, Greschus S et al. Acute rat lung injury: feasibility of assessment with micro-CT. Radiology 2004; 233(1): 165–71.

11. Langheinrich AC, Ritman EL. Quantitative imaging of microvascular permeability in a rat model of lipopolysaccharide-induced sepsis: evaluation using cryostatic micro-computed tomography. Invest Radiol 2006; 41(8): 645–50.

12. Burke AP, Farb A, Malcom GT et al. Plaque rupture and sudden death related to exertion in men with coronary artery disease. JAMA 1999; 281(10): 921–6.

13. Goldstein JA, Demetriou D, Grines CL et al. Multiple complex coronary plaques in patients with acute myocardial infarction. N Engl J Med 2000; 343(13): 915–22.

14. Rioufol G, Finet G, Ginon I et al. Multiple atherosclerotic plaque rupture in acute coronary syndrome: a three-vessel intravascular ultrasound study. Circulation 2002; 106(7): 804–8.

15. Goubergrits L, Affeld K, Fernandez-Britto J, Falcon L. Atherosclerosis in the human common carotid artery. A morphometric study of 31 specimens. Pathol Res Pract 2001; 197(12): 803–9.

16. Paigen B, Morrow A, Holmes PA, Mitchell D, Williams RA. Quantitative assessment of atherosclerotic lesions in mice. Atherosclerosis 1987; 68(3): 231–40.

17. Burke AP, Kolodgie FD, Farb A, Weber D, Virmani R. Morphological predictors of arterial remodeling in coronary atherosclerosis. Circulation 2002; 105(3): 297–303.

18. Langheinrich AC, Michniewicz A, Sedding DG et al. Correlation of vasa vasorum neovascularization and plaque progression in aortas of apolipoprotein E(–/–)/low-density lipoprotein(–/–) double knockout mice. Arterioscler Thromb Vasc Biol 2006; 26(2): 347–52.

19. Moreno PR, Purushothaman KR, Fuster V et al. Plaque neovascularization is increased in ruptured atherosclerotic lesions of human aorta: implications for plaque vulnerability. Circulation 2004; 110(14): 2032–8.

20. Moulton KS, Vakili K, Zurakowski D et al. Inhibition of plaque neovascularization reduces macrophage accumulation and progression of advanced atherosclerosis. Proc Natl Acad Sci USA 2003; 100(8): 4736–41.

21. Langheinrich AC, Michniewicz A, Bohle RM, Ritman EL. Vasa vasorum neovascularization and lesion distribution among different vascular beds in ApoE(-/-)/LDL(-/-) double knockout mice. Atherosclerosis 2007; 191(1): 73–8.

22. Moreno PR, Purushothaman KR, Fuster V et al. Plaque neovascularization is increased in ruptured atherosclerotic lesions of human aorta: implications for plaque vulnerability. Circulation 2004; 110(14): 2032–8.

23. Libby P, Ridker PM. Novel inflammatory markers of coronary risk: theory versus practice. Circulation 1999; 100(11): 1148–50.

24. Ross R. Atherosclerosis – an inflammatory disease. N Engl J Med 1999; 340(2): 115–26.

25. Fleiner M, Kummer M, Mirlacher M et al. Arterial neovascularization and inflammation in vulnerable patients: early and late signs of symptomatic atherosclerosis. Circulation 2004; 110(18): 2843–50.

26. Mazurek T, Zhang L, Zalewski A et al. Human epicardial adipose tissue is a source of inflammatory mediators. Circulation 2003; 108(20): 2460–6.

27. Zhang L, Zalewski A, Liu Y et al. Diabetes-induced oxidative stress and low-grade inflammation in porcine coronary arteries. Circulation 2003; 108(4): 472–8.

28. Moulton KS, Vakili K, Zurakowski D et al. Inhibition of plaque neovascularization reduces macrophage accumulation and progression of advanced atherosclerosis. Proc Natl Acad Sci USA 2003; 100(8): 4736–41.

29. Kolodgie FD, Gold HK, Burke AP et al. Intraplaque hemorrhage and progression of coronary atheroma. N Engl J Med 2003; 349(24): 2316–25.

30. Yuan XM, Anders WL, Olsson AG, Brunk UT. Iron in human atheroma and LDL oxidation by macrophages following erythrophagocytosis. Atherosclerosis 1996; 124(1): 61–73.

31. Lee TS, Lee FY, Pang JH, Chau LY. Erythrophagocytosis and iron deposition in atherosclerotic lesions. Chin J Physiol (China) 1999; 42(1): 17–23.

32. de Nooijer R, Verkleij CJ, von der Thusen JH et al. Lesional overexpression of matrix metalloproteinase-9 promotes intraplaque hemorrhage in advanced lesions but not at earlier stages of atherogenesis. Arterioscler Thromb Vasc Biol 2006; 26(2): 340–6.

33. Kolodgie FD, Gold HK, Burke AP et al. Intraplaque hemorrhage and progression of coronary atheroma. N Engl J Med 2003; 349(24): 2316–25.

34. Jeziorska M, Woolley DE. Neovascularization in early atherosclerotic lesions of human carotid arteries: its potential contribution to plaque development. Hum Pathol 1999; 30(8): 919–25.

35. Jeziorska M, Woolley DE. Local neovascularization and cellular composition within vulnerable regions of atherosclerotic plaques of human carotid arteries. J Pathol 1999; 188(2): 189–96.

36. Virmani R, Kolodgie FD, Burke AP et al. Atherosclerotic plaque progression and vulnerability to rupture: angiogenesis as a source of intraplaque hemorrhage. Arterioscler Thromb Vasc Biol 2005; 25(10): 2054–61.

37. Moreno PR, Purushothaman KR, Fuster V et al. Plaque neovascularization is increased in ruptured atherosclerotic lesions of human aorta: implications for plaque vulnerability. Circulation 2004; 110(14): 2032–8.

38. Langheinrich AC, Michniewicz A, Sedding DG et al. Quantitative X-Ray Imaging of Intraplaque Hemorrhage in Aortas of ApoE–/–/LDL–/–Double Knockout Mice. Invest Radiol 2007; 42(5): 263–73.

39. Kalender W, Felsenberg D, Suss C. [Material selective imaging and density measurement with the dual energy method. III. Determination of bone mineral of the spine with CT]. Digitale Bilddiagn 1987; 7(4): 170–6.

40. Marshall W, Hall E, Doost-Hoseini A et al. An implementation of dual energy CT scanning. J Comput Assist Tomogr 1984; 8(4): 745–9.

41. Goldberg HI, Cann CE, Moss AA et al. Noninvasive quantitation of liver iron in dogs with hemochromatosis using dual-energy CT scanning. Invest Radiol 1982; 17(4): 375–80.

42. Flohr TG, McCollough CH, Bruder H et al. First performance evaluation of a dual-source CT (DSCT) system. Eur Radiol 2006; 16(2): 256–8.

43. Leber AW, Knez A, Becker A et al. Visualising noncalcified coronary plaques by CT. Int J Cardiovasc Imaging 2005; 21(1): 55–61.

44. Virmani R, Burke AP, Farb A, Kolodgie FD. Pathology of the vulnerable plaque. J Am Coll Cardiol 2006; 47(8 Suppl): C13–C18.

Index

Notes: Page references in *italics* refer to Figures and Tables; CT = computed tomography